NUTRITION IN PUBLIC HEALTH
A Handbook for Developing Programs and Services
SECOND EDITION

Edited by

Sari Edelstein, PhD, RD
Simmons College
Boston, Massachusetts

Featuring

Security of Food Supply and Bioterrorism Preparedness
By Barbara Bruemmer, PhD, RD, CD

The importance of nutrition in maintaining good health and preventing disease is more clear than ever before, but translating this knowledge into public health practice remains a huge challenge. Nutrition in Public Health will provide an invaluable guide to those taking on this essential task.

Dr. Walter Willet
Harvard University
School of Public Health

JONES AND BARTLETT PUBLISHERS
Sudbury, Massachusetts
BOSTON   TORONTO   LONDON   SINGAPORE

World Headquarters
Jones and Bartlett Publishers
40 Tall Pine Drive
Sudbury, MA 01776
978-443-5000
info@jbpub.com
www.jbpub.com

Jones and Bartlett Publishers Canada
6339 Ormindale Way
Mississauga, ON L5V 1J2
CANADA

Jones and Bartlett Publishers International
Barb House, Barb Mews
London W6 7PA
UK

Jones and Bartlett's books and products are available through most bookstores and online booksellers. To contact Jones and Bartlett Publishers directly, call 800-832-0034, fax 978-443-8000, or visit our website at www.jbpub.com.

Substantial discounts on bulk quantities of Jones and Bartlett's publications are available to corporations, professional associations, and other qualified organizations. For details and specific discount information, contact the special sales department at Jones and Bartlett via the above contact information or send an email to specialsales@jbpub.com.

Library of Congress Cataloging-in-Publication Data
Nutrition in public health : a handbook for developing programs and services / edited by Sari Edelstein.-- 2nd ed.
     p. ; cm.
   Featuring a chapter on "Security of food supply and bioterrorism preparedness" by Barbara Bruemmer and Walter Willet.
   Includes bibliographical references.
   ISBN 0-7637-8358-7 (casebound)
   1. Nutrition--United States--Handbooks, manuals, etc. 2. Public health--United States--Handbooks, manuals, etc. 3. Nutrition policy--United States--Handbooks, manuals, etc.
   [DNLM: 1. Nutrition--United States. 2. Needs Assessment--United States. 3. Nutrition Policy--United States. 4. Public Health Practice--United States. 5. Risk Factors--United States. QU 145 N9752 2006] I. Edelstein, Sari.
   RA601.N84 2006
   362.17'6--dc22

                              2005008621

Production Credits
Acquisitions Editor: Michael Brown
Editorial Assistant: Kylah Goodfellow McNeill
Production Director: Amy Rose
Associate Production Editor: Kate Hennessy
Associate Marketing Manager: Marissa Hederson
Manufacturing Buyer: Therese Connell
Composition: Jason Miranda
Cover Design: Timothy Dziewit
Printing and Binding: Malloy Inc.
Cover Printing: Malloy Inc.

Printed in the United States of America
09 08 07 06 05   10 9 8 7 6 5 4 3 2 1

DEDICATION

I would like to thank all my wonderful colleagues at Simmons College who both contributed and supported this project.

Sari Edelstein

CONTENTS

CONTRIBUTORS

Deepa Arora, PhD
Fort Valley State University

Thelma B. Baker, PhD, RD, LD
Howard University

Elizabeth Barden, PhD
Simmons College

Jeanette Beasley, MPH, RD
University of North Carolina Chapel Hill
Johns Hopkins University

Margaret L. Bogle, PhD, RD, LD
United States Department of Agriculture

Barbara Bruemmer, PhD, RD, CD
University of Washington

Katherine Cairns, MPH, MBA, RD
Summit Health Group

Joseph M. Carlin, MS, RD, LDN, FADA
Administration on Aging

Shirley Chao, MS, RD, LDN
Office of Elder Affairs, Boston

Stacey Chappa, RD
WIC, Kalamazoo, MI

Rachel Colchamiro, MPH, RD
Massachusetts Department of
    Public Health

Pamella Darby, MS, MPH, RD
New York University

Sari Edelstein, PhD, RD
Simmons College

Teresa T. Fung, ScD, RD
Simmons College
Harvard University

Nancie Herbold, EdD, RD
Simmons College

Edna Harris-Davis, MS, MPH, RD, LD
Georgia Department of Public Health

David H. Holben, PhD, RD, LD
Ohio University

Jan Kallio, MS, RD, LDN
Massachusetts Department of
    Public Health

Patti S. Landers, PhD, RD, LD
University of Oklahoma

Beth Leonberg, MS, RD, CSP, LDN, FADA
Nutrition Outcomes, LLC

Beverly J. McCabe-Sellers, PhD, RD
United States Department of Agriculture

Shortie McKinney, PhD, RD, LDN, FADA
Drexel University

Elizabeth Metallinos-Katsaras, PhD, RD
Simmons College

Julie M. Moreschi, MS, RD, LDN
Benedictine University

Theresa A. Nicklas, DrPH
Baylor College of Medicine

Esther Okeiyi, PhD, RD, LDN
North Carolina Central University

Carol E. O'Neil, PhD, MPH, LDN, RD
Louisiana State University

Bruce Rengers, PhD, RD
Denver Public Health Department

Judith Sharlin, PhD, RD
Simmons College

Arlene Spark, EdD, RD, FADA, FACN
Hunter College

Bonnie Spear, PhD, RD
University of Alabama at Birmingham

Yeemay Su Miller, MS, RD
Simmons College

Inger Stallmann-Jorgensen, MS, RD, LD
Georgia Department of Public Health

Cynthia Taft Bayerl, MS, RD, LDN
Massachusetts Department of
    Public Health

Paul N. Taylor, PhD
Simmons College

Marcia Thomas, MS, MPH, RD
New York University

FOREWORD

The beginning of the 21st century is a time of contrasts. On one hand, our food supply continues to be reliable, abundant, and relatively cheap when compared with other countries. On the other hand, we are faced with a rapidly expanding epidemic of obesity in adults and children. Unfortunately, this problem is also emerging in many developing countries with increasing industrialization and adoption of industrialized lifestyle. Because of this, we will be facing a global problem of diseases related with obesity, such as type 2 diabetes and cardiovascular disease. In addition, we also face new challenges to safe guard our food supply, from emerging infectious organisms to contamination.

At the same time, a tremendous amount of data is available on how nutrients and other dietary factors can enhance wellness and prevent diseases. This together with sophisticated technology, we have the tools to turn around the nation's nutrition related health problems, and move forward towards the goals of Healthy People 2010. Although our society is filled with constant messages for consumption (hence the risk of over-consumption), many governmental and non-profit organizations have also launched efforts to curb over-consumption. This is the state of nutritional issue for the United States—a combination of problems and resources, and competing forces to influence the nation's consumption patterns.

In light of these issues, healthy eating and good nutrition need to be promoted in two fronts: personal knowledge of nutrition, skills, and responsibility to eat healthy, as well as a society that makes it easy to practice good nutrition for people at different stages in their lives. Both fronts are subjects of public health nutrition. The former should be taught in schools and other settings, the latter involves policymaking in various institution and also at the government level, and we need to seek cooperation from the food industry.

The knowledge of good health is not a secret, and the public health nutritionist plays a crucial role to steer a nation towards better health. Even for those who are not directly or primarily involved in this field, there is a little bit of public health nutritionist in all of us. We all can contribute to public health nutrition through civic involvement such as working with public schools to improve school meals, and making our voices heard to influence public policy. *Nutrition in Public Health* is of much importance as it empowers professionals involved in public health nutrition to perform their job better, and to make an important impact on people's health. But it is also useful to all those in health professions.

Dr. Sari Edelstein has been involved in various aspects of nutrition for many years. She is an experienced dietitian, educator, and leader. Her experience in this area, plus the expertise of the contributing authors, represents an enormous wealth of knowledge that they can share with the readers. The subjects discussed in this book are timely and significant, and make this text a must-have for both students and practitioners of public health nutrition.

Teresa T. Fung, ScD, RD
Assistant Professor in Nutrition
Simmons College, Boston, MA
Adjunct Assistant Professor in Nutrition
Harvard School of Public Health
Cambridge, MA

WHAT IS PUBLIC HEALTH NUTRITION?

Sari Edelstein, PhD, RD

Public Health Nutrition

Public health nutrition is a complex, multifaceted set of programs that are dedicated to improving the health of the population through improved nutrition. In more detail, public health nutrition primarily exists to[1]:

- Improve the health of the whole population and teach high-risk subgroups within the population improved nutrition;
- Emphasize health promotion and disease prevention through improved nutrition; and
- Provide integrated community efforts for improved nutrition with leadership demonstrated by government offices.

In order to accomplish the three primary elements of public health nutrition, as stated, the U.S. Public Health Service has delineated ten Essential Public Health Service Functions, as listed below.[2] Each of these ten elements will assist the reader in understanding the steps that must be taken by public health professionals to bring about definitive qualitative and quantitative results.

1. Monitor health status to identify and solve community health problems;
2. Identify and investigate the causes of health problems and health hazards in the community;
3. Mobilize community partnerships and action to identify and solve health problems;
4. Develop policies and plans that support individual and community health;
5. Enforce laws and regulations that protect health and ensure safety;
6. Link people to needed personal health services and assure the provision of healthcare when otherwise unavailable;
7. Inform, educate, and empower people about health issues;
8. Evaluate effectiveness, accessibility, and quality of personal and population-based health services;

9. Assure a competent public health and personal healthcare workforce; and,

10. Research for new insights and innovative solutions to health problems.

When these ten elements are expanded to full explanations for the reader, we create a compendium of information that mirrors the table of contents in this book. In this section, we recreate for the reader the organization of *Nutrition in Public Health, 2nd edition* that embraces the Essential Public Health Service Functions.

Part I Applying Nutrition in Public Health

Chapter 1 Understanding the Role of Nutrition in Public Health Service

Chapter 2 Applying Nutrition Science to the Public's Health

In Part I, the reader is introduced to the role of nutrition in public health service throughout American history, and is shown how science affected decisions that were made in the name of the public's health. From Chapter 1, we experience an America that is in need of a way to serve the less fortunate. Americans have little organized healthcare for the sick, including those at highest risk which are the young and the elderly. But, as America's public health service grows, so does the methods for ascertaining what nutritional information should be disseminated to the public. In Chapter 2, we experience the various studies that have brought public health nutrition to the standards we enjoy today. The authors of Chapter 2 bring the reader through each and every hallmark of nutritional science, explain how these standards were attained, and translate what these standards mean for the public health recipients of today.

Part II Assessing and Intervening in the Community's Nutrition Needs

Chapter 3 Community Needs Assessment

Chapter 4 Reaching Out to Those at Highest Nutritional Risk

Chapter 5 Addressing Overweight in Children: A Public Health Perspective

Chapter 6 Intervening to Change the Public's Eating Behavior

In Part II, the reader is introduced to how public health nutritionists target care for those at highest risk. In order to find those at highest risk, a needs assessment of the community must be performed. Chapter 3 describes the concepts and issues involved in needs assessment of the public health arena. It is through proper needs assessment that the public health nutritionist can serve those who need help in ways that are most useful. In Chapter 4, we see the results of more than a century of needs assessment, with the designation of the young and the old as being those groups we must serve. In addition, those with illness and disability must be supported by public health nutrition services. Perhaps, reaching those in need has been one of public health nutrition's most difficult challenges. In the 21st century, public health nutrition needs assessments have determined that America's indulgent eating habits have brought us to nutritional catastrophe. The epidemics of child (Chapter 5) and adult obesity (Chapter 6) are two additional areas that public health nutrition must find a way to intervene and provide solutions.

Part III Shaping the Policies that Affect the Public's Health

Chapter 7 Creating Public Policy
Chapter 8 Advocating and Influencing Health and Nutrition Policies
Chapter 9 The Role of the USDA in Public Health Nutrition

In Part III, we shift gears to investigate how science and needs assessment translate into public policy. It is through governmental policy that public health nutritionists are directed to educate and serve the public. Chapters 7 and 8 describe how nutrition policy is created, advocated, and influenced by the public, health practitioners, lobbyists, and legislators. What should be imparted to the reader in these chapters is the need for dietitians and nutritionists to get involved in advocating and influencing the passing of important nutrition policy. Chapter 9 demonstrates to the reader how the USDA acts on nutrition policy once it is made and illustrates the complexity of that role in fulfilling the challenges of public health nutrition.

Part IV Promoting the Public's Nutritional Health

Chapter 10 Growing a Healthier Nation: Maternal, Infant, Child, and Adolescent Nutrition
Chapter 11 The Importance of Public Health Nutrition Programs in Preventing Disease and Promoting Adult Health
Chapter 12 Assuring Nutrition Services for Older Adults
Chapter 13 Providing Nutrition Services in Public Health Primary Care
Chapter 14 The Baby Boomers: Identification of Wellness Needs
Chapter 15 Maintaining Nutrition and Food Service Standards in Group Care

Part IV includes those chapters that illustrate the programs and services public health nutrition provides for the differing groups of Americans. Through needs assessment, scientific study, and policy, many groups have been identified as recipients of public health nutrition. In Chapter 10, the programs and services, along with the challenges of serving children, adolescents, and women are discussed. While in Chapters 11 through 15, the reader is educated about the public health nutrition programs that affect adults, a special sub-set of adults such as the baby boomers, and the elderly. Each group differs in needs and challenges, but all will need to be provided for by public health nutrition now and in the future.

Part V Protecting the Public's Nutritional Health

Chapter 16   Safeguarding the Food Supply
Chapter 17   Securing Adequate Food for the Public
Chapter 18   Security of the Food Supply and Bioterrorism
             Preparedness

Part V includes *Nutrition and Public Health's* newest additions to the 2nd edition. While Chapter 16 had appeared in the first edition (which has now been greatly enriched), Chapters 17 and 18 bring us to a whole new frontier of public health nutrition. That new frontier is securing adequate food for those who still live in poverty in our great nation as discussed in Chapter 17, and in Chapter 18, the fact that we must be protected from potential bioterrorism plots directed at our food supply. Despite the present outreach of public health nutrition, a hefty percentage of Americans still live without adequate food and/or live in a constant state of fear of being without food, thus showing that we have far to go in reaching those at highest risk. Yet we still face the stinging realization that food, too, must be kept secure because it can be a potent avenue for terrorism. Public health nutrition will now have to meet the challenge of keeping food safe from many forms of invasion.

Part VI Managing the System

Chapter 19   Planning and Evaluating Nutrition Services for
             the Community
Chapter 20   Managing Data
Chapter 21   Managing Money

Part VI provides the reader with fundamental information for how public health nutrition is funded. Chapter 19 details how nutrition services are planned and evaluated, such that targeted funds can be delineated to effective programs. In order to evaluate the effectiveness and cost of a program, data must be collected and managed appropriately, as discussed in Chapter 20. And, lastly a discussion on how money is managed will help the reader take public health nutrition from funding to appropriations, as shown in Chapter 21.

Part VII Mobilizing Personnel

Chapter 22 Staffing Public Health Nutrition Programs and Services
Chapter 23 Managing Public Health Nutrition Personnel
Chapter 24 Leveraging Nutrition Education through the Public Health Team

Chapter 22 in Part VII reviews the core functions of the professionals that encumber the public health nutrition team and designates the number needed to carry out the programs and services. In addition, Chapter 23 educates the reader on effective management skills that enable the public health nutrition profession to work through the ranks and perform those services that are necessary. Nutrition education services, as is discussed in Chapter 24, is the final result of all the program planning, scientific data collection, nutrition policy, money appropriation, and safeguarding and distributing of the American public's food.

Part VIII Surviving in a Competitive World

Chapter 25 Networking for Nutrition
Chapter 26 Marketing Nutrition Programs and Services
Chapter 27 Earning Administrative Support
Chapter 28 Striving for Excellence and Envisioning the Future

Part VIII imparts important features to any program, that of networking, marketing, striving for excellence, and envisioning the future. For any program to be successful, these elements must be present and remain as one of public health nutrition's most daunting challenges. In order for programs to work and meet the needs of those targeted to receive help, networking and marketing must be carefully planned. Chapters 25 and 26 give the reader an insight to these tools. Chapter 27 instills in the reader the need to market nutrition programs within the organization of public health to assure survival. And, Chapter 28 reminds the reader that public health nutrition is a dynamic process and changes constantly. We must be able to anticipate needs and follow with provision of those needs to be successful.

Book Features

Nutrition in Public Health, 2nd Edition has maintained the cutting edge relevance of the 1st edition, but has added several enhancement features.

- *More in-depth information:* Each chapter from the 1st edition has been updated and enhanced to give the reader a vast supply of background information. By making each chapter very complete, the reader comes away with a full understanding of public health nutrition. In addition, new topics have been added to the 2nd edition to reflect today's public health issues. These include:
  - obesity in America
  - programs for the aged
  - demands of the baby boomers
  - food insecurity
  - food bioterrorism
  - the role of the USDA in public health nutrition
- *Section transitions:* The text is divided into eight sections that transcend the reader into the world of public health nutrition in a very organized fashion.

- *Text boxes:* Interesting websites, added information, and word definitions have been included in text boxes for easy reader viewing.

- *Websites:* The reader has been provided with an array of website addresses, so that more accurate information on any topic is accessible.
- *Relevant appendices:* The reader is given several public health nutrition foundational articles, as well as "how-to" guides. Appendix D: Guidelines for Community Nutrition Supervised Experiences, 2nd edition includes self-assessments for the public health nutritionist.
  - Appendix A: Public Health Nutrition: A Historical Perspective
  - Appendix B: Position of The American Dietetic Association: Providing Nutrition Services for Infants, Children, and Adults with Developmental Disabilities and Special Health Care Needs
  - Appendix C: Position of The American Dietetic Association: The Role of Dietetics Professionals in Health Promotion and Disease Prevention
  - Appendix D: Guidelines for Community Nutrition Supervised Experiences, 2nd edition
  - Appendix E: Helpful Nutrition Websites
  - Appendix F: State Health Department Websites

- Appendix G: 2004 Team Nutrition Training Grant Application
  - Appendix H: Learning Activities
- *Textbook website* at Jones & Bartlett Publishers (www.jbpub.com/catalog/0763783587/additional_resources.htm) for both the student and instructor.

For the student:
- chapter outlines,
- access to a PowerPoint presentation of each chapter, and
- website links to many of those noted in the textbook.

For the instructor:
- PowerPoint presentation of each chapter,
- test bank,
- curriculum recommendations, and
- quick access to most websites noted in the textbook.

References

1. Division of Epidemiology, School of Public Health, University of Minnesota. The LET Program, 1999.
2. U.S. Public Health Service Essential Public Health Services. Work Group of the Core Public Health Function Steering Committee, 1994.

ACKNOWLEDGMENTS

The editor and contributing authors of *Nutrition in Public Health: A Handbook for Developing Programs and Services, 2nd edition* would like to recognize the editor of the first edition, Mildred Kaufman, MS, RD. Mildred is an alumnus of Simmons College, which the majority of contributing authors call home, and a past Department Head of University of North Carolina Chapel Hill's School of Public Health. It is Mildred's pioneering spirit and fine efforts on the first edition of this book that have made the second possible. We are grateful to Mildred for this and her contribution to the field of nutrition, dietetics, and public health.

I would like to thank Lori DeCosta and Susan Savino, two wonderful teaching assistants at Simmons College, who helped with the administrative portions of this book. Also, many thanks to my publisher, Jones & Bartlett, Mike Brown, Kylah McNeill, Kate Hennessy, Marissa Hederson, Toni Zucarrini Ackley, and Jason Miranda for their patience and assistance with this project.

Sari Edelstein

PART I

APPLYING NUTRITION TO PUBLIC HEALTH

Chapter 1 Understanding the Role of Nutrition in
Public Health Service
Sari Edelstein, PhD, RD

Chapter 2 Applying Nutrition Science to the
Public's Health
Carol E. O'Neil, PhD, MPH, LDN, RD
Theresa Nicklas, Dr. PH

Part 1 introduces the reader to the role of nutrition in public health service throughout U.S. history and shows how science affected decisions that were made in the name of the public's health. Chapter 1 describes the United States' need to discover a way to serve the less fortunate. Americans had little organized healthcare for the sick, including those of highest risk, the young and the elderly. But, as the United States' public health service grew, so did the methods for ascertaining what nutritional information should be disseminated to the public. Chapter 2 describes the various studies that brought about the public health nutrition standards we enjoy today.

CHAPTER 1

UNDERSTANDING THE ROLE OF NUTRITION IN PUBLIC HEALTH SERVICE

Sari Edelstein, PhD, RD

Reader Objectives

After studying this chapter and reflecting on the contents, you should be able to:

1. Discuss the ethical foundation for public health nutrition.
2. Discuss the primary purpose of public health nutrition in history.
3. Define the populations who would be best served through public health nutrition.
4. Forecast the diversity and disability rate in the population and what they will mean in terms of providing nutritional services in the future.
5. Clarify the role of a public health nutritionist as the provider of care in preventing disease.
6. Describe an educational program that assists the student and practitioner in strengthening their public health nutrition competency.

The history of public health service is grounded in two basic ethical questions that citizens of every era have had to ask themselves: Who should be served? And how will this be financially supported? For most of public service, funds must be allocated from the whole society to help the few in need. Therefore, the practice of public health service involves, first and foremost, an ethical question concerning who to serve with resources that are never unlimited.

The pages of U.S. public health history are full of accounts of ethical decisions to help those in need. In the early years of the United States, society had little precedence to follow in feeding the poor or nourishing the disadvantaged, but made the decision to form centers or freestanding areas where they could provide aid. This chapter introduces the reader to the history of public health nutrition, where those ethical decisions were made and acted upon.

Currently, we face the challenge of educating those who have selected public health nutrition careers. We would be remiss not to include ethics and morality in the curriculum, as this is the foundation of all public service.

Ethics in Public Health Nutrition

In his book *Food Ethics*, Nigel Dower discusses human rights theory, which relates closely to public health nutrition and the responsibility to feed and nourish the population.[1] Dower reiterates Shue's theory defining the contents of human rights:

> There are three socially basic rights: subsistence, security and liberty. Three duties correspond to such rights: duties not to deprive, duties to protect from standard threats of deprivation, and duties to come to the aid of the deprived.[2]

This passage clarifies the type of morality that drives public health nutrition. In essence, the morality of a society to serve others, in terms of food subsistence, comes *before* societal law, legislation, money allocations, or political standing. The latter are all necessary functions of modern society, but do not represent the moral fibers that public health nutrition service was founded upon. An understanding of ethics in public health nutrition allows one to envision the following multi-layered process for providing services:

Layer 1: The altruism, prompted by ethics and morality, to feed and serve others in the name of human rights, as stated above

Layer 2: The assessment team that surveys, evaluates, and puts into place plans for service

Layer 3: The establishment of legislation and laws to decide how best to distribute equities to serve others

Layer 4: The establishment of agencies and departments to carry out public policy

Layer 5: The personnel to interpret public policy and finalize tasks that result in serving others

Note that layers 2 through 5 can be carried out in a variety of ways depending on societal politics and other factors.

The argument that public health, and specifically public health nutrition, is founded in ethics is demonstrated by the Public Health Leadership Society's publication titled *Principles of the Ethical Practice of Public Health*.[3] The society has developed 12 principles that reflect morality and human rights as a part of their framework. These principles are shown in Table 1-1.

TABLE 1-1   Principles of the Ethical Practice of Public Health

1. Public health should address principally the fundamental causes of disease and requirements for health, aiming to prevent adverse health outcomes.
2. Public health should achieve community health in a way that respects the rights of individuals in the community.
3. Public health policies, programs, and priorities should be developed and evaluated through processes that ensure an opportunity for input from community members.
4. Public health should advocate and work for the empowerment of disenfranchised community members, aiming to ensure that the basic resources and conditions necessary for health are accessible to all.
5. Public health should seek the information needed to implement effective policies and programs that protect and promote health.
6. Public health institutions should provide communities with the information they have that is needed for decisions on policies or programs and should obtain the community's consent for their implementation.
7. Public health institutions should act in a timely manner on the information they have within the resources and the mandate given to them by the public.
8. Public health programs and policies should incorporate a variety of approaches that anticipate and respect diverse values, beliefs, and cultures in the community.
9. Public health programs and policies should be implemented in a manner that most enhances the physical and social environment.
10. Public health institutions should protect the confidentiality of information that can bring harm to an individual or community if made public. Exceptions must be justified on the basis of the high likelihood of significant harm to the individual or others.
11. Public health institutions should ensure the professional competence of their employees.
12. Public health institutions and their employees should engage in collaborations and affiliations in ways that build the public's trust and the institution's effectiveness.

Source: Reprinted with permission from Public Health Leadership Society. *Principles of the Ethical Practice of Public Health,* Version 2.2, 2002.

The Public Health Leadership Society also offers 10 essential public health services, within which lie opportunities for the 12 ethical principles. Table 1-2 details where ethical principles can be demonstrated in the essential tasks of public health work.

TABLE 1-2   Correspondence of the 12 Ethical Principles with the 10 Essential Public Health Services

Essential Public Health Services[†]	Ethical Principle
1. Monitor the health status to identify community health problems	(5) collect information (7) act on information
2. Diagnose and investigate health problems and health hazards in the community	(5) collection information
3. Inform, educate, and empower people about health issues	(4) advocacy and empowerment (6) provide information
4. Mobilize community partnerships to identify and solve health problems	(12) collaboration
5. Develop policies and plans that support individual and community health efforts	(1) protect and promote health; address fundamental causes of health risks (3) feedback from the community (5) collect information
6. Enforce laws and regulations that protect health and ensure safety	(2) achieve community health with respect for individual rights (3) feedback from the community (7) act upon information
7. Link people to needed personal health services and assure the provision of healthcare when otherwise unavailable	(4) advocate for and empower; basic resources available to all (8) incorporate diversity
8. Assure a competent public health and personal health care workforce	(11) professional competence
9. Evaluate effectiveness, accessibility, and quality of personal and population-based health services	(3) community feedback (5) collect information
10. Research for new insights and innovative solutions to health problems	(5) collect information
No corresponding essential public health service	(9) enhance physical and social environments (10) protect confidentiality

[†]Developed by the Essential Public Health Services Work Group of the Public Health Functions Steering Committee, 1994.

Source: Reprinted with permission from Public Health Leadership Society. *Principles of the Ethical Practice of Public Health*, Version 2.2, 2002.

The History of Public Health Nutrition

The history of public health nutrition in the United States runs parallel to the other history-making events of the country's early years. However, one difference exists concerning public health history: As mentioned earlier, public health history is not just a series of events that occurred over time, but rather ethical decisions that were made throughout the ages based on human rights. For example, as the country faced public health ills, the public health services, whether voluntary or paid, responded to the needs of the nation. Although the founding societies of the United States faced high rates of morbidity and mortality caused by communicable diseases, poor hygiene, and poor sanitation, the public health service responded by establishing public health departments to assist with these problems. Later, in the late 19th and early 20th centuries, child labor and large numbers of people in poverty brought about federal-state partnerships and grants-in-aid for assistance to women, children, and disabled persons. As the 20th century rolled on, the United States experienced a rising prevalence of behavior-related problems such as substance abuse, adolescent pregnancy, sexually transmitted diseases, and a growing impoverished elderly population. Again, public health established many programs to feed and nourish those groups, such as Head Start and the Nutrition Program for the Elderly. In the present day, public health continues to provide nutritional programs that treat the population and create guidelines for disease prevention through better nutrition.

The following sections describe the status of public health in the United States during various eras and show how the nation ethically responded to those needs. For a more detailed explanation of the public health nutrition history of the United States, turn to Appendix A, which contains the full text of an article by M.C. Egan.[4]

Public Health Accomplishments: Mid to Late 1800s[4]

In this era, the United States had a high infant mortality rate, epidemics of communicable disease, and many other problems associated with poor hygiene and sanitation.

- Voluntary health agencies were organized in the 1850s (Visiting Nurse Association in New York and Boston).
- The first State Department of Health was established in Massachusetts in 1867.
- In 1872, the American Public Health Association was organized.
- By 1877, 14 states had Departments of Health.
- State government acted to control communicable diseases, improve sanitation, provide health and parent education, and address nutrition concerns.

- School lunch programs were initiated in Boston in 1894 and in New York City in 1889.
- In 1894, nutrition investigations were initiated in the Office of Experiment Stations of the U.S. Department of Agriculture.
- Milk stations were opened in New York City in 1895 and in Rochester, New York, in 1897.

Public Health Accomplishments: The Early Years (1900–1919)[4]

During these years, the United States saw high rates of morbidity and mortality, problems involving child labor, and large numbers of people in poverty.

- Pasteurized milk was introduced in 1910.
- In 1912, the U.S. Children's Bureau was created.
- Massachusetts employed its first nutritionist in 1917.
- Community nutrition work was being conducted by two pioneers, Frances Stern and Lucy Gillett.

Public Health Accomplishments: The Youthful Years (1920–1939)[4]

In these decades, the United States experienced the stock market crash and subsequent economic depression. These years were plagued with millions of people being poor, unemployed, and deprived. There also were high rates of immigration, which provided cultural challenges to providers.

- In 1920, the U.S. Children's Bureau launched studies of the nutritional status of children.
- In 1921, the Shepard-Towner Act was created. It provided the first federal-state partnership for health services and gave states grants-in-aid for maternal and child health.
- Many voluntary agencies, notably the American Red Cross, made major contributions to the development of public health nutrition.
- In 1924, iodine was added to salt in the first food fortification program.
- In 1935, Congress enacted the Social Security Act to combat the serious effects of the economic depression. This provided states with grants-in-aid for Maternal and Child Health and Crippled Children's Service (MCH) (Title V) and for Child Welfare (Title IV).
- The U.S. Children's Bureau employed its first nutrition consultant, Marjorie M. Heseltine, in 1936.
- By 1936, there were 11 positions for nutritionists in 4 states.
- By 1939, there were 39 positions for nutritionists in 24 states.

- The federal government created the Food Distribution Program in 1935 and an experimental Food Stamp Program in 1939.
- In 1937, the Milbank Memorial Fund supported the first roundtable on Nutrition and Public Health.
- The first qualifications for nutritionists in public health were published in 1938.

Public Health Accomplishments: The Middle Years (1940–1959)[4]

These two decades saw rapid changes in the United States, such as World War II. The war gave priority to nutritional aspects of national defense, and food supplies were rationed.

- Women moved into the workforce, and day care for children became necessary.
- The U.S. Children's Bureau (CB) added a second nutrition consultant, Helen Stacey, MS, to its staff in 1941. It also issued Food for Young Children in Group Care to assist day care providers.
- Antibiotics and the polio vaccine were discovered.
- In nutrition, advances were made in the enrichment of bread and flour and the fortification of milk and margarine.
- In 1942, the Public Health Service (PHS) began to conduct nutrition appraisals in selected states.
- Title V/MCH awarded a 3-year grant to the New York City Health Department to establish a nutrition division in 1943.
- In 1944, Normal Jolliffe, MD, began a diagnostic, treatment, and training clinic for nutritional deficiency diseases in New York City.
- By 1945, all but three states had at least one nutrition consultant position in their state health departments.
- The National Academy of Sciences established a Committee on Maternal Nutrition and Child Feeding in 1946.
- CB added three regional nutrition consultant positions in 1947.
- The Association of Faculties of Graduate Programs in Public Health Nutrition was formally organized in 1950.
- The Association of State and Territorial Public Health Nutrition Directors was formally organized in 1952.
- Public health nutritionists had a major role in the implementation of the new National School Lunch Program.
- The Special Milk Program followed in 1954.[5]

Public Health Accomplishments: The Maturing Years (1960–1979)[4]

During this era the United States endured considerable unrest as the nation struggled with civil rights, war, poverty and hunger, access to healthcare, increasing environmental pollution, and a rising prevalence of behavior-related problems such as substance abuse, adolescent pregnancy, and sexually transmitted diseases.

- President Johnson established many programs in the 1960s, including the special projects for Maternity and Infant Care (M & I) in 1963, the Comprehensive Health Projects for Children and Youth (C & Y) and community health center and migrant health programs in 1965, family planning programs in 1969, the Head Start program in 1965, the Medicare and Medicaid programs in 1965, and the University-Affiliated Centers program in 1963.
- The first conference on the role of the State Health Departments in Nutrition Research was held in 1961.
- The 1961 Survey of Home Care Programs indicated that part-time nutrition services were available in 34 of 37 programs.
- In 1963, the USDA and the Georgia Junior Chamber of Commerce launched a pilot program called the Surplus Food for Needy Expectant Mothers Program in three counties in Georgia.
- The Food Stamp Act passed in 1965.
- In 1967, Congress began a series of hearings on hunger, and created a Citizen's Board of Inquiry into the extent and nature of hunger.
- To provide more information about hunger and other nutritional problems, several studies and surveys were launched, including the Title V/MCH 1968 Study of Nutritional Status of Preschool Children in the United States, the PHS 1970 Ten State Survey, and the 1971 National Health and Nutrition Examination Survey.
- Public health nutritionists worked to improve food assistance to the needy, which led to the development of the Special Supplemental Food Program for Women, Infants and Children (WIC).
- Title V/MCH awarded a grant to the National Academy of Sciences (NAS) to support the work of the Committee of Maternal Nutrition in 1968.
- The first White House Conference on Food, Nutrition and Health was called in 1969.
- In 1970, the NAS published *Maternal Nutrition and the Course of Pregnancy*, which revolutionized nutrition care practices during pregnancy.
- A White House Conference on Aging was convened in 1971, which led to the establishment of the Nutrition Program for the Elderly in 1973.
- Dietary Goals for the United States were issued in 1977.

Public Health Accomplishments: Recent Years (1980–1994)[4]

During these decades, the United States saw an increase in the number of immigrants, as well as an increase in the number of elderly persons. New challenges included the rise of AIDS and Alzheimer's disease and the return of tuberculosis.

- Many national conferences, such as the Surgeon General's 1980 Conference on Breastfeeding and Human Lactation and the 1988 Conference on Nutrition and Health, had major impacts on the advance of public health nutrition.
- A few new sources of funding for nutrition became available, such as Medicaid funds, Education for Handicapped funds, and Risk Reduction grants.
- Nutrition services to children with special healthcare needs were expanded and improved.
- The National Academy of Sciences issued guidelines for nutrition services in perinatal care in 1981 and a revision in 1992.
- Legislation creating the National Nutritional Status Monitoring System was enacted.
- Human lactation and breast-feeding were successfully promoted.
- The National Academy of Sciences issued *Diet and Health: Implications for Reducing Chronic Disease Risk* in 1989 and *Improving America's Diet and Health: From Recommendations to Action* in 1991.
- The Institute of Medicine reports *Nutrition During Pregnancy* and *Nutrition During Lactation* were published in 1990 and 1991, respectively.[5]

Public Health Accomplishments: 1995–Early 21st Century[4]

Recently, the United States has been improving the nutritional status of the population. However, obesity is reaching a crisis point, especially in America's youth. Nutrition has been shown to have some proven disease prevention links, and applied science is being utilized to create guidelines for better health through nutrition.

- Healthy People 2000 and 2010
- Dietary Reference Intakes
- Dietary Guidelines for Americans (revised)
- National Cancer Institute's 5-A-Day Program
- National Nutrition Monitoring and Related Research Program
- Healthy Eating Index

The Changing Population of the 21st Century

The history of public health and public health nutrition has given us insight into where we have been, but where are we going in the 21st century? Who will public health nutrition serve now? To answer these questions, we turn to the demographics of the disadvantaged in our population. Figure 1-1 shows a U.S. Census Bureau graph that depicts the number of people in the United States who lived in poverty between 1959 and 2003.[6] Note that the poverty level in the United States in 2003 rose to a similar level as seen in 1959. This translates into real challenges for public health nutrition for the 21st century.

> See Chapter 4 to read about those at highest nutritional risk in America.

Public Health Nutrition and Persons of Diversity

The population of the United States continues to grow increasingly diverse in the 21st century. Hispanic Americans and other minority groups have grown faster than the rest of the population as a whole. These groups have grown from 16% of the U.S. population in 1970 to 27% in 1998, and are predicted to reach 50% by the year 2050.[7]

> Among the minority groups in America are non-Hispanic African Americans, Asian Americans, and Native Americans. Each ethnic group and its subgroups will have preferences as to how they are named, and this will change from time to time.

Statistical data from the Census Bureau indicates that growing immigration and diversity have important effects on social and economic status. Social and economic status can define household structure, age distribution, child poverty, and the prevalence of single-parent families. Since 1970, single-parent households have increased for all groups, as follows:[7]

- 38% African Americans
- 26% Native Americans
- 26% Hispanic Americans

Poverty rates are highest among children, and rates of criminal activity are highest among young adults, indicating the effect of age on social and economic status. Populations with a large percentage of people younger than 18 years of age have been linked to increased incidences of poverty. The following are the percentages of people under 18 in each ethnic group:[7]

- 24% non-Hispanic Caucasians
- 30% non-Hispanic African Americans and Asian Americans
- 35% Native Americans
- 35% Hispanic Americans

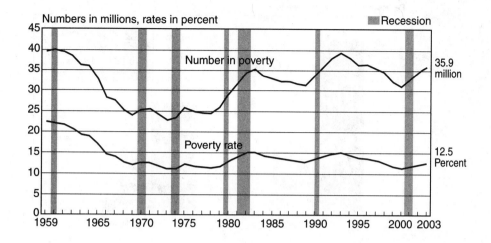

FIGURE 1-1 Number of People Living in Poverty and the Poverty Rate: 1959–2003
Source: U.S. Census Bureau. Available at: www.census.gov.

Public Health Nutrition and Persons with Disabilities and Special Needs

The chapters that follow include information about nutritional programs for those with disabilities and special healthcare needs. As of 1997, 1 in 5 Americans had a disability, which constitutes 12% of the population. The U.S. Census Bureau estimates that this number will rise to 1 in 10 Americans by the year 2030. This correlates directly to the number of people who will be 65 years or older in the United States by that year.[8] Figure 1-2 gives percentages of the population with disabilities, as measured in 1994–1995.

Legislative support for persons with disabilities began with the Developmental Disabilities Assistance and Bill of Rights Act of 1963. Nutritional training and service were a part of this program. In the 21st century, the need for legislation for disabled people continues. Examples of public health nutrition programs are included in many of the chapters of this book. The following lists just a few of those programs that provide nutritional assistance to the public:

- Elderly Nutrition Program
- Cooperative Extension Service
- American Cancer Society
- American Heart Association
- March of Dimes
- 5-A-Day for Better Health
- WIC (Supplemental Nutrition Program for Women, Infants and Children)

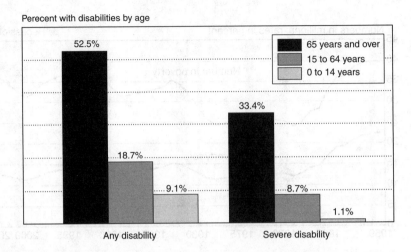

FIGURE 1-2   Disabilities and Age: October 1994–January 1995
Source: Department of Commerce. *Disabilities affect one-fifth of all Americans.* Census Briefs, December 1997, p. 1. Available at: www.census.gov.

- Food Stamp Program
- School Breakfast and Lunch Program
- Child and Adult Care Food Program

For more information on defining disabilities and the different disabilities that have a nutrition component, see Appendix B[9]; for the role of dietetic professionals, see Appendix C.[10] Appendices D and E provide a list of state Public Health Department websites and other helpful websites for accessing agencies and organizations that provide public health nutrition services.

The Education of Public Health Practitioners

It is hoped that those who have entered the field of public health nutrition understand the ethical principles behind feeding the population. One can now see how important educating public health nutritionists or any service-oriented personnel must be in terms of understanding the most primary of ideals. These ideals should be intertwined with the foundation of all education programs, and is apparent in the recommended guidelines available in Appendix F. Guidelines for Community Nutrition Supervised Experiences, 2nd edition,[11] provides curriculum content for training future public health nutritionists. Additionally, the guidelines provide a "Self Assessment Tool for the Public Health Nutritionist," which assists public health nutrition practitioners in assessing their skills in five areas:

1. Nutrition and dietetic practice
2. Communications

3. Public health science and practice
4. Management
5. Legislation and advocacy

All five curriculum units contain ethical components.

Issues for Discussion

1. Should the curriculum for public health practitioners have more explicit instruction and discussion of ethics?
2. The population is aging and becoming increasingly larger. Discuss the economic burden versus ethical responsibility of those who may have to fund their public health services.

References

1. Dower, N. (1996). Global hunger: Moral dilemmas. In B. Mepham (ed.), *Food Ethics* (pp. 3). New York: Routledge.
2. Shue, H. (1980). *Basic rights: Subsistence, affluence and U.S. foreign policy.* Princeton, NJ: Princeton University Press.
3. Public Health Leadership Society. (2002). *Principles of the ethical practice of public health* (version 2.2). Chicago, IL: American Public Health Association.
4. Egan, M. C. (1994). Public health nutrition: A historical perspective. *Journal of the American Dietetic Association*, 94(3), 298–305.
5. Compiled by the author with permission from M. C. Egan. Egan, M. C. (1994). Public health nutrition: A historical perspective. *Journal of the American Dietetic Association*, 94(3), 298–235.
6. U.S. Census Bureau. (n.d.). Number in poverty and poverty rate: 1959 to 2003. Retrieved February 28, 2005, from http://www.census.gov/hhes/poverty/poverty03/pov03fig03.pdf.
7. U.S. Department of Commerce. (December 1997). Disabilities affect one-fifth of all Americans. *Census Briefs*, p. 1. Retrieved February 28, 2005, from http://www.census.gov/prod/3/97pubs/cenbr975.pdf.
8. Council of Economic Advisers for the President's Initiative on Race. (June 1999). Changing America: Indicators of social and economic well-being by race and Hispanic origin. U.S. society & values. *Electronic Journal of the U.S. Information Agency*, 4(2). Retrieved August 27, 2004, from www.jsmccarthy.com.
9. Cloud, H. H. & Posthauer, M. E. (2003). Position of the American Dietetic Association: Providing nutrition services for infants, children, and adults with developmental disabilities and special healthcare needs. *Journal of the American Dietetic Association*, 11(2), 97–107.
10. Hampl, J. S., Anderson, J. V., & Mullis, R. (2002). Position of the American Dietetic Association: The role of dietetics professionals in health promotion and disease prevention. *Journal of the American Dietetic Association*, 102(11), 1680–1687.
11. Mixon, H., Dodds, J., & Haughton, B. (2003). *Guidelines for community nutrition supervised experiences* (2nd ed.). Chicago: IL: Public Health/Community Nutrition Practice Group, American Dietetic Association.

CHAPTER 2

APPLYING NUTRITION SCIENCE TO THE PUBLIC'S HEALTH

Carol E. O'Neil, PhD, MPH, LDN, RD

Theresa A. Nicklas, DrPH

Reader Objectives

After studying this chapter and reflecting on the contents, you should be able to:

1. Explain why nutrition policies and recommendations must be grounded in science.
2. Discuss how to evaluate scientific studies that are used in generating nutrition policies and recommendations.
3. Describe how each type of research study might be used to generate data for or monitor nutrition policy or programs.
4. Discuss how and why nutrition policies, recommendations, and programs are changed at regular intervals.
5. Debate the uses and misuses of nutrition policies and recommendations.
6. Outline resources that public health nutritionists might use to keep pace with current research or available programs that are grounded in research.

Introduction

> If we could give every individual the right amount of nourishment and exercise, not too little and not too much, we would have found the safest way to health.
>
> —Hippocrates 460–377 BCE

Hippocrates had it right, but appreciation of this relationship was a long time in coming for the rest of us. Before the 1970s, public health nutrition was focused primarily on preventing nutrient deficiency diseases. Early in the 20th century, there was a general lack of understanding of the relationship between diet and disease, and diseases such as pellagra and rickets were common. As deficiency diseases became less common, there was growing awareness that dietary excess and imbalance increased the risk of developing chronic disease, such as coronary heart disease (CHD) and hypertension.[1]

In 1977, the U.S. Senate Select Committee on Nutrition and Human Needs, under the leadership of Senator George McGovern, issued *Dietary Goals for the U.S.*[2] The goals engendered controversy among health professionals and the food industry because of the way they were conceived and presented. At that time, there was also a lack of consensus on the impact of food/nutrients on chronic disease risk. In retrospect, the authors of these dietary goals were remarkably perspicacious in their understanding of the relationship between diet and chronic disease. The statement by Dr. C. Edith Weir, Assistant Director of the Human Nutrition Research Division, U.S. Department of Agriculture (USDA), that "Most all of the health problems underlying the leading causes of death in the U.S. could be modified by improvements in diet"[2] remains the cornerstone of public health nutrition and nutrition policy in the United States.

Today, the preponderance of epidemiologic, clinical, and laboratory data clearly link diet and physical activity with disease, including chronic disease. Four of the leading causes of death—heart disease, malignant neoplasms, cerebrovascular disease, and diabetes mellitus—are related directly to diet. Although the actual numbers of individuals dying from these diseases may have changed over the last 20 years—for example, there has been a decline in heart disease over the past 20 years—the rank order of these diseases as causes of mortality has not changed (www.cdc.gov/nchsfastats/lchod.htm).[3] These diseases cost society over $200 billion a year in medical expenses and lost productivity.

> A PowerPoint presentation showing obesity trends in the United States between 1985 and 2003 can be found at http://www.cdc.gov/nccdphp/dnpa/obesity/trend/maps/index.htm.

Not included among the four major causes of death, but a major contributor to these and other health problems, is obesity. Obesity has reached epidemic proportions. National Health and Nutrition Examination Survey (NHANES) data from 1999–2000 and 2001–2002[4] showed that among adults[5] in those time periods, 65.1% of the population was overweight, 30.4% were obese, and 4.9% were extremely obese. In 1999–2002, 31.0% of children aged 6 through 19 years were at risk for being overweight, and 16.0% were overweight.[6,7] Data from 195,005 adults aged 18 years or older participating in the Behavioral Risk Factor Surveillance System (BRFSS) demonstrated that, in 2002, the prevalence of obesity was 22.1% versus 21.0% in 2001, and 11.6% in 1990. Over 2% of adults had a body mass index (BMI) of 40 or higher in 2001.[8] One caveat to the BRFSS data is that the data are self-reported. *The Surgeon General's Call to Action to Prevent and Decrease Overweight and Obesity*, published in 2001 (www.surgeongeneral.gov/topics/obesity), estimated the cost of obesity, separate from the chronic diseases with which it is associated, as $117 billion a year. Other investigators have placed this cost slightly lower, at $75 billion (in 2003 dollars); approximately half the cost of obesity is paid by Medicare or Medicaid.[9] Obesity has surpassed tobacco, alcohol, and poverty as a public health risk.[10,11]

These health problems are not unique to the United States. Globally, largely preventable chronic diseases account for 59% of deaths and 46% of the global disease burden. By 2020, it is estimated that nearly 75% of deaths worldwide will result from these diseases, with 60% occurring in developing countries that are experiencing rapid health transitions (www.who.int/nut/documents/trs_916.pdf). The World Health Organization (WHO) has compared the spread of chronic diseases to that of communicable diseases; however, chronic diseases appear to be spread by the Westernization of diets and a decline in physical activity associated with increasing industrialization, rather than by infectious or parasitic agents. In May 2004, the WHO finalized its global strategy for diet, physical activity, and health (www.who.int/dietphysicalactivity/strategy/eb11344en). This strategy was formulated carefully to reduce the risk of chronic noncommunicable diseases while continuing to carry forward long-term WHO goals on other nutrition-related areas, including undernutrition.

Relatively few modifiable risk factors, such as obesity, smoking, alcohol, and lack of physical activity, cause the majority of the chronic disease burden. Changes in diet and physical activity patterns can significantly reduce disease risk, often in a surprisingly short time period. It is estimated that a 1% reduction in the intake of fat and saturated fat and a 0.1% reduction in the intake of cholesterol would, over 20 years, prevent over 56,000 cases of CHD,[12] avoid over 18,000 deaths, and save over 117,000 life-years. Improved dietary patterns could save $43 billion in medical care costs and lost productivity resulting from CHD, cancer, stroke, and diabetes, and prevent over 119,900 premature deaths among individuals from 55–74 years of age. As the average life expectancy in the United States continues to rise, and if current dietary and physical activity patterns continue as they are, the incidence and prevalence of chronic diseases will continue to increase.

Public Health Nutritionists and the Science Behind Them

Public health nutritionists or registered dietitians working in public health settings can play decisive roles in improving our nation's health.[13] The Institute of Medicine's (IOM) *Future of Public Health* states that the mission of public health is to assure conditions where people can be healthy.[14] Over the past decades dramatic changes have occurred in the field of public health that both help and hinder this mission. There are changes in demographic profiles and differences in eating patterns (including the fact that more people are eating away from home); and, for consumers and health professionals alike, there is a bewildering array of information available. Information is available on the Internet and in peer-reviewed journals, as well as through standard media channels.[15-17] It is a challenge to understand, evaluate, or even generate the science behind nutrition programs and policies, and to be able to "translate" the science into nutrition messages for non-nutrition-trained health professionals and clients. In this chapter, we will look at examples of how nutritional science can be translated into messages, and how decisions can be made concerning the science behind legislation and policy.

> Anybody can put anything on the Internet—and very little information is removed. Get into the habit of evaluating websites to determine whether the site you've chosen for information is accurate, reliable, and timely. Need help? Learn how to evaluate all websites from a reliable website: http://www.library.cornell.edu/olinuris/ref/research/webeval.html.

Public health nutritionists need to have a broad understanding of the sciences, including the pathophysiology of disease, genetics, biotechnology and its impact on sustainable agriculture, nutritional biochemistry and molecular biology, biostatistics, epidemiology, and of course, nutritional sciences. Epidemiologic studies are particularly important for public health nutritionists and range from federal nutrition monitoring programs to studies such as the Bogalusa Heart Study and the Framingham Heart Study, both discussed later in this chapter. Table 2-1 more fully describes design strategies of epidemiologic studies and their uses. Metabolic diet studies and animal studies are also important in nutrition and health research.

> **Biotechnology**—The simplest definition is "applied biology." Today we think of it as cloning animals or gene splicing, but it's as old as man. Did you know that making wine and beer was an early form of biotechnology?

When doing or evaluating a study using either human subjects or laboratory animals, it is important to understand the ethical issues involved and to be sure that all federal guidelines, as well as any institutional guidelines, are met. Information concerning the use of human subjects in research can be found at www.nihtraining.com/ohsrsite; information about animals in research can be found at www.nal.usda.gov/awic/legislat/usdaleg2.htm.

The body of scientific literature available can be confusing, contradictory, and difficult to understand—especially for students as they begin to read and use it. The reasons why revolve around seemingly subtle *differences*. Different study designs may have been

TABLE 2-1   Epidemiologic Design Strategies

Descriptive Studies[1]: Hypothesis Generating

Population or Correlational Studies

These use data from entire populations to compare event (such as disease) frequencies with an exposure in different groups during the same time period or in the same group at different time points. These studies look at whole populations rather than individuals, so that it's impossible to link an individual exposure with the occurrence of disease in that individual.

Individual Studies

Case reports are careful, detailed reports of a patient. Case reports can be suggestive, but it's often difficult to exclude alternative explanations for a condition. These studies are usually used to study rare diseases.

Case series are compiled from multiple case reports describing the same conditions. Routine surveillance programs can often be used to compile case series.

Cross-sectional surveys look at individuals with respect to both exposure and disease at a point in time. Since both exposure and disease are assessed at the same time, it can be difficult to determine whether exposure pre-dated disease.

Analytical Studies: Hypothesis Testing

Observational Studies

Case control studies are a case series of individuals who have the disease of interest and a group of similar individuals who do not have the disease—exposure comparisons are made.

Cohort studies, such as the Nurses' Health Study, classify participants based on the presence or absence of exposure and follow them over time to assess disease development. In a *retrospective cohort study*, the disease of interest has already occurred at the time the study begins; in a *prospective cohort study*, the disease has not yet occurred.

Intervention studies are a type of prospective cohort study where the exposure is controlled by the investigator. These studies can be considered therapeutic (secondary prevention) or preventative. DASH and DASH sodium were intervention studies.

Randomized design is when individuals are randomly assigned to a treatment or control group.

Double-blind placebo-controlled design is when neither the individuals nor the investigator knows whether participants are assigned to a treatment or a placebo group. This study design is usually considered to provide the most compelling evidence of a cause and effect relationship.

[1]All epidemiologic studies have a descriptive element.

Source: Compiled by the authors.

used, and if different statistical analyses were used, the authors may have drawn different conclusions from apparently similar data. Different readers may have interpreted conclusions from articles differently. Different assessments may have been made on similar literature or different criteria may have been used to assess outcomes in similar articles. So, evaluation of the literature is difficult; however, the strength of scientific evidence for possible diet-disease relationships should be graded and assessed prior to setting pubic health goals (i.e., Healthy People 2010), developing dietary recommendations (e.g., Dietary Reference Intakes [DRI]), mandating nutrition policy (e.g., Dietary Guidelines for Americans [DGA]), or designing nutrition interventions (National Cancer Institute's 5 A Day Program [www.5aday.gov]). Epidemiologic studies, animal studies, metabolic diet studies, randomized clinical trials, and behavioral intervention studies (Figure 2-1) provide the science base that is used in legislation and policy.

To evaluate the strength of a body of scientific evidence, the following must be taken into account:

1. The quality of the studies, including the extent to which bias was minimized.
2. The quantity of the studies, including the magnitude of effect, the number of studies conducted, and the sample size and statistical power of the studies.

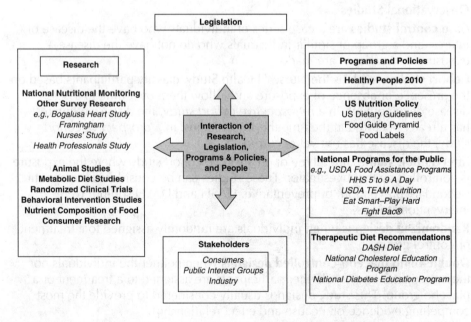

FIGURE 2-1   The Relationships Among Nutrition Research, Legislation, Stakeholders, and Nutrition Programs and Policies
Source: Adapted from Kuczmarski MF, Moshfegh A, Briefel R. Update on nutrition monitoring activities in the United States. *J Am Diet Assoc* 1994;94:753–760. Reprinted with permission.

3. The consistency of results—whether similar studies produce similar results and conclusions.

4. The study design—type of study used to produce the test results and the relevance to the disease under study.

The National Heart, Lung, and Blood Institute (NHLBI) uses a four-point scale to grade the scientific evidence from different study types (Table 2-2). Other types of evidence may also be available, but they are weaker and should be considered less definitive.

Cooper and Zlotkin[18] outlined a six-step framework by which nutrition guidelines can be developed (Table 2-3). Their method is similar to that of the NHLBI, but emphasizes nutrition information. The Agency for Healthcare Research and Quality (AHRQ) (www.ahrq.gov) provides additional information about evidence-based practice, outcomes and other types of research, technology assessment, and clinical practice guidelines. The AHRQ provides information to professionals and to the public. This review of systems to rate the strength of scientific evidence is available from the National Library of Medicine (http://www.ncbi.nlm.nih.gov/books/bv.fcgi?rid=hstat1.chapter.70996). Reports that promulgate the use of evidence-based treatments are available for the treatment of hypertension, CHD, obesity, dietary supplement use, and use of glycated hemoglobin and microalbuminuria in monitoring individuals with diabetes mellitus.

> **Glycated hemoglobin**, also known as glycosylated hemoglobin or HgA1c, is a measure of the level of glucose in the blood that binds to red blood cells. It is used to assess glycemic control over approximately a 90-day period.

Nutrition Monitoring

Collecting nutrition and health-related information from a population is critical for designing and evaluating policies and programs that improve health status and decrease risk factors. To be useful, information must be collected in a timely manner and presented to scientists, policymakers, and the public in readily understandable forms. Without current monitoring, decisions may be made using insufficient information or incorrect assumptions; further, important problems may not be addressed.

> Stay on top of nutritional monitoring and other events in public health; subscribe online to the Morbidity and Mortality Weekly Report: http://www.cdc.gov/mmwr/mmwrsubscribe.html.

Nutrition and health-related information can be obtained using several methods, notably nutrition assessment, nutrition screening, and nutrition surveillance; these are often collectively referred to as nutrition monitoring.

TABLE 2-2   National Heart, Lung, and Blood Institute's Evidence Categories

Category	Sources of Evidence	Definition
Category A	Randomized controlled trials (rich body of data)	Well-designed, randomized clinical trials that provide a consistent pattern of findings in the population for which the recommendation is made. Category A requires substantial numbers of studies involving substantial numbers of participants.
Category B	Randomized controlled trials (limited body of data)	Limited randomized trials or interventions, post-hoc subgroup analyses, or meta-analyses of randomized clinical trials are used when there are a limited number of existing trials, study populations are small or provide inconsistent results, or when the trials were undertaken in a population that differs from the target population.
Category C	Observational or non-randomized studies	Evidence is from outcomes of uncontrolled or non-randomized trials or from observational studies.
Category D	Panel consensus judgment	Expert judgment is based on the panel's synthesis of evidence from experimental research described in the literature or derived from the consensus of panel members based on clinical experience or knowledge that does not meet the criteria described in the above categories. This category is used only where the provision of some guidance was deemed valuable but an adequately compelling clinical literature addressing the subject of the recommendation was deemed insufficient to place in one of the other categories.

Source: Adapted from the National Heart, Lung, and Blood Institute. Available at: http://www.nhlbi.nih.gov/guidelines/obesity/ob_gdlns.pdf, with permission.

Nutrition assessment uses indicators of dietary status, including such methods as 24-hour dietary recalls,[21] food frequency questionnaires (FFQs), or other indicators of intake and nutrition-related health status, such as anthropometry or biochemical testing, to identify possible risk factors for chronic disease in individuals or populations, as well as the nature and extent of impaired nutritional status in individuals. Accurate assessment of intake is crucial[22]; thus, it is important to use multiple 24-hour dietary recalls, a multiple pass method for the recalls, and validated instruments to obtain this information. It is also important that ethnic, religious, and regional differences in food preferences and food availability be considered when designing FFQs or other instruments.[23] Measurement error has important implications; therefore, whenever possible dietary intake should be confirmed using appropriate biomarkers.[24,25] Nutrient intake is assessed by measuring specific foods or food groups, or individual nutrients using tools such as the USDA Nutrient Database for Standard Reference (www.nal.usda.gov/fnic/foodcomp). Intake can then be compared with recommended values for specific populations, and, in turn, with the prevalence or incidence of chronic disease.

TABLE 2-3   A Six-Step Methodology for the Creation of an Evidence-Based Nutrition Guideline

---

Step 1: Preliminary Decisions

Select the diet/disease relationship.

Determine study selection criteria.

Create an analytic framework.

Frame the question or problem to be addressed.

Step 2: Literature Search

Determine a strategy for choosing search keywords.

Retrieve the literature,

Step 3: Selection of Eligible Studies

Create literature retrieval instruments to filter eligible studies.

Filter the literature.

Step 4: Rate the Quality of Evidence Reviewed

Create instrument(s) to rate the quality of individual studies.

Perform a quality rating of individual studies.

Step 5: Generate the "Totality of Evidence"

Summarize the research findings from each of the scientific links in the analytic framework.

Step 6: Guideline Development

Summarize the evidence from all of the links to form the guideline.

Source: Reprinted with permission from Cooper MJ, Zlotkin SH. *J Am Diet Assoc.* 2003. Dec;103(12 Suppl 2):S28–33.

Nutrition screening is a systematic approach to quickly identify nutrition problems or individuals at nutritional risk who need further assessment or an intervention. The Nutrition Screening Initiative's (www.aafp.org/x16081.xml) DETERMINE questionnaire, used in screening elderly populations, is one well-recognized instrument.

Surveillance comes from the French word meaning "to watch over." In 1968, the World Health Assembly described surveillance as "the systematic collection and use of epidemiologic information for planning, implementation, and assessment of disease control."[26] Collection of demographic data, such as registration of live births not linked with prevention or control programs, does not constitute a surveillance program. Surveillance, in contrast to surveys, is continuous, and data that are collected can be used to provide the framework for public health policies and rationale for intervention. Surveillance also provides a way to monitor the effectiveness of specific interventions. This completes the loop; surveillance studies can be used to determine nutritional problems or nutritional needs, and after an intervention they can be used to determine whether the problems remain or if the intervention was effective.

Most governments track the health and nutrition status of their population. The U.S. federal government has tracked information on food and the food supply for nearly 100 years, starting with the USDA's Food Supply Series in 1909. The first USDA Household Food Consumption Survey (known as the Nationwide Food Consumption Survey after 1965) was conducted in the 1930s. In 1960, the National Health Examination Survey was begun; however, it did not include information on nutrition and its link with diet. Thus, federal officials could not provide information on diet and disease or undernutrition to Congress. The nation's first comprehensive nutrition survey was the Ten-State Nutrition Survey, conducted between 1968 and 1970 in 10 states—California, Kentucky, Louisiana, Massachusetts, Michigan, New York, South Carolina, Texas, Washington, and West Virginia. NHANES (National Health and Nutrition Examination Survey) I and II and the Pediatric Nutrition Surveillance Systems were initiated in the 1970s.

In 1990, the National Nutrition Monitoring and Related Research Program (NNMRRP) (PL 101–445) established a comprehensive, coordinated program for nutrition monitoring and related research to improve health and nutrition assessment in U.S. populations. The NNMRRP requires a program to coordinate federal nutrition monitoring efforts and assist states and local governments in participating in a nutrition monitoring network, to create an interagency board to develop and implement the program, and to create a nine-member advisory council to provide scientific and technical advice and to evaluate program effectiveness (caselaw.1p.findlaw.com/casecode/uscodes/7/chapters/84/subchapters/ii/sections/section_5331.html and caselaw.1p.findlaw.com/casecode/uscodes/7/chapters/84/subchapters/ii/sections/section_5332.html). The NNMRRP also requires that dietary guidelines (Dietary Guidelines for Americans [DGA]) be issued every 5 years, and that any dietary guidance issued by the federal government for the general public be reviewed by the Secretaries of Agriculture and Health and Human Services (HHS).

The NNMRRP encompasses more than 50 surveillance activities that monitor and assess health and nutritional status in the United States. Monitoring efforts are divided into five overarching areas: 1) nutrition and related health measurements; 2) food and nutrient consumption; 3) knowledge, attitude, and behavior assessments; 4) food composition and nutrient databases; and 5) food supply determinants. The directory is available as an Internet resource (http://www.cdc.gov/nchs/data/misc/direc-99.pdf), and important studies are summarized in Table 2-4. Many of the datasets generated through this program are available to the public. Datasets that are restricted, due to confidentially or disclosure rules/regulations, can be accessed by researchers through the Research Data Center (RDC) in the National Center for Health Statistics (NCHS) headquarters in Hyattsville, Maryland. All submitted proposals are reviewed by the RDC staff, and data are released to scientists for appropriate studies.

In 1998, the leadership of the Department of Health and Human Services (DHHS) and USDA integrated NHANES and the Continuing Survey of Food Intakes by Individuals (CSFII), the two major diet and health surveys, into a continuous data collection system, allowing diet and nutrition information to be linked directly to health status information. The NCHS will release public use datasets from the continuous NHANES in 2-year cycles.

Data collection for NHANES occurs at three levels: a brief household screener interview, an in-depth household survey interview, and a medical examination. Because detailed interviews and clinical, laboratory, and radiological examinations are conducted, participants' response burden is significant. The 1999–2004 survey content is available online (www.cdc.gov/nehs/data/nhanes/comp3.pdf). For the 1999–2000 and 2001–2002 time periods, the interview sample size was 21,004 and the Mobile Examination Center sample size was 19,759.

> Take a virtual tour of the NHANES Mobile Examination Center at http://www.cdc.gov/nchs/about/major/nhanes/mectour.htm.

NHANES is the only survey that collects biologic specimens from a representative sample of the U.S. population. During the second phase of NHANES III (1991–1994), lymphocytes from 7,000 participants aged 12 years and older were collected and stored frozen in liquid nitrogen or in cell culture immortalized with Epstein-Barr virus to create a DNA bank. In 2002, NCHS issued a call in the *Federal Register* (www.gpoaccess.gov/fr) for use of these samples. (Read more about the *Federal Register* in Chapters 7 and 8.) In 1999, 84% of eligible participants agreed to have their blood samples included in a repository for genetic research; in 2000, 85.3% consented.

TABLE 2-4 National Nutrition Related Health Assessments[1]

Nutritional and Related Health Measurements

Survey Name	Date	Target	Data Collected	Dept/Agency
NHANES[2]	1999–2004	Civilian, noninstitutionalized persons 2 months or older; oversampling of adolescents, African Americans, Mexican Americans, and adults >60 years	Survey elements are similar to NHANES III & NHIS[3]	NCHS, CDC (HHS)
NHANES III	1988–1994	Civilian, noninstitutionalized persons 2 months or older; oversampling of adolescents, non-Hispanic African Americans, Mexican Americans, children <6 years and adults >60 years	Demographics, dietary intake (24-hour recall and food frequency), biochemical analysis of blood and urine, physical examination, anthropometry, blood pressure, bone densitometry, diet and health behaviors, health conditions	NCHS, CDC (HHS)
NHANES III Supplemental Nutrition Survey of Older Persons	1988–1994	Representative U.S. elderly population	See NHANES III	NCHS, NIH/NIA
HHANES	1982–1984	Civilian, noninstitutionalized Mexican Americans in five southwestern states; Cuban Americans in Dade County, Florida; and Puerto Ricans in New York, New Jersey, and Connecticut, aged 6 months to 74 years	Demographics, dietary intake (24-hour recall and food frequency), biochemical analysis of blood and urine, physical exam, anthropometry, blood pressure, diet and health behaviors, health conditions	NCHS (HHS)

Survey Name	Date	Target	Data Collected	Dept/Agency
NHANES II	1976–1980	Civilian, noninstitutionalized persons aged 6 months to 74 years	Demographics, dietary intake, biochemical analysis of blood and urine, physical exam, anthropometry	NCHS (HHS)
NHANES I	1971–1974	Civilian, noninstitutionalized population of the conterminous states, ages 1 to 74 years	Demographics, dietary information, biochemical analysis of blood and urine, physical exam, anthropometry	NCHS (HHS)
PedNSS	1973, continuous	Low-income, high-risk children, birth to 17 years; emphasis on birth to 5 years	Demographics, anthropometry, birthweight, hematology	NCCDPHP, CDC (HHS)
PNSS	1973, continuous	Convenience sample of low-income, high-risk pregnant women	Demographics, pregravid weight and maternal weight gain, anemia, behavioral risk factors, birth weight, and formula-feeding data	NCCDPHP, CDC (HHS)
Food and Nutrient Consumption				
CSFII[4]	1994–1996 1989–1991 1985–1986	Individuals of all ages with oversampling in low income households	One- and three-day food intakes, times of eating events, sources of food eaten away from home	ARS, HNIS
TDS	1961, annual	Specific age and gender groups	Determines levels of nutrients and contaminants in the food supply—analyses are performed on foods that are "table-ready"	FDA (HHS)

(Continues)

TABLE 2-4 National Nutrition Related Health Assessments (Continued)

Survey Name	Date	Target	Data Collected	Dept/Agency
Consumer Expenditure Survey	1980, continuous	Noninstitutionalized population and a portion of the institution-alized population in the U.S.	Demographics, food stamp use, average annual food expenditures	U.S. Bureau of Labor Statistics
NFCS	1987 1977–1978	Households in the conterminous states—all income and low income	Households: quantity (pounds), money value (dollars), and nutritive value of food eaten Individuals: food intake, times of eating events, and sources of foods eaten away from home	HNIS (USDA) ARS (USDA)
SNDA II	1998	Public schools in the 48 contiguous states and the District of Columbia that participate in the National School Lunch Program	School and food service characteristics, nutrients by food group and relationship to the RDA and DGA by meals, source of meals, and nutrient content of USDA meals	FNS/USDA
WIC Feeding Practices Study	1994–1995	Pre- and post-natal women and their children who participate in WIC	Demographics, rates of breast and formula feeding, factors associated with breast-feeding.	FNS/USDA
5 a Day for Better Health Baseline Survey	1991	Adults 18 years and older	Demographics; fruit and vegetable intake; and knowledge, attitudes, and practices regarding intake	NCI (HHS)

Knowledge, Attitude, and Behavior Assessments

Survey Name	Date	Target	Data Collected	Dept/Agency
YRBBS	Biennial	Civilian, noninstitutionalized adolescents aged 12 to 18 years	Demographics, diet and weight; drug, alcohol, and tobacco use; seat belt and bicycle helmet use; behaviors that contribute to violence; suicidal tendencies[5]	CDC (HHS)/ NCCDPHP
BRFSS	1984, continuous	Adults 18 years and older in households with telephones located in participating states	Demographics, questions that assess risk factors associated with leading causes of death: alcohol and tobacco use, weight, seat belt and helmet use, use of preventative medical care[6]	CDC (HHS)/ NCCDPHP
DHKS	1994–1996	Adults 20 years of age and older who participated in CSFII 1994–1996	Demographics, self-perceptions of relative intake, awareness of diet and health relationships, food label use, perceived importance of following diet and health recommendations, beliefs about food safety, and knowledge of sources of nutrients—data can be linked with intake through CSFII data	ARS/USDA
Infant Feeding Practices Survey	1993–1994	New mothers and healthy infants up to 1 year of age	Demographics, prior infant feeding practices, baby's social situation, characteristics associated with breast feeding, development of allergies	FDA

(Continues)

TABLE 2-4   National Nutrition Related Health Assessments (Continued)

Survey Name	Date	Target	Data Collected	Dept/Agency
Consumer Food Handling Practices	1998 1992–1993	Civilian, noninstitutionalized over 18 years of age with telephones	Demographics, prevalence of unsafe food handling practices, knowledge of ood safety principles, use of sources of information about safe food handling, incidence of food borne illnesses	FDA
Food Composition and Nutrient Data Bases				
National Nutrient Data Bank	—	—	This is the repository for values of approximately 7,100 foods and up to 80 components. Essentially all food composition databases are derived from this data bank.	ARS (USDA)
Food Label and Package Survey	1977–1996, biennially	All brands of processed foods regulated by the FDA	Prevalence of nutrition labeling, declaration of select nutrients, prevalence of label claims and other descriptors	FDA (HHS)

Survey Name	Date	Target	Data Collected	Dept/Agency
Food Supply Determinations				
AC Nielsen SCANTRACK	1985, monthly	~3,000 U.S. supermarkets	Sales and physical volume of specific market items, selling price, percent of stores selling the product	ERS/USDA
U.S. Food & Nutrient Supply Series	1909, annually	U.S. population	ERS = Amount of food commodities that disappear into the food distribution system CNPP = nutrient levels of food supply Results are totaled for each nutrient and converted to per-day basis.	ERS/CNPP/USDA

[1]A complete guide to nutrition monitoring in the United States can be found at: http://www.cdc.gov/nchs/data/misc/nutri98.pdf

[2]ARS = Agricultural Research Service; BRFSS = Behavioral Risk Factor Surveillance System; CDC = Centers for Disease Control and Prevention; CNPP = Center for Nutrition Policy and Promotion; CSFII = Continuing Survey of Food Intakes by Individuals; DHKS = Diet and Health Knowledge Survey; ERS = Economic Research Service; FDA = Food and Drug Administration; HHANES = Hispanic Health and Nutrition Examination Survey; HHS = Health and Human Services; HNIS = Human Nutrition Information Service; NFCS = Nationwide Food Consumption Survey; NCCDPHP = National Center for Chronic Disease Prevention and Health Promotion; NCHS = National Center for Health Statistics; NCI = National Cancer Institute; NHANES = National Health and Nutrition Examination Survey; NHIS = National Health Interview Survey; NIA = National Institute on Aging; NIH = National Institutes of Health; PedNSS = Pediatric Nutrition Surveillance System; PNSS = Pregnancy Nutrition Surveillance System; SNDA = School Nutrition Dietary Assessment Study; TDS = Total Diet Study; USDA = United States Department of Agriculture; WIC = Women, Infants and Children; YRBSS = Youth Risk Behavioral Surveillance System

[3]http://www.cdc.gov/nchs/data/nhanes/comp3.pdf contains the complete survey content of NHANES 1999–2004/

[4]CSFII and NHANES have now been combined into a single survey.

[5]http://www.cdc.gov/mmwr/PDF/SS/SS5302.pdf contains the YBRSS report for 2004; MMWR summary reports available through CDC website.

[6]http://www.cdc.gov/brfss/#about_BRFSS contains full information for the Behavioral Risk Factor Surveillance System.

Source: Reprinted with permission from the CDC.

It's clear that genetics and the environment interact to modify risk factors for chronic disease (e.g., cholesterol levels or weight) and, therefore, to change the incidence of disease. Thus, genetic studies should ultimately allow us to individualize nutrition and diet recommendations,[27] which is leading to an incredibly exciting time in nutrition research and nutrition intervention.

It's important to note that there are ethnic differences among individuals not consenting to future genetic research. McQuillan and associates examined sociodemographic variables associated with consent for storage of DNA for future research, and they demonstrated using logistic regression that non-Hispanic African-American race/ethnicity was a predictor for not consenting for this research.[28] These findings suggest that ethnic minorities/groups may be underrepresented in studies; thus it is important to maximize strategies to be sure that all groups are represented when planning epidemiologic studies.

Criteria used to select genes for the study in NHANES included the following: known or hypothesized association with diseases of public health importance, role in pathways affecting multiple diseases, identified functional variants, relatively common variants (prevalence > 2%), previously described gene-environment or gene-gene interactions, relevant phenotypic data available in NHANES datasets, and no current use for clinical risk assessment or intervention. The final proposal included 87 variants of 57 genes known to be important in at least 6 major pathways: nutrient metabolism (e.g., folate and homocysteine), immune and inflammatory responses (e.g., cytokines), activation and detoxification pathways (e.g., drugs), DNA repair pathways (e.g., ionizing radiation), hemostasis and renin/angiotension pathways, and developmental pathways (www.cdc.gov/genomics/activities/ogdp/2003/chap01.htm).

It's difficult to quantify the tremendous impact that NHANES and related surveys have had on health policy and health research in the United States.[29] One way to quantify the impact is to look at the number of publications generated using NHANES data; a MedLine (www.nlm.nih.gov) search in January 2005 using the term "NHANES" produced nearly 8,800 articles on topics as diverse as late bottle weaning and obesity, urinary cadmium levels in a U.S. working population, alcohol consumption and periodontal disease, and blood pressure trends in children and adolescents. Other evidence of the importance of NHANES and similar studies is that in the 5-year period ending in 2003, 8 final rules and 89 proposed rules citing NNMRRP data were published in the *Federal Register* by federal agencies that were responsible for nutrition and food safety programs; these have had more than a $100 million economic impact.[29] Examples of major rules include Environmental Protection Agency (EPA) rules regarding pesticides in food and water that rely on dietary exposure, and the Food Safety and Inspection Service rule on nutrition labeling of chopped meat and poultry products. NHANES has provided data used to construct pediatric growth charts (www.cdc.gov/growthcharts).

NHANES data also are used to monitor serum cholesterol levels and have had an impact on community education programs. Surprisingly, data from NHANES have lead to lead-free gasoline, when survey information showed that Americans had high serum lead levels!

> If you're confused about nutrition information, or just want to find the most cutting-edge information, go to the peer-reviewed literature to find out about any nutrition and health issue: http://www.nlm.gov/entrez/query.fcgi.

NHANES has also shown that there are ethnic differences in dietary intake[30,31]; food sources for different nutrients are different in separate ethnic groups[32]; cardiovascular risk factors cluster according to socioeconomic status[33]; and hypertension varies according to geographical region.[34] These findings demonstrate that data cannot be generalized for state or local areas without considering age, gender, ethnicity, or socioeconomic status in the particular area, and that these data have important implications for intervention strategies.

Epidemiologic Studies

In addition to the NCHS data, a number of long-term, primarily government-funded, epidemiologic studies on adults and children/adolescents have provided critical information used to guide the nation's health policies. The Bogalusa Heart Study and Framingham Heart Study are leading examples. Other important epidemiologic studies in the United States that have contributed to our knowledge of risk reduction and disease prevention are the Nurses' Health Study (n = ~170,000 female registered nurses between the ages of 30 and 55 years at the beginning of the study), the Nurses' Health Study II (established in 1989, n = ~117,000 female nurses, between the ages of 25 and 42 years), and the all-male Health Professional Follow-up Study (initiated in 1986 with 2-year scheduled follow-ups), which was designed to complement the Nurses' Health Study in relating nutritional factors to the incidence of serious illnesses, such as cancer, heart disease, and other vascular diseases in 51,529 male health professionals. Also of import is the Iowa Women's Health Study, with a cohort of 41,837 postmenopausal women who have been followed since 1985. Combined, these studies have yielded more than 2,000 scientific publications and have helped shape medical care, risk reduction and health promotion, and public policy.

Bogalusa Heart Study

The Bogalusa Heart Study (BHS)[35–37] was designed initially to examine the early natural history of coronary heart disease and essential hypertension in a biracial (African-American/Caucasian) pediatric population. The BHS population consists of approximately 5,000 individuals who have been studied at various growth phases and have been followed for as long as 15 years. The overall study design of the BHS is presented in Figure 2-2. The mixed epidemiologic design of the study included cross-sectional and longitudinal surveys to provide information on three questions:

1. What is the distribution and prevalence of cardiovascular disease (CVD) risk factors in a defined pediatric population, and how are abnormal serum lipid levels, blood pressure, and other risk factors defined?
2. Do cardiovascular risk factors track and change over time?
3. What is the interrelationship among these risk factors?

Other questions—notably, the interaction of genetics and the environment—also had to be posed.

Data from the BHS have contributed significantly to our knowledge and understanding of cardiovascular risk factors in children. For example, information on children, adolescents, and young adults from birth to 31 years of age has provided the framework to establish desirable cholesterol levels in children, and has led investigators to recommend screening of cardiovascular risk factors for all children, not only those with a parental history, beginning at pre-school age. Data have also suggested that risk factors for cardiovascular disease "track"; that is, they remain in a rank relative to peers. For example, children with elevated serum total cholesterol or low-density lipoprotein (LDL) cholesterol levels are likely to become adults with dyslipidemia. BHS data has been used to characterize children's diets and secular trends in children's diets for more than 20 years.[38] BHS data were used by the American Academy of Pediatrics as part of the rationale for its recommendation that the DGA could apply to healthy children aged 2 years and older. The data were also used to develop the American Dietetic Association's position paper on dietary guidance for healthy children aged 2 to 11 years.[39] (Read more about public health problems concerning children in Chapter 5.)

One of the major accomplishments of the BHS comes not from the epidemiologic data per se, but from autopsy studies of participants,[40] usually those killed in accidents. BHS data confirmed and extended earlier studies[41] that showed aorta fatty streaks are evident in the first decade of life and that the extensiveness of these lesions is highly associated with serum total cholesterol and LDL levels. Principal accomplishments of the BHS are presented in Table 2-5.

Framingham Heart Study

The Framingham Heart Study has been described as "one of the most impressive medical works in the 20th century."[42] The Framingham Study has provided information critical to the recognition and man-

Bogalusa Heart Study: Overall Design

Experimental Design—Bogalusa Heart Study
Bogalusa 1973–1977

YEAR	PRESCHOOL AGE	SCHOOL AGE	POST HIGH SCHOOL
1973–74	0	2 3 4 5 6 7 8 9 10 11 12 13 14	
1974–75	6 MO 1	6 9 12 15	
		SPECIAL BLOOD PRESSURE STUDY	
1976–77	2	7 10 13 16	
1976–77	3	5 6 7 8 9 10 11 12 13 14 15 16 17	
1977–78	4	SUBSTUDY*	18 SUBSTUDY
1978–79		5 6 7 8 9 10 11 12 13 14 15 16 17	
1979–80		FRANKLINTON BLOOD PRESSURE SUBSTUDY	18 19 20
1980–81		FRANKLINTON BLOOD PRESSURE SUBSTUDY 17	GENETIC BIOBEHACIORAL STUDIES
1981–82		5 6 7 8 9 10 11 12 13 14 15 16 17	
1982–83		SPECIAL GENETIC BIOBEHAVIORAL	18 19 20 21 22 23
1983–84		SUBSTUDIES** BIOBEHAVIOR STUDIES**	
1984–85		5 6 7 8 9 10 11 12 13 14 15 16 17	
1985–86			18 19 20 21 22 23 24 25 26
1986–87		POST HIGH SCHOOL REGISTRY UPDATE	ECHOCARDIOGRAPHY SUBSTUDY
1987–88		5 6 7 8 9 10 11 12 13 14 15 16 17	20 21 22 23 24 25 26 27 28 29
1988–89		AMBULATORY BLOOD PRESSURE STUDY	21 22 23 24 25 26 27 28 29 30
1989–90			22 23 24 25 26 27 28 29 30 31
1990–91			
1992–March		SUBSTUDIES (Diabetes Substudy—Family Pedigree)	UPDATE REGISTRY
1992–93		5 6 7 8 9 10 11	
1993–94		11 12 13 14 15 16 17	EXPAND AND UPDATE REGISTRY
1994–95		SUBSTUDIES (Exercise, Heart Rate Varability)	YOUNG ADULT HEALTH SURVERY—Questionnaire (18–35 YEAR OLDS)
1995–96			19 20 21 22 23 24 25 26 27 28 29 30 31 32 33 34 35 36 37
1996–97			19 20 21 22 23 24 25 26 27 28 29 30 31 32 33 34 35 36 37 38

*Test new blood pressure instrument, biobehavior questionnaire and dietary workbook 24-hour recall
**Coordinated with cross-sectional screenings
***Diabetes—Obesity
****Exercise, blood pressure, heart rate variability

FIGURE 2-2
The Overall Study Design of the Bogalusa Heart Study. Courtesy of Dr. Gerald S. Berenson, Principal Investigator of the Bogalusa Heart Study.

agement of atherosclerosis, as well as its causes and complications. Initiated under the auspices of the National Heart Institute (now the National Heart, Lung, and Blood Institute) in 1948, 1,980 men and 2,421 women were enrolled originally in a 3-year observational study in Framingham, Massachusetts, which at the time was a novel idea. The first report, *Factors of Risk in the Development of Coronary Heart Disease—Six-Year Follow-up Experience; The Framingham Study*, published in 1961, identified high blood pressure, smoking, and high cholesterol levels as major factors in heart disease and conceptualized them as risk factors.[43] Continued study of the population has provided health professionals with multifactorial risk profiles for cardiovascular (CV) disease that have assisted in identifying individuals at high risk, as well as providing the basis for preventative measures.

TABLE 2-5   Principal Bogalusa Heart Study Accomplishments

- Observations clearly show that the major etiologies of adult heart disease, atherosclerosis, coronary heart disease, and essential hypertension begin in childhood. Documented anatomic changes occur by 5 to 8 years of age.
- CV risk factors can be identified in early life. Methods to study CV risk factors are now developed, and normative values from a large biracial (African-American/Caucasian) population (approximately 10,000 individuals) are available for comparison.
- The levels of risk factors in childhood are different than those in the adult years. Levels change with growth phases, i.e., in the first year of life, during puberty and adolescence, in the transition to young adulthood, and in adulthood. National Institute on Aging is now funding observations related to aging and longevity.
- Autopsy studies show atherosclerotic lesions in the aorta and coronary vessels, and changes in the kidney vasculature relate strongly to clinical CV risk factors, clearly indicating that atherosclerosis and hypertension begin in early life. Imaging studies of the heart, carotid, and femoral arteries are extending these findings.
- Gender and race contrasts are a major contribution to the research findings. It is well known that African-Americans have more, and a more severe form of, hypertension, and more diabetes; caucasian males have early coronary artery disease; and women show a lag in the development of heart disease. Subtle changes of aging are reflecting a life-long burden of CV risk factors.
- Environmental factors are significant and influence dyslipidemia, hypertension, and obesity. Those that are controllable include diet, exercise, and cigarette smoking.
- Lifestyles and behaviors that influence CV risk are learned and begin early in life. Healthy lifestyles should be adopted in childhood, because they are critical to modulation of risk factors later in life. Primary care physicians, pediatricians, and cardiologists can play a major leadership role in the prevention of adult heart diseases beginning in childhood. Physicians are encouraged to obtain risk factor profiles on children, along with a family history of heart disease.

Source: Used with permission of Dr. Gerald S. Berenson and available at: http://www.som.tulane.edu/cardiohealth/bog.htm.

During its more than 50-year history (Table 2-6), the Framingham Study has introduced the concept of biologic, environmental, and behavioral risk factors; identified major risk factors associated with heart disease, stroke, and other diseases; revolutionized preventive medicine; and changed how the medical community and general population regard disease pathogenesis. The *Detection, Evaluation, and Treatment of High Blood Cholesterol in Adults* report[12] uses the Framingham risk scoring system to determine the 10-year risk of CHD in adults. The Framingham Study has also supplied valuable information to the *Seventh Report of the Joint National Committee on the Prevention, Detection, Evaluation, and Treatment of High Blood Pressure* (http://www.nhlbi.nih.gov/guidelines/hypertension).

In 1971, the Framingham Heart Offspring Study (www.nhlbi.gov/ resources/deca/descriptions/framoff.htm), consisting of 5,124 men and women, ages 5–70 years, who were offspring and spouses of the offspring of the original Framingham cohort, began. The objectives of this study were to study the incidence and prevalence of CVD and its risk factors, trends in CVD incidence and its risk factors over time, and family patterns of CVD and risk factors. The Offspring Study provided the opportunity to evaluate a second generation of participants, assess new or emerging risk factors and outcomes, and provide a resource for future genetic analyses.

The quality of data from surveys and epidemiologic studies depends on the training of personnel and adherence to rigid protocols. It also depends on the validity and reliability of the test instruments used, as well as on the responses of the subjects. Instruments may need to be modified for specific populations. For example, in the BHS the 24-hour diet recall method had to be adapted for use with children.[44] To improve the reliability and validity of the diet recall, quality controls included the use of a standardized protocol that specified exact techniques for interviewing, recording, and calculating results; standardized graduated food models to quantify foods and beverages consumed; a product identification notebook for probing of snack consumption and foods and beverages most commonly forgotten; school lunch assessment to identify all school lunch recipes, preparation methods, and average portion sizes of menu items reflected in each 24-hour dietary recall; follow-up telephone calls to parents to obtain information on brand names, recipes, and preparation methods of meals served at home; and products researched in the field to obtain updated information on product cost, ingredients, and their weights (primarily snack foods and fast foods).[45] All interviewers participated in rigorous training sessions and pilot studies before the field surveys to minimize interviewer effects. One 24-hour dietary recall was collected on each study participant, and duplicate recalls were collected from a 10% random subsample to assess interviewer variability.[46]

TABLE 2-6   Timeline of Framingham Heart Study

Date	Event
1948	Start of the study
1956	Rheumatic heart disease progression
1959	Factors found that increased risk of heart disease; silent heart attacks discovered
1960	Cigarette smoking found to increase risk of heart disease
1961	"Cholesterol level, blood pressure, and ECG abnormalities found to increase risk of heart disease"
1965	First Framingham report on stroke
1967	Physical activity found to reduce risk of heart disease; obesity increases the risk of heart disease
1970	High blood pressure increases stroke risk
1971	Framingham Offspring Study begins
1974	Overview of diabetes and complications
1976	Menopause found to increase risk of heart disease
1977	"Effects of triglycerides, and LDL and HDL cholesterol described"
1978	Psychosocial factors found to affect heart disease; atrial fibrillation found to increase the risk of stroke
1981	Filter cigarettes found to give no protection against CHD; major report issued on the relationship between diet and heart disease
1983	Reports on mitral valve prolapse
1986	First report on dementia
1987	High blood cholesterol found to correlate directly with risk of death in young men; fibrinogen found to increase the risk of heart disease; estrogen therapy found to reduce risk of hip fractures in post-menopausal women
1988	High HDL levels found to reduce risk of death; association of type "A" behavior with heart disease reported; isolated systolic hypertension found to increase risk of heart disease; cigarette smoking found to increase the risk of stroke
1990	Homocysteine found to be a possible risk factor for heart disease
1993	Mild isolated hypertension shown to increase risk of heart disease; major reports predict survival after diagnosis of heart failure

Date	Event
1994	Enlarged left ventricle shown to increase risk of stroke; lipoprotein (a) identified as possible risk factor for heart disease; risk factors for atrial fibrillation described; lipoprotein (a) and apolipoprotein E found to be possible risk factors for heart disease
1995	First Framingham report on diastolic heart failure published; OMNI study of minorities begins
1996	Progression from hypertension to heart failure described
1997	Cumulative effects of smoking and high cholesterol on the risk of atherosclerosis reported; impact of an enlarged left ventricle and risk for heart failure in asymptomatic individuals investigated
1998	New risk prediction formulas to calculate patients' risk of developing coronary disease over the next 10 years published; work identifying a gene associated with hypertension in Framingham men published
2003	"Genetic studies suggest gene associated with nicotine dependence, HDL levels, and BMI; single determinant of inflammatory risk factors—especially IL-6 associated with increased CHF in people without prior MI; blood pressure associated with CHF"
2004	Alcohol (> 3 drinks/d) correlated with atrial fibrillation; plasma natriuretic peptide levels associated with cardiovascular events and death

Source: Compiled by the authors from http://www.framingham.com/heart/timeline.htm.

Regardless of the quality and extent of surveys and epidemiologic studies, they can only be used to accrue demographics on a population; to generate hypotheses, which in turn need to be investigated using other types of studies; or to look at temporal trends, tracking, and associations. Surveys cannot be used to determine cause and effect relationships. The gold standards for these relationships are metabolic diet studies, clinical trials, or laboratory animal studies.

Metabolic Diet Studies

Metabolic diet studies are conducted in clinical research centers where study participants are randomized into test or control groups and are fed an experimental diet or "normal" diet, respectively. Different designs are available for metabolic diet studies[47]; the one that provides the most valid results is a double-blind, placebo-controlled study. In these studies, neither the investigator nor the participant knows whether the test or control diet is being consumed. Since it is difficult and expensive to do these studies, they are usually short term and have a small sample size; compliance and drop-out rates are problems.

The Dietary Approaches to Stop Hypertension (DASH)[48] and DASH Sodium[49] trials are examples of metabolic diet studies. Epidemiologic studies, clinical trials, and studies using experimental animals showed that consumption of nutrients, notably sodium, potassium, and calcium, lowered blood pressure; people, however, eat food, not isolated nutrients. Thus, to test the impact that combination diets incorporating foods high in these nutrients had on blood pressure, the DASH study was performed. DASH was conducted at four academic medical centers with 459 adult participants; inclusion criteria were untreated systolic blood pressure less than 160 mm Hg and diastolic blood pressure 80 to 95 mm Hg. For 3 weeks, participants ate a "control" diet. They were then randomized to 8 weeks of a control diet; a diet rich in fruits and vegetables; or a combination diet rich in fruits, vegetables, and low-fat dairy foods, and reduced in saturated fat, total fat, and cholesterol. Salt intake and weight were held constant, and diets were isoenergic. All food was prepared in a metabolic kitchen and was provided to participants. The combination diet or "DASH diet" quickly (within 2 weeks) and substantially lowered blood pressure.

In DASH Sodium, a subsequent study, 412 participants were assigned to a control diet or a DASH diet; within the assigned diet, participants ate foods with high (3,450 mg/2,100 kcals), intermediate (2,300 mg/2,100 kcals), or low levels (1,150 mg/2,100 kcals) of sodium for 30 consecutive days each, in random order. Reduction of sodium intake to levels below the current recommendation of 100 mmol per day, combined with the DASH diet, substantially lowered blood pressure, with the low-sodium DASH diet lowering blood pressure most effectively. The DASH diet has been widely embraced for the treatment of hypertension, and nutrition education materials (www.nhlbi.nih.gov/health/public/heart/hbp/dash/new_dash.pdf) are widely available. As elegant and persuasive as the DASH studies were, one drawback to feeding studies is that participants receive all foods; thus, the studies do not assess how compliant people will be after the study.[47]

Clinical Trials

Clinical trials are commonly used to determine the effectiveness or efficacy of drugs or other pharmacologic agents; however, they can also be used to assess diet or dietary interventions. They have many of the same advantages and disadvantages as metabolic studies. Since clinical trials with different diets may involve pharmacologic intervention, they carry a risk that is not usually seen with metabolic diet studies. The classic example of this was seen in the Alpha-Tocopherol, Beta-Carotene Cancer Prevention Study (ATBC Study)[50] and the Beta-Carotene and Retinol Efficacy Trial (CARET).[51] Based on epidemiologic data that showed a relationship between dietary intake of fruits and vegetables,[52,53] or, specifically, of beta-carotene,[54] and a reduced risk of developing lung cancer, especially in smokers,[55] the ATBC and CARET studies used high-dose beta-carotene in major cancer chemopreventive trials. Investigators expected to see reductions in lung cancer by as high as 49% in some high-risk groups.[51] In actuality, the opposite was seen; beta-carotene increased the risk of lung cancer, forcing the CARET study to be stopped early.[56] These studies clearly point to the necessity of additional research, and have important public health implications.[57]

Animal Studies

Animal studies are important in nutrition research for many reasons. Animals that are genetically identical and exposed to the same environmental conditions can be fed carefully characterized diets with different combinations of nutrients; thus, the number of variables in a study are limited. Special treatments—for example, ovariectomies to mimic the physiologic state of postmenopausal women[58]—can be performed on animals. Since the lifespan of most laboratory animals is short, the effects of dietary manipulation can be followed over several generations. Animals can be sacrificed at the end of the experiment, and the effect of the treatment can be examined closely at the organ, tissue, or cellular level. Animal studies can explore molecular mechanisms behind a given observation in humans. For example, ferrets were used to determine that high doses of beta-carotene caused keratinized squamous metaplasia in lung tissues, which was exacerbated by exposure to cigarette smoke.[59] This explains the paradoxical relationship between beta-carotene and smoking seen in the clinical trials discussed earlier. It also points out another use of animal studies—that the metabolism of natural products should be investigated using animal models *before* beginning intervention trials, particularly if doses exceed normal dietary levels.[60]

Animals most commonly used in nutrition research are rats, mice, rabbits, guinea pigs, dogs, sheep, and monkeys. The species selected for a given experiment should be that which is the most similar to human metabolism for a particular nutrient. The importance of this is illustrated in the classic studies of vitamin C metabolism, where guinea pigs are the only laboratory animal that, like man, has an obligatory requirement for this nutrient; thus, a review of the literature shows that only guinea pigs are used for this research.

Many of the elements that make animal studies so appealing in nutrition research are also drawbacks. With the exception of monozygotic twins, humans are not genetically identical; thus, no matter how carefully a human experiment is controlled, responses to dietary manipulations may be different due to individual genetic backgrounds. Interactions between genetics and the environment are easy to study in animals, but difficult to translate into humans.

Healthy People 2010

Individual health is closely linked to *community* health; that is, the health aspects of the environment in which individuals live, work, and play. Community health, in turn, is profoundly affected by the collective beliefs, attitudes, and behaviors of everyone who lives in the community.

The underlying premise of Healthy People (HP) 2010 (www.healthypeople.gov) is that the health of the individual is almost inseparable from the health of the larger community, and that the health of every community in every state and territory determines the overall health status of the nation. That is why the vision for Healthy People 2010 is "Healthy People in Healthy Communities."

HP 2010, published jointly by DHHS and USDA, is the comprehensive health promotion and disease prevention agenda for the nation. HP 2010 goals and objectives are, in part, driven by the 10 leading health indicators: physical activity, overweight and obesity, tobacco use, substance abuse, responsible sexual behavior, mental health, injury and violence, environmental quality, immunization, and access to healthcare. These leading health indicators were chosen because of their ability to motivate action, the availability of data to measure progress, and their importance as public health issues.

HP 2010 grew out of health initiatives pursued over the last 25 years. In 1979, *Healthy People: The Surgeon General's Report on Health Promotion and Disease Prevention*[61] provided nutritional goals for reducing premature deaths and preserving older adults' independence. In 1980, *Promoting Health/Preventing Disease: Objectives for the Nation* targeted 226 health objectives for the nation to achieve over the next 10-year period.[62] These were followed by HP 2000 and HP 2010. During the development of HP 2010, there were two public comment periods, in 1997 and 1998, and over 11,000 comments were received.

HP 2010 has two overarching goals: 1) increase the quality and years of healthy life, and 2) eliminate health disparities. Progress toward these goals is measured through 467 objectives in 28 focus areas. Focus Area 10 is Food Safety (discussed in Chapter 16). Focus Area 19 is Nutrition and Overweight (Table 2-7), and its goal is to promote health and reduce chronic disease associated with diet and weight. In addition, other HP 2010 goals (Table 2-8) are related directly to nutrition, diet, and weight. The nutrition and overweight goals of HP 2010 are derived from nutrition monitoring data and parallel the nutrition recommendations promulgated by the DGA, FGP, and NCI. At the time HP 2010 was written, it was also consistent with the RDA (DRI) and the National Cholesterol Education Program's (NCEP) recommendation for total fat and saturated fat intake. Changes in recommendations for these nutrients will likely be included in the next set of Healthy People goals.

The NCHS is responsible for coordinating efforts to monitor progress toward the HP 2010 objectives. National data are gathered from more than 190 different data sources, from more than 7 federal government departments (DHHS, as well as the Departments of Commerce, Education, Justice, Labor, and Transportation, and the EPA), and from voluntary and private non-governmental organizations. As appropriate, data for the objectives are provided for subgroups defined by relevant dimensions (such as sociodemographic subgroups of the population, health status, or geographic classifications) through DATA 2010 (wonder.cdc.gov/data2010), an interactive database system, and the CDC Wonder System (wonder.cdc.gov). Quarterly reports are made available to the public (www.cdc.gov/nchs/hphome.htm). An example of what is available on the NCHS site is the data presented at the January 2004 progress review meeting regarding Focus Area 19 (www.cdc.gov/nchs/about/otheract/hpdata2010/focusareas/fa19-nutrition.htm).

Many states have developed their own healthy people plans (www.healthypeople.gov/implementation/stateplans.htm). Development of state-specific plans allows states to prioritize health problems, address the needs of specific ethnic groups, and develop solutions that are economically feasible for state budgets. Other specific interest groups have developed similar plans; for example, Healthy Workforce 2010 (www.prevent.org/publications/healthy_workforce_2010.pdf) provides a resource for large and small employers and Rural Healthy People 2010, a companion document for rural areas (www.srph.tamushsc.edu/rhp2010/publications.htm), focuses on health problems and solutions of rural Americans. The NHLBI's HP 2010 Cardiovascular Gateway (hp2010.nhlbihin.net/cvd_frameset.htm) illustrates how this agency links goals from HP 2010, the DGA, and the NCEP to provide information and ideas to the public and health professionals. The program Improving Health/Changing Lives: Communities Taking Action illustrates effective health campaigns in America. Programs of excellence funded by the NHLBI are the Healthy Heart Project in rural West Virginia and the Helping Educators Attack Cardiovascular Risk Factors Together (HEART) program. To support HP 2010, the NHLBI also has nutrition education material available, as well as access to conferences, meetings, exhibits, and distance learning opportunities.

TABLE 2-7 Healthy People 2010—Objectives Related to Nutrition and Overweight (Developmental Goals Not Included)

Goal: Promote health and reduce chronic disease associated with diet and weight.

Weight Status and Growth

19-1. Increase the proportion of adults who are at a healthy weight from 42% to 60%.[1]

19-2. Reduce the proportion of adults who are obese from 23% to 15%.[1]

19-3. Reduce proportion of children and adolescents (aged 6 to 19 years) who are overweight or obese to 5%.[1]

19-4. Reduce growth retardation among low income children under age 5 years from 8% to 5%.[2]

Food and Nutrient Consumption

19-5. Increase the proportion of persons aged 2 years and older who consume at least two daily servings of fruit from 28% to 75%.[3]

19-6. Increase the proportion of persons aged 2 years and older who consume at least three daily servings of vegetables, with at least one-third being dark green or deep yellow vegetables, from 3% to 50%.[3]

19-7. Increase the proportion of persons aged 2 years and older who consume at least six daily servings of grain products, with at least three being whole grains from 7% to 50%.[3]

19-8. Increase the proportion of persons aged 2 years and older who consume less than 10% of calories from saturated fat from 36% to 75%.[3*]

19-9. Increase the proportion of persons aged 2 years and older who consume no more than 30% of calories from fat from 33% to 75%.[3*]

19-10. Increase the proportion of persons aged 2 years and older who consume 2,400 mg or less of sodium daily from 21% to 65%.[1]

19-11. Increase the proportion of persons aged 2 years and older who meet dietary recommendations for calcium from 46% to 75%.[1]

Iron Deficiency and Anemia

19-12. Reduce iron deficiency among young children and females of childbearing age from 9% to 5% (children aged 1 to 2 years), 4% to 1% (children aged 3 to 4 years), and non-pregnant females aged 12 to 49 years from 11% to 7%.[1]

19-13. Reduce anemia among low-income pregnant females in their third trimester from 29% to 20%.[4]

Schools, Worksites, and Nutrition Counseling

19-16. Increase the proportion of worksites with 50 or more employees that offer nutrition or weight management classes or counseling from 55% to 85%.[5]

19-17. Increase the proportion of physician office visits made by patients with a diagnosis of cardiovascular disease, diabetes, or hyperlipidemia that include counseling or education related to diet and nutrition from 42% to 75%.[6]

Food Security

19-18. Increase food security from 88% to 94% of all U.S. households and in so doing reduce hunger.[7]

[1]Data source: NHANES, CDC, CCHS

[2]Data source: Pediatric Nutrition Surveillance System, CDC, NCCDPHP

[3]Data source: CSFII (2-day average), USDA

[4]Pregnancy Nutrition Surveillance System, CDC, NCCDPHP

[5]National Worksite Health Promotion Survey, Association for Worksite Health Promotion

[6]National Ambulatory Medical Care Survey, CDC, NCHS

[7]Current Population Survey, U.S. Department of Commerce, Bureau of the Census; National Food and Nutrition Survey, DHHS, and USDA

*NCEP ATP III recommendations have changed.

Source: Reprinted from the Department of Health and Human Services.

Nutrient Requirements

The first RDAs were published in 1941 "as a guide for advising on nutrition problems in connection with national defense."[63] The first edition included recommendations for only nine nutrients: protein, thiamine, riboflavin, niacin, ascorbic acid, vitamins A and D, calcium, and iron. In the 7th edition (1968), additional nutrients were included: folate, vitamins B_6 and B_{12}, vitamin E, phosphorous, magnesium, and iodine. This edition continued to use the recommendation for an Estimated Safe and Adequate Daily Dietary Intake. The last edition of the RDAs (1989) added vitamin K, zinc, and selenium. The RDAs were geared to healthy populations, such as those in the military or schoolchildren, rather than to individuals. However, they were often used to assess the adequacy of an individual's diet.

In 1993, the Food and Nutrition Board faced the question of whether the RDAs should be changed. Support for change included that:

1. Sufficient new scientific information had accumulated to substantiate reassessment of these recommendations.
2. Where sufficient data for efficacy and safety existed, reduction in the risk of chronic diet-related diseases should be considered. Previously, the RDA had focused on preventing deficiency diseases.
3. Upper levels of intake should be established where there were data concerning risk of adverse effects.
4. Components of food of possible benefit to health, although not meeting the traditional concept of a nutrient, should be reviewed, and if adequate data exist, reference intakes should be established.

TABLE 2-8　Nutrition-Related Objectives from HP 2010 Focus Areas

1. Access to quality health services
   1-3. Counseling about health behaviors
2. Arthritis, osteoporosis, and chronic back conditions
   2-9. Cases of osteoporosis
3. Cancer
   3-1. Cancer deaths
   3-3. Breast cancer deaths
   3-5. Colorectal cancer deaths
   3-10. Provider counseling about preventive measures
4. Chronic kidney disease
   4-3. Counseling for chronic kidney failure case
5. Diabetes education
   5-1. Diabetes education
   5-2. Prevent diabetes
   5-6. Diabetes-related deaths
7. Educational and community-based programs
   7-2. School health education
   7-5. Worksite health promotion programs
   7-6. Participation in employer-sponsored health promotion activities
   7-10. Community health programs
   7-11. Culturally appropriate community health promotion programs
10. Food safety
    10-4. Food allergy deaths
    10-5. Consumer food safety practices
11. Health communication
    11-4. Quality of Internet health information sources
12. Heart disease and stroke
    12-1. Coronary heart disease (CHD) deaths
    12-7. Stroke deaths
    12-9. High blood pressure
    12-11. Action to help control blood pressure
    12-13. Mean total cholesterol levels
    12-14. High blood cholesterol levels
16. Maternal, infant, and child health
    16-10. Low birth weight and very low birth weight
    16-12. Weight gain during pregnancy
    16-15. Spina bifida and other neural tube defects
    16-16. Optimum folic acid
    16-17. Prenatal substance abuse
    16-18. Fetal alcohol syndrome
    16-19. Breast feeding

18. Mental health and mental disorders

18-5. Eating disorder relapses

22. Physical activity and fitness

22-1. No leisure-time physical activity

22-2. Moderate physical activity

22-3. Vigorous physical activity

22-6. Moderate physical activity in adolescents

22-7. Vigorous physical activity in adolescents

22-9. Daily physical activity in schools

22-13. Worksite physical activity and fitness

26. Substance abuse

26-12. Average annual alcohol consumption

Source: Reprinted from the Department of Health and Human Services.

Since 1994, the Institute of Medicine's (IOM) Food and Nutrition Board's Dietary Reference Intakes (DRI) have extended and replaced the former RDAs and the Canadian Recommended Nutrient Intakes (RNI). Conceptually, the DRIs differ from the original RDAs because they incorporate the concepts of disease prevention, upper levels of intake and potential toxicity, and non-traditional nutrients. The latter establishes a precedent; as scientists learn more about the relationships among phytochemicals, herbals, or botanicals and health, these too can be incorporated into the recommendations. Conceptually, the DRIs are the same as the RDAs in that their formulation relies on the best scientific evidence available at the time of issuance,[64] are designed for healthy individuals over time, and can vary depending on life cycle stage or gender. The reference values for heights and weights of adults and children that are used in the DRIs are from NHANES III.

> **Phytochemicals** are chemicals found in plants that may have non-nutritive health benefits—for example as antioxidants (e.g., carotenoids) or antibacterials (e.g., garlic).

Where scientific evidence is available, each DRI is a set of at least four nutrient-based reference values (Table 2-9). Briefly, the four reference values are: the estimated average requirement (EAR), RDA, tolerable upper intake level (UL), and adequate intake (AI). The EAR is the median usual intake value estimated to meet the requirements of half of healthy individuals; it is based on specific criteria of adequacy and careful review of the scientific evidence. Not all nutrients have an EAR, because there may not be an acceptable science base on which to define one. The EAR is used to calculate the RDA (RDA = EAR + 2 SD [standard deviations] of the requirement), which is the average daily dietary intake level sufficient to meet the nutrient requirement of approximately 98% of individuals. Clearly, if there is no EAR for a nutrient, there can be no RDA. If this is the case, an AI is provided. This value is determined by experts and is intended to meet or exceed the needs of a healthy population. The AI can be used as a guide for intake, but cannot be used for all the applications for which the EAR can; it is also an indication that additional research is required for a nutrient. The assumption is that when this research is completed and evaluated, the AI can be replaced by an EAR and RDA. The UL is the highest level of continued daily nutrient intake that is unlikely to pose an adverse health effect. It's interesting to note that the word *tolerable* was chosen to avoid implying a possible beneficial effect.

The IOM has published DRIs and related information for electrolytes and water (2004); energy, carbohydrates, fiber, fat, fatty acids, cholesterol, protein, and amino acids (2002); vitamin A, vitamin K, arsenic, boron, chromium, copper, iodine, iron, manganese, molybdenum, nickel, silicon, vanadium, and zinc (2001); dietary antioxidants and other related compounds (2000); folate and other B vitamins (1998); and calcium, phosphorus, magnesium, vitamin D, and fluoride (1997). A complete set of the updated DRIs is available online (www.iom.edu/object.file/master/21/372/0.pdf) or can be ordered in book form.

The DRIs are not simply tables to be referred to occasionally; they have many applications, as indicated by other related works—*Applications in Dietary Planning* (2003), *Dietary Reference Intakes: Pro-*

TABLE 2-9 Dietary Reference Intakes

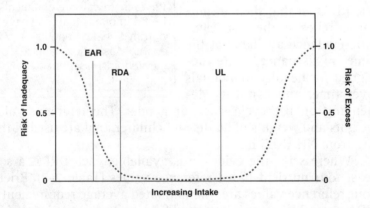

Estimated Average Requirement (EAR): The average daily nutrient intake level estimated to meet the requirement of half the healthy individuals in a particular life stage and gender group.

Recommended Dietary Allowance (RDA): The average daily nutrient intake level sufficient to meet the nutrient requirement for nearly all (97–98%) of healthy individuals.

Adequate Intake (AI): A recommended average daily nutrient intake level based on observed or experimentally determined approximations or estimates of nutrient intake by a group (or groups) of apparently healthy people that are assumed to be adequate—when an RDA cannot be determined.

Acceptable Macronutrient Distribution Range (AMDR): The range of intakes for carbohydrates, fat, and protein that provides adequate intake of essential nutrients, but is associated with reduced risk of chronic disease.

Upper Tolerable Intake Level (UL): The highest average daily nutrient intake level likely to pose no risk of adverse health effects to almost all individuals in the general population. As intake increases above the UL, the potential for adverse effects increases.

DRIs. Note the EAR is the intake at which risk of inadequacy is 50% for an individual. The RDA is the intake that meets the needs of 97–98% of healthy adults. AI does not bear a consistent relationship to the EAR or RDA since it is set without being able to estimate the requirement. At intakes between the RDA and UL, risk of inadequacy and excess are close to zero. At intakes above the UL, risk of adverse effects increases.

Source: Reprinted from the IOM.

posed *Definition of Fiber* (2001), *Dietary Reference Intakes: Guiding Principles for Nutrition Labeling and Fortification* (2003), and *Dietary Reference Intakes: Applications in Dietary Assessment* (2000)—that provide guidance on the interpretation and uses of the DRIs for individuals and groups (www.iom.edu/project.asp?id=4574). Important uses of the DRIs include individual diet planning, dietary guidance, institutional food planning, military food and meal planning, planning for food assistance programs, food labeling and fortification, developing new or modified food products, and guaranteeing food safety. In planning diets, for individuals or groups, it is important to meet the RDA or AI without exceeding the UL. Summaries of the development of the DRI,[65] as well as the uses of the DRI to assess dietary assessment[66,67] and to plan menus,[68] can be found in the literature.

The Center for Nutrition Policy and Promotion (CNPP)

The CNPP was created in December 1994 and is the office within the USDA where scientific research is linked with the nutritional needs of the American public. The CNPP also provides insight for nutrition professionals who teach nutrition/diet to the public. The CNPP carries out its mission (www.usda.gov/cnpp/aboutCNPP.html) by:

- Developing and coordinating nutrition policy within the USDA
- Assessing the cost-effectiveness of government-sponsored nutrition programs on food consumption, food expenditures, food-related behavior, and nutritional status

- Preparing periodic updates on the cost of family food plans and of raising children
- Investigating techniques for effective nutrition communication for Americans
- Evaluating the nutrient content of the U.S. food supply

The projects of the CNPP are the Dietary Guidelines for Americans (DGA), MyPyramid (the old Food Guide Pyramid [FGP] and the FGP for Young Children), USDA Food Plans (thrifty, low-cost, moderate cost, and liberal), Expenditures on Children by Families, web-based training on the Dietary Guidelines for professionals, USDA Healthy Eating Index (HEI), Interactive HEI, Nutrient Content of the U.S. Food Supply, Nutrition Insights, and the *Family Economics and Nutrition Review.*

The *Dietary Guidelines for Americans* are the foundation of federal nutrition policy, nutrition education programs, and information activities. The DGA provide nutrition and dietary advice designed to promote health and reduce the risk of chronic disease for healthy Americans aged 2 years and older. By law (PL 101-445), the DGA are developed and published jointly by the DHHS and USDA every 5 years. The sixth edition was released on January 12, 2005 (earlier editions were published in 1980, 1985, 1990, 1995, and 2000 [www.nal.usda.gov/fnic/dietary/12dietappl.htm]). Changes in the DGA must reflect current scientific and medical knowledge available at the time of publication.[69] Two important documents demonstrate the necessity of relying on a science base: The 1988 *Surgeon General's Report on Nutrition and Health*[70] and the 1989 National Research Council's report, *Diet and Health: Implications for Reducing Chronic Disease Risk.*[1]

The DGA affects U.S. federal nutrition policies in that 21.4 million Americans receive food stamps; 28 million children participate in USDA Child Nutrition Programs; approximately 7.4 million women, infants, and children receive benefits under the Women, Infants and Children (WIC) program; and potentially all adults over the age of 60 years receive assistance through the Elderly Nutrition Program. The DGA also affects information policy, as evidenced in MyPyramid, food labels, and federal nutrition education programs, such as the Expanded Food and Nutrition Education Program (EFNEP) of the Cooperative Extension Service. This pivotal use of the DGA assures that all nutrition information promulgated by the government is consistent. Although not mandated, the DGA also provide the foundation for nutrition recommendations and programs from non-federal agencies, such as the American Heart Association and the American Cancer Society.

An example of how the DGA were used to affect a policy change was seen in 1995, when the USDA published the School Meals Initiative for Healthy Children final rule. That ruling mandated that school meals be brought into compliance with the 1990 guidelines to "Choose a diet low in fat, saturated fat, and cholesterol." The rule stated that school meals, averaged over a 1-week period, would provide not more than 30% of energy from fat and 10% of energy from saturated fat. (Note: These recommendations are no longer current.) School meals also had to meet current recommendations for vitamins, minerals, and energy. These changes were heralded as the most substantive changes in the Child Nutrition Program in 50 years.[71]

Most consumers are familiar with the DGA as a graphic with succinct statements of nutrition advice for the public; however, much more information is available to consumers and to nutrition educators. The entire DGA report is available through the CNPP website (the report's key recommendations are in Table 2-10, and a picture of the cover is shown in Figure 2-3). In addition, this site allows people to access the consumer brochure, *Finding Your Way to a Healthier You*; a Toolkit for Health Professionals; a list of key recommendations; the chronology of the development of the DGA; frequently asked questions; media graphics; archived webcasts; and links to other resources, including MyPyramid. A PowerPoint presentation titled *Dietary Guidelines: Role in Nutrition Policy and Programs* by Eric J. Hentges, of the CNPP, also can be downloaded.

The DGA committee spent over a year formulating the DGA for 2005 (www.usda.gov/cnpp/aboutcnpp.html). This was the first time that an evidence-based approach was used to formulate the DGA committee's recommendations. To learn more about the process and who was on the committee, see Table 2-11.

What are the key 2005 revisions to the dietary guidelines? They revolve around these central tenets:

1. Make smart choices from every food group.
2. Find your balance between food and physical activity.
3. Get the most nutrition out of calories.

The 2005 guidelines are different from previous editions. The USDA website, http://www.usda.gov/cnpp/Pubs/DG2000/Dgover.pdf, provides notably more specific information, including key recommendations for special populations such as pregnant women or people with hypertension. The 2005 DGA quantifies physical activity recommendations more fully, and food servings have been converted to household measures, such as cups. Further, the new guidelines discuss specific food groups or nutrients, like grains and potassium, respectively. The guidelines also include a recommendation for trans-fat, and increase the recommended consumption of low-fat or fat-free milk (or equivalents) to 3 cups daily. The amount of fruits and vegetables was increased, based on a 2,000 kilocalorie diet, to 2 cups of fruit and 2 $\frac{1}{2}$ cups of vegetables. One other notable difference between the 2005 guidelines and the 2000 guidelines is that the 2005 guidelines recommend adopting a balanced eating program, such as the U.S. Food Guide or the DASH Diet, rather than using the old Food Guide Pyramid. As discussed in the next section, MyPyramid descends directly from the new DGA.

TABLE 2-10   The 2005 Dietary Guidelines for Americans

ADEQUATE NUTRIENTS WITHIN CALORIE NEEDS

Key Recommendations

Consume a variety of nutrient-dense foods and beverages within and among the basic food groups while choosing foods that limit the intake of saturated and trans-fats, cholesterol, added sugars, salt, and alcohol.

Meet recommended intakes within energy needs by adopting a balanced eating pattern, such as the USDA Food Guide or the DASH Eating Plan.

WEIGHT MANAGEMENT

Key Recommendations

To maintain body weight in a healthy range, balance calories from foods and beverages with calories expended.

To prevent gradual weight gain over time, make small decreases in food and beverage calories and increase physical activity.

PHYSICAL ACTIVITY

Key Recommendations

Engage in regular physical activity and reduce sedentary activities to promote health, psychological well-being, and a healthy body weight.

To reduce the risk of chronic disease in adulthood, engage in at least 30 minutes of moderate-intensity physical activity, above usual activity, at work or home on most days of the week.

For most people, greater health benefits can be obtained by engaging in physical activity of more vigorous intensity or longer duration.

To help manage body weight and prevent gradual, unhealthy body weight gain in adulthood, engage in approximately 60 minutes of moderate- to vigorous-intensity activity on most days of the week while not exceeding caloric intake requirements.

To sustain weight loss in adulthood, participate in at least 60 to 90 minutes of daily moderate-intensity physical activity while not exceeding caloric intake requirements. Some people may need to consult with a healthcare provider before participating in this level of activity.

Achieve physical fitness by including cardiovascular conditioning, stretching exercises for flexibility, and resistance exercises or calisthenics for muscle strength and endurance.

FOOD GROUPS TO ENCOURAGE

Key Recommendations

Consume a sufficient amount of fruits and vegetables while staying within energy needs. Two cups of fruit and 2 ½ cups of vegetables per day are recommended for a reference 2,000-calorie intake, with higher or lower amounts depending on the calorie level.

Choose a variety of fruits and vegetables each day. In particular, select from all five vegetable subgroups (dark green, orange, legumes, starchy vegetables, and other vegetables) several times a week.

Consume 3 or more ounce-equivalents of whole-grain products per day, with the rest of the recommended grains coming from enriched or whole-grain products. In general, at least half the grains should come from whole grains.

Consume 3 cups per day of fat-free or low-fat milk or equivalent milk products.

FATS

Key Recommendations

Consume less than 10% of calories from saturated fatty acids and less than 300 mg/day of cholesterol, and keep trans-fatty acid consumption as low as possible.

Keep total fat intake between 20 and 35% of calories, with most fats coming from sources of polyunsaturated and monounsaturated fatty acids, such as fish, nuts, and vegetable oils.

When selecting and preparing meat, poultry, dry beans, and milk or milk products, make choices that are lean, low-fat, or fat-free.

Limit intake of fats and oils high in saturated and/or trans-fatty acids, and choose products low in such fats and oils.

CARBOHYDRATES

Key Recommendations

Choose fiber-rich fruits, vegetables, and whole grains often.

Choose and prepare foods and beverages with little added sugars or caloric sweeteners, such as amounts suggested by the USDA Food Guide and the DASH Eating Plan.

Reduce the incidence of dental caries by practicing good oral hygiene and consuming sugar- and starch-containing foods and beverages less frequently.

SODIUM AND POTASSIUM

Key Recommendations

Consume less than 2,300 mg (approximately 1 tsp of salt) of sodium per day.

Choose and prepare foods with little salt. At the same time, consume potassium-rich foods, such as fruits and vegetables.

ALCOHOLIC BEVERAGES

Key Recommendations

Those who choose to drink alcoholic beverages should do so sensibly and in moderation—defined as the consumption of up to one drink per day for women and up to two drinks per day for men.

(Continues)

TABLE 2-10   The 2005 Dietary Guidelines for Americans (Continued)

Alcoholic beverages should not be consumed by some individuals, including those who cannot restrict their alcohol intake, women of childbearing age who may become pregnant, pregnant and lactating women, children and adolescents, individuals taking medications that can interact with alcohol, and those with specific medical conditions.

Alcoholic beverages should be avoided by individuals engaging in activities that require attention, skill, or coordination, such as driving or operating machinery.

FOOD SAFETY

Key Recommendations

To avoid microbial foodborne illness:

Clean hands, food contact surfaces, and fruits and vegetables. Meat and poultry should not be washed or rinsed.

Separate raw, cooked, and ready-to-eat foods while shopping, preparing, or storing foods.

Cook foods to a safe temperature to kill microorganisms.

Chill (refrigerate) perishable food promptly and defrost foods properly.

Avoid raw (unpasteurized) milk or any products made from unpasteurized milk, raw or partially cooked eggs or foods containing raw eggs, raw or undercooked meat and poultry, unpasteurized juices, and raw sprouts.

Note: Key recommendations for special groups were omitted from this table, but are available from the website.

Source: Reprinted with permission and available at http://www.health.gov/dietaryguidelines/dga2005/document/html/executivesummary.htm.

Food Group Plans

In the United States, food group plans have provided dietary guidance based on current scientific knowledge for almost 100 years.[72] The USDA published its first recommendations in 1916. Between 1916 and the 1940s, plans had between 5 and 16 separate food groups and were published by various government agencies. In 1943, as part of the wartime effort, the USDA published the *National Wartime Nutrition Guide. The Basic Seven Food Guide*, derived from the *Wartime Guide*, was issued in the late 1940s and was used until 1955, when the Department of Nutrition at the Harvard School of Public Health recommended collapsing the groups to four. This format was accepted by the USDA in 1956; in 1979, a fifth group containing fats, sweets, and alcohol was added. These plans had one thing in common: they were designed to meet nutrient requirements and to prevent nutritional deficiencies. With the recognition of the relationship between diet and chronic disease risk and the develop-

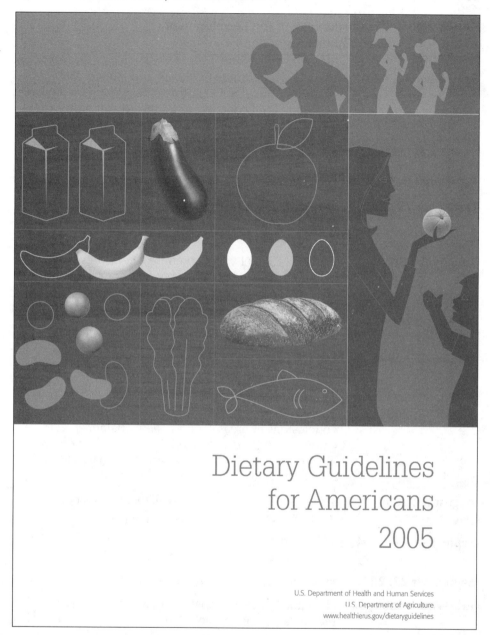

Dietary Guidelines
for Americans
2005

U.S. Department of Health and Human Services
U.S. Department of Agriculture
www.healthierus.gov/dietaryguidelines

FIGURE 2-3   2005 Dietary Guidelines for Americans Cover
Source: Reprinted with permission from the Center for Nutrition Policy
and Promotion.

ment of the DGA, it was important to design a way to help people
implement these guidelines.[73] These efforts culminated with the
Food Guide Pyramid (FGP).[74-79]

The Food Guide Pyramid was the most recognized nutrition education tool in the United States. Like the DGA, it emphasized overall
health, was based on current scientific research, addressed the total

**TABLE 2-11   The Chronology of the Development
of the 2005 Dietary Guidelines**

September 4, 2003	The U.S. Department of Health and Human Services (HHS) and the U.S. Department of Agriculture (USDA) publish in the Federal Register the official notice of the first meeting of the Dietary Guidelines Advisory Committee (DGAC) and solicit written comments on the review of the Dietary Guidelines for Americans.
September 24, 2003	The advisory committee holds its first meeting.
December 29, 2003	HHS and USDA provide notice of the second meeting of the committee, and request oral testimony and written comments.
January 8, 2004	The DGAC meets. The committee considers issues including energy balance, fatty acids, nutrient adequacy, food safety, and alcohol.
March 30–31, 2004	The DGAC meets to consider issues including energy balance, physical activity, and fluids and electrolytes.
May 26–27, 2004	The DGAC meets and formulates major conclusions in areas including food choices, energy balance, fats, fruits and vegetables, whole grains, and dairy.
August 11, 2004	The DGAC meets. The committee formulates major conclusions in areas such as energy balance, carbohydrates, fats, selected fluids and electrolytes, alcohol, selected food groups, discretionary calories, and food safety.
August 27, 2004	The DGAC report is made available in the Federal Register. Public comment period begins.
September 21, 2004	Oral comments from the public are presented at HHS Headquarters in Washington, D.C.
September 27, 2004	Final written public comments are received.
Fall/Winter 2004	HHS and USDA conduct internal scientific review of the advisory committee's report.
January 12, 2005	HHS Secretary Tommy G. Thompson and USDA Secretary Ann M. Veneman release the final 2005 Dietary Guidelines for Americans.

Who was on the 2005 Dietary Guideline Advisory Committee? Go to http://www.usda.gov/cnpp/DG2005/PressRelease081203.htm to find out. Check them out, along with their fields of expertise. To learn more about the procedure, including viewing meeting minutes, go to http://www.health.gov/dietaryguidelines/dga2005/default.htm.

Source: Reprinted with permission and available at
http://www.health.gov/dietaryguidelines/dga2005/chronology.htm.

diet, and was built on successful elements of previous food plans.[74] Consumer testing prior to its original release showed a pyramid was the most effective graphic. The shape helps to convey key dietary concepts of variety, proportionality, and moderation.[75] It is not surprising, therefore, that when the decision to revise the pyramid was made, the new recommendations remained in this shape.

MyPyramid (Figure 2-4), a new symbol and interactive food guidance system, was released by Mike Johanns, the Secretary of Agriculture, on April 19, 2005. Its message is simple: "Steps to a Healthier You." MyPyramid also sends the message that one size does not fit all; this new pyramid can be customized based on the consumer's age, gender, and activity level. This is a major advantage over the old FGP, which left consumers guessing whether 6 servings of grain were enough, or if they needed 11, or if they needed something in between. MyPyramid also stresses the importance of physical activity—this is consistent with the more fully developed recommendations for physical activity promulgated by the DGA. MyPyramid also introduces the concept of discretionary calories and that each person has a total calorie budget for the day—exceeding this budget can lead to overweight and obesity.

The MyPyramid website (included in Table 2-12) provides consumers and health professionals with a wealth of information, including a personalized assessment of food intake and physical activity, how to track compliance with this assessment (Figure 2-5), and how to implement the plan (e.g., suggestions for physical activity or how to choose vegetables with high nutritional content). For professionals, there's a 19-page downloadable booklet that provides the educational framework of MyPyramid. Much of the information is available in English and Spanish. One drawback is that it is unclear how this interactive experience can be made available to people without computer access.

The United States is not the only country to have a food group plan.[80] Many other countries have several, and not all are in a pyramid form. These include various cultural food pyramids and pyramids for different age groups. Food plans should be appropriate for each nation and be based on its national food supply, food consumption pattern, nutrition status of individuals and populations, and nutritional standards.

Although the FGP has been replaced by MyPyramid, it's still something that nutritionists need to be familiar with—especially because there is a substantial body of literature linking dietary intake with the pyramid recommendations. It's important to be able to understand this literature and its significance. The FGP has generally been shown to be a good indicator of dietary adequacy.[81-83] Intake of food groups, consistent with the recommendations in the pyramid, is related to blood lipid levels[84] and may reduce risk factors for obesity[85] and chronic disease.[86] Compliance with dietary recommendations, such as the DGA and FGP, is associated with a decrease in all

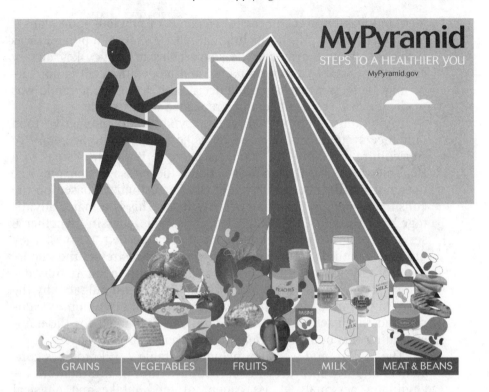

FIGURE 2-4   MyPyramid
Source: Reprinted with permission from the U.S. Department of Agriculture and
the U.S. Department of Health and Human Services, Center for Nutrition Policy
and Promotion.

causes of mortality.[87] Despite the widespread recognition of the
FGP, many Americans do not follow its recommendations; CSFII
data from 1994–1996 and 1998 (see Figure 2-6) illustrate this
(www.ba.ars.usda.gov/cnrg/services/tables.pdf). Evaluation of the
average number of servings can be misleading, because individuals
with high intakes may skew results. For example, individuals over
the age of 20 years consume an average of 3.3 servings of vegetables, but only 42% of females and 60% of males meet the FGP recommendation for vegetables. Averages can also obscure other
important information, such as that Americans consume an average
of only 0.2 servings each of dark green and deep yellow vegetables.

Why is the low intake of vegetables important? The inverse relationship between intake of fruit and vegetables and the development of cancer is one of the best established tenets in nutritional
epidemiology.[88,89] Plant-based diets are also used to lower blood
pressure and reduce serum lipid levels.[90] How is this information
used in public health nutrition? Data like these provide the foundation science for the DGA, and the 2005 guidelines specify increased
intake of vegetables and emphasize the importance of vegetable
color. Goal 19-6 for HP 2010 (shown earlier in Table 2-7) is to in-

USDA RELEASES MYPYRAMID TRACKER

A tool to help consumers evaluate their daily food choices and physical activity level

MyPyramid Tracker is a web-based interactive tool that helps consumers compare their diet and physical activity to current health recommendations. Individuals can enter the foods they eat and their physical activities for a day and obtain the energy balance between them. MyPyramid Tracker provides each user with detailed, personalized results.

By using MyPyramid Tracker consumers can:

➢ Compare their food choices for a day to current nutrition recommendations from the Dietary Guidelines.

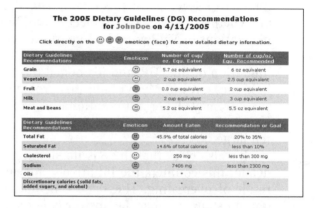

➢ See if they are eating the right amount of foods from each of the MyPyramid food groups.

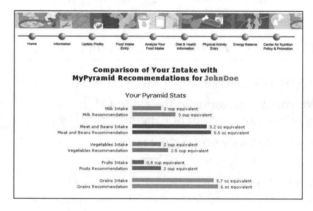

Get Tracking Today — at MyPyramid.gov!

FIGURE 2-5 MyPyramid Tracker
Source: Reprinted with permission from the U.S. Department of Agriculture and the U.S. Department of Health and Human Services, Center for Nutrition Policy and Promotion.

crease from 3% to 50% the proportion of the population of persons aged 2 years and older who consume at least three daily servings of vegetables, with at least one-third being dark green or deep yellow. Programs such as the National Cancer Institute's 5 A Day Program (www.5aday.gov) provide the public and health professionals with specific information on why and how to increase the intake of fruits and vegetables.

Despite the failure of many Americans to follow the FGP, the media has criticized it as being responsible for the obesity epidemic. The FGP provided a convenient focus for an overwhelming public health problem. But, let's look at the science: The majority of Americans do not follow the dietary advice promulgated by either the DGA or the FGP[75]; either they fail to meet the recommended number of servings[91,92] or they exceed the recommendations for the number of servings of fats/oils or added sugars.[93] (It's not known yet whether Americans will meet or will be able to meet the recommendations in MyPyramid.) In part, this could be the result of consumers not recognizing what a serving size is. This was a recognized limitation of the FGP, and it's hoped that by using common household measures in MyPyramid this problem will be overcome. Consumers may have unintentionally exceeded recommendations, especially when eating away from home where serving sizes are often large.[94]

It's also clear that there is no simple answer to the obesity epidemic; this counters the intuitively appealing thought that it's the result of overeating. The *science* behind evaluating the causes of obesity shows us that the answer is not simple and is not the result of the FGP. Although individual nutrients and foods have been im-

---

TABLE 2-12   Internet Sites for Community Nutritionists

NATIONAL NUTRITION MONITORING

Nutrition Monitoring in the United States
http://www.cdc.gov/nchs/data/misc/direc-99.pdf

National Center for Health Statistics
http://www.cdc.gov/nchs/Default.htm

NHANES1999–2004 Survey Content
http://www.cdc.gov/nchs/data/nhanes/comp3.pdf

Healthy Women
http://www.cdc.gov/nchs/healthywomen.htm

National Health Interview Survey
http://www.cdc.gov/nchs/nhis.htm

Behavioral Risk Factor Surveillance System
http://www.cdc.gov/brfss

SMART BRFSS
http://apps.nccd.cdc.gov/brfss-smart/index.asp

Youth Risk Behavior Surveillance System
http://www.cdc.gov/HealthyYouth/yrbs/index.htm

Food Surveys Research Group
http://www.barc.usda.gov/bhnrc/foodsurvey/home.htm

Pediatric and Pregnancy Nutrition Surveillance System
http://www.cdc.gov/nccdphp/dnpa/PedNSS.htm

NUTRITION RECOMMENDATIONS

Center for Nutrition Policy and Promotion
http://www.cnpp.usda.gov/index.html

Dietary Guidelines 2005 (6th edition)
http://www.cnpp.usda.gov/DG2005/index.html

Development of the 2005 Guidelines
http://www.health.gov/dietaryguidelines/dga2005/default.htm

Dietary Guidelines 2000 (5th edition)
http://www.cnpp.usda.gov/DietGd.pdf

History of the Dietary Guidelines
http://www.nutriwatch.org/05Guidelines/dgahistory.html

MyPyramid
http://www.mypyramid.gov

MyPyramid Education Framework
http://www.mypyramid.gov/downloads/MyPyramid_education_framework.pdf

Food Labeling
http://www.nal.usda.gov/fnic/etext/000027.html

Food Labeling Requirements
http://www.access.gpo.gov/nara/cfr/waisidx_01/21cfr101_01.html

Food Labeling Questions and Terms
http://vm.cfsan.fda.gov/~dms/flg-6c.html

Dietary Reference Intakes
http://www.iom.edu/project.asp?id=4574

Healthy People 2010
http://www.healthypeople.gov/default.htm

Food and Nutrition Information Center
http://www.nal.usda.gov/fnic/index.html

HEALTH GUIDELINES

National Cancer Institute 5-A-Day
http://www.5aday.gov

National Cholesterol Education Program
http://www.nhlbi.nih.gov/chd

NCEP Adult Treatment Panel III
http://www.nhlbi.nih.gov/guidelines/cholesterol/index.htm

National Diabetes Education Program
http://ndep.nih.gov

(Continues)

TABLE 2-12   Internet Sites for Community Nutritionists (Continued)

DASH Eating Plan
http://www.nhlbi.nih.gov/health/public/heart/hbp/dash

American Heart Association Diets
http://www.americanheart.org/presenter.jhtml?identifier=851

3-A-Day of Dairy
http://www.3aday.org

OTHER RESOURCES

Healthier US.gov
http://www.healthierus.gov

Nutrition.gov
http://www.nutrition.gov

Food & Nutrition Information Center
http://www.nal.usda.gov/fnic/index.html

Office of Disease Prevention & Health Promotion
http://odphp.osophs.dhhs.gov

National Health Information Center
http://www.health.gov/nhic

Beltsville Human Nutrition Research Center
http://www.barc.usda.gov/bhnrc

National Institute of Medicine
http://www.iom.edu

National Center for Chronic Disease Prevention & Health Promotion
http://www.cdc.gov/nccdphp/about.htm

International Food Information Council
http://www.ific.org/index.cfm

Healthy Eating Index
http://warp.nal.usda.gov/fnic/HEI/hlthyeat.pdf

World Health Organization
http://www.who.int

Food and Agricultural Organization of the United Nations
http://www.fao.org

National Library of Medicine
http://www.ncbi.nlm.nih.gov/pubmed

AGRICOLA
http://agricola.nal.usda.gov

DataFerrett
http://ferret.bls.census.gov/cgi-bin/ferret

Source: Compiled by the authors.

plicated in obesity, few attempts have been made to identify eating patterns that could contribute to the problem. Because foods are generally not eaten in isolation, the overall pattern of consumption may have a greater cumulative impact on obesity than any single nutrient or food. Nicklas et al. have begun using BHS data to examine this problem in children.[95,96] Figure 2-7 illustrates the factors that may be influencing the prevalence of obesity in children. (Read more about children and obesity in Chapter 5.)

Healthy Eating Index

The USDA's CNPP developed the Healthy Eating Index (HEI) to assess and monitor the dietary status and dietary changes of Americans.[97] The HEI was originally developed in 1995 using 1989–1990 CSFII data, and was updated using 1994–1996 data and 1999–2000 NHANES data. The HEI, the sum of 10 components representing aspects of a healthy diet, is a summary measure of overall dietary quality (Table 2-13). Components have a maximum score of 10 and a minimum score of 0; intermediate scores are computed proportionally. High component scores indicate being close to recommendations. (Note: The HEI does not reflect the updated DRIs for fat, saturated fat, or cholesterol intake[103] or the recommendations promulgated by the Third Report of the National Cholesterol Education Program's Adult Treatment Panel.[12]) An HEI score over 80 suggests a "good" diet, a score between 51 and 80 suggests the diet "needs improvement," and an HEI score less than 51 suggests a "poor" diet. As valuable as the HEI is as an assessment, it's an example of why these tools need to be updated and revised regularly, as it has not been updated to reflect the new recommendations for saturated fat and cholesterol.[12]

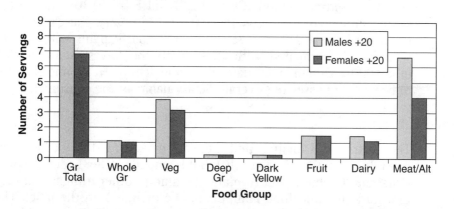

FIGURE 2-6 Average Number of Servings from the Food Guide Pyramid Consumed by Males and Females over the Age of 20 Years from CSFII 1994–1996, 1998
Source: Adapted from USDA, Agricultural Research Service (ARS) Reprinted with permission from the USDA. Available at http://www.barc.suda.gov/bhnrc/chrg; accessed May 17, 2005.

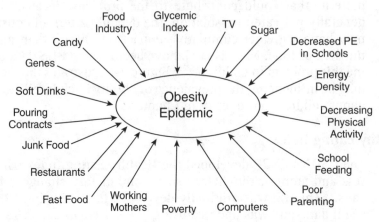

FIGURE 2-7   Factors That May Be Influencing Obesity in Children
Source: Courtesy of Theresa Nicklas, DrPH.

Since its release, the HEI has been used to examine demographics and healthful eating,[98] to study consumer understanding of diet quality,[99] to evaluate dietary interventions in schools,[100] and to look at the diet quality of people throughout the life span.[101,102] These data, in turn, can be used to make specific recommendations. The percentage of children's diets that were reported to "need improvement" ranged from 60% (ages 2–3 years) to 80% (ages 7–9 years)[101]; this information was used to make specific recommendations for improving the diets of children in the American Dietetic Association's position paper on diets of children.[39]

Recently, using NHANES III data,[104] a statistical correlation was shown between HEI scores and serum ($r = 0.25$) and red cell folate ($r = 0.27$), serum vitamins C ($r = 0.30$) and E ($r = 0.30$), and all the serum carotenoids except lycopene ($r = 0.17$ to 0.27). These blood nutrient levels were 21% to 175% higher for participants with an HEI score > 80, compared with those with the lowest score (< 50) ($p < 0.0001$). Other studies have also validated the HEI[105] and found it to be useful in assessing overall dietary habits of the consumer.[97]

Food Labels

The Nutrition Labeling and Education Act of 1990 (the 1990 amendments) (Public Law 101-535) amended the Federal Food, Drug, and Cosmetic Act to mandate, among other things, that certain nutrients and food components be included on the label. The regulatory authority for the food label rests with the Food and Drug Administration (FDA) and the Federal Trade Commission. The Secretary of HHS (and by delegation, the FDA) can add or delete nutrients included in the food label, if this action is necessary to assist consumers in maintaining healthy dietary practices. In response to

TABLE 2-13 Components of the Healthy Eating Index and Scoring System

	Score Ranges	Criteria for Maximum Score of 10	Criteria for Minimum Score of 0
Grain consumption	0–10	6–11 servings	0 servings
Vegetable consumption	0–10	3–5 servings	0 servings
Fruit consumption	0–10	2–4 servings	0 servings
Milk consumption	0–10	2–3 servings	0 servings
Meat consumption	0–10	2–3 servings	0 servings
Total fat intake	0–10	30% or less energy from fat	45% or more energy from fat
Saturated fat intake	0–10	10% or less from saturated fat	15% or more from saturated fat
Cholesterol intake	0–10	300 mg or less	450 mg or more
Sodium intake	0–10	2400 mg or less	4800 mg or more
Variety	0–10	8 or more different items/day	3 or fewer different items/day

Source: Adapted with permission from USDA, CNPP-12. http://www.usda.gov/cnpp/Pubs/HEI/HEI99-00report.pdf.

these provisions, the FDA published a proposed rule entitled "Food Labeling; Reference Daily Intakes and Daily Reference Values; Mandatory Status of Nutrition Labeling and Nutrient Content Revision" in the *Federal Register* of November 27, 1991. In that document, the agency proposed a requirement that foods bear nutrition labels listing certain nutrients and the amount of those nutrients found in a serving of the food.

Under the Nutrition Labeling and Education Act (NLEA), some foods are exempt from the food labeling laws: food served for immediate consumption, such as that served in hospital cafeterias and airplanes, and food sold by food service vendors. These include, for example, mall cookie counters, sidewalk vendors, and vending machines; ready-to-eat food that is not for immediate consumption, but is prepared primarily on site (for example, bakery, deli, and candy store items); food shipped in bulk, as long as it is not for sale in that form to consumers; medical foods, such as those used to address the nutritional needs of patients with certain diseases; plain coffee and tea and some spices; and other foods with no significant amounts of any nutrients.

Placement of information on the label, type size, manufacturer name and contact information, and other information related to content are also mandated. Special requirements exist to accommodate foods sold in small packages. The USDA also regulates poultry in accordance with the Poultry Products Inspection Act and meat under the Federal Meat Inspection Act.

Daily values (DV) are one of the key elements of the food label; these are the daily dietary intake standards used for nutrition labeling. The first daily intake standards for the nutrition label, referred to as the U.S. Recommended Daily Allowances (U.S. RDAs), were established in 1973 and were based on the RDAs.[106,107]

The food label is a good way for most consumers to evaluate their eating habits and how their food patterns meet national recommendations for nutrients and energy. Many consumers, however, do not look past one or two points on the label, often just sodium and cholesterol. Helping clients to understand food labels and how they may relate to disease prevention, how the information is important to individuals with certain disease states, and how the food in question integrates into a total food plan is clearly within your purview as a nutrition professional.

As mandated by the Nutrition Labeling and Education Act of 1990, the Food and Drug Administration has issued final food labeling rules for health claims. More recent information released in 2003 qualifies and explains claims that can be made for convention food and dietary supplements. The claims fall into three major categories: 1) health claims; 2) nutrient content claims; and 3) structure function claims.

The rules published in the January 6, 1993, *Federal Register*, and amended in June 1999 and November 2000, allow the following health claims on food labels (In October 2002, Oatrim [amylase-hydrolyzed whole oat flour or oat bran] was added to the eligible sources of oat soluble-fiber):

- Calcium and a reduced risk of osteoporosis (a condition of lowered bone mass)
- Sodium and an increased risk of hypertension (high blood pressure)
- Dietary saturated fat and cholesterol and an increased risk of coronary heart disease
- Dietary fat and an increased risk of cancer
- Fiber-containing grain products, fruits, and vegetables and a reduced risk of cancer
- Fruits, vegetables, and grain products that contain fiber, particularly soluble fiber, and a reduced risk of coronary heart disease

Before a company can place such a claim on a label, stringent requirements must be met; there are also criteria that all foods allowed such health claims must fulfill. An example of the final listing of an approved health claim can be seen in Table 2-14 (www.cfsan.fda.gov/ndms/flg-6c.html).

The food label is being changed to meet current scientific research and public demand. In 1991, when label information was modified as stated above, there was insufficient scientific knowledge about trans-fatty acids and their potentially adverse affects on health to mandate their inclusion on the label. Since that time, however, the inverse relationship between dietary trans-fats and increased LDL cholesterol levels has been clearly demonstrated.[108–110] In July 11, 2003, the *Federal Register* printed the final rule on requiring the trans-fat content of foods be added to labels. Effective January 1, 2006, labels must have, on a separate line immediately under that for saturated fatty acids, the trans-fat content of food. Confirmation of the relationship between trans-fat and heart disease has resulted not only in changes to food labels, but also in recommendations from the National Academy of Science's IOM to "keep trans fatty acid consumption as low as possible while consuming a nutritionally adequate diet" (www.iom.edu/object.file/master/13/083/0.pdf). There was no way

TABLE 2-14   Sample Claims and FDA Requirements for Labels

Example of an Approved Claim	Food Requirements	Claim Requirements	Model Claim, Statements
Dietary saturated fat & cholesterol and Risk of Coronary Heart Disease— 21 CFR 101.75	– Low saturated fat – Low cholesterol – Low fat (Fish & game meats: "Extra lean")	Required terms: "Saturated fat and cholesterol," "Coronary heart disease," or "Heart disease." Includes physician statement (individuals with elevated blood total—or LDL— cholesterol should consult their physicians) if claim defines high or normal blood total—and LDL— cholesterol.	While many factors affect heart disease, diets low in saturated fat and cholesterol may reduce the risk of this disease.

Note: Terms incorporated into these requirements are also defined by the FDA; for example the term "low" is used above. For saturated fat, "low" means that the food must have 1g or less per reference amount and 15% or less of calories from saturated fat, whereas for cholesterol, "low" means 20 mg or less per reference amount.

Source: Reprinted with permission from the FDA.

for consumers to follow this recommendation without knowing how much trans-fat they were actually eating. Hence, the change in the food label. Comments in the *Federal Register* about the food label can be found at: http://www.foodriskclearinghouse.umd.edu/ fedregistervol58part4.htm.

In part, the changes in the food label resulted from a 1994 citizen petition from the Center for Science in the Public Interest (CSPI). In 2004, the CSPI submitted another petition that would prohibit the use of partially hydrogenated oils, the major source of dietary trans-fat, as a food ingredient (cspinet.org/new/pdf/trans_fat_petition.pdf). There are no known requirements for trans-fats, nor are there any data that suggest they confer a health benefit.

The ripple effect of science impacting the labeling law can be seen in food companies that are reformulating products with no or lower amounts of trans-fats. Frito-Lay™, a manufacturer of chips and other snack foods, was the first to announce it would remove trans-fats from its products and was also the first to voluntarily and proactively list the trans-fat content of its products.

Campbell's™, Kraft™, and Crisco™ are also developing trans-fat-free or trans-fat-reduced foods. Corporate responsibility plays a pivotal role in assuring a safe and healthful food supply. To come full circle with this story, ongoing nutrition monitoring and food composition studies will determine how these changes affect intake of trans-fats and the trans-fat levels of food and whether these changes impact coronary heart disease morbidity and mortality.

Questions remain in the trans-fat saga. If trans-fats have no known health benefit and pose a clear-cut health risk by increasing LDL levels, why didn't the IOM set the UL at zero (www.iom.edu/ object.file/master/13/083/0.pdf), rather than recommending that trans-fat intake be "kept as low as possible"? The answer is that it's only possible to remove up to 80% of trans-fat from a typical diet, the percentage reportedly due to consumption of partially hydro-genated vegetable oils. With changes in menu items available to the public, such as described above, it should be relatively easy to reduce trans-fat intake. However, eschewing the approximately 20% of naturally occurring trans-fats would require extraordinary dietary changes, and would limit intake of nutrient-dense foods, like meat and milk.

Bringing Nutrition Recommendations to the Public

There are a number of existing programs designed to improve the health of the nation that have a science base. The NCI's 5 A Day program, which was designed to encourage people to eat 5 to 9 servings of fruit and vegetables daily, serves as a model program.

The Science Behind the Program

The inverse relationship between eating fruits and vegetables and reducing the risk of some types of cancer is one of the best established tenets of nutritional epidemiology.[52-54,89,111-124] It's important to understand, however, that the studies supporting this finding are not consistent for all types of cancer.[112,125-126] Other studies have shown that consuming fruit[114,127] but not vegetables reduced the risk of some types of cancer; others showed the effect was linked with vegetable intake only.[114] Some studies have shown no association or only a weak one.

Intake of fruits and vegetables also reduces the risk of other chronic diseases, notably cardiovascular disease and stroke.[123,128-129] The importance of including fruits and vegetables in the diet is underscored by their prominent position in HP 2010, DGA, FGP, and MyPyramid. Every major diet and health organization recommends a diet rich in fruits and vegetables for prevention of chronic disease. Therapeutic diets and programs, including the DASH and the NCEP, also recommend diets rich in fruits and vegetables.

The NCI's 5 to 9 a Day program (Table 2-15) provides health professionals and consumers alike with information on how and why to include fruits and vegetables in their diet. This program has ideas and materials that target high-risk groups, such as men (www.5aday.gov/9aday/index.html). The 5 to 9 a Day program also has information geared to state coordinators, and makes available brochures, posters, retail merchandise (including those in Spanish), teaching aids, recipes, and other products needed to conduct a nutrition intervention.

TABLE 2-15   The 5–9 a Day for Better Health Campaign

The Science Behind the Program	Comment
5–9 servings of fruits and vegetables a day reduce the risk of certain types of cancer. Block and co-workers published the seminal study in 1992[52] looking at cancer risk and fruit and vegetable intake.	Different studies have produced different results, both from a standpoint of the presence or level of risk reduction[112] and the different types of cancers that may be affected.[111,113] This may result from different populations, different study designs, and different study instruments to assess the populations.[22, 114-118] There is no consensus about which specific plant products or combinations reduce cancer risk—candidates are antioxidants, fiber, and phytochemicals.[119-122]

Source: Reprinted with permission from The National Cancer Institute and National Institutes of Health. Available at: http://www.5aday.gov.

Is this program effective in helping Americans meet program and national recommendations? Yes. Studies have suggested that the 5 a Day campaign is successful in increasing intake of fruits and vegetables by low-income individuals[130,131] and at worksites.[132, 133] In fact, no studies have suggested that the program did not increase fruit and vegetable intake.[134] Studies have indicated, however, that it is important to consider characteristics of the specific target population, including barriers to consumption and stages of change, and to deliver positive messages.[135-137]

Conclusions

There is a bewildering array of nutrition information available to the public and to professionals. Nutrition messages are often conflicting, confusing, and often simply rhetoric. More consumer research is needed to understand more fully the best way to communicate health messages, recommendations, and dietary guidance to the public. The challenge for nutritionist professionals is to evaluate critically the scientific evidence before it is translated into public health practice. Nutrition professionals need to bring positive recommendations to the public in a unified way to assure that consumers are getting the best possible information available that allows them to make positive lifestyle changes.[138]

Issues for Discussion

1. Dietary recommendations for the public change as scientific studies discover new information. How can these changes be brought to the public in a way that doesn't confuse them or make them resentful?

2. What ethical responsibility, if any, does industry or the media have in assuring the public's health?

3. The Dietary Guidelines for Americans and MyPyramid promulgate prudent diets, but Americans clearly have difficulty following these recommendations. Why?
   If people can't follow them, should we continue to make these recommendations?

References

1. National Academy of Sciences, National Research Council, Food and Nutrition Board. *Diet and Health: Implications for Reducing Chronic Disease Risk.* Washington, DC: National Academy Press; 1989.

2. U.S. Senate Select Committee on Nutrition and Human Needs. *Dietary Goals for the U.S.* 2nd ed. Washington, DC: U.S. Government Printing Office; 1977.

3. American Heart Association. *Heart and Stroke Statistical Update*. Dallas, TX: American Heart Association; 2005. Available at: www.cdc.gov/nchs/fastats/icod.htm

4. Hedley AA, Ogden CL, Johnson CL, et al. Prevalence of overweight and obesity among US children, adolescents, and adults, 1999–2002. *JAMA*. 2004;291:2847–2850.

5. National Institutes of Health, National Heart, Lung, and Blood Institute. *Clinical Guidelines on the Identification, Evaluation, and Treatment of Overweight and Obesity in Adults, The Evidence Report*. 1998. NIH Publication No. 98–4083.

6. Dietz WH, Bellizzi MC. Introduction: the use of body mass index to assess obesity in children. *Am J Clin Nutr*. 1999;70:123S–125S.

7. Himes JH and Dietz WH. Guidelines for overweight in adolescent preventive services: recommendations from an expert committee. The Expert Committee on Clinical Guidelines for Overweight in Adolescent Preventive Services. *Am J Clin Nutr*. 1994;59:307–316.

8. Mokdad AH, Ford ES, Bowman BA, et al. Prevalence of obesity, diabetes, and obesity-related health risk factors, 2001. *JAMA*. 2003;289:76-79.

9. Finkelstein EA, Fiebelkorn IC, Wang G. State-level estimates of annual medical expenditures attributable to obesity. *Obes Res*. 2004;12:18–24.

10. Sturm R. The effects of obesity, smoking, and problem drinking on chronic medical problems and healthcare costs. *Health Affairs*. 2002;21:245–253.

11. Sturm R, Wells KB. Does Obesity Contribute As Much to Morbidity As Poverty or Smoking? *Public Health*. 2001;115:229–295.

12. National Institutes of Health, National Heart, Lung, and Blood Institute. *Third Report of the Expert Panel on: Detection, Evaluation, and Treatment of High Blood Cholesterol in Adults (Adult Treatment Panel III)*. Final Report, 2002. Available at: http://www.nhlbi.nih.gov/guidelines/cholesterol/atp3full.pdf. Accessed July 4, 2004.

13. Hampl J, Anderson JV, Mullis R. The role of dietetics professionals in health promotion and disease prevention. *J Am Diet Assoc*. 2002;102:1680–1687.

14. Institute of Medicine. *The Future of Public Health*. Washington DC: National Academy Press; 1989.

15. Borra ST, Earl R, Hogan EH. Paucity of nutrition and food safety "news you can use" reveals opportunity for dietetics practitioners. *J Am Diet Assoc*. 1998;98:190–193.

16. Keenan DP, AbuSabha R, Robinson NG. Content Analysis of Media Coverage of the 1995 Dietary Guidelines for Americans. *Journal of Extension* 2001;39. Available at: http://www.joe.org/joe/2001october/rb5.html. Retrieved March 10, 2005.

17. Shine A, O'Reilly S, O'Sullivan K. Consumer attitudes to nutrition labeling. *British Food Journal*. 1997;99:283–289.

18. Cooper MJ, Zlotkin SH. An evidence-based approach to the development of national dietary guidelines. *J Am Diet Assoc*. 2003;103(Suppl 2):S28–S33.

19. Dourson ML, Andersen ME, Erdreich LS, MacGregor JA. Using human data to protect the public's health. *Regul Toxicol Pharmacol*. 2001;33:234–256.

20. Kroke A, Boeing H, Rossnagel K, Willich SN. History of the concept of "levels of evidence" and their current status in relation to primary prevention through lifestyle interventions. *Public Health Nutr.* 2004;7:279–284.

21. Jonnalagadda SS, Mitchell DC, Smiciklas-Wright H, et al. Accuracy of energy intake estimated by a multiple pass, 24-hour dietary recall technique. *J Amer Diet Assoc.* 2000;100:303–308.

22. Kipnis V, Midthune D, Freedman L, et al. Bias in dietary-report instruments and its implications for nutritional epidemiology. *Public Health Nutr.* 2002;5:915–923.

23. Shahar D, Shai I, Vardi H, et al. Development of a semi-quantitative Food Frequency Questionnaire (FFQ) to assess dietary intake of multiethnic populations. *Eur J Epidemiol.* 2003;18:855–861.

24. Bingham SA. Biomarkers in nutritional epidemiology. *Public Health Nutr.* 2002;5:821–827.

25. Kaaks RJ. Biochemical markers as additional measurements in studies of the accuracy of dietary questionnaire measurements: conceptual issues. *Am J Clin Nutr.* 1997;65(4 Suppl):1232S–1239S.

26. World Health Organization. *Report of the technical discussions at the twenty first World Health Assembly on "national and global surveillance of communicable diseases."* A2.1. 18-5-1968. Geneva, Switzerland: Author; 1968.

27. Stover PJ, Garza C. Bringing individuality to public health recommendations. *J Nutr.* 2002;132(8 Suppl):2476S–2480S.

28. McQuillan GM, Porter KS, Agelli M, Kington R. Consent for genetic research in a general population: The NHANES experience. *Genet Med.* 2003;5:35–42.

29. Woteki CE. Integrated NHANES: uses in national policy. *J Nutr.* 2003;133:582S–584S.

30. Arab L, Carriquiry A, Steck-Scott S, Gaudet MM. Ethnic differences in the nutrient intake adequacy of premenopausal US women: results from the Third National Health Examination Survey. *J Am Diet Assoc.* 2003;103:1008–1014.

31. Ford ES, Ballew C. Dietary folate intake in US adults: findings from the third National Health and Nutrition Examination Survey. *Ethn Dis.* 1998;8:299–305.

32. Looker AC, Loria CM, Carroll MD, et al. Calcium intakes of Mexican Americans, Cubans, Puerto Ricans, non-Hispanic whites, and non-Hispanic blacks in the US. *J Am Diet Assoc.* 1993;93:1274–1279.

33. Sharma S, Malarcher AM, Giles WH, Myers G. Racial, ethnic and socioeconomic disparities in the clustering of cardiovascular disease risk factors. *Ethn Dis.* 2004;14:43–48.

34. Hicks LS, Fairchild DG, Cook EF, Ayanian JZ. Association of region of residence and immigrant status with hypertension, renal failure, cardiovascular disease, and stroke, among African-American participants in the third National Health and Nutrition Examination Survey (NHANES III). *Ethn Dis.* 2003;13:316–323.

35. Berenson GS, ed. *Causation of Cardiovascular Risk Factors in Childhood: Perspectives on Cardiovascular Risk in Early Life.* New York, NY: Raven Press; 1986.

36. Berenson GS, McMahan CA, Voors AW, et al. *Cardiovascular Risk Factors in Children—The Early Natural History of Atherosclerosis and Essential Hypertension.* New York, NY: Oxford University Press; 1980.

37. Berenson GS, Wattigney WA, Bao W, et al. Rationale to study the early natural history of heart disease: The Bogalusa Heart Study. *Am J Med Sci.* 1995;310(Suppl 1):S22–S28.

38. Nicklas TA, Demory-Luce D, Yang SJ, et al. Children's food consumption patterns have changed over two decades (1973–1994): The Bogalusa heart study. *J Am Diet Assoc.* 2004;104:1127–1140.

39. Nicklas T, Johnson R. Dietary guidance for healthy children aged 2 to 11 years. *J Am Diet Assoc.* 2004; 104:660–677.

40. Berenson GS, Wattigney WA, Tracy RE, et al. Atherosclerosis of the aorta and coronary arteries and cardiovascular risk factors in persons aged 6 to 30 years and studied at necropsy (The Bogalusa Heart Study). *Am J Cardiol.* 1992;70:851–858.

41. Strong JP, McGill HC Jr. The natural history of coronary atherosclerosis. *Am J Pathol.* 1962;40:37–49.

42. Metha NV, Khan, AI. Cardiology's 10 greatest discoveries of the 20th century. *Tex Heart Inst J.* 2002;29:164–171.

43. Kannel WB, Dawber TR, Kagan A, Revotskie N, Stokes J 3rd. Factors of risk in the development of coronary heart disease—six-year follow-up experience. The Framingham Study. *Ann Intern Med.* 1961;55:33–50.

44. Farris RP, Nicklas TA. Characterizing children's eating behavior. In: Suskind RM, Suskind LL, eds. *Textbook of Pediatric Nutrition.* New York, NY: Raven Press; 1993.

45. Nicklas TA, Forcier JE, Webber LS, Berenson GS. School lunch assessment as part of a 24-hour dietary recall for children. *J Am Diet Assoc.* 1991;91:711–713.

46. Frank GC, Hollatz AT, Webber LS, Berenson GS. Effect of interviewer recording practices on nutrient intake—Bogalusa Heart Study. *J Am Diet Assoc.* 1984;84:1432–1436.

47. Most MM, Ershow AG, Clevidence BA. An overview of methodologies, proficiencies, and training resources for controlled feeding studies. *J Am Diet Assoc.* 2003;103:729–735.

48. Appel LJ, Moore TJ, Obarzanek E, et al. A clinical trial of the effects of dietary patterns on blood pressure. DASH Collaborative Research Group. *N Engl J Med.* 1997;336:1117–1124.

49. Sacks FM, Svetkey LP, Vollmer WM, et al. Effects on blood pressure of reduced dietary sodium and the Dietary Approaches to Stop Hypertension (DASH) diet. DASH-Sodium Collaborative Research Group. *N Engl J Med.* 2001;344, 3–10.

50. Albanes D, Heinonen OP, Taylor PR, et al. Alpha-tocopherol and beta-carotene supplements and lung cancer incidence in the alpha-tocopherol, beta-carotene cancer prevention study: effects of base-line characteristics and study compliance. *J Natl Cancer Inst.* 1996;88:1560–1570.

51. Omenn GS, Goodman G, Thornquist M, et al. The beta-carotene and retinol efficacy trial (CARET) for chemoprevention of lung cancer in high risk populations: smokers and asbestos-exposed workers. *Cancer Res.* 1994;54(7 Suppl):2038s–2043s.

52. Block G, Patterson B, Subar A. Fruit, vegetables, and cancer prevention: a review of the epidemiological evidence. *Nutr Cancer.* 1992;18:1–29.

53. Steinmetz KA, Potter JD. Vegetables, fruit, and cancer. I. Epidemiology. *Cancer Causes Control.* 1991;2:325–357.

54. Le Marchand L, Hankin JH, Kolonel LN, et al. Intake of specific carotenoids and lung cancer risk. *Cancer Epidemiol Biomarkers Prev.* 1993;2:183–187.

55. Steinmetz KA, Potter JD, Folsom AR. Vegetables, fruit, and lung cancer in the Iowa Women's Health Study. *Cancer Res.* 1993;53:536–543.

56. Smigel K. Beta carotene fails to prevent cancer in two major studies; CARET intervention stopped. *J Natl Cancer Inst.* 1996;88:145.

57. Pryor WA, Stahl W, Rock CL. Beta carotene: from biochemistry to clinical trials. *Nutr Rev.* 2000;58(2 Pt 1):39–53.

58. Roy HJ, Keenan MJ, Zablah-Pimentel E, et al. Adult female rats defend "appropriate" energy intake after adaptation to dietary energy. *Obes Res.* 2003;11:1214–1222.

59. Wolf G. The effect of low and high doses of beta-carotene and exposure to cigarette smoke on the lungs of ferrets. *Nutr Rev.* 2002;60:88–90.

60. Russell RM. The enigma of beta-carotene in carcinogenesis: what can be learned from animal studies. *J Nutr.* 2004;134:262S–268S.

61. U.S. Department of Health and Human Services. *Healthy People: The Surgeon General's Report on Health Promotion and Disease Prevention.* Washington, DC: Government Printing Office; 1979: section 25.

62. Perspectives in Disease Prevention and Health Promotion Implementing the 1990 prevention objectives: Summary of CDC's seminar. *MMWR.* 1983;32:21–24.

63. Food and Nutrition Board. *Recommended Dietary Allowances*, 10th ed. Washington, DC: National Academy Press; 1989.

64. Yates AA. National nutrition and public health policies: issues related to bioavailability of nutrients when developing dietary reference intakes. *J Nutr.* 2001;131:1331S–1334S.

65. Yates AA. Process and development of dietary reference intakes: basis, need, and application of recommended dietary allowances. *Nutr Rev.* 1998 Apr;56(4 Pt 2):S5–9.

66. Murphy SP, Poos MI. Dietary Reference Intakes: summary of applications in dietary assessment. *Public Health Nutr.* 2002;5:843–849.

67. Murphy SP, Barr SI, Poos MI. Using the new dietary reference intakes to assess diets: a map to the maze. *Nutr Rev.* 2002;60:267–275.

68. Barr SI, Murphy SP, Agurs-Collins TD, Poos MI. Planning diets for individuals using the dietary reference intakes. *Nutr Rev.* 2003;61:352–360.

69. Dwyer JT. Nutrition guidelines and education of the public. *J Nutr.* 2001;131(11 Suppl):3074S–3077S.

70. U.S. Department of Health and Human Services, Public Health Service. *The Surgeon General's Report on Nutrition and Health.* DHHS (PHS) Publication No. 88-50215;1988.

71. Merrill D. The new dietary guidelines and kids: Will they sit at the same table? *School-Business-Affairs.* 1997;63:22–26.

72. Welsh S, Davis C, Shaw A. A brief history of food guides in the U.S. *Nutrition Today.* 1992;November/December:6–11.

73. Cronin FJ, Shaw AM, Krebs-Smith SM, et al. Developing a food guidance system to implement the dietary guidelines. *J Nutr Ed.* 1987;19:281–302.

74. Davis CA, Britten P, Myers EF. Related articles, Past, present, and future of the Food Guide Pyramid. *J Am Diet Assoc.* 2001;101:881–885.

75. Goldberg JP, Belury MA, Elam P, et al. The obesity crisis: don't blame it on the pyramid. *J Am Diet Assoc.* 2004;104:1141–1147.

76. Welsh S, Davis C, Shaw A. Development of the Food Guide Pyramid. *Nutrition Today.* 1992;November/December:12–23.

77. Dixon LB, Cronin FJ, Krebs Smith SM. Let the pyramid guide your food choices: capturing the total diet concept. *J Nutr.* 2001;131:461S–472S.

78. Davis CA, Britten P, Myers EF. Past, present, and future of the Food Guide Pyramid. *J Am Diet Assoc.* 2001;101:881–885.

79. Nestle M. Dietary advice for the 1990s: the political history of the Food Guide Pyramid. *Caduceus.* 1993 Winter;9(3):136–153.

80. Painter J, Rah J-H, Lee Y-K. Comparison of international food guide pictorial representations. *J Am Diet Assoc.* 2002;102:483–489.

81. Foote JA, Murphy SP, Wilkens LR, Basiotis PP, Carlson A. Dietary variety increases the probability of nutrient adequacy among adults. *J Nutr.* 2004;134:1779–1785.

82. Falciglia GA, Troyer AG, Couch SC. Dietary variety increases as a function of time and influences diet quality in child. *J Nutr Educ Behav.* 2004;36:77–83.

83. Tavelli S, Beerman K, Shultz JE, Heiss C. Sources of error and nutritional adequacy of the food guide pyramid. *Am J Coll Health.* 1998;47:77–82.

84. Tande DL, Hotchkiss L, Cotugna N. The associations between blood lipids and the Food Guide Pyramid: findings from the Third National Health and Nutrition Examination Survey. *Prev Med.* 2004;38:452–457.

85. Newby PK, Muller D, Hallfrisch J, et al. Dietary patterns and changes in body mass index and waist circumference in adults. *Am J Clin Nutr.* 2003;77:1417–1425.

86. Gambera PJ, Schneeman BO, Davis PA. Use of the Food Guide Pyramid and U.S. Dietary Guidelines to improve dietary intake and reduce cardiovascular risk in active-duty Air Force members. *J Am Diet Assoc.* 1995;95:1268–1273.

87. Kant AK, Graubard BI, Schatzkin A. Dietary patterns predict mortality in a national cohort: the National Health Interview Surveys, 1987 and 1992. *J Nutr.* 2004;134:1793–1799.

88. Cooper DA. Carotenoids in health and disease: recent scientific evaluations, research recommendations, and the consumer. *J Nutr.* 2004;134:221S–224S.

89. Key TJ, Schatzkin A, Willett WC, et al. Diet, nutrition, and the prevention of cancer. *Public Health Nutr.* 2004;7:187–200.

90. Kris-Etherton PM, Etherton TD, Carlson J, Gardner C. Recent discoveries in inclusive food-based approaches and dietary patterns for reduction in risk for cardiovascular disease. *Curr Opin Lipidol.* 2002;13:397–407.

91. Cleveland LE, Moshfegh AJ, Albertson AM, Goldman JD. Dietary intake of whole grains. *J Am Coll Nutr.* 2000;19(3 Suppl):331S–338S.

92. USDA/Agricultural Research Service. *Pyramid Servings Intakes by U.S. Children and Adults, 1994–1996, 1998.* ARS Community Nutrition Research Group. Available at: http://www.barc.usda.gov/bhnrc/cnrg. Accessed July 15, 2004.

93. Putnam J, Allshouse J, Kantor LS. U.S. per capita food supply trends: more calories, refined carbohydrates, and fats. USDA, Economic Research Service. *Food Rev.* 2002;25:2–15.

94. Young LR, Nestle M. Expanding portion sizes in the U.S. marketplace: implications for nutrition counseling. *J Am Diet Assoc.* 2003 Feb;103(2):231–234.

95. Nicklas TA, Baranowski T, Cullen KW, Berenson G. Eating patterns, dietary quality and obesity. *J Am Coll Nutr.* 2001;20:599–608.

96. Nicklas TA, Yang SJ, Baranowski T, Zakeri I, Berenson G. Eating patterns and obesity in children. The Bogalusa Heart Study. *Am J Prev Med.* 2003;25:9–16.

97. Kennedy ET, Ohls J, Carlson S, Fleming K. The Healthy Eating Index: design and applications. *J Am Diet Assoc.* 1995;95:1103–1108.

98. Variyam JN, Blaylock J, Smallwood D, Basiotis PP. *USDA's Healthy Eating Index and Nutrition Information.* Washington, DC: Economic Research Service, U.S. Department of Agriculture; 1998. Technical Bulletin No. 1866.

99. Variyam JN, Shim Y, Blaylock J. Consumer misperceptions of diet quality. *J Nutr Educ.* 2001;33:314–321.

100. Dwyer J, Cosentino C, Li D, Feldman H, et al. Evaluating school-based interventions using the Healthy Eating Index. *J Am Diet Assoc.* 2002;102:257–259.

101. Carlson A, Lino M, Gerrior S, Basiotis P. *Report Card on the Diet Quality of Children Ages 2 to 9: Nutrition Insights, USDA Center for Policy and Promotion, 2001*; September 2001. Available at: http:// www.cnpp.usda.gov/Insights/Insight25.pdf. Accessed May 17, 2005.

102. Tangney CC, Evans DA, Bienias JL, Morris MC. Healthy eating index of black and white older adults. *Nutr Res.* 2001;21:1411–1423.

103. Institute of Medicine of the National Academies. *Dietary Reference Intakes for Energy, Carbohydrate, Fiber, Fat, Fatty Acids, Cholesterol, Protein, Amino Acids (Macronutrients).* Washington, DC: National Academies Press; 2002.

104. Weinstein SJ, Vogt TM, Gerrior SA. Healthy Eating Index scores are associated with blood nutrient concentrations in the third National Health and Nutrition Examination Survey. *J Am Diet Assoc.* 2004;104:576–584.

105. Hann CS, Rock CL, King I, Drewnowski A. A validation of the Healthy Eating Index with use of plasma biomarkers in a clinical sample of women. *Am J Clin Nutr.* 2001;74:479–486.

106. Pennington JA, Hubbard VS. Derivation of daily values used for nutrition labeling. *J Am Diet Assoc.* 1997 Dec;97(12):1407–1412.

107. Origin and framework of the development of dietary reference intakes. *Nutr Rev.* 1997;55(9):332–334.

108. Judd JT, Clevidence BA, Muesling RA, et al. Dietary trans fatty acids: effects on plasma lipids and lipoproteins of healthy men and women. *Am J Clin Nutr.* 1994;59:861–868.

109. Kris-Etherton PM, Yu S. Individual fatty acid effects on plasma lipids and lipoproteins: human studies. *Am J Clin Nutr.* 1997;65(5 Suppl): 1628S–1644S.

110. Lichtenstein AH, Ausman LM, Jalbert SM, Schaefer EJ. Effects of different forms of dietary hydrogenated fats on serum lipoprotein cholesterol levels. *New Engl J Med.* 1999;340:1933–1940.

111. Chainani-Wu N. Diet and oral, pharyngeal, and esophageal cancer. *Nutr Cancer.* 2002;44:104–126.

112. Key TJ, Schatzkin A, Willett WC. Diet, nutrition and the prevention of cancer. *Public Health Nutr.* 2004;7(1A):187–200.

113. Steinmetz KA, Potter JD. Vegetables, fruit, and cancer prevention: a review. *J Am Diet Assoc.* 1996;96:1027–1039.

114. Riboli E, Norat T. Epidemiologic evidence of the protective effect of fruit and vegetables on cancer risk. *Am J Clin Nutr.* 2003;78(3 Suppl): 559S–569S.

115. Kampman E, Arts IC, Hollman PC. Plant foods versus compounds in carcinogenesis; observational versus experimental human studies. *Int J Vitam Nutr Res.* 2003;73:70–78.

116. Temple NJ, Gladwin KK. Fruit, vegetables, and the prevention of cancer: research challenges. *Nutrition.* 2003;19:467–470.

117. Smith-Warner SA, Spiegelman D, Yaun SS, et al. Intake of fruits and vegetables and risk of breast cancer: a pooled analysis of cohort studies. *JAMA.* 2001;285:769–776.

118. Kim DJ, Holowaty EJ. Brief, validated survey instruments for the measurement of fruit and vegetable intakes in adults: a review. *Prev Med.* 2003;36:440–447.

119. Ziegler RG. Vegetables, fruits, and carotenoids and the risk of cancer. *Am J Clin Nutr.* 1991;53(1 Suppl):251S–259S.

120. Duthie GG, Gardner PT, Kyle JA. Plant polyphenols: are they the new magic bullet. *Proc Nutr Soc.* 2003;62:599–603.

121. La Vecchia C, Altieri A, Tavani A. Vegetables, fruit, antioxidants and cancer: a review of Italian studies. *Eur J Nutr.* 2001;40:261–267.

122. Reddy L, Odhav B, Bhoola KD. Natural products for cancer prevention: a global perspective. *Pharmacol Ther.* 2003;99:1–13.

123. Van Duyn MA, Pivonka E. Overview of the health benefits of fruit and vegetable consumption for the dietetics professional: selected literature. *J Am Diet Assoc.* 2000;100:1511–1521.

124. van't Veer P, Jansen MC, Klerk M, Kok FJ. Fruits and vegetables in the prevention of cancer and cardiovascular disease. *Public Health Nutr.* 2000;3:103–107.

125. Bazzano LA, Serdula MK, Liu S. Dietary intake of fruits and vegetables and risk of cardiovascular disease. *Curr Atheroscler Rep.* 2003;5:492–499.

126. Hu FB. Plant-based foods and prevention of cardiovascular disease: an overview. *Am J Clin Nutr.* 2003;78(3 Suppl):544S–551S.

127. Joshipura KJ, Ascherio A, Manson JE, et al. Fruit and vegetable intake in relation to risk of ischemic stroke. *JAMA.* 1999;282:1233–1239.

128. Feldman EB. Fruits and vegetables and the risk of stroke. *Nutr Rev.* 2001;59(1 Pt 1):24–27.

129. Bazzano LA, He J, Ogden LG, et al. Fruit and vegetable intake and risk of cardiovascular disease in U.S. adults: the first National Health and Nutrition Examination Survey Epidemiologic Follow-up Study. *Am J Clin Nutr.* 2002;76:93–99.

130. Anderson JV, Bybee DI, Brown RM, et al. 5 a day fruit and vegetable intervention improves consumption in a low income population. *J Am Diet Assoc.* 2001;101:195–202.

131. Havas S, Anliker J, Damron D, et al. Final results of the Maryland WIC 5-A-Day Promotion Program. *Am J Public Health.* 1998;88:1161–1167.

132. Sorensen G, Stoddard A, Peterson K, et al. Increasing fruit and vegetable consumption through worksites and families in the Treatwell 5-a-day study. *Am J Public Health.* 1999;89:54–60.

133. Beresford SA, Thompson B, Feng Z, et al. Seattle 5 a Day worksite program to increase fruit and vegetable consumption. *Prev Med.* 2001;32:230–238.

134. Stables GJ, Subar AF, Patterson BH, et al. Changes in vegetable and fruit consumption and awareness among U.S. adults: results of the 1991 and 1997 5 A Day for Better Health Program surveys. *J Am Diet Assoc.* 2002;102:809–817.

135. Havas S, Treiman K, Langenberg P, et al. Factors associated with fruit and vegetable consumption among women participating in WIC. *J Am Diet Assoc.* 1998;98:1141–1148.

136. Langenberg P, Ballesteros M, Feldman R, et al. Psychosocial factors and intervention-associated changes in those factors as correlates of change in fruit and vegetable consumption in the Maryland WIC 5 A Day Promotion Program. *Ann Behav Med.* 2000;22:307–315.

137. Campbell MK, Reynolds KD, Havas S, et al. Stages of change for increasing fruit and vegetable consumption among adults and young adults participating in the national 5-a-Day for Better Health community studies. *Health Educ Behav.* 1999;26:513–534.

138. Patterson RE, Satia JA, Kristal AR, et al. Is there a consumer backlash against the diet and health message? *J Am Diet Assoc.* 2001;101:37–41.

PART II

ASSESSING AND INTERVENING IN THE COMMUNITY'S NUTRITION NEEDS

Part II introduces the reader to how public health nutritionists target care for those at highest risk. Chapter 3 explains the role of needs assessment in public health and how it helps Americans. Proper needs assessment allows the public health nutritionist to serve most usefully those who need help. In Chapter 4, we see the results of more than a century of needs assessment, with the designation of the young and the old, as well as people coping with illness and disability, as those who must be supported by public health nutrition services. Reaching those in need has been one of public health nutrition's most difficult challenges.

In the 21st century, public health nutrition needs assessments have determined that the United States' indulgent eating habits have brought about a nutritional catastrophe. The epidemics of overweight in children (Chapter 5) and adult obesity (Chapter 6) are two additional areas in which public health nutrition must find a way to intervene and provide solutions.

CHAPTER 3

COMMUNITY NEEDS ASSESSMENT

Elizabeth Metallinos-Katsaras, PhD, RD

Reader Objectives

After studying this chapter and reflecting on its contents, you should be able to:

1. Define community in the context of public health nutrition.
2. Explain the rationale for community needs assessment.
3. Define the terms used in community needs assessment.
4. Describe the steps to follow when conducting a community needs assessment.
5. Describe the types of data that can be collected about a community and how these data can be obtained.
6. Identify existing sources of data that can be used.
7. Describe the types of data that can be used to assess the nutritional status of the target population.
8. Compare assessed needs with the capacity of existing services to meet these needs.

The commissioner of public health in your town has come to you with the following question: "What are the major nutritional problems of our community that are currently not being addressed effectively?" Embedded within this question are several additional queries, including: "Who is most affected by the nutritional problems? What are some of the barriers to their improvement? What is the healthcare system doing about them?" The overarching goal of the task you have been handed is to develop new programs or to identify ways in which existing public health nutrition programs can address the most pressing nutritional needs of a community. Such a request from a high-ranking official may sound a bit far-fetched; however, in an era in which the obesity epidemic is at the forefront of not only scientific inquiry, but also the media, there is a renewed interest in prevention. Prevention is, after all, the hallmark of public health nutrition.

How would you go about responding to this inquiry? What would you do first? What information or data would you need and where would you get it? This chapter describes the process you can use to determine the unmet nutrition-related needs of a community.

Both hypothetical and actual needs assessment examples are used to exemplify both nutritional status and community resource data.

Community Needs Assessment: Definition and Overview

An integral step in the public health process is determining the nutritional needs of the community and population with which you are working. Accurate and focused needs assessment is an essential step in the planning, implementation, and evaluation of public health programs for several reasons. First, public health departments and agencies must know about the primary problems and unmet needs of the community prior to developing a new program, modifying existing programs, or distributing resources. Second, in order to allocate resources to program development and implementation, it is essential to also determine the most important and pressing needs. Although we as community and public health nutritionists are committed to improving all aspects of nutrition-related community health, resource constraints underlie most programmatic decisions. Thus, one needs to identify the most pressing nutrition-related problems, the underlying causes in the specific group in question, and which problems are not being met by existing resources in order to prioritize and distribute resources.

Equally important in the identification of the nutrition problems is who will be affected in order to address their issues. A community can be defined broadly as *a group of people with common characteristics*. The individuals within the community, who are the focus of the needs assessment, comprise the target population. For example, Roxbury is a low-income, inner-city neighborhood of Boston, Massachusetts. In recognition of the importance of obesity prevention, you as the public health nutritionist would like to conduct a community needs assessment of school-age children living in Roxbury, Massachusetts. Therefore, the community is Roxbury, while the target population is school-age children.

> A community is a group of people with common characteristics. These can include a location or region; sociodemographic characteristics such as ethnicity, age, education, or occupation; a nutritional problem (e.g., obesity); or a common bond (e.g., members of an organization) (McKenzie, Pinger, & Kotecki, 2002).

Community needs assessment includes both an assessment of the community resources and an assessment of the nutritional status/concerns of the target population. The scope of the community needs assessment can be large (e.g., a nationwide maternal and child nutrition needs assessment) or small (e.g., determining the need for breast-feeding

> A target population is the group that is the focus of an assessment, a study, an intervention (Boyle, 2003), or a program (McKenzie, Pinger, & Kotecki, 2002).

support among Laotian American participants of a specific Special Supplemental Nutrition Program for Women, Infants and Children [WIC] program).

The types of data and methods of obtaining data vary greatly as well. The foundation of some needs assessments is the collection, compilation, and interpretation of existing (i.e., secondary) data, whereas others incorporate a primary data collection component. Which data collection route should be taken depends on the purpose of the needs assessment, but it is important to note that numerous existing data sources are publicly available to the public health nutritionist. Table 3-1 lists some of these. Some public health nutritionists may embark on primary data collection prematurely, unknowingly ignoring existing data pertinent to their needs assessment. Thus, we cannot overstate the importance of investigating existing data sources and research in the published literature that may be relevant to your specific needs assessment.

Who will conduct the community needs assessment? You might envision a lonely public health nutritionist setting out to complete all the phases of the assessment. In reality, in most cases a team is assembled to conduct the assessment. The desirability of this approach is underscored by the fact that numerous and varied skills are needed to effectively conduct a community needs assessment. The public health nutritionist is the nutrition expert, but may not be a data or survey development expert. Nor can public health nutritionists alone represent the stakeholders. Thus, others on the team will complement the public health nutritionist with their expertise in qualitative or quantitative research methods, data analysis, and interpretation.

> **Qualitative research:** Any method of data collecting that generates narrative data or words rather than numerical data or numbers. The words must reflect the study participant perspective (Achterberg & Shepherd, 2003).
>
> **Quantitative research:** Hypothesis-testing research that gathers numerical data or data that can be quantified.

As some have noted (Peterson & Alexander, 2001), needs are in the eye of the beholder, and many decisions can be based on value judgments about the problems that exist in a target population. For example, most consider obesity to be a serious public health problem, but there are some who disagree (Campos, 2004). The fact that a public health nutritionist's perceived need may not be met with unanimous agreement by the public makes it important to engender community support for the findings of the needs assessment (Peterson & Alexander, 2001). Thus, the needs assessment process includes not only a scientific and analytic component, but also a political one. Therefore, it is important to include those individuals or groups in the needs assessment process who will be affected by the findings (Peterson & Alexander, 2001). These stakeholders include:

TABLE 3-1   Examples of Secondary Datasets That Could Be Sources for a Community Needs Assessment

Description	Website
2000 Census Datasets	ftp://ftp2.census.gov/census_2000/datasets
DataWarehouse for NCHS public use data files for: • National Health and Nutrition Examination Survey • National Health Care Survey • National Health Interview Survey • National Immunization Survey • Longitudinal Studies on Aging	http://www.cdc.gov/nchs/datawh/ftpserv/ftpdata/ftpdata.htm
Youth Risk Behavior Surveillance System: Monitors priority health risk behaviors that contribute markedly to the leading causes of death, disability, and social problems among youth and adults in the United States. Data files and documentation.	http://www.cdc.gov/HealthyYouth/yrbs/about_yrbss.htm
DataFerrett System: NCHS and the Bureau of the Census collaborated to provide NCHS datasets in the Census's DataFerrett system. It is a unique data mining and extraction tool that allows you to select a data basket full of variables, recode those variables as needed, and then develop and customize tables and charts.	http://www.cdc.gov/nchs/datawh/ferret/ferret.htm
United States Department of Agriculture (Economic Research Service): Early Childhood Longitudinal Survey's Food Security in the United States	http://www.ers.usda.gov/data/foodsecurity/ECLSK

Source: Compiled by the author.

- Consumers/program recipients
- Policymakers
- The target population
- Nutrition program providers
- Nutrition program funders

The individuals represented within each of these groups provide a unique perspective, not only in developing the needs assessment process but also in addressing the nutrition problem in question.

Steps to Conduct a Community Needs Assessment

The community needs assessment includes a planning phase in which the public health nutritionist makes a case for the needs assessment, a methodology development phase, a data collection and analysis phase, and a utilization phase (Boyle, 2003 and Peterson & Alexander, 2001).

Phase 1: Needs Assessment Planning

In the first phase of the needs assessment, the public health nutritionist must not only make a case for the needs assessment in a specific community, but also lay out the organizational framework that will guide the process. The following sections describe the steps necessary to achieve this.

Step 1: Identify the Community of Interest

At this initial stage of the needs assessment, you need to articulate which community is of concern. This community can include the group of people who are the focus of your needs assessment (i.e., the target population) or a specific region or neighborhood in which they live (e.g., Roxbury, MA), the nutritional problem of concern (e.g., obesity), or all of the above (e.g., overweight children living in Roxbury, MA). It is important to be as specific as possible in order to focus your needs assessment efforts.

Step 2: Describe the Problem, Research Its Underlying Causes, and State Why a Needs Assessment Is Necessary

In this step, you as the public health nutritionist prepare a brief, but compelling, statement of the problem (Boyle, 2003). It should include a description of the nutritional problem of concern, who is affected, the magnitude of the problem, what is known about its causes, and why there is justification for the needs assessment. An essential component of this step is to comprehensively review the research in the published literature in terms of both underlying causes and public health impact. Fortunately, the Internet can be used to identify relevant research articles; in many cases, full text articles are available online. In order to minimize the possibility that you are missing important research in this area, you should utilize a reference librarian to guide you in your use of key words and finding the best databases for your topic. Public health nutritionists are often not in a position to conduct scientific research into the underlying causes of nutrition-related problems; however, the wealth of published research available precludes the need for them to do so.

To return to the former example regarding the nutrition-related problem of overweight children in Roxbury, one needs to examine the literature regarding:

- *The magnitude of the problem:* This includes determining the percentage of children who are overweight or at risk of becoming overweight, and identifying which specific groups of children are most at risk.
- *The importance of addressing this problem in children:* This includes the tracking of overweight people from childhood to adulthood; chronic disease consequences, both in childhood and adulthood; and cost to the healthcare system.
- *The known causes of children being overweight:* What is known about how overweight indices have increased among children in general? These include increases in sedentary behavior (e.g., TV watching), reductions in physical activity, and increased consumption of specific types of food (e.g., fast food, soft drinks).
- *Gaps in the scope of influence:* This refers to those individuals living in a community in which there are gaps in nutrition knowledge relevant to the identification and resolution of the nutritional problem in the target population. In this case this would include parents, teachers, school administrators, and other community members who can influence children's macro- or micro-environment.

Step 3: Define the Target Population

At this point, you have research and data that identify which groups are most at risk for a specific nutritional problem or overall poor nutritional status, and in which groups the nutritional problem has the greatest effect on public health. This will guide you to define more clearly the target population for your needs assessment. For example, in the case of overweight children in Roxbury, you may have found from your review of the published literature that the prevalence of obesity increases substantially during adolescence. This provides the justification for choosing pre-teens living in Roxbury as the target population, if your needs assessment is for obesity prevention programs.

> Prevalence, also called *prevalence proportion,* is the proportion of people in a population who have a disease (Rothman, 2002, p. 41).

Step 4: Determine the Purpose, Goals, and Objectives of the Community Needs Assessment

The purpose is a general description of the intent of the needs assessment. A community needs assessment may be conducted for any of the following reasons:

- To identify groups of people in the community who are at nutritional risk (Boyle, 2003)
- To discover the community's or target population's most critical unmet nutritional needs and prioritize them (Boyle, 2003)
- To assess the degree to which existing programs and services meet the needs of the target population (Boyle, 2003)
- To distribute resources either within a program (regionally) or between different types of programs based on nutrition needs in the community
- To identify factors in the community that contribute to the nutritional problem within the target population

It is important to note that the last example listed must be distinguished from the research question, which is often epidemiological in nature regarding what causes a disease or condition. Although, for example, in the case of the community needs assessment, there is evidence that TV watching may contribute to the development of obesity in children, a nutrition needs assessment will ascertain: a) whether TV watching is high among children in that community, and b) the factors in the community that may contribute to this behavior. As part of the community needs assessment, factors such as unsafe neighborhoods, lack of parks, and lack of affordable after school and summer youth programs may all be factors contributing to the high TV watching among children in this community and subsequent childhood obesity.

Goals and objectives lay the foundation for all activities subsequently conducted for the needs assessment, including data gathering, analysis, and utilization. Goals drive the type of data that will be needed and how it will be used. As McKenzie et al. (2002) note, goals will be the basis for all subsequent activities and is the "hoped for end result." There may be more than one goal for the needs assessment. Objectives, on the other hand, are statements that describe the specific result or outcome that will be achieved or activity accomplished (one result or activity per statement). As Boyle (2003) notes, strong verbs should be used in objective statements; examples of such verbs are *increase, decrease, reduce, assess,* and *identify*. What is described in each objective should be measurable in some way; thus, by collecting data you should be able to assess the degree to which you were successful at achieving each specific objective. There are usually two or more objectives per goal.

Step 5: Determine the Organizational Structure for the Needs Assessment

It is important that the organizational structure for the needs assessment be determined at the outset (Peterson & Alexander, 2001). This includes identifying who will direct the needs assessment and all agency and non-agency members of the needs assessment team. What resources will be assigned to this activity, including dedicated staff? How will community members be involved? The composition of the team responsible for conducting the needs assessment depends on the goals and objectives of the needs assessment. Some important members of the needs assessment team include a nutrition professional, staff responsible for nutrition program service delivery and program administration, and someone with expertise in quantitative or qualitative data collection/management/analysis methods (depending on the data needed, expertise will vary). In order for the needs assessment to be conducted thoroughly and effectively, resources need to be allocated consistent with the scope of the needs assessment. This can be a challenge for public health agencies at times, and this is one of the underlying reasons for determining resource allocation at the outset. If adequate resources cannot be allocated, then the scope of the needs assessment may need to be curtailed.

Phase 2: Methodology Development

In this phase of the community needs assessment process, the team will lay out in detail which data will be needed to meet each objective of the needs assessment and how they will obtain the data. Although time-consuming, this type of planning in advance will facilitate all activities related to the needs assessment. As with the literature review, careful and systematic attention to completeness and detail will minimize surprises and ensure that all data that are needed can be obtained.

Step 6: Specify the Data Needed and Design a Plan for Acquiring the Data

The data that may be needed for a nutrition needs assessment will likely fall under one or more of the following four categories.

- Community data
  - *Community organizational structure and authorities:* Data related to how the community is organized politically and socially
  - *Community services and usage:* Data related to nutrition-related programs, services, and usage in the community
  - *Community demographics and health:* The overall health of the community
  - *Community environment:* Includes local, state, and national policies and systems, as well as the specific community's

physical environment that can affect the nutritional status of the target population
- Target population data
  - Data related to the nutritional status of the target population
  - Lifestyle factors affecting nutritional status
  - Sociodemographic factors; living and working conditions
  - Data related to attitudes, perceptions, and opinions of the target population
- As noted by Peterson and Alexander (2001), the wealth of data potentially available can be both advantageous and disadvantageous. Having numerous indicators implies that the degree to which nutrition-related needs/status is measured is improved (as opposed to having only a few indicators available). Conversely, having too many indicators available can be overwhelming for data management, and tabulation can become unmanageable. Thus, it is important to carefully choose the best indicators that relate to the objectives of your nutrition needs assessment. The following specific criteria can be used to assess the potential costs and benefits of choosing indicators (Peterson & Alexander, 2001):
  - *Simplicity:* An indicator needs to be conceptually straightforward, be well defined, and be a valid and reliable measure of what it purports to represent. Both the public and policy makers should be able to understand it.
  - *Stability:* Estimates derived from these indicators should be based on large enough numbers so that they do not fluctuate dramatically due to small sample size.
  - *Availability:* Ideally the indicator is available at national, state, and local levels, so that even if your needs assessment is conducted on a local community, it is possible to examine relative health as compared to state and national status.
  - *Broad representation:* An indicator should reflect the potential nutrition-related concerns of most of the target population as well as higher risk groups within the target population.
  - *Political feasibility:* Although the public health impact of the nutrition-related problem is one of the most important considerations, one must also consider whether the political environment will facilitate or hinder an intervention to deal with this problem.
- The types of data that will be obtained for the needs assessment fall under two general categories: qualitative data and quantitative data. In addition, there are two types of data: data already collected and in a database or report (i.e., secondary data sources) and data that must be collected directly from the community or target population as part of the needs assessment (i.e., primary data collection).

Plan to Obtain Community Data

1. Community data, including the organizational structure and authorities: How the community's governmental agencies and healthcare organizations are organized and who is in power can affect the healthcare as well as the preventative service delivery for the target population. Community leaders are also important to identify because not only will they be invaluable sources of information about the unmet needs in the community, but also they will be essential to any successful strategy to address the unmet need identified by the needs assessment. One method that can be used to identify such individuals is obtaining organizational charts of government offices and healthcare organizations, either through the Internet or through visiting the offices. In addition, reading the local newspapers and listening to local radio stations will provide information on both community and business leaders, as well as influential media groups. Finally, those who have particular influence on, involvement with, or a vested interest in the well-being of the target population (i.e., stakeholders) should be identified and included.

2. Community services and usage: Information on which nutrition-related services and programs are available in the community can be obtained from local health organizations, government agencies and civic groups, the yellow pages, and voluntary health organizations such as the American Heart Association, the American Red Cross, the American Diabetes Association, and the United Way directories. Usage data includes the number of

> American Heart Association is available at www.americanheart.org.
>
> American Red Cross is available at www.redcross.org.
>
> American Diabetes Association is available at www.diabetes.org.
>
> United Way is available at www.national.unitedway.org.

people using services, as well as segments of the target population that are more or less likely to use specific services. This type of information can be obtained from the agencies and programs delivering the services; however, this may not be public information. Thus, involving key personnel who are involved in delivering programs relevant to the specific goals of the nutrition needs assessment facilitates access to such data.

3. Community demographics and health: Demographic data and health data can be obtained from a variety of sources (see Table 3-2). Some important demographic data include ethnicity, age distribution, gender, marital status, income, and poverty statistics. These all provide a description of who lives in the community. A variety of health statistics reflect overall health of the community, and these can point to segments of the population that are at risk for malnutrition. The following are some health statistics, most of which are available at the national and state level; some may be available for the local level as well (Boyle, 2003):

- *Age-adjusted mortality:* These include overall rates of death, both in general and from specific diseases.
- *Natality statistics:* These include the percent of mothers with adequate prenatal care, the infant mortality rate, average birth weights, and the percent of unmarried mothers.
- *Leading causes of death:* This is a rank order list of those causes to which deaths are most frequently attributable.
- *Morbidity statistics:* These include rates of nutrition-related diseases such as obesity, hypertension, and diabetes (as well as complications from diabetes).
- *Health risk behaviors:* These include sedentary activities, smoking, serum cholesterol concentration, lead exposure, and iron deficiency anemia.

TABLE 3-2   Sources for Demographic and Health Statistics for the Community Needs Assessment

Source Description	Website with Link to Statistical Information
Census Data: Statistical Abstract of the U.S. 2004–2005.	www.census.gov/prod/www/statistical-abstract-04.html
Census Data: American Community Survey. Includes state and county data.	www.census.gov/acs/www/
National Health statistics produced in report format by the National Center for Health Statistics (2004). Comprehensive report drawing from a variety of data sources.	www.cdc.gov/nchs/data/hus/hus04.pdf
FastStatsAtoZ provides state-specific natality and mortality statistics as well as health and health risk behavior data.	www.cdc.gov/nchs/fastats/map_page.htm
National Health and Nutrition Examination Survey (NHANES) results.	www.cdc.gov/nchs/about/major/nhanes/survey_results_and_products.htm
Links to NCHS surveys related to health and health care.	www.cdc.gov/nchs/default.htm
National Vital Statistics system: Annual reports that present detailed vital statistics data, including natality, mortality, marriage, and divorce.	www.cdc.gov/nchs/products/pubs/pubd/vsus/vsus.htm
The Behavioral Risk Factor Surveillance System (BRFSS) is the world's largest telephone survey and tracks health risks in the United States.	www.cdc.gov/brfss/

(Continues)

TABLE 3-2   Sources for Demographic and Health Statistics for the Community Needs Assessment (Continued)

Source Description	Website with Link to Statistical Information
Includes national and state statistics as well as statistics on selected metropolitan areas.	
Youth Risk Behavior Surveillance System: The YRBSS was developed in 1990 to monitor priority health risk behaviors that contribute markedly to the leading causes of death, disability, and social problems among youth and adults in the United States.	www.cdc.gov/HealthyYouth/yrbs
The Pediatric Nutrition Surveillance System (PedNSS) and the Pregnancy Nutrition Surveillance System (PNSS) are program-based surveillance systems that monitor the nutritional status of low-income infants, children, and women in federally funded maternal and child health programs.	www.cdc.gov/pednss/
Data Warehouse for NCHS data: Includes links to detailed statistical tables on a variety of health topics.	www.cdc.gov/nchs/datawh.htm
United States Department of Agriculture: International Food Consumption Patterns.	www.ers.usda.gov/data/ InternationalFoodDemand/
United States Department of Agriculture: Economic Research Service	www.ers.usda.gov
United States Department of Agriculture: Food Stamp Program statistics.	www.fns.usda.gov/pd/fspmain.htm
United States Department of Agriculture: WIC Program statistics.	www.fns.usda.gov/pd/wichome.htm
United States Department of Agriculture: Food Security in the United States. Links to a variety of statistics on food security.	www.ers.usda.gov/Data/foodsecurity/

Source: Compiled by the author.

Some of these statistics are also stratified by demographic characteristics, which can then be more accurately compared to the target population demographics. This is particularly useful if local data on a particular health outcome is not available for the specific community.

4. Environmental conditions within the community: This includes availability of food, access to medical care, access to preventative services, transportation, parks, walkways, and bicycle paths. All of these factors comprise the environment of the community that can affect the nutritional status of the target population. Availability of food, for example, is determined by what community grocery stores, supermarkets, co-ops, farmer's markets, or garden supply stores are in the area. For many community residents, food availability within the specific community determines what they can buy and have in their homes. How can we ascertain food availability? One of the best ways, if logistically possible, is to walk around the community and visit supermarkets and grocery stores, also noting types of restaurants and transportation availability. Visiting stores and noting food quality, availability, and cost will provide valuable qualitative information on what the target population faces in their food procurement on a day-to-day basis. In addition, it would also provide an opportunity for you to get a true feel of the community, the ethnic groups represented, and the physical surroundings that can affect opportunities for physical activity.

Plan to Obtain Data on the Target Population

Data on the nutritional status of the target population can be obtained through either secondary data sources or primary data collection. The former is desirable, if it is appropriate for the needs assessment, because it requires much fewer resources and can be obtained much more quickly. The National Nutrition Monitoring and Related Research Program publishes statistics at the national and state levels. In addition, you can obtain some of these datasets and conduct further analyses as part of the needs assessment. For example, it may be that your target population is Puerto Rican, but the statistics you identify are described for those of Hispanic descent as a whole. If the data set is available, then the member of your team who is responsible for data management and analysis can analyze the data for Puerto Ricans, specifically.

> The National Nutrition Monitoring and Related Research Program (www.cdc.gov/nchs/about/otheract/nutrishn/nutrishn.htm) includes all data on the collection and analysis activities of the federal government related to measuring the health and nutritional status, food consumption, dietary knowledge, and attitudes about diet and health of the U.S. population, and measuring food consumption and quality of the food supply.

Thus, existing datasets, if they include the indicators pertinent to the nutrition needs assessment, can be used to describe the target population's health and nutritional status. These can also be used as a basis to compare the target population's nutritional status with national and state statistics.

Nutritional status indicators fall under one of the following four categories (Gibson, 1990):

- Dietary assessment
- Laboratory/biochemical assessment
- Anthropometric assessment
- Clinical assessment

1. *Dietary assessment:* Dietary assessment methods are used to collect data on usual food and nutrient intake of individuals. Some frequently used dietary assessment methods are 24-hour recalls (single or repeated), estimated or weighed food records, dietary history, and food frequency questionnaires (Gibson, 1990). All of the aforementioned methods have systematic errors (Gibson). The goal is to minimize these errors as much as possible. There is an extensive literature in the area of dietary assessment, and many research articles that describe improved methodology (Jonnalagadda et al., 2000) and their validity and reliability in various populations. Therefore, the following is simply a summary of the most important points to consider.

There are various challenges to obtaining dietary data that reflect usual diet, not the least of which is that among free-living individuals, dietary intake exhibits variation from day to day. This variation is superimposed on a consistent pattern (Willett, 1998, p. 33). What the researcher is attempting to ascertain is that consistent pattern. Depending on the dietary assessment method used, the accuracy of intake data often reflects a person's literacy and educational level (for all methods, but especially food records), memory (24-hour recall and food frequency questionnaire), and ability to accurately quantify foods (24-hour recall and food frequency questionnaire). Another source of error is that individuals often alter their dietary intake while undergoing the assessment, thus reducing the accuracy with which the foods reflect what is usually eaten.

If you are considering collecting dietary data, you need to consider several factors. First, who is your population and what method is most appropriate? If your population is a well-educated one, then using food records (Willett, 1998) may be a good choice. On the other hand, if the population has limited literacy, then repeated 24-hour recalls may be a better choice.

Second, the number of days of dietary intake affects the validity with which the data reflects the individual's usual intake. A single day, whether it be a 24-hour recall or a food record, is not adequate to estimate a person's true usual intake for any macro- or micro-nutrient (Willett, 1998, p. 41); a single day, however, can provide an estimate of the average usual nutrient intake of a large population group if all the days of the week are represented (Gibson, 1990, p. 50). The degree of day-to-day variability affects the number of days needed, and this also depends on the nutrient under examination. For example, it has been stated that in order to obtain an estimate of an individual's vitamin A intake, such that 95% of observed values are within 10% of the true mean, one needs 105 days of dietary intake data (Willett, 1998, p. 44). This may seem absurd, but this example illustrates that it is virtually impossible to estimate an individual's intake based on one 24-hour recall. However, by administering repeated 24-hour recalls, you can improve the validity with which they represent the individual's usual diet.

The third issue is how the data will be analyzed. For 24-hour recalls and food records, you need to use a nutrient analysis program to assess the macro- or micro-nutrient content of the diet. If using a validated food frequency questionnaire, such as the Harvard semi-quantitative food frequency questionnaire (FFQ), then often the nutrient analysis is provided for a fee by the institution that sponsors that FFQ.

The following are generally recommended methods based on the objective of the dietary assessment:

> For a description of the semi-quantitative food frequency questionnaire used in the Nurses Health Study at the Harvard School of Public Health, visit the following website:
>
> http://www.hsph.harvard.edu /Academics/nutr/department/ Nurses%20Study.html.

- *Average usual intakes of a population group:* Can use a single 24-hour recall or food record (Gibson, 1990), although repeated measures are always better.
- *Proportion of the population "at risk" for a nutrient deficiency or excess:* Repeated 24-hour recalls or food records (Gibson, 1990). The number of days depends on the nutrient(s) that are the focus of the needs assessment (Gibson; Willett, 1998).
- *Usual nutrient intakes of individuals:* Repeated 24-hour recalls or food records (Gibson, 1990). The number of days depends on the nutrient(s) that are the focus of the needs assessment (Gibson; Willett, 1998).
- *Pattern of food use for a group or individual or ranking of individuals:* Food frequency questionnaires (Gibson, 1990).

To summarize, if a dietary assessment is needed as a part of the needs assessment, you should choose the method that will produce the most valid and reliable data for the target population that will meet the objectives of the needs assessment in the most succinct manner. Ideally, someone on the needs assessment team should have expertise in the area of dietary assessment, and a review of the literature should be conducted prior to choosing a method.

2. *Laboratory/biochemical assessment:* This is an objective measure of subclinical nutrient deficiency; it involves measurement of nutrient level, a nutrient's metabolite, or functional tests that measure nutrient-dependent enzyme activity or concentrations (Gibson, 1990, pp. 285–295). The aforementioned may be measured in blood, urine, hair, fingernails, or toenails. Many other functional tests exist as well, but are likely beyond the scope of a public health nutrition needs assessment. One of the most common laboratory tests used in nutritional surveillance is hemoglobin or hematocrit, which is used as an indicator of iron deficiency anemia. Note, however, that hemoglobin is a relatively insensitive indicator and nonspecific; this means that a significant proportion of people may truly have iron deficiency anemia, but be classified as having normal hemoglobin (insensitivity), while others may be diagnosed with iron deficiency anemia based on their hemoglobin levels, but are not truly anemic (nonspecific). Part of the problem is that hemoglobin (and hematocrit) is affected by many factors other than iron, including inflammation, infections, protein energy malnutrition, thalassemia minor, vitamin B12, or folate deficiencies, to name a few (Gibson, 1990, p. 352). Thus, in order to more accurately identify those who have iron deficiency anemia, other indicators of iron status (e.g., transferrin saturation, serum ferritin) should also be collected.

3. *Anthropometric assessment:* This type of nutritional assessment includes all measures of physical dimensions and body composition (Gibson, 1990). The two general objectives of anthropometric assessments are to assess growth and body composition (Gibson). The most commonly used indices of linear growth are recumbent length (in those under 2 years of older) and standing height (in those 2 years of age or older). Head circumference in children under 3 years of age is related to brain size. Weight along with height is used to calculate body mass index (BMI), which is used as an indirect measure of obesity (Gibson, p. 178). Other anthropometric measurements used to assess body composition are skinfold (e.g., triceps skinfolds) and circumferences (waist and mid-arm). Note that interpretation

$$\text{Body mass index (BMI)} = \frac{\text{weight (kg)}}{\text{height (m)}^2}$$

of these data requires a comparison to reference data and/or prediction equations to calculate body composition from the data. The Centers for Disease Control and Prevention has released updated reference growth charts for infants and children (2000 CDC Growth Charts, see below) and a module for using the BMI for age growth charts.

Whether you use secondary or primary data, it is essential for the needs assessment that you use standardized protocols to collect these data (usually height/length or weight). If you use reference data to convert raw data into either percentiles or z-scores, these must be based on the CDC 2000 growth curves. The Health Resources and Services Administration (HRSA) has produced a training module, available on the Web, that describes how to accurately measure height and weight in children and adolescents.

4. Clinical assessment: Clinical assessment occurs via a physical examination and medical history in order to detect physical signs and symptoms of under- or overnutrition (Gibson, 1990, p. 577). This requires expertise and training on the part of the examiner in order for him or her to accurately associate these signs with a nutritional deficiency. These signs are generally nonspecific, so they should be used in conjunction with one or more of the other nutritional assessment methods (Gibson). Note that by the time clinical signs develop there will already be a manifestation of an advanced stage of nutrient deficiency, because clinical signs occur when malnutrition

> For a copy of the 2000 CDC growth charts, along with a comprehensive description, see:
> http://www.cdc.gov/growthcharts/
>
> For a module on using the BMI-for-age growth charts for infants and children, see:
> http://www.cdc.gov/nccdphp/dnpa/growthcharts/training/modules/module1/text/intro.htm
>
> For training on accurate measurement in children and adolescents, see the HRSA training module:
> http://depts.washington.edu/growth/module5/text/page7b.htm

is chronic in nature. An example of a clinical sign of vitamin C deficiency is swollen red gums (Gibson, p. 583); however, swollen red gums also could be due to various non-nutritional problems (e.g., periodontal disease). Combined with other information (such as a dietary assessment showing a low intake of vitamin C–containing foods), however, the accurate attribution of this clinical sign to vitamin C deficiency may be made.

The following types of data regarding other behaviors can affect nutritional status and health:

- *Health risk behaviors:* This includes tobacco or alcohol use and drug abuse.
- *Use of healthcare:* This includes disease screening, annual physical exams, and frequency of visits to a healthcare professional.
- *Physical activity:* This includes structured physical activities, as well as leisure time activities.
- *Sedentary behavior:* This includes the amount of time spent in sedentary activities such as TV watching, computer use, and video/computer game use.

Data on socioeconomic status and living and working conditions include factors that may directly or indirectly affect nutrition and health status, as well as need in the community. The following subcategories are listed along with some examples of what type of data would be obtained. These can be important determinants of health (Boyle, 2003).

- *Income:* Income distribution and percentage of population living below the poverty level
- *Educational level:* Distribution and percentage attaining specific levels of education
- *Household composition and size:* Who lives in the household (e.g., mother, father, grandmother, 3 children) and how many people live in the household
- *Occupation:* Can refer to the occupation of any or all the adults living in the household
- *Working conditions:* Hours of work, job benefits, and job stress
- *Living conditions:* Potential health risks associated with the housing (e.g., lead paint)
- *Primary social groups:* Family, friends, and work groups (Boyle, 2003)
- *Healthcare access:* Health insurance coverage, level of coverage, and other means by which individuals and families obtain healthcare

Data on attitudes, perceptions, and opinions can be a critical component of the needs assessment data collection plan because it is often the lack of insight into the target population's attitudes and perceptions about a nutrition or health problem, the contributing factors, and workable solutions that hinder the successful implementation of an effective plan of action. This type of data can be qualitative in nature.

Methods for Obtaining Data on the Target Populations (Primary Data Collection)

Surveys   Surveys can be used to obtain data about health risk behaviors, such as use of healthcare; physical activity and sedentary behaviors; socioeconomic factors; working and living conditions; and attitudes, perceptions, and opinions. Although many set out to develop their own surveys, this is not recommended unless there are survey development experts on the needs assessment team. Although it may seem simple enough, survey development is complicated and time consuming, and if it is not done correctly, the derived data may be unusable. Thus, if you are going to use a survey to collect primary data for the needs assessment, you can use the following series of steps that prioritize validated and extensively used surveys over survey development. Note that some resources include copies of existing health surveys (Aday, 1996).

1. Identify surveys in the research literature or those used in the National Nutrition Monitoring and Related Research Program (NNMRRP) that address the question of interest.
2. Give preference to those surveys that have strong evidence of validity (i.e., construct and predictive validity) and reliability.

3. If there is no strong evidence of survey validity, give preference to those existing surveys used in national nutrition surveillance or monitoring. Although formal validation may not have been done, the questions have been used on large population groups and the data have been analyzed and utilized; this implies that the data were usable for the purpose intended. In addition, this will enable comparison of your local or regional needs assessment data to national statistics.

4. If a set of survey questions comprise a scale (e.g., body image), it is important to use the entire set of questions that form that scale.

Detailed guidance for survey development is beyond the scope of this chapter; however, there are several excellent reference books that provide guidance in developing surveys (Fowler, 1993, 1995). Drafting questions for a survey seems deceptively simple; in fact, writing questions that are straightforward, are universally understood by all respondents, and result in the data that answer the question the researcher sets out to answer is complicated. The final wording (and formatting) of the question and response categories evolve from a process of obtaining input from experts, pre-testing, and reliability and validity testing. For many, resource constraints preclude such survey development. Unfortunately, what results from hurried attempts at drafting questions are data of questionable quality that may not prove to have been worthwhile to collect using such a survey. Exhibit 3-1 is a compilation of some important points to consider when drafting your own survey. In addition, if the instrument that you select has been used in samples that are sociodemographically or ethnically different from your target population, you need to test it with your target population prior to its use for the needs assessment.

EXHIBIT 3-1 Survey Checklist

This checklist is intended to be a guide for you in the development of your survey. However, following all of these recommendations cannot replace extensive pre-testing of your survey instrument to determine what is working and what isn't. In addition to wording and formatting, pre-testing can help you determine optimal question and response order. This list combines and summarizes Fowler's guidelines for conducting survey research and improving survey questions (Fowler, 1993, 1995) along with the author's observations regarding common errors made when reviewing surveys that students as well as non-survey experts attempt to draft. It is not intended to be an exhaustive list, nor can it be used in lieu of the guidance of survey development experts. It also does not address other aspects such as mode of administration, training of interviewers, and other facets of collecting high-quality survey data.

(Continues)

EXHIBIT 3-1 Survey Checklist (Continued)

Questions: Wording, Content, and Order

- Use full sentences.
- Define all words that people may interpret differently (Fowler, 1995).
- Be as specific as possible. For example, if asking about smoking, you need to specify the type, and what you are defining as a smoker.
- Language level should match respondent ability.
- Avoid hypothetical questions, avoid asking about causality, ask only one question at a time, and so on. See Fowler's books, listed in the References.
- Include all the domains laid out in your conceptual framework in your survey.
- Avoid words like *typical, usually,* and *on average.* Use a specific time frame whenever possible.
- If using a self-administered survey, it is very important that you place the most critical information needed for your research near the beginning. This is also important in an interviewer-administered survey, but less so.
- Place sensitive questions appropriately. For an interviewer-administered survey they need to be near the end. For a self-administered survey they can be closer to the beginning.
- Avoid derogatory or negative terms/words that may cause bias in response. If there is something threatening or negative in your survey, attempt to neutralize it by inserting an introductory sentence acknowledging that some people do this behavior or have this problem.

Response Categories

- List all possible responses, but only once.
- If you determine that a respondent can accurately provide a relatively accurate quantitative response, then ask for the actual number instead of selecting categories. This is desirable as long as it doesn't make completing the survey more difficult for the respondent. For example, if you want to know how many siblings a person has, simply leave a space or two (depending on how many siblings you think he or she has) and let them give you the actual number.
- Specify the response format (e.g., if you want years, include that in the response).
- If only one answer is required, make response categories mutually exclusive.
- Ensure that the number of response categories captures the full range of possible responses, including adequate variability (e.g., if most people are going to check the last category, then you need to break down that category further so that you can differentiate better among people).
- Make the order of responses consistent throughout the survey. For example, if numerical categories are listed, then they all need to be listed in the same order (lowest to highest is most common).
- Use specified frequencies whenever possible instead of the words *like, often, sometimes,* and *so on.*
- Make sure there is a space for the respondent to respond. For example, if you say "check off one answer," then you need a space (__) or check-off box.

Introductions and Transition Statements and Instructions

- Provide an introduction to the survey itself. Here you generally describe the purpose of the survey, what you expect the respondent to do, and what she or he should do if they don't understand something or have questions. Also, this is where you should assure the respondent of confidentiality or anonymity (whichever applies in your case).
- If the survey is broken up into sections (which it should be if the survey is longer than a few pages), then number and label the sections with section headings, and have a brief introduction to each section.
- Although you may have instructed the respondent at the beginning of a section or at the beginning of the survey, you still need to provide instructions to tell the respondent exactly what to do for every question. The instructions should be in a different font than the question (they can be italicized or bolded or capped). Be consistent throughout in terms of how you want the person to respond—circle or check off responses. In the instructions, also include how many they can choose (i.e., all that apply or one).
- If you have an "other" option, then ask respondents to specify or describe what that is.

Survey Format and Layout

- General rule: Avoid crowding and maximize white space.
- There should be space between questions and between questions and response categories.
- Provide plenty of space for the responses (whether it be a number written in or room for them to check something off).
- If you have contingency questions (i.e., questions that depend on a response to another question) and it is a self-administered questionnaire, it is best to use arrows to actually lead the person to the next question. The arrow normally stems from the response. If it is an interviewer-administered survey, it is OK to say "Go to question __," but these instructions should also be adjacent to the response category.
- However you decide to lay out your response categories, be consistent (columnar or in rows).
- If you have a series of questions with the same response categories and decide to lay them out in a tabular format, shade every other row so that people won't lose their place.
- Make sure that the question and the response categories are on the same page.

General

- Number all pages.
- Each page should have a place for an ID number.
- At the end of each page note that there are more pages to the survey. You can say "Next page" with an arrow or something else that will tell the respondent that there is more to complete. On the next to the last page of the survey, note "only one more page left." This is essential for any survey that is more than two pages long.

Source: Compiled by the author.

Focus Groups   A focus group usually consists of 7 to 10 people who are relatively homogeneous and whose input or opinion is sought through broad open-ended questions about a research topic (Morse & Field, 1995). Focus group participants are selected because they are considered knowledgeable about the topic. Focus groups are often used to obtain qualitative data on perceptions, attitudes, or opinions about a specific issue or product. This can be an extremely important method in the work of needs assessment because it can provide a method for eliciting opinions from the target population on their perceived needs, barriers to preventing disease, or even why certain programs are not working. For example, in the case of the nutrition problem of childhood obesity in Roxbury, a focus group of teenagers may provide insight as to why they choose what they do after school, why they don't use certain after school programs, and what kinds of activities they would participate in that would get them moving.

Key Informant Interviews   Key informant interviews consist of structured or unstructured interviews (phone or face to face) of individuals (i.e., key informants) who have been identified as having specific knowledge about the topic of interest. In this case it would be someone who has knowledge about the community, target populations, services, or other efforts (past or present) to address health- or nutrition-related problems, or stakeholders who may have important insights about the needs of the community or target population.

Phase 3: Data Collection and Analysis

By the time this phase is reached, all the methods for the needs assessment, including indicators, datasets that will be used, and the methods for primary data analysis, will have been determined. This is the phase in which data will be collected, either directly from participants or from existing reports, or additional analysis will be completed from secondary data sets.

Step 7: Collect Data on the Community and the Target Population
Irrespective of the methods used for the needs assessment data collection, it is imperative that someone be responsible for overseeing the following:

- Data collection progress and troubleshooting
- Data entry and cleaning (if primary data collection)
- Data management in terms of how databases will be designed and what software will be used
- Quality or limitations of the data

Step 8: Analyze and Interpret Data
In this stage, the pertinent data will be summarized for the community and target population. As Boyle (2003, p. 430) notes, the following steps must be undertaken in the analysis stage in order to

"diagnose" the community; that is, to describe the unmet needs in the community:

- Interpret the health status of the target population that lives in the community.
- Interpret the pattern of health care, health services, and nutrition- or health-related programs that are designed to reach the target population.
- Assess the relationship between the health/nutrition needs of the target population and the pattern of services available in the community.

The results of the needs assessment should then be summarized in a report. The summary should include the needs assessment methods used, a description of the nutritional problems, their severity and prevalence, their distribution across the community and target population (e.g., is it worse in urban areas or in specific age or ethnic groups?), causes specific to that target population and community, and the consequences in terms of morbidity and mortality (Boyle, 2003, p. 430). In addition, you should prepare an executive summary, no longer than one to two pages, that highlights the key points of the needs assessment.

Phase 4: Using the Needs Assessment Results

Step 9: Share the Findings of the Assessment

The findings of the needs assessment must be shared not only with others in the agency that undertook the lead for the needs assessment and participating agencies and organizations, but also with the stakeholders who either provided advice and key information or work with the target population. An example of those who should be informed is shown in Table 3-3; this list was developed and used by the Iowa Department of Public Health for a needs assessment of WIC nutrition education and for program planning. Note that many different organizations are included in the sharing of WIC nutrition education needs assessment data.

Step 10: Prioritize the Needs of the Community and Target Population

Many unmet needs may be identified as a result of the needs assessment; however, resource limitations often constrain the degree to which all unmet needs can be addressed. Thus, it is essential that needs be prioritized. Various methods of prioritization have been proposed (Gilmore & Campbell, 2005, pp. 37–40); two will be reviewed here.

In their seminal book, *Community Nutritional Assessment*, Jelliffe and Jelliffe (1990) laid out five principles that can be used to set priorities. First, priority should be given to what the community identifies as its priorities, preferences, or concerns. Second, common

TABLE 3-3   Possible Stakeholders to Share Information

Agency

- WIC staff
- Agency staff
- Agency board of directors

Community

- Area education agencies
- Child health, maternal health, and family planning programs
- Churches
- Civic and business organizations
- Community action agencies
- Community health planning groups
- County public health nursing agencies
- Empowerment areas
- Government officials
- Hospitals and other health organizations
- Local boards of health
- Local press (editors, editorial boards, health reporters)
- Public/private school districts

Source: Reprinted with permission from Iowa Department of Public Health.

problems should be given priority over rare ones. Third, serious problems should be prioritized over less critical ones. Fourth, easily preventable problems should have higher priority than those for which prevention is more difficult. Finally, those health problems that have exhibited increases over time should be given preference over those whose frequencies are decreasing or have stabilized.

Another simple method of prioritization is to use members of the target population and program providers who may have been included on the needs assessment team to rank the top five needs. The series of rankings assigned to each need is reverse-scored (i.e., if a need is ranked as 1, it is given a score of 5); scores are then summed, and those with the highest numbers are given priority (Gilmore & Campbell, 2005, pp. 37–38).

Step 11: Develop a Plan of Action to Use the Needs Assessment Findings to Improve the Nutritional Status of the Target Population

Once the needs assessment is completed and unmet needs are identified and prioritized, a plan of action to address the priority needs must be developed. This may involve modifying an existing program or programs to better meet the need or developing new programs, or advocating for funding to address the unmet need, utilizing the needs assessment results as ammunition. The team needs to include stakeholders in the process of developing this plan of action.

Needs Assessment in Practice:
Massachusetts WIC Needs Assessment

The Massachusetts WIC Needs Assessment (WIC NA) was developed in 1983 by the Massachusetts Department of Public Health (MDPH) Advisory Committee in order to guide the allocation of caseload and resources (i.e., the statewide distribution of funds). Some of the methodology was derived from a broader needs assessment process whose goal was to distribute funds statewide for primary prenatal and pediatric care services (Guyer et al., 1983). In 1993, MDPH revised the WIC needs assessment in order to: 1) to compensate for the reported 1990 census undercount and to update economic indicators (e.g., poverty); 2) to compensate for economic changes that have occurred since the release of the 1990 poverty data; and, 3) to better account for variation in ethnicity distribution by communities.

The methodology is composed of what is referred to as both a *qualitative score* for ranking cities and towns, in terms of variables correlated with the need for WIC services (considered indicators of risk) and a *quantitative estimate* of the number of people eligible for WIC services at the local level.

The methodology takes into consideration the eligibility requirements of the WIC program. In Massachusetts, infants and children under five 5 years of age, and pregnant and post-partum women whose household income is below 185% of the poverty line, are eligible to receive WIC services. This plan

> Read more about the Special Supplemental Nutrition Program for Women, Infants and Children in Chapters 4 and 5.

is the result of a well thought out and detailed methodology that is still in use. A person with strong quantitative, programming, and data skills is needed to conduct this needs assessment.

For the qualitative indicator of overall need for nutrition services, various health and socioeconomic indicators are used in a principal component analysis to produce composite z-scores, which reflect risk. Cities and towns are then ranked according to the magnitude of these scores. The following health and socioeconomic indicators comprise this score.

Health Indicators for the Five Most Recent Years

All the health indicators are taken from the birth file, which includes all birth data for the entire state. Because MDPH is the agency responsible for the birth data, WIC does not have to wait for the public release of these data, and therefore has access to the most current data (i.e., the open surveillance file). The following up-to-date data were available:

- Neonatal mortality rate
- Proportion of adolescent pregnancies
- Percent low birth weight

The birth file data were chosen over the census data because these data are timelier and have been shown to be a better reflection of the true population of infants, children, and mothers (Massachusetts Public Health Department, 1993).

Socioeconomic Indicators

The following socioeconomic indicators are used:

- *Unemployment rate for the current year:* This information is obtained from the Department of Education and Training.
- *Percentage of the population under 5 years old who are living under 100% of the poverty line:* This information is obtained from the most current census poverty file (from the Census Bureau).
- *Percentage of the population that is a minority (using race/ethnicity):* This is based on the race/ethnic distribution of births as indicated by the city and town birth data.

  The estimate of the number of WIC-eligible individuals is derived from the sum of eligible mothers (pregnant and postpartum) and eligible children (children 0–5 years of age). Birth certificate data is again used because it is considered to be a more accurate reflection of the population than the census data for reasons previously noted. The following are used to estimate the total number of eligible people:

  - Total eligible number of infants and children: This is calculated using the 5-year birth totals multiplied by the percent below 200% of poverty. The percent of those under 5 years of age living below 200% of poverty could not be derived directly from the census data because only the percent of those living under 100% of poverty is available. Information about children 0 to 5 years old living between 100% and 200% of poverty are not available, so the percentage of the total population that lived between 100% and 200% of poverty had to be used instead. Thus, the estimate of the number of 0 to 5-year-olds who were eligible for WIC was calculated by adding together the following two estimates:
    - Number of children living below 100% of poverty = 5-year birth totals (proportion of 0 to 5-year-olds < 100% of poverty)
    - Number of children living between 100% and 200% of poverty = 5-year birth totals (proportion of total population who lived between 100% and 200% of poverty)

- Total number of pregnant women: This was calculated using the total number of unborn eligible infants and women who knew that they were pregnant. It was assumed that a woman can begin to receive WIC services when she is 1-month pregnant, or alternatively for 8 months of her pregnancy (i.e., 66.7% of the year).
  - Estimate of number of eligible pregnant women = eligible infants $\times$ 0.667
- Total number of postpartum women: This was considered equal to the number of eligible infants.

In order to combine the socioeconomic and health risk factors with the size of the population who are in need of WIC services into a single indicator that would be used to guide caseload allocation decisions, the qualitative needs assessment z-score is combined with the quantitative measure of estimated eligible individuals; this combines to produce the "risk-adjusted" eligible population by city and town.

In summary, the WIC NA is the result of a well thought out, complex methodology developed by an advisory group for allocating caseload and resources for the WIC program statewide. It estimates the numbers of individuals eligible for WIC and adjusts for other health and socioeconomic risk factors, using a variety of internal (e.g., birth data) and external (e.g., census data) data sources and has allocated appropriate staff to carry it out. It was developed and continues to be carried out through a collaborative effort between administrative, management, and other personnel with strong data and analytic skills. It exemplifies the best of public health needs assessment efforts.

Conclusions

This chapter provided an overview of community needs assessment, an integral component of the pubic health process in general, and public health nutrition in particular. This overview is intended to act as a starting point for those planning to undertake a community needs assessment. The aspiring public health nutritionist is encouraged to use the more detailed references noted in this chapter at the early stages of the needs assessment planning process in order to obtain more detail on the many steps involved in this process.

Unmet need should be at the forefront of public health consciousness, and designing the strategy and obtaining the tools to identify this need in a specific community and target population lay the foundation for its identification. The scope of a community needs assessment can be broad or limited in nature; its success doesn't lie in its breadth, but rather in its ability to meet its objectives, identify unmet need within the scope defined, and design effective action plans that are inclusive of the public health program personnel, community, and stakeholders. After all, effective teamwork is both the challenge and reward of public health.

Issues for Discussion

1. Why would it be important to include program providers as part of your needs assessment team?
2. What is the rationale for examining the leading causes of death as a measure of the community's health? In relation to mortality, what else could you examine?
3. If the purpose of the Roxbury example provided in the text is to identify the causes of the high prevalence of obesity among children living in Roxbury, lay out one goal and at least two objectives for such a needs assessment.

References

Achterberg C.L. & Shepherd S.K. (2003) The philosophy and role of qualitative inquiry in research. IN: *Research Successful Approaches,* 2nd ed. Elaine Monsen, editor, pp. 120–128.

Aday, L. A. (1996). *Designing and conducting health surveys,* 2nd ed. San Francisco, CA: Jossey-Bass.

Boyle, M. (2003). *Community nutrition in action: An entrepreneurial approach,* 3rd ed. Belmont, CA: Wadsworth, pp. 411–465.

Campos, P. (2004). *The obesity myth: Why America's obsession with weight is hazardous to your health.* New York, NY: Gotham.

Gibson, R. S. (1990). *Principles of nutritional assessment.* Oxford: Oxford University Press.

Gilmore, G. D. & Campbell, M. D. (2005). *Needs assessment capacity assessment strategies for health education and health promotion,* 3rd ed. Sudbury, MA: Jones and Bartlett.

Fowler, F. J., Jr., (1993). *Survey research methods,* 2nd ed. Applied Social Research Methods Series, vol. 1. Newbury Park, CA: Sage.

Fowler, F. J., Jr. (1995). *Improving survey questions, design and evaluation.* Applied Social Research Methods Series, vol. 38. Newbury Park, CA: Sage.

Guyer, B., Schor, L., Messenger, K., Prenney, B., & Evans, F. (1984). Needs assessment under the Maternal and Child Health Services block grant: Massachusetts. *American Journal of Public Health,* 74, 1014–1019.

Jonnalagadda, S. S., Mitchell, D., Smickilas-Wright, H., Meaker, K., Van Heel, N., Karmally, W., Ershow, A., & Kris-Etherton, P. M. (2000). Accuracy of energy intake data estimated by a multi-pass, 24 hour recall technique. *Journal of the American Dietetics Association,* 100, pp. 303–308, 311.

Jelliffe D. B., Jelliffe E. F. P., Community (1989) nutritional assessment: with special reference to less technically developed countries. New York: Oxford Medical Publications, pp. 452–453.

Massachusetts Public Health Department. (July 15, 1993). Internal memo.

McKenzie, J. F., Pinger, R. R., & Kotecki, J. E. (2002). *An introduction to community health,* 4th ed. Sudbury, MA: Jones & Bartlett, pp. 3, 123.

Morse, J. M. & Field, P. A. (1995). *An overview of qualitative methods.* In Qualitative research methods for health professionals, 2nd ed. (pp. 31–32). Chapman and Hall, Thousand Oaks, CA.

Peterson, D. J. & Alexander, G. R. (2001) *Needs assessment in public health: A practical guide for students and professionals*. New York: Kluwer Academic/Plenum Publishers, pp. 15–37.

Rothman, K. J. (2002). *Epidemiology: An introduction.* Oxford: Oxford University Press.

Willett, W. (1998). *Nutritional epidemiology.* Oxford: Oxford University Press.

CHAPTER 4

REACHING OUT TO THOSE AT HIGHEST NUTRITIONAL RISK

Jan Kallio, MS, RD, LDN

Rachel Colchamiro, MPH, RD

Reader Objectives

After studying this chapter and reflecting on the contents, you should be able to:

1. List social and environmental factors that contribute to nutritional risk in communities, families, and individuals.
2. Describe the extent to which these factors affect various populations in the United States and how these factors impact nutritional status in families and individuals.
3. Describe information needed by nutritionists to assess and effectively respond to factors in communities, families, and individuals that increase nutritional risk.
4. Describe the community services available to provide food, nutrition education, education, financial assistance, and health insurance to at-risk populations in the United States.

Defining High-Risk Factors

A high-risk factor is a biological, economic, environmental, or social insult that increases risk. Factors that place individuals, families, and communities at risk must be investigated and described in the community needs assessment. Social, economic, and environmental factors that contribute to nutritional risk include, but are not limited to:

- Poverty
- Unemployment and underemployment
- Inadequate education and literacy
- Immigration and cultural background
- Substandard housing and homelessness
- Hunger and food insecurity

- Geographic or social isolation
- Limited or inadequate healthcare

These complex societal issues require the concerted attention of all those who are concerned about the nutritional health and well-being of community members. The immediate needs of families and individuals are a shared responsibility of the interdisciplinary teams and networks that provide health and human services. Many clients and their families are known to multiple programs and agencies. Assessment and eligibility information should be shared among service providers, and services should be coordinated to ensure comprehensive, unduplicated efforts.

Poverty

Poverty income guidelines were first set in 1964, using the index developed by Mollie Orshansky of the Social Security Administration. Findings of the 1955 U.S. Department of Agriculture (USDA) *National Food Consumption Study* indicated that at that time the average American family spent approximately one-third of its net income for food. In the early 1960s, the USDA developed cost-specific, nutritionally balanced food plans and designated the *Economy Food Plan* as the least expensive food purchasing plan to meet a family's nutritional needs. Therefore, the poverty line was established at three times the cost of the Economy Food Plan for a family of four.

In 1975, the USDA replaced the Economy Food Plan with the similarly cost-defined Thrifty Food Plan, which became the national standard for a low-cost nutritious diet. The Thrifty Food Plan (also used to calculate food stamp allowances) is still multiplied by three and adjusted for the size of the family unit and the current consumer price index, in order to calculate the official poverty income guidelines each year. These guidelines are used by federal agencies as criteria for eligibility for various federal assistance programs and as a basis for compiling data on poverty.[1] Table 4-1 shows the 2004 poverty income guidelines used by federal government agencies.

Unfortunately, the current poverty guidelines may no longer accurately measure poverty. Since the creation of the original poverty thresholds in the 1960s, the relative prices of the basic necessities of life for a family have changed considerably. Housing, transportation, child care, and healthcare now comprise a larger proportion of a family's budget, while the relative cost of food has declined. It is estimated that today's families spend less than one-fifth of their incomes on food; therefore, a more appropriate poverty guideline would be more than five times the cost of the Thrifty Food Plan.[2]

> Poverty guidelines are set annually by the U.S. government. Check www.nutrition.gov for current guidelines.

TABLE 4-1   2004 Poverty Guidelines for the 48 Contiguous States and the District of Columbia*

Size of Family Unit	Poverty Guideline
1	$9,310
2	$12,490
3	$15,670
4	$18,850
5	$22,030
6	$25,210
7	$28,390
8[†]	$31,570

*There are separate poverty guideline figures for Alaska and Hawaii that reflect the Office of Economic Opportunity administrative practice, which began in the 1966–1970 period.

[†]For family units with more than eight members, $3,180 is added for each additional member.

Source: Reprinted with permission from: Nord, M., Andrews, M., Carlson, S. *Household Food Security in the United States., 2002.* Washington, DC: Economic Research Service, U.S. Department of Agriculture; October 2003.

In 2002, an estimated 12.1% of the U.S. population lived in poverty (34.6 million individuals), defined that year for a family of four, including two children under the age of 18, as having an annual income of less than $18,244. For African Americans, 24.1% lived in poverty, and 21.8% of Hispanic Americans lived in poverty. The poverty rate for Americans over the age of 65 was 10.4% (3.6 million individuals), which included nearly one in four older African Americans and more than one in five older Hispanic Americans.[3]

A disproportionate number of children live in poverty. Children represent 25% of the total population, but 35% of the poor population. In 2002, 16.7% of children (12.1 million children) lived in poverty, 40% of whom (5 million) lived in extreme poverty (less than half the federal poverty level). Child poverty rates are highest for African American children (32.3%) and Hispanic American children (28.6%). The most at-risk children are those under the age of 6 and living in single female-headed households. Although 17.3% of families with children younger than 6 lived in poverty, 44.9% of female-headed families with children younger than 6 lived in poverty.[3]

Thirty-eight percent of children (27.8 million) lived in households at 200% of the federal poverty line, which is the amount identified as needed to meet basic family necessities. These families are considered "low-income." For African American children, 59.5% live in low-income families, as do 62% of Hispanic American and 33.9% of Caucasian children.[3]

Poverty is a clear predictor of health status. The infant mortality rate is more than 50% higher among poor families than among families living above the poverty line.[4] Low-income children with chronic health conditions, such as asthma or diabetes, have worse overall health, spend more days in bed, and face more hospitalizations than do higher-income children with the same conditions.[5] A recent survey showed that whereas 2.6% of children of higher income were reported to have a fair or poor health status, 8.3% of low-income children were reported to have the same.[6]

The health disparities associated with poverty grow more apparent with age and persist through adulthood. Nearly 25% of poor individuals report limitation of activity caused by chronic health conditions, whereas less than 10% of the non-poor report the same.[7,8]

Assessing an individual's or family's income with the poverty guidelines can give initial critical information regarding the ability to meet immediate basic needs. Even if a family does not meet the definition of poverty, their housing and utility costs may use up the major portion of their income. Therefore, they are left with little or no money for food and other basic household essentials. To determine an individual's or family's ability to buy food, nutritionists must compare total net income with fixed costs for housing, utilities (heat, gas, electricity, water, telephone), medical care, transportation to and from work, and child care. This calculation will identify their needs for financial and food assistance, healthcare, and social service programs.

Unemployment and Underemployment

The economic downturn of the last few years has resulted in higher numbers of unemployed individuals, as well as underemployed persons, who are working in jobs below their job training or work experience, part-time, or in low-paying jobs. When the United States entered a recession in March 2001, labor force participation rates fell at a steeper rate than during the labor market downturn of the 1990s.[9] The unemployment rate in early 2004 was at 5.6%, accounting for 8.2 million Americans. Unemployment rates for African Americans and Hispanic Americans were higher at 9.8% and 7.4%, respectively.[10] In 2002, 14% (3.7 million) children lived in households with no employed parent.[3]

Although most policy and service planners focus on issues related to unemployment, underemployment is a hidden issue and rarely recognized. Individuals employed in low-paying jobs, particularly at minimum wage, do not earn a "living wage," which is a wage that can provide for basic household needs. An individual earning the minimum wage of $5.15 per hour, working 40 hours a week, 52 weeks a year, will earn only $10,712 annually, about 57% of the 2004 poverty level for a family of four. Almost two-thirds of the 7.2 million families living in poverty in 2002 had at least one family member that worked during the year. Nearly 2 million families had one family member that worked full-time year-round.

With the rapid advances of technology in the United States, there are fewer blue-collar jobs (industrial or factory jobs with unskilled or skilled manual labor) than ever before. Recent years have experienced instability of high-tech jobs, resulting in workers who once thought they had secure jobs being laid off. Service jobs (maids, housecleaning, janitorial, maintenance, food service) continue to be low paying and very often inadequate to meet family household needs.

Assessment of the food intake of the unemployed and underemployed may show consistent inadequacy or an episode when the individual or family had little or no food and nutrient intake was poor. Surveys indicate that an initial consequence of unemployment is to cut back on the spending for food, as well as to postpone medical or dental treatment, as reported by half of survey respondents.[11]

It must be realized that the needs of the newly unemployed differ from the needs of those who have been unemployed for extended periods of time. For the newly unemployed, it is important to know if their income prior to unemployment was moderate, low, or below the poverty level; if their previous work had been continuous or sporadic; and if there is another wage earner in the household. First-time unemployed individuals and families working in low-paying jobs are less likely to know about available food and financial assistance programs and services and may not be familiar with their eligibility and the application processes.

Inadequate Education and Literacy

According to 2002 U.S. Census data, 17% of adults in the United States have an 11th-grade education or less. This varies widely by ethnicity; 12% of Caucasians, 22% of African Americans, and 43% of Hispanic Americans have not graduated from high school. Poor people, regardless of ethnicity, are more likely to drop out of school.[12]

Twenty percent of adult Americans read at less than a fifth-grade level. It is estimated that nearly 50% of Americans do not have the literacy proficiency considered the minimum standard to be employable in today's labor market.[13] These adults generally have sufficient skills to cope with their usual daily activities, but are not eligible for jobs that require reading and writing proficiency.

Most jobs require basic skills in reading, writing, and mathematics. Additionally, many require computer skills. As the educational requirements of jobs increase, people with less education do not qualify. In 2000, 31.4% of job applicants lacked the basic skills necessary to perform the jobs they sought.[14] Clearly, poor literacy is tightly linked to poverty. According to the most recent National Adult Literacy Survey (NALS) performed in 1992, 43% of people with the lowest literacy skills lived below the poverty line. For families in the cycle of inadequate education, unemployment, and poverty, improving the education of one or more family members can be the key to breaking the cycle.

Refugees and immigrants may have limited literacy in their own language, making learning to communicate in a new language even more difficult. They may learn to understand some English to meet basic needs for daily living before they learn to speak, read, and write this new language.

Low literacy affects the nutritional health of individuals and families by limiting access to the understanding of basic nutrition and health information, including food labels, medical or food preparation instructions (e.g., infant formula preparation), and dietary plans. Nutritionists should provide educational interventions and materials that consider the clients' ability to speak, read, write, and comprehend English. Many tools are available, including the SMOG Readability Formula and the Fry Graph Reading Level Index, which can be utilized to evaluate written materials to determine the appropriateness of their reading level.

> The SMOG (Simplified Measure of Gobbledygoop Grading) Readability Formula is a method for determining the reading level of written materials. It is based on how many three-syllable words you use in your writing. See the website www.med.utah.edu/pated/authors/readability.html for more information.

Programs presented to non-English-speaking populations must build on their cultural food preferences and customs. Written materials should use pictorial graphics to communicate nutrition messages. Pictures and text should be field tested with the target audience to assure that the materials are acceptable and easy to understand.

Data regarding educational attainment and language spoken is collected by many public health assistance programs. This information can be utilized to plan and respond more effectively to the needs of the populations served.

In most cases, nutritionists will not be assessing an individual's literacy level. However, it should not be assumed that all clients are able to read either in English or in their native language. There are simple, informal methods to easily identify individuals with low literacy skills, without causing embarrassment to the client. Methods include asking open-ended questions about the materials received or handing written materials to clients upside down to observe if they turn it right side up to read. Nutritionists should also listen for comments commonly given to mask the inability to read, such as "I left my reading glasses at home" or "I'll read this later."

Cultural Barriers

During the past three decades, political, social, cultural, religious, and economic oppression in Central America, South America, the Caribbean Islands, Eastern Europe, Africa, and Southeast Asia has brought an influx of refugees into the United States. Approximately 1,064,000 immigrants entered the United States legally in 2002.[15] It is estimated that half of those migrating to the United States between 1997 and 2003 entered the country illegally.[16] An estimated 11.5% of the U.S. population (approximately 32.5 million people) are now foreign-born.[17] New immigrants need guidance and support as they resettle in an adopted land.

Citizenship status affects family members' employability, income, and eligibility for tax-supported services. Immigrants and refugees, who are not naturalized citizens or legal residents, may have difficulty finding jobs with adequate pay or even finding work at all. They may hesitate to follow through on referrals to government assistance programs, because they fear deportation or future problems in obtaining citizenship.

Within each cultural group, patterns and practices of families and individuals differ according to their socioeconomic status, religion, education, and age when they immigrated to the United States. Immigrants face an unfamiliar choice of foods in large and impersonal supermarkets, more "high-tech" kitchen equipment, and high prices for their traditional foods. They frequently give up their more nutrient-dense traditional foods in favor of U.S. snack foods and fast foods. Many choose to feed their babies formula instead of following traditions of breast-feeding.

Religion, tradition, beliefs, taboos, medical uses and philosophies, and the traditional roles of family members influence food habits. Nutritionists should be knowledgeable about common cultural food patterns and should complete an individual assessment to determine the core foods that are a regular part of a client's daily diet, considering the nutrient contributions and typical preparation of these foods. This knowledge should serve as the beginning point for nutrition education, suggesting more emphasis on familiar or similar foods before introducing new foods.

When working with undocumented clients, their fears and concerns must be respected. Professionals must know about program eligibility, make referrals on a case-by-case basis, and maintain the family's confidentiality.

Substandard Housing and Homelessness

The dramatic rise in rents and housing costs, the decreased availability of newly built government-subsidized housing, and condominium conversion of much of the rental property during the last few decades have made housing unavailable or unaffordable to families who must live on a fixed income, limited budget, or public assistance allowance. The cost of renting a two-bedroom apartment rose 37% between 1999 and 2003, a pace not matched by increases in income. Ninety percent of all renter households in the United States must earn more than twice the minimum wage to afford housing in their community, while still having money to meet other basic household needs.[18]

As housing costs rise beyond the means of low-income families and as affordable rental units are more difficult to obtain, many move in with friends and extended family. Families who are guests in someone else's household have little or no control over the kinds or quality of foods purchased or how foods are prepared.

Although they may have a roof over their heads, many poor families live in substandard housing, lacking an adequate refrigerator, range, oven, or running water to prepare foods. Facilities to wash dishes, pots, and pans may be inadequate. There may be improper food storage or trash and garbage disposal, with rampant rodent and insect infestation. Older housing may have lead-containing paint that is peeling, cracked, or chipped. Lead poisoning can result in impaired growth, learning disabilities, and even mental retardation for infants and children if the peeling paint is ingested.

For some families the housing crisis has resulted in homelessness, which is a growing problem among women, children, and young families. Approximately 600,000 individuals in the United States are homeless on any given night. Eight percent are temporarily homeless, 10% experience episodic homelessness, and 10% are chronically homeless.[19] Recent estimates suggest that 1 in 50 children are homeless at some point during the course of a year.[20] Homeless children are 2.5 times more likely to have a health problem than housed children and more than 6 times as likely to have multiple health problems versus a single health problem.[21]

Many homeless families are housed temporarily in hotels, motels, or shelters, while some find themselves on the street. Often mothers who live in shelters or on the streets feel guilty when they are not able to prepare adequate and nutritious meals for their children. Some shelters for the homeless serve meals or provide refrigerators and possibly hot plates. However, many of the hotels and motels do not provide refrigerators, hot plates, group kitchens, or any place to store food, and they may even prohibit the use of small appliances to cook food in the rooms. These hotel and shelter residents may need to choose between spending their few dollars on high-priced restaurants or ready-to-eat foods and not eating.

Nutritionists should assess the housing issues in their community and identify potential problems experienced by families or individuals that relate to food access. Nutritionists should be aware of the food storage and food preparation resources available to individuals and families living in hotels, motels, or shelters. Nutritionists must identify potentially malnourished children and adults in the homeless population. They must advocate and assist in improving the availability of nutritious food for homeless individuals and families and those living in substandard housing. Nutrition education and food assistance should be responsive to the particular needs and resources of the individual or family.

Hunger and Food Insecurity

Food insecurity and hunger are persistent problems in our society. Food security is defined as the assured access at all times to enough food for an active, healthy life, as well as access to enough food that is safe, nutritious, and acquired in socially acceptable ways.[1,22] Hunger is an outcome of limited or uncertain access to food.

Nutritionists can help families to achieve food security by assuring that all eligible families utilize the federally funded Food Stamp, Child Nutrition, Special Supplemental Nutrition Program for Women, Infants and Children (WIC), and elderly meal programs in combination with local food banks, soup kitchens, and food pantries. The federal food assistance programs are described in Table 4-2. The Food Stamp and Child Nutrition programs are federally funded entitlement programs that are available in every community to serve all people who meet the income eligibility criteria. The Summer Food Service Program, School Breakfast, WIC, and Nutrition Services Incentive Program (formerly the Elderly Nutrition Program) are available when a service provider in a community establishes, implements, and directs the programs. Household income is used to determine eligibility for all of the federally funded food assistance programs except the Nutrition Services Incentive Program.

Participation in one or more food assistance programs extends the family's food purchasing power to better meet the nutritional needs of family members. In assessing family needs, each household member's participation in or eligibility for food assistance programs must be determined. When their household incomes are very low, families may not be able to meet their food needs even when they participate in one or more federal food assistance programs. In these cases, families may turn to emergency food assistance programs such as food pantries and soup kitchens. The community needs assessment should include the number of requests to food pantries and visits to soup kitchens, particularly by families with children. Although these emergency food assistance programs provide food to satisfy immediate needs, they are not designed to provide food for extended periods of time.

Over the long term, increased utilization of the federal food programs could decrease the need for families to regularly use emergency food programs and reduce the growing burden on private food assistance programs. In addition, increased utilization could improve the stability of meeting basic food and nutritional needs of communities, families, and individuals. Many families still do not know about these programs or have inaccurate or insufficient information regarding their eligibility requirements. Complicated application forms and procedures, excessive eligibility documentation, and/or inconsistent administrative operations deter many families from applying for food assistance. Nutritionists must know eligibility requirements and be aware of administrative barriers so that they

TABLE 4-2   Food Assistance Programs

Program	Services/Benefits	Who Qualifies	Funding and Administration
Special Supplemental Nutrition Program for Women, Infants and Children (WIC)	Provides supplemental food, nutrition education, referrals, and access to health-care to low-income pregnant, postpartum, and breastfeeding women; infants; and children to 5 years of age at nutritional risk. Monthly foods include milk, cheese, eggs, fruit juice, cereal, peanut butter or legumes, tuna, carrots, infant formula, and infant cereal.	Pregnant women, postpartum women (6 months), breast-feeding women (up to 1 year), infants, and children (up to 5 years); must be certified to be at nutritional risk; household income determined to be at or below 185% of poverty level.	Funded by USDA (some states offer supplemental funding) Administered by state health agencies Services provided by state or local agencies
Food Stamps	Provides low-income households with coupons and electronic benefit transfer (EBT) cards to purchase eligible foods for a nutritionally adequate diet at authorized food stores.	U.S. citizen; limited benefits to legal immigrants and to able-bodied adults without dependents; eligibility and allotments are based on household size, income, assets, and other factors.	Funded by USDA Administered by state welfare, social service, or human service agency Services provided by local welfare, social service, or human service offices
National School Lunch Program	Provides nutritious low-cost lunch at full or reduced prices, or free to children enrolled in school.	All children attending school may participate: free meals to children from families with incomes at or below 130% of poverty level; reduced-price meals to children	Funded by USDA Administered by state department of education and local school districts Services provided by all public schools; voluntary in private schools

Program	Services/Benefits	Who Qualifies	**Funding and Administration**
		from families with incomes between 131% and 185% of poverty level; full price meals to children from families with incomes over 185% of poverty.	
School Breakfast Program	Provides nutritious low-cost breakfast at full or reduced prices, or free to children in participating schools or institutions.	All children attending schools where the breakfast program operates may participate: free breakfast to children from families with incomes at or below 130% of poverty level; reduced-priced breakfast available to children from families with incomes between 131% and 185% of poverty level; full price to children with family incomes over 185% of poverty.	Funded by USDA Administered by state department of education and local school districts Services provided by all public schools; voluntary in private schools
Summer Food Service for Children	Provides free nutritious meals and/or snacks to children as a substitute for the National School Lunch and School Breakfast programs during summer vacation.	Children under 18 years who come to an approved site; persons over 18 years who are enrolled in school program for persons with disabilities.	Funded by USDA Administered generally by state department of education, but state health or social service department or an FNS regional office may be designated Services provided by public and nonprofit private schools, public— local, municipal, county, tribal, or

(Continues)

TABLE 4-2   Food Assistance Programs (Continued)

Program	Services/Benefits	Who Qualifies	Funding and Administration
			state—government; nonprofit private organizations; public or private nonprofit camps
Special Milk Program	Provides milk to children in schools, summer camps, and child care institutions that have no federally supported meal program.	Children attending schools or half-day pre-kindergarten programs and institutions with special milk program; milk is free to child from family eligible for free meals.	Funded by USDA Administered by state department of education Services provided by public or nonprofit private schools of high school grade and under, eligible camps, and public or nonprofit private child care institutions not participating in other federally supported meal programs
WIC Farmers Market Nutrition Program	Provides coupons to WIC participants to purchase fresh, unprepared, locally grown fruits and vegetables at approved farmers and farmers' markets.	Women, infants (over 4 months), and children who have been certified to receive WIC program benefits or who are on a waiting list for WIC certification. States may serve some or all of these categories.	Funded by USDA Administered by state agencies such as state agriculture departments, health departments, or Indian tribal organizations Services provided by state or local agencies
Senior Farmers Market Nutrition Program	Provides coupons to low-income seniors to purchase fresh, unprepared, locally grown fruits and vegetables at approved farmers' markets, roadside stands, and community-supported agriculture programs.	Individuals who are at least 60 years old and who have household incomes at or below 185% of poverty.	Funded by USDA Administered by state agencies such as state agriculture departments, health departments, U.S. territories or Indian tribal organizations Services provided by state or local agencies

Program	Services/Benefits	Who Qualifies	Funding and Administration
Child and Adult Care Food Program	Provides cash reimbursements and commodity foods for meals served in child and adult day care centers, and family and group day care homes, homeless shelters, and approved after-school care programs. *Adults who are functionally impaired and are enrolled in adult day care centers or who are 60 years of age or older.*	Children 12 years and under and adults who attend eligible day care programs; children of migrant workers 15 years and younger; physically/mentally handicapped individuals provided care in a center where the majority are age 18 or younger; children residing in homeless shelters; snacks and suppers to youths participating in eligible after-school care program; income eligible for free or reduced-priced meals.	Funded by USDA Administered by state department of education or alternate state agency (state health or social service department) Services provided by public and nonprofit private licensed child and adult day care centers and homes, outside after-school-hours care centers, Head Start, other licensed/approved day care centers, homeless shelters
The Emergency Food Assistance Program (TEFAP)	Provides commodity foods to low-income persons, including elderly people, food banks, food pantries, and soup kitchens.	Each state sets criteria for household eligibility; households may participate in another federal, state, or local food health or welfare program for which eligibility is based on income; homeless, including low-income seniors, can receive meal in congregate setting. There are no eligibility criteria for using a soup kitchen.	Funded by USDA Administered by state agencies Services provided by food banks, food pantries, soup kitchens, and other public and private nonprofit organizations that distribute food to the needy through the distribution of food for home use or the meal preparation

(Continues)

TABLE 4-2   Food Assistance Programs (Continued)

Program	Services/Benefits	Who Qualifies	Funding and Administration
Food Distribution Program on Indian Reservations	Provides commodity foods and nutrition education to low-income families who live on Indian reservations and to Native American families who live in approved areas near reservations. Serves as an alternate to the Food Stamp Program.	Low-income households, including American Indian and non-Indian, living on a reservation or households who live in approved areas near reservations or in Oklahoma with at least one person who is a member of a federally recognized tribe. Must meet income and resource eligibility standards. Food package selected from over 70 food products. Cannot participate in the Food Stamp Program in the same month.	Funded by USDA Administered by Indian tribal councils or state agency Services provided by Indian tribal councils or state agency
Nutrition Assistance Program: Puerto Rico, American Samoa, and the Commonwealth of the Northern Marianas Islands	Block grant program to provide cash and coupons to participants to buy nutritious foods in place of food stamps and commodities.		Funded by USDA
Nutrition Services Incentive Program (Nutrition Program for the Elderly)	Provides meals for senior citizens at senior citizen centers or delivered by meals-on-wheels programs through the receipt of cash and/or commodities from USDA; nutrition screening and assessment; nutrition	People age 60 or older with greatest economic or social need, with special attention given to low-income minorities and rural older people; spouses of eligible people; disabled persons under age 60 who reside in housing facilities occupied primarily	Funded by DHHS, Administration on Aging (AoA); private donations Administered by state Units on Aging funded through Title III of the Older American Act (OAA); Indian tribal organizations funded through Title VI of OAA

Program	Services/Benefits	Who Qualifies	**Funding and Administration**
	education; links to other in-home and community-based services, transportation, and home repair programs.	by the elderly where congregate meals are served, disabled persons who reside at home and accompany older persons to meals; nutrition service volunteers.	Services provided by senior centers, faith-based settings, schools, homes of homebound older adults
Head Start, Early Head Start	Provides comprehensive medical, educational, nutrition, social, and dental services, referrals to social services, and other services to low-income children from birth to age 5, pregnant women and their families through assessment, early intervention, and prevention; provides nutritious meals and snacks	Children birth to 5 years, pregnant women and their families from low-income families receiving public assistance (TANF—Temporary Assistance for Needy Families or SSI—Supplemental Security Income) or total annual income not more than 100% of poverty level; children in foster care; at least 10% of total enrollment available for handicapped children	Funded by DHHS—Administration for Children & Families

Administered by DHHS regional offices

Services provided by local public agencies, private non-profit and for-profit organizations, Indian Tribes, and school systems |

Source: Compiled by the authors.

can assist potentially eligible clients in applying for benefits and navigating the food assistance system. Nutritionists should also advocate, both locally and nationally, for measures that make it easier for individuals and families to use these services.

Some families feel that there is a stigma attached to the use of government assistance programs. The negative perceptions and attitudes associated with these programs may foster shame and embarrassment, and prevent families in need from applying for food assistance.

> Chapter 17 discusses food insecurity in the United States in more depth.

Nutritionists should be sensitive to these feelings so that they can support clients and break down negative stereotypes attributed to people using public assistance programs.

Geographic and Social Isolation

Families who live in remote areas, distanced from settled communities or blocked from social support systems, are considered isolated. A family who does not have transportation, or the money to pay for it, may not be able to obtain adequate food at affordable prices or be able to access and/or utilize food assistance or healthcare programs. The geographically isolated include migrant and seasonal farm workers, mountain families, the rural poor, Native Americans on reservations, and homeless, displaced families without access to public transportation, even in urban areas.

Social isolation occurs when individuals or families are unable to establish supportive relationships with others. Social isolation is more subtle and difficult to recognize, as well as to overcome, than geographic isolation. Socially isolated individuals have difficulty establishing or maintaining supportive interpersonal relationships, within either their community or their family. This may occur when people move to new communities or when their cultural or ethnic background and/or their primary language differs from that of the community. Individuals and families experiencing homelessness, unemployment, marriage dissolution, mental illness, emotional breakdowns, or depression often distance themselves from their friends and family. Drug use, alcoholism, violence, and abuse dramatically change family dynamics and communication.

Social isolation may prevent an individual from seeking healthcare, food, financial or housing assistance, or other services they need. Social isolation has been identified as a contributor to inadequate food consumption for the elderly. Fewer calories are consumed at meals when eating alone than when eating with others.[25] In addition, an individual who lacks social support may find it difficult to continue ongoing healthcare or follow through on care plan recommendations. It may be difficult for individuals and families to access services when one family member or community decision maker, often referred to as the "gatekeeper," controls the use of assistance programs.

Single and/or teen parents are often overwhelmed by parenting responsibilities, limited employment opportunities, low incomes, and lack of transportation, child care, and family support. Parents caring for a handicapped or chronically ill child, or adults caring for a disabled or homebound spouse or parent, are also stressed emotionally, physically, and often financially. As such, these individuals may be socially isolated and less likely to seek services. In addition, they may be unable to cope with buying and preparing nutritious meals for themselves and their children.

Nutritionists should not expect to be able to single-handedly address or resolve the social issues of isolation that may affect their clients. Nutritionists must identify the immediate needs of the individual or family and be sensitive and supportive in their response. They must gain the approval and support of family gatekeepers so that the use of services and ability to follow recommendations can be improved. The community needs assessment must identify other health and social services available in their community so that nutritionists can make appropriate and timely referrals. Additionally, nutritionists must recognize an individual's or family's ability to navigate service delivery systems to receive needed services and provide assistance as considered necessary. Most importantly, nutritionists must work with other members of the health and human service agency teams to address the multiple and often long-standing problems faced by many families and advocate, both locally and nationally, for solutions.

Limited or Inadequate Healthcare

Regular medical care helps individuals avoid health crises, and ultimately protects their nutritional status. Although it is well established that early and ongoing prenatal care is associated with positive pregnancy outcome, many pregnant women do not seek adequate prenatal care. In addition, some children and adults go without needed treatment, as well as ongoing preventive care. This is most often a result of no insurance, not enough money to pay physicians or hospitals, or

> **Medicaid**—A U.S. government program that pays for medical assistance for certain individuals and families with low incomes. Learn more at: http://www.cms.gov/medicaid/
>
> **Medicare**—A U.S. government medical benefit program for certain individuals when they reach age 65. Learn more at: http://www.medicare.gov

providers not willing or unable to provide free care or accept Medicaid or Medicare payments that are less than their usual fees.

The most recent *Pregnancy Risk Assessment Monitoring System* (PRAMS) data, evaluating maternal behavior trends from 1993 to 1999, found that up to 30% of women reported receiving late or no entry into prenatal care. The prevalence of inadequate prenatal care was much higher among low-income Medicaid recipients than among higher-income prenatal women.[29]

A survey conducted in 2002 found that while 9.5% of all children in the United States did not have health insurance, 16.1% of low-income children were uninsured. Approximately 570,000 children were both uninsured and in either fair or poor health. More than two-thirds of those children were Hispanic American, yet less than one-fifth of all children in the United States in 2002 were of Hispanic descent. The same survey reported that while 17% of all American adults did not have health insurance, more than twice that many (36.8%) low-income adults were uninsured.[6]

Nutritionists should know the availability of medical care services in the community and the barriers low-income families face in accessing these services. They need to work with health providers and community members to support regular medical care, including nutrition services, and ensure that it is accessible and responsive to the needs of at-risk families. It is essential to advocate for nutrition intervention, referral, and follow-up to be integrated into medical services.

Improving Services to At-Risk Families

Community needs assessment is key in providing targeted nutrition services that will support and respond to the needs of at-risk individuals and families, as was discussed in Chapter 3. Table 4-3 presents key factors to include in the assessment. This information documents needs and suggests priorities for developing community services and determining family and individual care plans. Identification of nutrition-related risk factors can be used to plan professional in-service training, mobilize resources, develop and implement health and nutrition programs, and ensure policies that respond to the nutritional needs of at-risk individuals and families and community nutrition efforts.

Action to improve services to at-risk families should be well integrated into the healthcare and nutrition service delivery system. Ideas to consider include:

- Recruit health or nutrition aids, lay health advisors, peer counselors, or volunteers that represent the populations and cultural groups in the community and train them to provide services to at-risk families.
- Coordinate one-stop service delivery by arranging with food stamp, public assistance, and social services agencies to enroll eligible clients in health and social services.
- Address specific barriers that prevent eligible individuals/ families from participating in assistance programs and design outreach strategies and methods to overcome these barriers.
- Streamline application processes of all programs targeting at-risk populations and utilize electronic data systems to eliminate duplication in data collection, including eligibility determination criteria.
- Schedule clinic hours so families do not need to take time off from work and lose pay to obtain services; offer locations that are accessible to clients with limited/no transportation.
- Enlist volunteer groups or clubs to adopt a service project to provide layettes, clothing, diapers, nutritious foods, or other essentials for at-risk families.
- Apply for grants to research and provide innovative services that help at-risk families work toward self-sufficiency.

Concerned health professionals, in conjunction with political leaders and concerned citizens, can collaborate with and mobilize community partners to provide integrated, comprehensive, and coordinated services to at-risk clients and families. They can partici-

TABLE 4-3 Assessing At-Risk Factors in the Community, Families, and Individuals

At-Risk Factor	Community Assessment	Family/Household Assessment	Individual Assessment
Income	Median family income; per capita income; % of population below 100% of poverty level; % of population below 200% of poverty level; TANF benefit levels; availability of community-based assistance programs for food, child care, fuel, etc.; housing and basic household costs (utilities, healthcare, etc.)	Family/household income; family size; # of wage earners; participation in federal/state nutrition programs; income supplements such as TANF, unemployment benefits, fuel assistance; educational expenses; childcare costs; housing and household costs	Individual's monthly income; lives alone or with others; household expenses, child support; participates in federal/state food assistance; income supplement such as TANF, unemployment benefits, fuel assistance; educational expenses; child care; single parent; homebound; disabled; elderly
Employment opportunities	State or local unemployment rate; median wage; predominance of minimum-wage, service-sector jobs; layoff or strike in community; jobs available; seasonal jobs (e.g., agriculture, construction, tourism)	Household member laid off or on strike	Individual unable to find work at a wage that meets basic needs; recently laid off or on strike; barriers that prevent individual from finding adequate employment (lack of child care, job opportunities)
Educational level/literacy	% of adults over age 18 with less than eighth grade education; % of adults over age 18 who are functionally illiterate; % of teen high school dropouts (by ethnicity)	Education level of head of household and mother; education obtained in country of origin	Education level; education obtained in country of origin; ability to read, speak, or write English; if in school, grade level

(Continues)

TABLE 4-3   Assessing At-Risk Factors in the Community, Families, and Individuals (Continued)

At-Risk Factor	Community Assessment	Family/Household Assessment	Individual Assessment
Cultural or language barriers	Ethnic/cultural distribution in community; languages spoken, read, and/or written; availability of services representing the ethic community; signs and information in appropriate languages; availability of traditional foods; prevailing community attitudes	Ability of head of household to speak, read, or write English; ability to read/write native language; use of traditional foods; use of traditional healers, folk medicine; power structure in family; degree of acculturation	Ability to speak, read, or write English; ability to read/write native language; use of traditional foods; use of traditional healers, folk medicine
Housing	Rental unit vacancy rate; % of substandard housing (lacking indoor plumbing, electricity, kitchen facilities with working refrigerator, stove, oven); % of rental units built before 1950 (risk of lead paint); availability of subsidized housing and length of waiting list; average and range of rents for 1-, 2-, and 3-bedroom units; median purchase price for a house; condo conversion in community; estimated number of homeless individuals and families	Family lives in substandard housing; problems with rodents, roaches, chipping or peeling paint or plaster; family living in a hotel, motel, shelter, car, or on the street; recently moved in with friends or relatives due to the inability to obtain adequate housing; % of the family/household income spent on rent and utilities	Individual lives in substandard housing; living in hotel, motel, shelter, car, or on the street; lives in room without cooking facilities or without working refrigerator or stove; % of income spent on rent/utilities; inability to pay rent; evicted for nonpayment of rent

At-Risk Factor	Community Assessment	Family/Household Assessment	Individual Assessment
Food availability, food costs, accessibility of grocery stores	Supermarkets/grocery stores in the neighborhood offer a variety of nutritious, good-quality foods at competitive prices; number of "mom and pop" neighborhood markets; availability of culturally preferred foods at a reasonable price; accessible by public transportation or within walking distance; food delivery or shopping services available; availability of farmers' markets; average cost of full market basket of food	Family access to transportation to available grocery stores; cultural foods available at reasonable price	Individual's food needs met by himself/herself or other household members; elderly or disabled individual able to arrange for assistance with shopping for food
Geographic or social isolation	Public transportation available; dispersed rural community; geographic barriers; condition of roads; cultural, ethnic, rural hostilities; immigrant, refugee, or migrant community; highly transient community	Supportive relationships; transportation or money for transportation; cultural or language barrier; victim of cultural, ethnic, or racial prejudice; immigrant refugee, migrant family; mobile family; homeless family; family stress, unstable family, alcoholism, drug abuse, domestic abuse, violence	Single parent; teen parent; homebound living alone; physical or mental disability; lack of supportive relationships; lack of transportation or money for transportation; victim of cultural, ethnic, or racial prejudice; immigrant, refugee, migrant; mobile; alcoholic, drug abuser

(Continues)

TABLE 4-3   Assessing At-Risk Factors in the Community, Families, and Individuals (Continued)

At-Risk Factor	Community Assessment	Family/Household Assessment	Individual Assessment
Access to health services	Public health, health centers, and medical practices available (e.g., obstetrics, pediatrics, family practice); sliding fee scale; number of persons receiving and eligible for Medicare and Medicaid; services near public transportation; % of no-show in a clinic or health program; preventive programs offered at no cost or reasonable cost; Medicaid payments accepted	Satisfaction of family with health services available; family members go without needed care	Satisfaction of individual with health services available; perceived barriers to utilization of services; repeatedly misses scheduled appointments
Health insurance coverage	Health insurance coverage provided by employers includes maternity care; Medicaid available to low-income married couples; coverage for prenatal care for low-income teens living with parents; % of jobs with no health insurance benefits; sliding fee scale or free healthcare available; Medicaid payment accepted by physicians	Household members covered by health insurance, HMO, or Medicaid coverage; uninsured families have access to sliding fee scale or free healthcare; Medicaid unavailable because teen lives in parents' household; family's insurance covers preventive care, well-child care	Individual has health insurance, HMO, Medicaid coverage; types of services covered; amount of deductible; denial of healthcare due to lack of medical coverage or Medicaid

At-Risk Factor	Community Assessment	Family/Household Assessment	Individual Assessment
Health status	Infant mortality rate; hospital discharge data; leading causes of death and disability; nutritional status and nutrition-related health measurements—% of population by age groups with anemia, high serum cholesterol levels, overweight/obesity, high lead levels, cardiovascular disease, cancer, diabetes, stroke, hypertension; smoking rates; breastfeeding rates	Nutrient content of diet; knowledge, attitude, and behavior related to healthy behaviors (e.g., breast-feeding, physical activity, fat intake, fruit/vegetable intake); family history of nutrition-related health conditions (cardiovascular disease, cancer, diabetes, stroke, hypertension); smoking in household	Nutrient content of diet—intake of key nutrients (calcium, iron, vitamin C, folate, etc.) and intake of fat, sugar, and salt; intake of fruits, vegetables, and whole grains; knowledge, attitude, and behavior related to healthy behaviors (e.g., breast-feeding, physical activity, fat intake, fruit/vegetable intake); health parameters—weight, hemoglobin/hematocrit, cholesterol level, blood glucose, blood pressure, dental health; tobacco/alcohol/drug use

TANF = Temporary Assistance for Needy Families
Source: Compiled by the authors.

pate in policy development and plans to increase awareness of problems; identify short- and long-term goals; allocate resources; and define, implement, and assess strategies to address the many complex economic and social issues that today's families face. Community coalitions can recommend and advocate for state and federal legislation that will address universal food access, housing, job training, healthcare, and employment.

Community needs assessment data can be presented in public meetings, legislative hearings, or other forums. An ongoing surveillance system can be used to monitor hunger, malnutrition, diet-related health problems, and utilization of food assistance programs. Grant funding can be sought to implement outreach and nutrition education projects and to improve access to and use of various food assistance programs.

The nutritionist has a vital and critical role in effectively reaching out to those at highest risk and must take on leadership to promote, implement, and evaluate effective services to meet the needs of at-risk populations.

Issues for Discussion

1. Discuss the impact of federal cuts to those at highest risk.
2. Determine how you might set up a public health nutrition assistance program considering:
   a. income level
   b. minority status
   c. single parent families
3. Discuss why and whether other taxpayers should pay for those who cannot provide for themselves.
4. Discuss the pros and cons of one or more federal nutrition programs.
5. Forecast what you believe to be the future for those at the highest nutritional risk in the United States.

References

1. Nord M, Andrews M, Carlson S. *Household Food Security in the United States, 2002*. Washington, D.C.: Economic Research Service, U.S. Department of Agriculture; October 2003.
2. Economic Policy Institute. *EPI Issue Guide: Poverty and Family Budgets Issue Guide*. Washington, D.C.:Economic Policy Institute; 2004.
3. Proctor BD, Dalaker J. *Poverty in the U.S.: 2002*. Washington, D.C.: U.S. Census Bureau, U.S. Department of Commerce; September 2003.
4. Annie E. Casey Foundation. *Kids Count Data Book: State Profiles of Child Well-being*. Baltimore, MD: Annie E. Casey Foundation; 2003.
5. Case A, Lubotsky D, Paxson C. Economic status and health in childhood. *Poverty Research News*. September/October 2001;55:3–5.
6. Finegold K, Wherry L. *Race, Ethnicity and Health*. Snapshots of America's Families III, No. 20. Urban Institute, March 2004.
7. Freid VM, Prager K, MacKay AP, Xia H. *Chartbook on Trends in the Health of Americans. Health, U.S., 2003*. Washington, D.C.: National Center for Health Statistics; 2003.
8. Pamuk E, Makuc D, Heck K, Ruben C, Lochner K. *Socioeconomic Status and Health Chartbook. Health, U.S., 1998*. Washington, D.C.: National Center for Health Statistics; 1998.
9. *Issues in Labor Statistics: Labor Force Participation During Recent Labor Market Downturns*. Washington, D.C.: Bureau of Labor Statistics, U.S. Department of Labor; September 2003.
10. *Labor Force Statistics from the Current Population Survey*. Washington, D.C.: Department of Labor Statistics, U.S. Department of Labor; March 2004.
11. Shapiro I. *Unmet Need Hits Record Level for the Unemployed*. Washington, D.C.: Center on Budget and Policy Priorities; February 2004.
12. U.S. Census Bureau. *Educational Attainment in the U.S.: Detailed Tables*. Washington, D.C.: U.S. Census Bureau; March 2002.

13. Sum A, Kirsch I, Taggart R. *The Twin Challenges of Mediocrity and In-equality: Literacy in the U.S. from an International Perspective.* Princeton, NJ: Policy Information Service, Educational Testing Service; February 2002.

14. American Management Association. *Research Survey: Corporate Concerns 2001.* New York, NY: American Management Association; 2001.

15. U.S. Department of Homeland Security. *2002 Yearbook of Immigration Statistics, Immigration Information.* Washington, D.C.: U.S. Department of Homeland Security; 2002.

16. Camarota S. *Immigration in a Time of Recession: An Examination of Trends Since 2000.* Washington, D.C: Center for Immigration Studies; November 2003.

17. *Foreign-Born Population in the U.S.: March 2002.* Washington, D.C.: U.S. Department of Commerce, Economics and Statistics Administration, U.S. Census Bureau; February 2003.

18. Pitcoff W, Pelletiere D, Crowley S, Shaffer K, Treskon M, Vance C, Dolbeare C. *Out of Reach 2003: America's Housing Wage Climbs.* Washington, D.C.: National Low-Income Housing Coalition; 2003.

19. Secretary's Work Group on Ending Chronic Homelessness. *Ending Chronic Homelessness: Strategies for Action.* Washington, D.C.: U.S. Department of Health and Human Services; March 2003.

20. Burt MR, Laudan YA. *America's Homeless II: Populations and Services.* Urban Institute; January 2000.

21. Berti LC, et al. Comparison of health status of children using a school-based health center for comprehensive care. *Journal of Pediatric Healthcare.* 2001;15:244-250.

22. *Paradox of Hunger and Obesity in America.* Waltham, MA: Center on Hunger and Poverty and the Food Research and Action Center; July 2003.

23. Andrews MS, Prell MA. *Second Food Security Measurement and Research Conference, Volume I: Proceedings.* Washington, D.C.: Economic Research Service, U.S. Department of Agriculture; February 2001.

24. Ribar DC, Hamrick KS. *Dynamics of Poverty and Food Sufficiency.* Washington, D.C.: Economic Research Service, U.S. Department of Agriculture; September 2003.

25. *Hunger Issue Brief, Hunger and Food Insecurity among the Elderly.* Waltham, MA: Food Security Institute, Center on Hunger and Poverty, Brandeis University; February 2003.

26. Hofferth SL. *Persistence and Change in the Food Security of Families with Children, 1997-99.* Washington, D.C.: Economic Research Service, U.S. Department of Agriculture; March 2004.

27. *Consequences of Hunger and Food Insecurity for Children, Evidence from Recent Scientific Studies.* Waltham, MA: Center on Hunger and Poverty, Brandeis University; June 2002[TZA1].

28. Brown JL. *Statement on the Link between Nutrition and Cognitive Development in Children.* Medford, MA: Center on Hunger, Poverty and Nutrition Policy, Tufts University; 1998.

29. Centers for Disease Control and Prevention. *MMWR Surveillance Summaries. 2002* Apr;51(SS02):1-26.

Portions of this chapter were reprinted or compiled with permission from the publisher from the first edition of (Kaufman M.) *Nutrition in Public Health,* 1990.

CHAPTER 5

ADDRESSING OVERWEIGHT IN CHILDREN: A PUBLIC HEALTH PERSPECTIVE

Edna Harris-Davis, MS, MPH, RD, LD

Inger Stallmann-Jorgensen, MS, RD, LD

Reader's Objectives

After studying this chapter and reflecting on the contents, you should be able to:

1. List the growing problems related to overweight in children.
2. Describe the paradigm shift that occurred over the years to cause overweight in children.
3. Describe economic impacts of overweight in children on society.
4. Identify essential skills or tools that a public health nutritionist may need to help prevent or control overweight in children.
5. Describe the importance of recommendations and policy and environmental interventions.
6. Describe opportunities for public health nutritionists to address overweight in children in existing programs.
7. List three evidence-based practices to prevent or control overweight in children.
8. List some steps that families can take to help prevent overweight in children.
9. List prevention strategies that could be incorporated into existing federal programs.

Obesity and obesity-related diseases are some of the largest public health challenges of the 21st century. The rapidly increasing rate of overweight in children is especially alarming. Historically, public health has been in disarray because the medical treatment model has dominated the healthcare system and failed to provide a proactive stance to support a prevention-based model.[1] The saying that "an ounce of prevention is worth a pound of cure" needs to be taken more seriously by the food and advertising industry, community planners, school systems, businesses, public health leaders, policy-makers, the health industry, and other stakeholders. Ultimately, the cry for partnerships and resources to prevent overweight and obesity will be heard because of the unparalleled rise in U.S. medical and healthcare costs for treatment of obesity and related conditions. Thus, now is the time for public health nutritionists to accept the urgent challenge of addressing overweight and obesity through prevention-based approaches. To maximize effectiveness, overweight and obesity prevention efforts must target children and their families and focus on policy and environmental interventions.

The topic of overweight in children is a large and complex issue, and it is not possible to address every aspect of the problem and its prevention and treatment in this chapter. Rather, the aim of this chapter is to provide an overview of overweight in children and to guide the public health nutritionist student and entry-level practitioner in addressing this challenging public health issue. Thus, the authors will review various aspects of the problem of overweight in children and obesity, such as the health consequences, economic impact, environmental factors, and nutrition and physical activity issues. We hope that the reader will acknowledge the changes in the environment that contribute to the development of the current epidemic of overweight in children. Due to the important role of environmental interventions, we also hope that the reader will see that one-on-one interventions alone will not arrest this epidemic. Rather, population-based interventions will be needed to achieve the greatest effect. The authors will also discuss skills important to public health nutritionists, such as developing partnerships, writing grants, using media resources, and keeping current with the scientific literature. In addition, overweight in children will be addressed using a *prevention-based approach* by applying the *public health model* (assessment, policy development, and assurance) and evidence-based efforts (increase physical activity and healthy eating, and decrease television viewing). Finally, one community's experience in addressing overweight in children will be discussed.

The magnitude of the current problem of overweight in children is unprecedented; public health nutrition professionals have limited past experience with community-based interventions to address this issue comprehensively. In fact, effective strategies are few compared to the enormity of the challenge. New approaches must be conceived, tested, and applied without delay. Careful analysis of surveillance data, sound research, community resources, and priorities must be considered when problem-solving and producing effective interventions. Advocacy and education will be crucial to sound the alarm for community stakeholders and gain their support. The authors hope that public health nutritionists become empowered with the information presented and will apply this information to develop, implement, and evaluate innovative prevention-based approaches for overweight in children.

Assessment of Overweight in Children

In the pediatric population, the Body Mass Index (BMI) is used as a screening tool and is not a diagnosis for overweight in children. The Centers for Disease Control and Prevention (CDC) have revised and published growth charts for children 2–20 years of age: BMI-for-Age, Weight-for-Age, and Stature-for-Age. The BMI-for-Age nutrition status indicators for At-Risk for Overweight Children are ≥ 85th percentile to < 95th percentile and ≥ 95th percentile, respectively.[2] There is documentation supporting that many overweight children will become obese adults.[3,4] However, the BMI-for-Age assessment should be applied carefully so as to not label children as obese in error. It is important to determine whether a child indeed has extra fat mass and not extra muscle mass, particularly across genders and ethnicity.[5,6] In addition, labeling as "obese" carries a stigma for many people. Therefore, as defined by the CDC, the terms "overweight" and "at-risk for overweight" should be used when addressing the pediatric population and to establish some consistency when making comparisons between various groups of children, particularly in research literature.

Currently, the terms "at-risk for overweight" and "overweight" are preferred to the terms "at-risk for obesity" and "obese." However, the authors recognize the widespread use of the terms "obese" and "obesity" throughout the overweight in children literature and that sometimes the two sets of terms are synonymous and at other times they have different meanings. Both sets of terms will be used throughout the chapter and when citing other literature to reflect the meaning intended by the original author.

Overweight in Children in a Public Health Perspective

Overweight Rates in the United States

There has been a rapid increase in our nation's rates of obesity in adults over the past two decades. The United States is not alone in facing this serious public health problem. Obesity has been declared one of the top 10 risk conditions in the world and one of the top 5 in the developed world by the World Health Organization (WHO). Recent data from the 1999–2000 National Health and Nutrition Examination Survey (NHANES) found almost 65% of the U.S. adult population to be overweight, as defined by a BMI of greater than 25 kg/m^2.[7] This is an increase from an already high obesity prevalence of 56% shown by NHANES III data collected during the period 1988–1994.

The trend of overweight in children has increased to an even greater degree. Between NHANES I (1971–1974) and NHANES II (1976–1980) the prevalence of overweight in children was unchanged overall; however, between NHANES II and NHANES III (1988–1994) the prevalence rose within all age and gender groups. A comparison between NHANES III and the NHANES 1999–2000 data shows these trends continuing their upward trajectory for all groups, except boys aged 6–23 months, who showed a 0.1% (nonsignificant) decrease in prevalence. Thus, the latest data show overweight rates for 6–23-month-old children to be 11.6%, and for 2–5-year-old, 6–11-year-old, and 12–19-year-old children to be 10.4%, 15.3%, and 15.5%, respectively. These data represent increases in prevalence rates of 30%, 44%, 35%, and 48% for these respective age groups, occurring in less than two decades (see Tables 5-1 and 5-2). The increases in overweight status have not occurred to the same extent among all age groups; neither are the various ethnic groups affected equally. Most affected by the rising trend in rates of obesity are Mexican American males ages 6–11 and 12–19, followed by non-Hispanic African American females ages 12–19 and 6–11. For these groups, about one in five youths is classified as overweight. When both those overweight and those at-risk for overweight are included in the prevalence data, non-Hispanic African American females, ages 12–19, lead the epidemic of obesity with a rate of nearly 45.5%; nearly half of these adolescents weigh too much.[8] (See Figure 5-1.)

TABLE 5-1   Trends in Overweight in Children, Birth through 19 Years, by Gender and Age Group

	NHES 2 (1963–1965)	NHES 3 (1966–1970)	NHANES I (1971–1974)	NHANES II (1976–1980)	NHANES III (1988–1994)	NHANES 1999–2000	P Values for NHANES III vs. NHANES 1999–2000
6–23 mo.[+]							
Total				7.2 (1.0)	8.9 (0.7)	11.6 (1.9)	.09
Male				8.2 (1.4)	9.9 (0.8)	9.8 (2.2)	.48
Females				6.1 (1.3)	7.9 (1.0)	14.3 (3.5)	.04
2–5 yrs.[#]							
Total		5.0 (0.6)	5.0 (0.6)	7.2 (0.7)	10.4 (1.7)	.04
Boys		5.0 (0.9)	4.7 (0.6)	6.1 (0.8)	9.9 (2.2)	.06
Girls		4.9 (0.8)	5.3 (1.0)	8.2 (1.1)	11.0 (2.5)	.16
6–11 yrs.[#]							
Total	4.2 (0.4)		4.0 (0.5)	6.5 (0.6)	11.3 (1.0)	15.3 (1.7)	.02
Boys	4.0 (0.4)		4.3 (0.8)	6.6 (0.8)	11.6 (1.3)	16.0 (2.3)	.05
Girls	4.5 (0.6)		3.6 (0.6)	6.4 (1.0)	11.0 (1.4)	14.5 (2.5)	.11
12–19 yrs.[#]							
Total		4.6 (0.3)	6.1 (0.6)	5.0 (0.5)	10.5 (0.9)	15.5 (1.2)	< .001
Adolescent boys		4.5 (0.4)	6.1 (0.8)	4.8 (0.5)	11.3 (1.3)	15.5 (1.6)	.02
Adolescent girls		4.7 (0.3)	6.2 (0.8)	5.3 (0.8)	9.7 (1.1)	15.5 (1.6)	.002

Values are expressed as percentage (SE).
[+]A weight-for-length at the 95th percentile or higher is considered overweight.
[#]A body mass index for age at the 95th percentile or higher is considered overweight.
Source: Reprinted with permission from C. Ogden. Prevalence and trends in overweight among U.S. children and adolescents, 1999-2000. *JAMA*, October 9, 2002, vol. 288, no. 14, pp. 1728–1732.

TABLE 5-2   Prevalence of Overweight or At Risk for Overweight in Children by Sex, Race/Ethnicity, and Age Group: NHANES 1999–2000

Sex	Age, yrs.	All[§]	Overweight or at Risk[†] Non-Hispanic White	Non-Hispanic Black	Mexican American	All[§]	Overweight[‡] Non-Hispanic White	Non-Hispanic Black	Mexican American
Both sexes	2–5	20.6(1.8]	20.5(2.7)	19.3(3.5)	22.7 (3.0)	10.4(1.7)	10.1 (2.4]	8.4 (2.3)	11.1 (2.5)
	6–11	30.3 (2.4]	26.2 (3.6)	35.9 (3.0)	39.3 (3.0)	15.3(1.7)	11.8 (2.4)	19.5(2.0)	23.7 (2.0)[#]
	12–19	30.4(1.9)	26.5 (2.4)	40.4 (2.2)	43.8 (2.6)	15.5(1.2)	13.7(1.7)	23.6(2.1)[#]	23.4 (2.1)[#]
Male	2–5	20.9 [2.4]	21 .4 (3.7)	12.6(3.1)	26.0 (4.9)	9.9 (2.2)	8.8(3.2)[ǁ]	5.9(2.4)[ǁ]	13.0(3.9)
	6–11	32.7 (3.7)	29.4 (5.7)	34.5 (3.6)	43.0 (4.2)	16.0(2.3)	12.0(3.0)	17.1 (2.8)	27.3 (3.1)[#]
	12–19	30.5(2.1)	27.4 (3.0)	35.7 (2.8)	44.2 (3.0)	15.5(1.6)	12.8(2.4)	20.7 (2.6)	27.5 (3.0)[#]
Female	2–5	20.4 (3.0)	19.7(4.1)	26.6(6.4)	19.5(4.0)	11.0(2.5)	1 1.5 (3.3)	11.2(3.8)ǁ	9.2 (2.9)ǁ
	6–11	27.8 (3.2)	22.8 (4.7)	37.6 (3.6)	35.1 (4.4)	14.5(2.5)	11.6(3.5)ǁ	22.2 (3.3)	19.6(3.1)
	12–19	30.2 (2.8)	25.4 (3.3)	45 5 (3.0)	43.5 (4.2)[¶]	15.5(1.6)	12.4(2.1)	26.6 (2.7)[#]	19.4 (2.8)

Values are expressed as percentage (SE). NHANES indicates National Health and Nutrition Examination Survey.
[†]Body mass index for age is at the 95th percentile or higher.
[‡]Body mass index is at the 95th percentile or higher.
[§]Includes racial/ethnic groups not shown separately (e.g. other category).
[ǁ]Does not meet standard of statistical reliability and precision (relative SE > 30%).
[¶]Includes one influential observation. When this observation is deleted, the prevalence (SE) is 39.6 (2.3).
[#]Significantly different from non-Hispanic whites at P < .05 (with Bonferroni adjustment).
Source: Reprinted with permission from C. Ogden. Prevalence and trends in overweight among U.S. children and adolescents, 1999-2000. *JAMA*, October 9, 2002, vol. 288, no. 14, pp. 1728–1732.

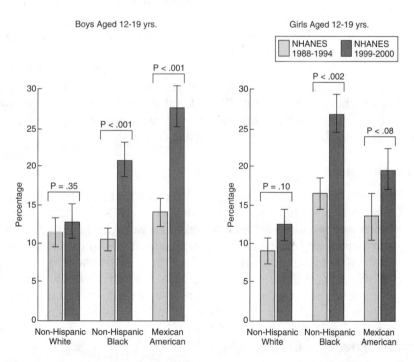

FIGURE 5-1   Overweight Prevalence by Race/Ethnicity for Adolescent Boys and Girls
Source: Reprinted with permission from C. Ogden. Prevalence and trends in overweight among U.S. children and adolescents, 1999–2000. *JAMA*, October 9, 2002, vol. 288, no. 14, p. 1731.

Health Effects of Overweight

The recent trends of overweight in children are especially disturbing because of the predicted health consequences of being overweight later in life. Freedman et al. studied the longitudinal relationship between children's BMI and their adult levels of lipids, insulin, and blood pressure. The mean time interval between first and follow-up measurements was 17 years. Over this time period, 77% of overweight children remained overweight as adults.[9] The persistence of being overweight, once it occurs, is of great concern because being overweight is more strongly linked to chronic disease than living in poverty, smoking, or drinking. The impact of obesity on overall health has been likened to aging by 20 years[10]: ". . . childhood obesity precedes insulin resistance/hyperinsulinemia and strongly predicts the risk of developing a constellation of metabolic, hemodynamic, thrombotic, and inflammatory disorders of syndrome X".[11]

Although there is well-justified concern for overweight in children tracking into adulthood and increasing the risk of adult health problems, one must not ignore the acute physical and psychological health issues that affect the overweight child. Many body functions are affected by being overweight, including the nervous, pulmonary, cardiovascular, skeletal, gastrointestinal, endocrine, and reproductive systems. In addition, overweight children suffer from mental health problems such as depression, anxiety, lowered self-esteem, and sometimes eating disorders.[12–14]

Pediatricians are diagnosing the most obese children and adolescents with hypertension, dyslipidemia, and non-insulin-dependent diabetes mellitus (NIDDM). Even if the overweight status does not track into adulthood, there may be long-lasting medical and psychosocial effects for overweight children.[15]

Health Disparities

Ethnic, cultural, gender, genetic, socioeconomic, and regional differences exist that influence which children are at greater risk for being overweight. Hispanic American boys, African Americans, and those residing in the South are especially likely to experience higher rates of being overweight.[16,17] The ethnic differences in the degree to which certain population groups are affected by overweight prevalence may exacerbate long-term health outcomes and economic disparities that already exist in the United States.[17]

Economic Effects of Overweight

If the trend of overweight in children continues on its present course, the United States will be overwhelmed by the healthcare expenditures required to treat acute and long-term complications of this condition. Hospital costs related to overweight in children have increased from an annual cost of $35 million in 1979–1981 to the latest data (1997–1999) from the CDC of $127 million dollars.[18] A cost estimate from 2003 data suggests that each U.S. taxpayer pays $175 a year for obesity-related illnesses (heart disease, cancer, diabetes, gallbladder disease) via Medicare and Medicaid programs.[19] Hospital discharges for youths, ages 6–17, have doubled from 1.43% to 2.36% for obesity-related conditions such as diabetes, while obesity and gall bladder disease tripled from 0.36% to 1.07% and from 0.18% to 0.59%, respectively, within two decades (1979–1999). When diagnoses such as asthma and certain mental disorders are listed as the primary discharge diagnosis, it is not unusual to see overweight or obesity listed as a secondary diagnosis.[18] The choice of primary discharge diagnosis may be influenced by which diagnosis will result in higher hospital reimbursements for healthcare services. Such tactics could contribute to an underestimate of the weight-related causes for hospitalization, as healthcare institutions may seek to maximize reimbursements for care.

The 2000 Actual Causes of Death report from the CDC found the leading cause of death to be tobacco use, at 435,000 annual deaths (18.1% of all deaths).[20] However, death resulting from poor diet and physical inactivity was the second-leading cause of death at 365,000, or 15.2% of all deaths per year.[20,102] Assuming that the obesity-related disease trends will continue to increase with the rise in the number of overweight children, poor diet and lack of exercise may soon be the number one cause of death in the United States. The economic cost of obesity will be increasingly challenging when considering the healthcare needs of the aging population, the already strained healthcare systems, and budget crises. Compounding these problems is society's new task of providing care for young people affected by overweight and related health problems.

The burden of being overweight stresses individuals, families, and society. For the individual, quality of life issues such as family income, rates of marriage, and educational attainment were all lower, while poverty rates were higher for women who had been obese in late adolescence and young adulthood.[13] Financially, child hospitalizations for conditions related to obesity cause parents or caregivers to be absent from work, stressing family budgets and causing loss of productivity for the parents' employer(s).

The full economic consequences of our overweight children cannot yet be known with certainty. For example, type 2 diabetes historically has been considered an adult onset condition, with negative effects on a person's health generally limited to the adult years. In adults, type 2 diabetes may show a certain pattern of development of health complications, such as peripheral neuropathy and impaired vision. The onset of such diabetic complications appears to depend to some extent on the length and severity of exposure to the diabetes condition. Thus, weight-related type 2 diabetes, which begins in youth, has the potential to cause excess morbidity, mortality, and diminished quality of life and productivity for many.

It is reasonable to expect that the longer the duration of complications of being overweight, the greater the healthcare costs incurred with their treatment.[21]

On a societal level, healthcare costs related to childhood obesity could have serious implications. The new generation of young adults that is expected to "carry" the nation's productivity and pay into social security, Medicare, Medicaid, and support federal and state social programs with their tax dollars may find themselves disabled or with limited earnings potential due to overweight-related impairments in health. National and state budgets will be doubly strained as healthcare payouts to program recipients soar while the funds supplying the coffers are diminishing by a less productive workforce. In the private sector, health insurance premiums can be expected to increase to keep pace with the increased costs of healthcare associated with treatment for overweight and its complications. Also important are the "opportunity costs" of society not being able to fund other important social, educational, and public programs due to the drain on budgets from the healthcare costs of treating overweight individuals.

Environmental Influences on Children who Are Overweight

Societal Factors Influencing Children who Are Overweight

Some overweight people have experienced discrimination because of the negative attitudes and judgmental behaviors of others who may see them as lazy and lacking willpower. Such attitudes have contributed to a social stigma and caused psychological pain for those suffering from the condition. Viewing overweight in children within a construct of "personal responsibility" has allowed past treatment interventions to focus on the child and, perhaps, the family unit. Experience has shown that this treatment model used by itself often has failed as many overweight children have grown up to be overweight adults.

Today, it is widely recognized that the micro-environment (home and family setting) and the macro-environment (the setting in which the family is imbedded) promote either healthy weight or overweight. The mission of public health is to fulfill society's interest in assuring conditions in which people can be healthy.[1] Thus, altering both the micro- and macro-environments to prevent or treat overweight in children is vital to the mission of public health.

The dynamics among individuals and their near, intermediate, and distal environments influence their food choices and physical activity levels, both of which play important roles in the development of obesity. A framework for understanding these interactions between individuals and their environment were discussed in detail in a report by a group of experts.[22] The figure in the report illustrates the determinants of food choice and physical activity behaviors within this framework (see Figure 5-2a). The reader should keep this framework in mind when reading the remainder of this chapter. Figure 5-2b provides an explanation for understanding the framework.

Overweight and Energy Balance

The environmental factors underlying the recent increase in obesity rates in the United States are multiple; however, diet and physical activity play a crucial role. Basic to this concept is the fact that to maintain a stable weight, energy intake and output must be balanced. Thus, when physical activity level is low, weight status can be maintained with a diet appropriately lower in calories. However, if an adjustment is not made by either increasing physical activity or decreasing energy intake, energy intake will exceed expenditure and will result in weight gain. The alarming rise in overweight among U.S. children begs the question: What changes have occurred in our lifestyles that could have contributed to this rapid rise in the prevalence of overweight in children?

> The 2005 Dietary Guidelines Advisory Committee recommends that children engage in at least 60 minutes of physical activity on most (preferably all) days of the week. Physical activity may include short bouts (i.e., 10 minutes each) of moderately intense activity. In this way, exercise can be accumulated through three to six bouts over the course of the day. The accumulated total of physical activity is what is important for health.

Dietary Trends Affecting Overweight Status in Children

Historical Perspective

Today's lifestyles are very different from the lifestyles of our hunter-gatherer ancestors. Genetically, we humans evolved during the Paleolithic period 2.6 million to 10,000 years ago, and were biologically adapted to survive under the prevailing conditions of that time. Today's Western-style diet is in sharp contrast to the diet of the hunter-gatherers, yet our human genome has changed little since that

> **n-6 fatty acid**—A polyunsaturated fatty acid in which the first double bond is six carbons from the methyl end of the carbon chain. Found in soybean and corn oils, and margarines and dressings made with vegetable oils.
>
> **n-3 fatty acid**—A polyunsaturated fatty acid in which the first double bond is three carbons from the methyl end of the carbon chain. Found in certain fish tissues, and in vegetable sources such as flax seeds, walnuts, and canola oil.

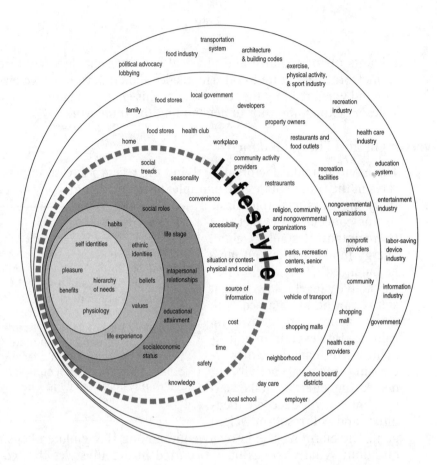

Psychobiologic Core: Genetically programmed metabolism and behavior—instinctive behavior, innate values related to survival, which are essentially immutable. Early conditioned behaviors (e.g., positive and negative reinforcement of pleasure, pain, etc.) and experiential learning, physiologic state; these are behavioral and metabolic phenotypes expressed within a given environment. The psychobiologic core also includes current health status.

Cultural: Personal life experienced, "inherited" values and beliefs (e.g., ethnic and cultural identity), self-identity within immediate social/cultural surroundings.

Societal: Roles and relationships, "acquired" values and beliefs, how society views the individual and vice versa, i.e., self-identity within broader social/cultural environment, broader societal values (e.g., social trends). This layer interacts with the cultural layer: how society views you affects how you view yourself.

Enablers of Choice: Most proximal factors affecting choices that are commonly identified as enhancers or barriers to change. These factors tend to be the ones most focused on in order to facilitate change.

Lifestyle: Visible physical activity and eating behavior choices made by the individual, may be a mix of who they are and who they would like to be.

Behavior Settings: Physical and social settings in which physical activity and eating behaviors take place and choices are made—the situational context within which behavior takes place.

Proximal Leverage Points: Controllers of the structure and features of the microenvironment that affect the physical activity and eating behavior choices.

Distal Leverage Points: All beahvior settings and macroenvironments are influenced by additional layers of factors, either directly or indirectly (e.g., controllers of the raw materials and finished goods that consumer purchase or are exposed to, along with the laws, policies, economics, politics, etc. that affect the controllers). The distal leverage points also include some multidimensional factors that pervade all levels and that shape attitudes, beliefs, and knowledge, e.g., media.

FIGURE 5-2A   Framework for Determinants of Physical Activity and Eating Behavior
FIGURE 5-2B   Layers of the Framework.
Source: Figures 5-2a and 5-2b are reprinted with permission from S. Booth. Environmental and societal factors affect food choice and physical activity: rationale, influences, and leverage point. *Nutrition Reviews*, vol. 59, no. 3, 2001, pp. S23–24.

period to help us adapt to our present-day lifestyles. Now, most of us "dwell in mechanized urban settings, leading sedentary lives and eating a highly processed, synthetic diet".[23] Some differences in our diets were that hunter-gatherers consumed foods higher in fiber content and lower in energy density, and with a different diet composition of the long chain fatty acids. The long chain fatty acids of the n-6 and n-3 families were consumed in a ratio of about 1:1. Today's Western-type diet can provide less of the omega-3 fatty acids with an n-3:n-6 ratio of 1:15–17.[24] The diet of the hunter-gatherer was rich in plant foods, supplemented by fish and lean meats and nuts. Indications are that these early ancestors did not experience obesity. Changes in agricultural practices, as well as food processing and manufacturing, have resulted in a vastly different food supply that has evolved over a relatively short time, historically. The development of agricultural societies led to diets based on grains. With this change, from a plant-based to a grain-based diet, vitamin and mineral deficiencies began to appear, as evidenced by studying bones and teeth. Our natural preference for foods that are calorically dense is rooted in the conditions of our ancestors, who required high levels of physical activity and high energy expenditures to obtain food for survival through hunting, fishing, and gathering.

In contrast, obtaining food today means a car ride to the grocery store and little connection between energy intake and expenditure.[23] The typical American diet today may be lower in fiber and plant foods, higher in meat, high in highly refined carbohydrates (high glycemic load), and possibly contain a much higher ratio of the n-6 relative to the n-3 long chain fatty acids. Sources of n-3 fatty acids that are possibly diminished in our diet include fish, shellfish, wild game, and plant foods. Potassium intakes are much lower today, while sodium intakes are much higher than the intakes of our ancestors. In short, most people consume a diet they were not genetically designed to eat. Calcium is an important mineral to human health, yet calcium intakes are not adequate for adolescent girls, older women, and older males. Although calcium intake has increased a little for females ages 20–74 since NHANES III, recommendations for milk and dairy intake are not met by 70% of the population over 2 years of age according to the NHANES 1999–2000 data.[25] Researchers contend that these dietary changes, combined with sedentary lifestyles, play a significant role in the etiology of chronic diseases affecting developed countries: heart disease, diabetes, cancer, and obesity.[26,27]

Changes in the Food Environment

One of the most noticeable changes affecting our food environment during the past two decades is the rapid growth in the number of restaurants and especially of fast food establishments which are currently approaching 250,000 outlets nationally. Fast food restaurants are found throughout our communities, even inside public schools and hospitals. The effective marketing and advertising of these restaurants to adults and children have fueled the growth of this industry. Unfortunately, fast food restaurant fare is usually high in calories, fat, salt, and sugars, while low in fiber content.[28] This is especially true for menu items offered as "special value" promotions. Often, the more healthful selections on fast food menus are more expensive and are not subject to the low price offers that might otherwise encourage customers to buy them.

Fast food items are convenient and relatively low cost. These factors appeal to working and single parents, and the percentage of children eating fast food meals will likely increase.[28] The amount of food dollars spent purchasing meals at dine-in and take-out restaurants has increased significantly to now comprise about 46% of total household food budgets. Fast food meals consume about 34% of the family food dollar. Meals eaten outside the home tend to have large portion sizes, have a higher energy content, and include fewer fruits and vegetables than meals eaten in the home. As a result, the increase in out-of-home meal consumption may have a negative impact on diet quality and on the obesity and health risk of children and their families.[29,30]

Product innovations launched during the past two decades have included many products designed to lower the fat content of popular foods to address consumers' concerns about dietary fat and unwanted weight gain. In spite of an explosive growth in low-fat food products in many food categories, these food supply changes have seemingly not had the desired effect on our obesity rates. Many food manufacturers offset the lower fat content of the reformulated foods by increasing sugar and carbohydrate contents to maintain product acceptance by consumers. In the end, the caloric content of the lower fat product is often similar to the original version. There is also concern that so-called low-fat foods may encourage the consumer to actually eat more calories overall because the low-fat food provides a "license to eat more."[31]

Energy intakes in children's diets have remained fairly stable since 1971–1974 (NHANES I), except for increases for children ages 1–2, and for adolescent females ages 12–19. The macronutrient composition of children's diets has changed, however, reflecting changes in the food supply. Fat intake as a percentage of energy intake fell from 38% to 33% since 1973, while carbohydrate and protein intakes increased. Still, about 75% of children did not meet the fat intake recommendations in 1994.[30,32]

Children's diets have changed in respect to the types of carbohydrate they consume. In a 1998 roundtable and national briefing on child nutrition, the Director of the National Institute of Child Health and Human Development was quoted as saying that children's diets are characterized by "too much energy . . . too much sugar, and too little fiber" (fruits and vegetables) and could be described as an inverted My Pyramid (formerly called the Food Guide Pyramid).[33] Easily digestible, highly refined carbohydrates from foods and beverage sources have increased in consumption recently. A lot of scientific interest has focused on the possible role of high glycemic index (GI) foods in the childhood and adult obesity epidemic. An effect of the GI of breakfast foods on subsequent unrestricted food intake at lunch has been studied. Lunch intake after a high-GI-load breakfast was greater than after a breakfast of low GI.[34] In a review of the high-GI foods and their connection to hunger and obesity, Roberts[35] concludes that compared to similar low-GI carbohydrates, high-GI carbohydrates promote a more rapid return of the hunger sensation and increase subsequent caloric intake. High-GI foods may, therefore, contribute to maintenance of excess weight in the obese, and weight gain in susceptible individuals. Many children start their day with high-sugar-content breakfast cereals of high-GI. Over the longer term, frequent intake of high-GI foods could lead to higher energy intake and contribute to excess weight gain.[36]

Glycemic index (GI) is the effect of carbohydrate in a food on blood glucose, as a percentage of the effect of an equal amount of glucose.

High-sugar beverage intake is linked with fast food consumption because soft drinks are usually marketed and bundled with meal packages in fast food restaurants. Twice as many children and adolescents drank carbonated soft drinks if they had consumed fast foods on one of two survey days than if they had not consumed fast foods.[37] The so-called "super-sized" meal offers upgrade beverage serving size along with food portions. "Super-sizing" of meal packages may have contributed to increased intakes of sweetened beverages by children. Between 1977–79 and 1994, the proportion of children who consumed soft drinks on a given day increased by 74% for boys and 65% for girls.[30] High consumption of soft drinks among children and adolescents has been shown to be associated with higher energy intakes.[38] An association between schoolchildren's sugar-sweetened drink consumption and their BMI has been demonstrated, although more research is ongoing. For example, a study conducted prospectively over 19 months showed that for each additional serving of sugar-sweetened beverage consumed, both BMI and propensity to become obese increased. This was after controlling for anthropometric, demographic, dietary, and lifestyle variables.[39]

The typical 12-fluid-ounce can of soda is rapidly being replaced by the 20-fluid-ounce bottle at convenience stores and in vending machines, encouraging increased consumption of these drinks. Many brands offer a 32-fluid-ounce version that is packaged in a bottle shape that is easy to tote around, thereby encouraging increased consumption. Average portion sizes of soft drinks have increased by 12–18% for persons ages 2 and older.[25] Soft drink consumption (per capita) has increased about 500% over the past 50 years, with adolescents consuming between 36 grams and 58 grams of sugar daily from this source.[39]

Food portions have increased as well. Most consumers recognize portion inflation among baked goods, such as bagels and muffins, and for hamburgers, which are both larger and offered with two or three servings of meat and cheese.

Regulation of Energy Intake

Although very young children possess innate abilities to regulate energy intake based on their needs, children tend to lose some of this ability as they age and become more responsive to environmental influences, increasingly taking their behavioral cues from their surroundings. Children vary in their ability to self-regulate energy intakes,[40] but children who have experienced so-called restrictive feeding practices appear to be less able to respond appropriately to internal signs of hunger and satiety, and may be more susceptible to overeating.[41] Also, as children learn from their environment, food portion sizes will influence their intake. Thus, children may over-eat when presented with excessive food and beverage portions, risking excessive weight gain over time.

The Family Eating Environment

Genetic differences are estimated to account for about 30%–50% of the variance of BMI within a population, but these estimates do not describe the complex interactions taking place between genetics and the environment.[42] For example, parents contribute both genetics and environment to the equation, and their own eating behaviors that help shape the child's eating environment may to an extent be influenced by genetics. In turn, the child or adolescent's eating environment will help shape the development of the child's own eating behaviors. These learned eating behaviors will again influence whether any genetic predispositions toward obesity will be expressed in the child.[41]

Parents who are struggling with personal weight issues may hamper their children's ability to self-regulate energy intake. Since many adults suffer from overweight or obesity,[7] some parents are understandably concerned about their children's risk of also becoming overweight or obese. Aiming to avoid overweight in their children, parents may impose greater restrictions on their children's intake. If these same parents exhibit uninhibited eating styles themselves, they will serve as poor role models. These behaviors in combination can cause the transfer of eating styles that pose an increased risk for the development of overweight in the child. As a result, well-intentioned parents may actually produce the very outcome they sought to avoid.[40] A common strategy employed to control children's intake is to restrict their access to high-calorie foods, or to use favorite foods as a reward to shape behavior. At first, these behaviors may seem reasonable enough; however, restricting certain foods has been shown to increase the child's desire to consume these foods. When available, these desirable foods will likely be consumed in greater amounts. Again, such family dynamics around food may set up patterns of poor self-control of energy intake in the child.[43]

An optimal environment for children to develop self-control of energy intake is when parents provide nutritious food and allow children to determine when and how much to eat. These principles of division of responsibility are discussed extensively in other resources.[44-47]

Household Food Insecurity

Although seemingly paradoxical, low income compared to higher income households appear to experience increased rates of overweight for some individuals. Proposed mechanisms for this effect include higher intakes of cheaper, more calorie dense foods, which may lead to excessive energy intakes.[48,49] Persons from low income, food insecure households may overeat during periods of relative abundance and gain weight as a result. Food insecurity in low-income households appears to play a role in

> **Retrospective studies**—These studies examine events that have occurred in the past or they represent attribute variables that cannot be manipulated; therefore, the researcher does not have direct control of the variables under study.
>
> **Longitudinal studies**—The researcher follows a cohort of subjects over time, performing repeated measurements at prescribed intervals.

the increased overweight rates among older Caucasian girls (8–16 years of age) compared to children from low-income households that do not experience food insecurity.[49] However, family participation in programs such as the National School Breakfast and Lunch Programs and Food Stamp Programs may be protective for these girls. Girls who participated in all three programs were 68% less likely to become overweight when compared to nonparticipants from families experiencing food insecurity.[50] On the other hand, a more recent study found a 42.8% increase for young girls and a 28.8% decrease for young boys in the predicted probability of obesity with participation in the Food Stamp Program for the previous 5 years. This study did not control for food insecurity within households, which may help to explain the differing results.[51] Additional studies that are retrospective, longitudinal, and include assessment of food security and hunger status of each household member are needed to help explain why some children are affected more than others. This is important because not all members of a household may be experiencing food insecurity to the same extent. Understanding these dynamics better will help to focus attention on those within a household who may be at a greater risk of being overweight. (Read more about food insecurity in Chapter 17.)

Breast-feeding

New mothers returning to work may decide against breast-feeding or nurse their infants for only a very limited time because of the real and/or perceived obstacles involved with breast-feeding their infants while holding a job. This is unfortunate, as breast milk is the ideal food for infants. Evidence is emerging that breast-feeding may offer some protection against obesity.[52] Proposed mechanisms for this effect include more normal growth patterns (lower early weight gain) possibly associated with lower basal insulin levels in the breast-fed infant compared with an infant fed formula, and the inherent control of food intake maintained by the breast-fed infant.[53] Breast-feeding on demand is thought to teach infants to regulate their intakes appropriately, based on internal cues for hunger and satiety, and in response to their individual growth needs. Formula-fed infants may have fewer opportunities to develop this important skill, perhaps because parents or caregivers want to follow a set feeding schedule or encourage the baby to consume a certain amount of formula. Both of these feeding behaviors override the infant's internal cues and may result in overfeeding and lessening of the infant's ability to self-regulate energy intake.[41]

Physical Inactivity Affecting Overweight Status in Children

Physical inactivity among children is one of the major public health concerns regarding overweight children. Children learn to be physically inactive by emulating adults who are inactive and having limited access to community recreation activities, unsafe neighborhoods, and perhaps, unlimited access to television viewing and other media outlets, including computers. In addition, many newly developed communities are poorly planned and don't include "built-in" access to physical activity. Often children are bused to school because walking to school is not an option due to safety issues and distance. In many towns and cities, sidewalks were once common, but now some urban and suburban developments have shaped many residential areas into "unwalkable" communities. Although further research is needed for a better understanding of the influence of the human-built environment on physical activity, it appears clear that urban sprawl has caused some relationship between land use, transportation, and health, particularly children's health.[54]

School Physical Education

At school, children are challenged to find opportunities to be physically active on a daily basis. Often, school academic curriculums and programs take priority over physical education and recess time. Physical education (PE) curriculums and recess have slowly diminished over the last few years.

The percentage of schools that require physical education in each grade declines from around 50% in grade one through five, to 25% in grade eight, to only 5% in grade 12. Although National Association for Sport and Physical Education (NASPE) and National Association of State Boards of Education (NASBE) discourage student exemption from physical education based on participation in other school and community activities, some states, districts, and schools allow such exemption from required physical education.[55]

Data from the Youth Risk Behavior Surveillance System (YRBSS) show that 55.7% of students nationwide were enrolled in PE classes one or more days in an average week, while only 28.4% of students nationwide attended PE classes 5 days in an average week. Of the 55.7% of students enrolled in PE classes nationwide, 80.3% of students actually exercised or played sports for more than 20 minutes. Improvements in PE are also needed to decrease inappropriate teaching practices, such as prohibiting physical activity as a form of punishment or physical activity games that may cause embarrassment or aggressive behavior (e.g., dodge ball).[55] Although some PE improvements are needed, a nationwide effort to establish laws or policies to increase student enrollment and participation in daily PE is desirable, especially in the older student population. The goal is for children to establish healthy lifestyle habits that may carry over into adulthood.

While the majority of children spend much of their waking hours in school, it is a threat to children's health and fitness when the school infrastructure does not mandate daily physical activity. Advocacy for increasing student participation in daily recess and physical activity should be a top priority of schools and health and community leaders to help prevent overweight in children.

Television Viewing

Television viewing and other media outlets to an extent have displaced a more natural environment of family interactions for growing children, such as learning and playing. Children who spend more time in sedentary activities tend to weigh more and be at greater risk of being overweight. Several studies conclude that children who watch 4 or more hours of TV are more likely to be overweight than those who watch less TV.[56-58] In addition, African American (30%) and Hispanic American (22%) children are both more likely than Caucasian (12%) children to spend more than 5 hours a day watching TV. Similarly, African American (69%) and Hispanic American (60%) children are more likely than Caucasian (48%) children to have a TV in their bedroom.[59] One cross-sectional study failed to find a relationship between TV viewing and overweight in adolescent girls.[60] There may be some question about leisure activities in the United States, indicating that U.S. children overall are less active than children in other countries and cultures. A participant in one focus group made a comparison between U.S. children and the children in her country. She stated that "one exercises three times a day, one goes to the river to swim in the afternoon, and here the children don't do that. They just sit to watch television and to eat."[61] The trend toward increasingly sedentary lifestyles is obvious to many older adults, as they compare the children's activity level in this current generation to that of children two or three generations earlier. Learning, playing, and being physically active were an integral part of family life, and television viewing was a special occasion. Today, television viewing, which is a sedentary behavior, is a prominent part of family life.

Not only will excessive television viewing leave less time for positive family interactions and activities, but the actual programs and advertisements may also be questionable for young viewers. Granted, there are many beneficial programs to watch on television. Unfortunately, not all programs and advertisements have children's health as a priority. One major challenge is the multimillion-dollar advertising industry that promotes products between and during television programming.[62] Appealing and enticing advertising segments are targeted at children to increase their desire to choose unhealthy foods. Food products advertised directly to young children during children's television programming have contributed to an impressive growth in sales of high-sugar breakfast cereals and snack foods. Young consumers predictably request the products or even purchase these themselves during trips to the grocery store, as they recognize their favorite cartoon characters on the colorful packages that are strategically placed at their eye level when riding in the grocery cart. Excessive television viewing by children creates a cycle of physical inactivity and high calorie consumption due to the influence of TV food advertising, which is a perfect formula for fueling the growth in numbers of overweight children.

An important part of treating overweight in children is to decrease sedentary behavior and increase physical activity.[63] This is an important factor in the treatment process; however, children are still challenged with real barriers that exist in their physical environment. As discussed, limited access to safe physical activity in the community, unlimited television viewing, decreased physical activities in the schools, and adults who may not view physical activity as a priority are important barriers to physical activity. Thus, U.S. children live in an obesigenic society in which they continually face barriers to making healthy living choices, such as daily physical activity.

> **Obesigenic**—An environment that encourages obesity through features such as unlimited quantities of a variety of foods high in caloric density together with minimal energy expenditure.

Addressing Childhood Obesity/Overweight as a Public Health Nutritionist

Public health nutritionists will soon experience a new role in their profession when addressing obesity in this nation, as the comfort level of doing what always has been done will not benefit the public. One recent study reported that the majority of health professionals working in obesity-related fields stated that they were most comfortable with education-based prevention strategies and less comfortable

> See Chapters 7 and 8 to learn about advocating for policies and resources. In addition, see Chapter 26 to learn about social marketing for programs needed for the health and welfare of the public.

with environmental-based strategies.[64] Clearly, many health education strategies have not been effective during the rise of childhood obesity due to many environmental conditions that require global and societal action.[65,66] Thus, public health nutritionists may need to go beyond the traditional practice and learn to apply policy- and environmental-based strategies.[67] Public health nutritionists must become assertive in learning and applying policy and environmental interventions and be aggressive enough to demand the resources and support to implement and evaluate them. Public health nutrition leaders will be the change agents that are needed in a society that some assert is in denial about overweight in children.[68]

Due to the low rate of overweight in children in the past, childhood obesity was not a high priority in the healthcare arena. Therefore, the traditional practice of a public health nutritionist, in addressing overweight in children, has been mostly reactive versus proactive. In the reactive mode, parents of an overweight child may or may not seek treatment and/or counseling depending on their cultural belief system, attitude, and knowledge. If treatment was sought, usually discussions occurred in medical offices with a doctor or nurse. In the past, public health nutritionists' roles were mostly as consultants to medical professionals and/or serving as nutrition educators or counselors to families on healthy eating and exercise.

Because obesity is a multifactor disease, public health nutritionists must be proactive in learning new skills and acquiring new tools to prevent and control weight-related problems in children. Effective treatment practices are necessary for the existing population of overweight children. Treatment practices must be reliable and tailored to individuals and populations in order to be effective at changing behavior and the health status of overweight in children. Some existing treatment practices are education, behavioral therapy, and surgical procedures; however, some of these are questionable for this population.[69] The primary focus should be a multifactor population-based approach of prevention, including assessment, policy and environmental interventions; support for healthy eating, physical activity, limited TV viewing, and breast-feeding promotion; and community planning within communities, schools, worksites, faith-based groups, medical facilities, and families. This multifactor population-based approach should be included in academia and training for public health nutrition students and professionals, respectively.[70] In addition, the public health nutritionist should be culturally competent and support the Healthy People 2010 Objectives (HP 2010) to eliminate health disparities in chronic illnesses, such as in overweight and obesity.[71]

> Read more about Healthy People 2010 at: www.healthypeople.gov.

Partnerships

Due to the complexity of population-based approaches in addressing overweight in children, it is essential for public health nutritionists to develop internal and external partnerships. Partnerships are useful because partners may adopt the vision of healthy children, expand resources, and build momentum and synergy to address the healthcare needs of target populations. Being aware of the knowledge, skills, and limitations of yourself and partners will enable you to close the gaps and accomplish goals set for the target population. Nutrition expertise is valuable; however, the focus must advance from educating, counseling, and telling people about the importance of healthy eating and physical activity to working with partners to change the environment so as to enable people, especially children, to eat healthy foods and to exercise or be physically active.[72,73]

Often, public health nutritionists encourage their target population to eat more fruits and vegetables, even when there are well-known barriers to consuming the recommended amount of these foods. Availability, accessibility, and affordability are real barriers to eating fruits and vegetables daily for many individuals, including children. Acknowledgement of these barriers and knowing partners who can help overcome them will help to increase fruit and vegetable intake among children. Local media may serve as an outlet to increase fruit and vegetable intake among children through social marketing campaigns. Meetings and discussions with local day care and school food service directors may lead to a policy change that promotes and serves more fresh fruits and vegetables during school meals and snacks. Cooperative Extension Agents may conduct classes on purchasing fruits and vegetables in season and preservation, thus increasing fruit and vegetable availability throughout the year. Local farmers and grocers may sell their produce at different locations throughout the community. Fruits and vegetables sold at annual events (e.g., sum-

> The 2005 Dietary Guidelines Advisory Committee has recommended the intake of fruits and vegetables, as well as non-fat/low-fat dairy products and whole grains for children.

mer and fall fests) or sporting activities may also promote healthy eating. Religious groups may encourage potluck lunches or dinners that include more fruits and vegetables. Restaurants may encourage children to eat healthier by featuring fruits and vegetables acceptable to children on the menu. Finally, after-school programs may serve fruits and vegetables as snacks more often.

The marketing that creates a high demand for soft drinks causes its main ingredient, corn syrup, to be produced at high volumes. Therefore, soft drinks are relatively cheap and readily available. This same principle may be applied to increasing the consumption of fruits and vegetables by producing them at high volumes that cause them to be relatively inexpensive and readily available. Partnerships with the media, local farmers, grocers, community planners, schools, extension services, and USDA Food Assistance Programs all have the ability to influence the way people view fruits and vegetables. Partnerships help to remove the barriers and enable people, especially children, to obtain and consume fruits and vegetables daily. Although it may be challenging to organize partnerships, develop policies, or change the environment to increase fruit and vegetable consumption, it can be rewarding.

Another potential partnership for the public health nutritionist is to collaborate with research universities and/or institutes. Such partnerships may offer opportunities to develop evidence-based interventions focused on prevention of obesity or promotion of a healthy weight from which both parties may benefit. For instance, the public health nutritionist may have an existing partnership in the school system that is interested in developing programs or interventions that prevent and control obesity in children. The public health nutritionist and research investigator may collaborate with the school partner and plan, develop, implement, monitor, and evaluate the intervention. As a result, the public health nutritionist's goals and objectives may be implemented and the investigator may assist with the development of monitoring systems and evaluation tools. The investigator may also serve as an independent reviewer of data, and do monitoring, data analysis, and evaluation. Once the program is complete, the public health nutritionist and investigator may submit abstracts and manuscripts to professional conferences and journals. Also, this valuable information should be shared with community leaders and those working with the target populations. Other partnerships may also be established with existing internal partners, such as an epidemiologist, community planner, or the like.

> **Evidence-based** is a concept whereby analysis is based on scientific proof.

Internal agency partnerships are also important. Often, internal partners do not know about their own agency's resources and services to the community. Sometimes internal partners may be territorial and work in silos. However, when working in the community or clinical settings, it is important to know about various internal programs and services. Hence, individuals and communities benefit when internal partners, including the public health nutritionist, are unified and present consistent, current resources and referrals.

Another responsibility of the public health nutritionist may be to form an internal or external coalition. There are a few important things to remember when forming a coalition:

1. Solicit key partners with a shared vision of the goals and objectives to accomplish.
2. Establish a mission, goals, and objectives that will advance a common vision and that benefit a majority of the goals of key partners. Often the momentum of the coalition diminishes when members are not focused, organized, or challenged with activities from which they and their constituents or target population may benefit.
3. Review the accomplishments and failures of the coalition at regular intervals and evaluate whether goals and objectives were met.

Developing partnerships is a process that demands a significant investment of time and attention. Therefore, it is essential to attend meetings, from the local town hall and county coalition meetings to state and professional meetings. At these meetings, the ultimate goal is to know the community leaders and health professionals. Leaders need to know your skills, as a public health nutritionist, and your goals and vision of healthy children and adults. Over time, relationships can be developed into strong partnerships that are essential for public health nutritionists to be effective in their communities.

> **Coalition**—An alliance, sometimes temporary, of people, factions, or parties.

Grant Writing

Many social programs have experienced budget constraints and/or cuts and are forced to become more creative with existing resources, or obtain grant funding to develop or even continue programs. Although doing more with less is the norm for many agencies, many are seeking grant funding to advance their programs. Therefore, grant applications have become very competitive, and the ability to write a favorable grant application is now an essential skill of the public health nutrition practitioner.

The public health nutritionist should possess some grant writing skills; however, working as a team to coordinate and complete the grant application is ideal. Completing a grant application is very time consuming and labor intensive. For this reason alone, a professional grant writer may be needed to coordinate the activities and gather materials needed to complete the grant. The role of the public health nutritionist should be to describe the vision for the project and to develop a plan of action of assessment, policy and environmental interventions, evaluation, and assurances. In addition, the public health nutritionist must act as a resource to obtain letters of support from internal and external partners. Development of a budget is also necessary, and should be a shared responsibility between the public health nutritionist and the agency accountant. The public health nutritionist will be able to describe staffing and salary requirements needed to complete the tasks required of the action plan, and the accountant will be able to provide technical assistance for the grant budget requirements. A grant steering committee is very helpful when submitting a grant application for a large sum of money. This committee may consist of the agency epidemiologist, nurse administrator, nutrition administrator, accountant, key health professionals that may work directly with the proposed grant activities, and grant writer. The public health nutritionist can be the primary person to determine the services needed to accomplish the goals and objectives of the project. However, it is equally important to solicit the opinions of people on the grant steering committee and internal and external partners. If possible, public health nutritionist positions and responsibilities should be included in the grant. Thus, the public health nutritionist should plan to write portions of the grant. See Appendix G for more on grant writing.

Private and public funding have various requirements; therefore, it is important to review the requirements and complete the application, as specified. Most grant applications have similar requirements. A *cover sheet* includes the title, the organization's information, and the budget requested. The *proposal abstract* provides a brief description of the project including the community problem, mission, goals, objectives, project strategies, past accomplishments, and support from internal and external partners. The *proposal narrative* describes the project in detail through the following: introduction, statement of community problem, project vision, mission and objectives, methods, evaluation plan, plan for financial sustainability, budget and budget justification, and overall significance.[74] Although all grant applications may not follow the same format, most applications targeted to prevent or control chronic diseases and/or illnesses require some basic information.

Many grant applications require letters of support. Sometimes public health nutritionists may appear as a salesperson when requesting a letter of support. In such cases, the request must offer a win-win solution for both parties involved. For instance, a school superintendent is asked to write a letter of support for a grant application on prevention and control of obesity in children. Before the school superintendent can write a letter of support, he or she should be able to visualize the benefits of the proposed project for the student population. Due to the existing trend of overweight in children, many leaders, including school superintendents, are eager to receive funding to address this public health issue, but are unsure of how to proceed. The public health nutritionist's role is to present the problem and some possible solutions (e.g., policy and environmental interventions), and provide suggestions as to how the school population and environment may be improved through proposed grant activities.

Advice

There are some pointers to keep in mind for each grant submitted. A peer should review the grant before you submit it. A good proofreader often catches errors or items not clearly defined. Although staffing, if allowed, may absorb most of the grant funding, it is important to establish program sustainability after the grant monies have ended. Therefore, sharing grant funding with the community and developing infrastructures to carry out the project activities after the funding has ended is ideal. In addition, many grant applications allow "matching" and in-kind contributions from various partners, which also encourage sustainability. A project should develop or enhance collaboration and partnerships, which will in turn develop momentum for the project. Also, as much as possible, the budget should be outcome driven. For instance, did the proposed project meet the objectives of decreasing the amount of fundraisers that sold high-calorie foods or increasing healthy food options in the vending machines? After 2 years, did students participate in more physical activity or eat healthier meals? Did students' BMI decrease and fitness level increase?

Finally, the application must follow the grant guidelines and be written concisely. This includes calling the grant agency to get technical assistance or to clarify what is required of the grant. The writing style should be clear, logical, concise, and professionally presented. A good grant application is one that shares resources, focuses on capacity building, encourages sustainability after the funding has ended, and is written concisely for grant application reviewers.

Media

Media professionals can be a useful resource for advancing the vision of healthy children. They can be seen as coworkers that present important health information to the public. Thus, establishing good media relationships can enhance media advocacy interventions targeted for overweight children. The media should not sensationalize overweight in children, but instead use this public health concern to increase people's awareness of the health problem. Therefore, it is the public health nutritionist's role to enlighten audiences about the actions being taken to combat the trend of overweight in children. Hence, the public health nutritionist should be available as a resource for current data on overweight in children. This data may be available from a variety of resources, such as the Youth Risk Behavior Surveillance System (YRBSS), Pediatric Nutrition Surveillance System (PedNSS), and pediatric surveillance research from local universities or school data from students' annual physical exams. In addition, public health nutritionists should be actively involved in project interventions that address overweight in children, such as the School Health Index (SHI). These activities may be discussed in newsprint, on television, on radio, or on websites as ways to lower the rate of overweight in children.

Also, public health nutritionists should provide some thought-provoking ideas or challenges for the intended audiences. For instance, the nutritionist can write an article for a school newsletter that may encourage parents to get involved with developing school menus by reviewing menu items and participating in taste testing. Or, a local newspaper article may encourage local vendors to get involved in fundraising activities that do not involve food. This may initiate creative fundraising activities and eliminate the traditional bake sales and candy sales.

Working with media professionals can be stressful, especially for an entry-level public health nutritionist. However, some of this stress may be alleviated with a proactive approach and attitude. When possible, the public health nutritionist should meet with local media professionals prior to a story. It helps to get to know media professionals and relate to them as professional colleagues.

Be prepared to discuss topics that you are most familiar with and don't be afraid to say, "I don't know" on topics that you are not. A folder containing current facts, statistics, and program interventions for your population, state, district/region, county, and town/neighborhood is a valuable tool to keep at hand. This folder should be updated regularly with the latest data, including bookmarked sites on your computer. An effective delivery of the information is as important as knowing the facts. Therefore, it is a good idea to attend workshops and training opportunities on public speaking and effective communication. One organization that can help enhance your communication skills is Toastmasters International.™

Ensure that your point gets across while addressing the media professional's agenda. With preparation and organization, the public health nutritionist can ensure that the message will not be lost in the excitement of obtaining the story and meeting deadlines.

There are advantages and disadvantages to working with the media. Doing a media segment on overweight in children and possible interventions will reach more people instantly than if you were working with a small community group. Also, media can be very resourceful when planning a social marketing campaign that encourages children to be physically active and to eat healthier foods. However, one should be mindful that everyone does not have access to television, radio, or print. Also, some people in target populations may have limited language or literacy skills.

Advice

Develop a partnership with your local media professional. Invite them to a coalition meeting and discuss ways they can develop a story on successful accomplishments. Become familiar with their schedules and deadlines. Being proactive rather than reactive gives you time to develop a story, instead of being called 30 minutes before a story is being aired or printed. Remember that most media segments are short; therefore, it's important to be concise and focused, and to avoid jargon, acronyms, and large words. If you are unfamiliar with a topic, you may offer to research that information and follow up with the media professional. Interviews are good, but media professionals love it when health professionals can tell a story through sounds and images (e.g., children eating and talking in the lunchroom, students making a decision on snacks at the vending machine, or students exercising or not exercising during PE class). Media professionals appreciate receiving a thank-you note after a story is completed, and this helps to extend your relationship.

Research in the Area of Overweight in Children

Overweight in children is an active area of current research. Numerous articles on the topic regarding all its many facets are published each year, adding to our body of knowledge and defining new questions in need of answers. To be effective in planning successful interventions, the public health nutritionist should be familiar with the childhood overweight literature through periodic literature reviews and attendance at professional meetings, where up-to-the minute research findings are presented, often before appearing in print.

A critical review of the literature will enable the practitioner to distinguish between studies that provide information and will be useful in his or her area of practice and those that may not. The public health nutritionist should consider issues such as these in making this judgment:

- *Study design:* What was the research question or objective? Was the study designed in such a way that the question could be answered or the objective obtained? If it was an intervention study, was there a control group? Were there confounding variables that could lead to inconclusive or erroneous findings, or were such confounders considered?
- *Study subjects:* Were the subjects part of a specific ethnic group? How were subjects recruited and selected? Was the study free of bias in recruitment and selection? Was bias introduced through subject self-selection? For intervention versus control subjects, was group assignment random? Was selection done at the individual level or group level (e.g., randomization is done for individual children within a school or setting, in contrast to

one or more schools being selected at random for intervention while other schools serve as the controls). Did a sufficient number of subjects participate to draw the stated conclusions? How does a given study sample compare to the population served by the public health nutritionist?

- *Outcomes/results:* What interventions were most effective? Most cost-effective? What failed to show the desired results?
- *Application/implications:* What lessons may be applied to intervention planning, policy development, and so on for a given population? What data does the public health nutritionist already have access to (PedNSS, YRBSS, HP2010, etc.) that can be studied with current research in mind?

Considering these issues and applying the deeper understanding in a thoughtful manner to public health activities will help ensure that our practice is evidence-based.

Being armed with a sound knowledge of the topic of childhood obesity will provide the public health nutritionist with the necessary confidence to seek and obtain support from government, community leaders, the medical community, stakeholders, the media, and community change agents, as well as from his or her own public health department and supervisor in advocating for obesity prevention. It would be most helpful to have a well-stocked inventory of successful research studies to draw upon for inspiration in planning evidence-based community interventions. However, to date, there is a lack of studies with highly successful outcome measures, for a variety of reasons. Some suggested reasons include lack of adequate funding, too short a duration of intervention, or insufficient skills of key implementers. Other reasons include the inherent difficulty in achieving an effect big enough in the study sample on an outcome-based study, such as BMI. BMI will increase normally as children grow, making an intervention on BMI difficult to measure. Interventions to address overweight in children are ongoing at this writing, and it is hoped that these studies-in-progress will have benefited from weaknesses in earlier studies, resulting in outcomes that clearly demonstrate effective strategies. CATCH (Child and Adolescent Trial for Cardiovascular Health), SPARK (Sports, Play, and Active Recreation for Kids), and Planet Health are examples of recent intervention studies that provide insights into the challenges and successes of childhood obesity intervention research.

Although obesity interventions typically have been a product of academic research centers, public health nutritionists may be able to become involved in investigations through cooperation and collaboration with academic researchers. Certain issues, such as logistics and funding assurance for protection of study subjects, will need to be addressed; these efforts may offer great learning opportunities for the public health nutritionist who is new to research. The public health nutritionist has a unique knowledge of the study population, its

CATCH:
http://www.childtrends.org/Lifecourse/programs/
ChildandAdolesentTrialforCardiovascularHealth.htm

SPARK: http://www.sparkpe.org

Planet Health:
http://www.hsph.harvard.edu/prc/proj_planet.html

barriers to a healthy lifestyle, and obesity prevention, which can contribute to the formulation of appropriate research questions, and often has access to large amounts of data. The investigator, in contrast, has the research experience, access to statistical analysis, and sometimes support staff and graduate students to assist in the investigation.

Public Health Model and Overweight in Children

In public health, assessment, policy development, and assurance are integral parts of any intervention plan.[1] The following sections will review each component as it relates to addressing overweight in children.

Assessment

CDC School Health Index

The School Health Index (SHI) is a self-assessment and planning guide developed for grades K-12 by the CDC in Atlanta, Georgia. It consists of eight modules based on the coordinated school health program model. The modules have assessment questions in health education, physical education, health services, nutrition services, counseling, psychological and social services, healthy school environment, health promotion for staff, and family/community involvement. The current version focuses on physical activity, nutrition, and tobacco use in elementary, middle, and high schools. It is a tool that identifies the strengths and weaknesses of a school's health promotion policies and programs. The SHI assists teachers, parents, students, and community members to develop an action plan for improving the health of the student population. Some improvements in the action plan can be implemented with little or almost no resources. Other improvements may require grant funding for implementation.[75]

The SHI is easy to administer and complete. The role of the public health nutritionist is to present current trends of poor eating habits and physical inactivity nationally, statewide, and locally. In addition, an existing partnership with local tobacco-use prevention educators is important because they may discuss trends of tobacco use in children. Once the evidence of health problems is described, the public health nutritionist should review resources, such as the SHI and examples of policy and environmental interventions for targeted schools. Some examples of policy interventions are: to serve breakfast to all students; to serve low fat milk, fresh fruits and vegetables, and whole grain products; to limit access to vending machines during school hours and/or provide healthy options in the vending machines; to provide opportunities for vigorous physical activity for all students; and, to offer healthy food options in school stores. Some examples of environmental interventions include: building a walking track for student, staff, and community members to use; purchasing playground equipment for students; and planning an annual community health event for community members, parents, teachers, and children.

The public health nutritionist acts as a consultant to the SHI site coordinator, who assembles and supports the SHI team members. Team members complete the assessment questions and planning guide. They develop an action plan with interventions tailored for their school. The role of the public health nutritionist is to ensure the development of an appropriate action plan that results in interventions of healthy eating practices and physical activity, especially among the student population.

The public health nutritionist should attend the planning meeting to assist SHI members in developing an action plan. Although the site coordinator should facilitate the meeting and solicit ideas and opinions, the public health nutritionist serves as a consultant by helping the team members to focus on healthy eating and physical activity. In addition, the public health nutritionist should seek, obtain, and disburse funding sources to implement some or all of the interventions. This is important because funding serves as an incentive to improve the school's health policies and programs. The SHI is an excellent tool in developing partnerships with local school staff and community, obtaining and dispersing grant funding to promote health, and monitoring and evaluating interventions that benefit children's health.

Policy Development

Recommendations, Policy, and Environmental Interventions

After an assessment is completed, areas that need improvement are identified. The next step is to develop interventions that actually empower a target population to accomplish a desired outcome. There are several types of interventions; however, for the purpose of this chapter, recommendations, policy, and environmental interventions will be discussed.

Recommendations

A recommendation is a course of action strongly advised by someone of authority, but not necessarily enforced. It is ideal to develop a policy after an assessment is complete. However, a recommendation may be used as a mechanism to get an actual policy written and/or established. A recommendation may follow the dictum of "first, do no harm." Although many people are reluctant to change, a recommendation allows them time to accept the ultimate goal of healthy children. For those who are involved, a recommendation gives people time to accept the new idea and adopt behaviors that support healthy children. In essence, this process is similar to the Diffusion of Innovation Theory, in that a new idea is disseminated throughout the invested population in the hope that they will adopt the projected behavior (i.e., healthy eating and physical activity).

Example   After completing an assessment in one school, it was determined that fund-raising activities (e.g., candies, bake sales, etc.) may contribute to children being overweight. Since this was identified, there was a great level of reluctance among staff and administrators to develop a policy due to the revenue and cultural norm of fund-raising activities. Thus, a compromise was made and a recommendation was established for staff. The recommendation pointed out the increased number of overweight children in their student population and encouraged staff to consider non-food items for fund-raising activities. Although this was only a school recommendation, it created awareness among staff and was an important first step in policy development.

Policy

Policy is a law, regulation, rule, or guiding principle. It is different from a recommendation in that a policy is a guiding principle that is enforced by administrators or others. Policy may be dispersed informally, such as in a memo. Or it may be formal, including a rationale, program policy, intent, evaluation, policy review, and determination as to how it will be enforced.[76] A policy demands and expects a certain behavior. Currently, a no-smoking policy in restaurants is the norm in many cities; a vending machine or a la carte service with healthy food selections will be the norm when policies are written and enforced in school settings.

Example   In one school, the school food service director developed a policy to serve low-fat milk during mealtime. This policy decreases the fat content of the student's diet at school. Although you would expect the children to complain, it was mostly the school staff that had a difficult time adjusting to the policy. The policy also saved the school some money because whole milk cost more than low-fat milk. The students benefited from consuming low-fat milk rather than the standard whole milk served.

Environmental Interventions

Environmental interventions include changes to the economic, social, or physical surroundings. This intervention changes the physical environment to make it convenient to adopt healthy behaviors. It is important to recognize barriers to making positive changes in health behaviors among the target population. For example, barriers to exercise could include unsafe neighborhoods, lack of sidewalks and parks, and so on. The building and refurbishing of walking or biking trails in the community is an intervention that helps the target population to adopt healthy physical activity behaviors.

Example   It was identified that a walking track was needed to encourage children to walk during recess and PE classes. As a result, a walking track was built in front of the elementary school. Many parents drive or bus their children to school, so walking on the track is a good physical activity outlet for the children. Children establish many behaviors during childhood. Children who are encouraged to walk and exercise increase their chances of being physically active in their adult years.[77] In addition, school staff and community members may use the walking track.

Assurance

Interventions are essential to implement change, particularly in overweight children. However, it is vital to evaluate the process and outcome of the interventions to assure that projected outcomes benefit the target population.

Evaluation

Evaluation is a systematic investigation of an object's merit, worth, or significance.[78] Major goals of evaluations are to assess the program's success in meeting stated objectives and identify potential improvements in program operation.[79] Process evaluation assesses the internal development of the project. It asks if certain protocols were followed, such as:

1. A school council made up of teachers, administrators, parents, health professionals, and community leaders was formed to address children's health and factors that caused them to be overweight.
2. All school nurses received training on how to measure students' BMI accurately and how to record and report data.
3. WIC nutritionists and/or Head Start providers received training on cultural issues regarding overweight in children, educating parents on feeding young children, and overcoming barriers to healthy living for families.

Outcome evaluation assesses the external results of the program. It asks whether the program was effective and whether it accomplished its goals and objectives. For instance:

1. After teachers attend a training session, 85% of them reported not using physical activity as a form of punishment.
2. Of students who participated in 30 minutes of vigorous activity, 90% of them increased from three times per week to five times per week.
3. Of the 15% of children who were overweight, 85% either maintained or lost up to 5 pounds in the last school year.

In major program interventions, evaluation tools should be standardized for several reasons.

- The tool may be used as a guide when collecting and analyzing data.
- It eliminates the use of various tools that may have insufficient analysis beyond the primary program.
- A standardized tool will be validated and, thus, measures what is supposed to be measured.
- A standardized tool is efficient to use because it eliminates time spent developing a new tool.

Overall, evaluation is important because it helps to determine the program's successes and failures, and it serves as a guide for future program planning.

Survey Development

In a small program, a public health nutritionist may be asked to develop a survey or evaluation tool to see how the program is progressing and the degree to which the goals and objectives were met. To this end, the public health nutritionist should review the program goals, objectives, and strategies. A *process objective* may be, for example, to ensure that a trained individual will determine students' BMI during certain timeframes. A *process evaluation* would measure how many school nurses or nutritionists successfully completed a training on assessing overweight in children and if a trained individual took their height and weight measurements during the specific timeframes. In the survey, a question may be "During the first, second, third, and fourth quarter, what percentage of students' heights and weights were screened?" The outcome objective may be to decrease the number of children with a BMI greater than the 85th percentile from 15% to 10%. An outcome evaluation would measure the percentage of children who have a BMI greater than the 85th percentile. In the survey, an appropriate question would be: "What is the percentage of students who had a BMI greater than the 85th percentile?"

Surveys, observations, and other assessment tools are essential in the evaluation process because they provide a final picture of the intervention. When developing a survey, avoid "yes" or "no" questions. Formulate questions into multiple choices, instead of "Do you exercise?" ask "How many times a week do you exercise for more than 20 minutes?" (See Table 5-3 for sample survey questions from the 2005 State and Local Youth Risk Behavior Survey.[80])

Surveys are also important because they may be included in grant applications and the data analyzed may be used as baseline data for the target population. Grant application reviewers like to see effective and successful programs. Without an evaluation, it is difficult to demonstrate effectiveness of an intervention in reaching

TABLE 5-3   Sample Survey Questions from the 2005 Youth Risk Behavioral Surveillance System

1. During the past 7 days, how many times did you eat fruit? (Do not count fruit juice.)
   A. I did not eat fruit during the past 7 days.
   B. 1 to 3 times during the past 7 days
   C. 4 to 6 times during the past 7 days
   D. 1 time per day
   E. 2 times per day
   F. 3 times per day
   G. 4 times per day

2. On how many of the past 7 days did you exercise or participate in physical activity for *at least 20 minutes that made you sweat and breathe hard*, such as basketball, soccer, running, swimming laps, fast bicycling, fast dancing, or similar aerobic activities?
   A. 0 days
   B. 1 day
   C. 2 days
   D. 3 days
   E. 4 days
   F. 5 days
   G. 6 days
   H. 7 days

3. On an average school day, how many hours do you watch TV?
   A. I do not watch TV on an average school day.
   B. Less than 1 hour per day
   C. 1 hour per day
   D. 2 hours per day
   E. 3 hours per day
   F. 4 hours per day
   G. 5 or more hours per day

Source: Reprinted from National Center for Chronic Disease Prevention and Health Promotion. 2005 State and Local Youth Risk Behavioral Survey. Available at www.cdc.gov/HealthyYouth/yrbs/pdfs/2005highschoolquestionaire.pdf. Accessed August 25, 2004.

desired outcomes for a population. Evaluation also provides feedback about weaknesses of the program or intervention that impede progress so that improvements can be made.

Surveys are not the only mechanism for evaluating an intervention. Observing and collecting anthropometric data are some other forms of evaluation. For instance, observing children while they eat or participate in physical activity or collecting weight and height measurements to assess BMI are some other ways to evaluate.

Opportunities for Public Health Nutritionists to Intervene and Prevent Overweight in Children

Public health nutritionists are challenged to think of new ways to address the problem of childhood obesity within existing venues and frameworks. To be most successful, the emphasis must be on population-based approaches and prevention, as traditional and clinical-based practices clearly have failed to adequately address the obesity epidemic. Thus, the public health nutritionist may examine existing nutrition, social, and other programs and seize opportunities to advance goals. Some suggestions for opportunities are listed in the following sections.

WIC

- Develop policies and provide outreach activities to recruit pregnant women into prenatal care during the first trimester. This may improve nutrition delivery to the unborn child to avoid pregnancy under- or over-nutrition, and thereby lower the risk of future obesity.[21] Grocery store tours are conducted in some clinics to teach shopping skills for healthy eating to program participants.
- Assess monitoring systems and develop policies or protocols to target high-risk children older than 2 who exhibit rapid weight gain, and ensure that they receive intensive guidance through culturally appropriate interventions.
- Train the healthcare team in anticipatory guidance and counseling, with regard to infant and child feeding and physical activity consistent with obesity prevention, to enable the team to serve as positive role models.
- Assess the clinic environment for inconsistencies (deliberate, as well as unintended) in the healthy eating and physical activity messages, and develop policies that promote a healthy environment for staff and program participants.
- Develop policies and environmental interventions that promote, support, and protect breast-feeding.

Head Start/Preschool/Day Care

- Develop policies that ensure healthy menu items and eating environments for children.
- Develop policies that ensure children participate in recommended physical activity daily.
- Train child care providers and the food service team in obesity prevention strategies through provision of nutritious food choices and daily physical activity appropriate for age and development.

- Assist with grant writing to fund environmental intervention (e.g., playground, equipment for physical activity) and policy interventions for staff and parents to attend training in healthy eating practices for children. In addition, sponsor community events that involve families and staff to adopt healthy living practices, such as reducing sedentary behavior and increasing physical activity.

School Systems

- Advocate for daily recess and active physical education for all children through school boards, parent and teacher organizations, and school administrators.
- Develop policies that limit competitive foods and beverages, and serve fresh fruits and vegetables daily on the breakfast and lunch menus.
- Develop nutrition standards for vending machines and school stores.
- Advocate for a unified message for healthy eating and physical activity throughout the school (no candy fund-raisers, no food and/or candy rewards for good behavior in the classroom, healthy snacks at parties and school events, and a campus that is friendly to physical activity, such as walkways, bicycle racks, and safe outdoor play equipment).
- Advocate for universal school breakfast and lunch program participation.
- Advocate for strengthening the nutrition education throughout the entire school curriculums, K-12, and make an impact on student behavior (50 hours/year minimum).[81]
- Develop monitoring systems to assess children's health and behaviors (e.g., height and weight, BMI, blood pressure, fruit and vegetable consumption, TV viewing, transportation modes to school, and actual physical activity during recess and PE classes).

After-School Classes

- Train staff to support obesity prevention efforts (healthy snacks, physical activity for all children).
- Survey the environment for consistency of the health messages, minimizing the availability of competitive foods of poor nutritional quality, and make the environment friendly to physical activity.
- Assist with obtaining grants to provide facilities and equipment to enable and encourage physical activity (e.g., walking track, basketball court, playground equipment, etc.).

Other Possible Venues

- Advocate for child participation in federal summer feeding programs for needy children.
- Advocate for a healthful environment at various settings for children, such as Boys and Girls Clubs, YMCA/YWCA, summer camps, and other programs through provision of training opportunities and materials in obesity prevention to directors and their staff.
- See the Resources section at the end of the chapter for examples and additional possible venues.

Programs and Resources That Support Evidence-Based Practices in Preventing Overweight in Children

The CDC's Nutrition and Physical Activity Program has established three evidence-based goals to prevent and control obesity:

- To increase physical activity
- To reduce television viewing
- To improve nutrition through increased breast-feeding, fruit and vegetable consumption, and healthy eating[82]

Although research is limited on successful practices in various settings, the following are a few programs and resources that may be used by a public health nutritionist when addressing overweight in children.

Physical Activity

KidsWalk-to-School

A community-based program developed by the CDC Nutrition and Physical Activity Program, *KidsWalk-to-School* ". . . encourages children to walk to and from school in groups accompanied by adults."[83] This program mobilizes community members such as school staff, the Parent Teacher Association, police departments, businesses, civic associations, and so on to work together to increase safe routes to and from school for children to walk or use their bicycles. Overall, the community becomes aware of the importance of children participating in daily physical activity, thereby changing an unwalkable community into a walkable community, which is an environmental intervention. This program supports the HP 2010 objectives related to children's trips to school by walking or bicycling.[71]

Television Viewing

TV Turnoff Network

The goal of *TV Turnoff Network* is to encourage children and adults to turn off the television and replace that time with quality life activities that promote healthier living and communities. It sponsors two programs: TV Turnoff Week and More Reading, Less TV. TV Turnoff Week is held during the last week of April of every year. It encourages physical activities, such as gardening, skating, dancing, walking, bicycling, or playing a sport, along with other non-physical activities. More Reading, Less TV encourages reading as a replacement to television viewing among children and adults. As mentioned earlier, there is a link between excessive TV viewing and increased BMI in children. Thus, decreasing TV viewing may encourage children to be more physically active.[84] These programs support the HP 2010 objectives related to increasing the number of adolescents watching 2 hours or less of television on school days.[71]

Nutrition

Breast-feeding

Since breast-feeding may be an early intervention to prevent childhood obesity, breast-feeding promotion can occur in various settings. For instance, the public health nutritionist may develop a breast-feeding coalition that focuses on developing breast-feeding policies in work sites, hospitals, or public areas. In addition, coalition members may monitor and evaluate the interventions implemented. Or, a public health nutritionist may collaborate with partners or participate in coalitions to increase breast-feeding awareness and promotion through World Breastfeeding Week, health fairs, or other community events. In addition, a public health nutritionist may train other nutritionists, nurses, doctors, or other medical professionals on breast-feeding management and support ways to increase breast-feeding initiation and duration rates. In a clinical setting, a public health nutritionist may provide one-on-one breast-feeding education, counseling, and support of pregnant and lactating women to increase the breast-feeding initiation and duration rates. This initiative supports the HP 2010 objectives related to increasing the proportion of women who breast-feed their babies.[71]

5 A Day

The Produce for Better Health Foundation is a consumer education foundation that chairs the National 5 A Day for Better Health Program. This program is the nation's largest public-private nutrition education initiative. National 5 A Day Month is observed in September and encourages people to consume 5–9 servings a day of colorful fruits and vegetables. Researchers have studied the relationship between fruit and vegetable intake and weight maintenance and loss in the pediatric population. Some found that it is possible to decrease overweight and to increase the consumption of fruits and vegetables. Strategies to decrease energy intake while increasing fruit and vegetable intake hold promise as a dietary approach to lowering risk of overweight. Additionally, a message to increase fruits and vegetable intake has the benefit of being positive and guiding people to eat healthy foods, rather than being negative as when recommending that people do not eat high fat and sugary foods.[98,99] In addition, 5 A Day campaigns are useful because they have adaptable toolkits and other promotional items that fit various settings. In particular, *There Is a Rainbow on My Plate* is a useful guide. It is designed to educate children on the importance of healthy eating by consuming a variety of colorful fruits and vegetables. This initiative supports the HP 2010 objective related to persons 2 years and older consuming two servings of fruit and three servings of vegetables daily.[71]

Other Programs

Beyond breast-feeding, healthy eating habits among toddlers and children are vitally important, as these lay the foundation for life-long eating habits. There are many good sources of information on healthy eating practices among toddlers. One example is Children's Healthcare of Atlanta's Stress-Free Feeding curriculum,[97] which advocates a healthy eating environment that includes patience and learning healthy eating habits for both the parent and child. This initiative supports the HP 2010 objective (developmental) related to increasing the proportion of children and adolescents who consume meals and snacks that are of good overall dietary quality.[71]

The programs and resources discussed above are only a few avenues to explore and suggest to partners and perhaps focus groups. To accomplish the ultimate goal of healthy children in healthy communities, the public health nutritionist should be resourceful when suggesting programs, initiatives, and campaigns related to overweight in children. He or she must have a toolbox of information ready when entering various settings: coalition, community, school, worksite, healthcare facility, or other organizations. This toolbox of information and resources will vary depending on the target population. Nevertheless, public health nutritionists must be creative and timely in sharing their vision and potential solutions to address childhood obesity. The authors encourage public health nutritionists and students to research other resources and participate in Internet listservs for best practices and new findings in preventing and controlling overweight in children.

One Community's Experience

A local university conducted a surveillance study on 4th, 8th, and 11th graders in a small southern rural county. After reviewing the process and conducting visual observations, it was evident to the public health nutritionist and county nurse that the student population had a large number of overweight children. When grants became available on preventing heart disease and overweight in children, the baseline data was available from the university.

The public health nutritionist reviewed the grant and its requirements, and discussed the grant application with key partners in the county (the county charge nurse, school superintendent and nurse, and community leaders). A grant application was submitted, describing the county demographics, assessment of the problem, goals, objectives, strategies, time frame, stakeholders, and budget along with letters of support. The grant was awarded to work with this school district. The goals were to conduct the School Health Index (SHI) and develop policy and environmental interventions related to physical activity and nutrition.

The public health nutritionist presented the problems of obesity in children and factors involved, such as soda consumption, decreased milk consumption, increased sedentary behavior and decreased PE, TV viewing, and computer games. In addition, possible solutions through the use of the SHI and policy and environmental interventions were presented. A SHI site coordinator was appointed and teachers were assigned to eight different teams. The SHI teams completed the SHI questionnaire and met with the public health nutritionist for technical assistance in developing an action plan. This action plan served as a guide when using grant funding to ensure expenditures were appropriate and related to the goals and objectives of the project.

Many interventions were developed from the SHI. A recommendation was developed to assess all fund-raising activities to ensure that items sold were non-food items and/or encouraged healthy eating. Second, a policy was developed to sell only low-fat milk and use whole-wheat bread on school menus. Third, an environmental intervention for the school was to build a walking track to be used by students, staff, and community members and encourage daily exercise. Finally, the SHI team established a county-wide community health day featuring several events including a 5K marathon run, a 1-mile fun walk, and a health fair that assessed community members' blood pressure, blood sugar, waist circumference, and BMI. In addition, children participated in a reading expo, and TV Turnoff Week was promoted. Local sponsors, including the school nutrition program, grocers, and a bottling company, donated fruits and vegetables and water, respectively. This community event involved a lot of partners from the hospital and health department as well as private and public donors. Television and print media promoted many activities related to healthy eating, physical activity, and the decrease of TV viewing, and covered the accomplishments of the local school staff and partners.

In addition, process and outcome evaluation tools were developed by the public health nutritionist to determine if the goals and objectives were met, as outlined in the grant application. The public health nutritionist developed an additional survey tool to capture the health status of adults who attended the health fair. The school principal developed and completed an evaluation tool to determine who used the track and how many miles were walked among students during the school year. For TV Turnoff Week, the public health nutritionist developed pre- and post-surveys to determine if participants changed their behavior during that week. From the series of events, baseline data were gathered, partnerships developed, and the potential to receive additional funds to address childhood obesity increased. A small grant mobilized the school and community to participate in healthy lifestyle choices that work toward preventing chronic diseases caused by obesity.

Summary

Public health nutritionists may use existing nutrition and social programs as opportunities to promote evidence-based strategies to prevent obesity in children.

However, many programs are designed for specific groups (such as WIC) and do not serve or reach all segments of the population that are involved in the care of children. Because many nutrition and social programs have a narrow focus, population-based services are essential to help communities, schools, worksites, other organizations, and families to adopt healthy behaviors. Healthy eating among children cannot be addressed without including the family as a whole and the environment. As discussed earlier, almost 65% of adults are overweight or obese, and this is a risk factor for their children becoming overweight.[7,100,101]

Overweight in children is a major public health concern; however, preventive efforts must target the parents and caregivers, as well as the children. "If obese parents of at-risk children reduce access to low-nutrient, calorically dense foods available in the shared family environment, model healthier eating and activity habits, and share positive food related family experiences that reinforce eating high nutrient-dense foods, the parents may reduce their risk of their child becoming obese as well as modify their own body weight."[98] Improving family interaction through healthy eating practices and physical activity is essential to preventing childhood obesity. Healthy lifestyle behaviors can be taught in parenting classes and discussed during doctor's office visits, at worksites, at health fairs, in parent-teacher organizations, and at other sites. In addition, population-based services and partners can develop and implement policy and environmental interventions that make it convenient for families to include healthy eating practices and daily physical activity.

Healthy eating practices and physical activity are interrelated when addressing childhood obesity. Both play an integral role in decreasing the rate of overweight in the United States. Although some traditional public health nutrition roles, as nutrition educator or a consultant to medical professionals, are still valuable; the new role of public health nutrition practitioners has expanded to include stepping outside of the office and into the community. Working with partners is essential, as is obtaining financial resources to implement programs in the community or schools. The media offers endless opportunities to reach target populations with various health messages and social marketing campaigns. Policy and advocacy will be crucial in developing standard nutrition and physical activity policies within various settings.

The prevention and control of overweight and obesity in this society will be one of the greatest public health challenges in the 21st century. Public health nutritionists have rich opportunities for innovation, creativity, and personal development as this challenge demands the use of each person's unique skills: up-to-date knowledge of evidence-based care, communication and media skills, grant writing and budget know-how, research and presentation skills, advocacy and policy development, cultural competency, and relationship and coalition building. Population-based approaches should be comprehensive so that environmental changes will support healthy eating and regular physical activity and encourage optimal health for people of all ages.

Picture a future where prenatal care is provided for all pregnant women in the first trimester and health professionals provide anticipatory counseling for families to encourage breast-feeding and prevent feeding problems. Working mothers are given adequate breast-feeding support before and after returning to work. Allowable WIC foods include fresh fruits and vegetables year-round in addition to the traditional WIC foods. Other food programs provide access to fresh produce at low cost for low-income families. Children learn early to love foods that will sustain their health, and feel secure that they will have enough to eat. Schools serve nutritious lunches that children enjoy, and recess time allows for daily physical activity for all children. Vending machines at school are stocked with healthful choices that supply nutrients important to children's health. After-school programs offer ample opportunities to play and consume nutritious snacks. Neighborhoods are planned with adequate green space for play and recreation, or parks are added during urban renewal projects. Children can walk or ride their bikes safely to and from school on walking trails and bike paths. Neighborhoods are planned for mixed use so that it is possible to walk to the store or other local businesses. Government agricultural support is increased for the growing of fruits and vegetables, while government subsidies for production of corn for high fructose corn syrup manufacturing decrease. Healthy foods are inexpensive, and high fat and sugar foods are expensive. Advertisers don't advertise high-fat and sweetened foods to children during and between children's TV programming. Children participate in daily activities and their weight gain is appropriate for their growth and development. Hopefully, healthy children will become healthy adults with many quality years of life.

Issues for Discussion

1. Why is it important to have internal and external partnerships? Why is it important for public health nutritionists and internal partners to be aware of their agencies' programs and services? Discuss programs or services of a local community that you may promote to a school board to prevent or control obesity in children.

2. Physical activity and exercise are as important as healthy eating in the pediatric population. How would you include physical activity as an intervention for children if you have limited training in this area?

3. List and describe other tools or resources that a public health nutritionist may use to address overweight in children.

4. Develop a sample survey for a Parent Teacher Association to determine children's and parents' eating habits and physical activity levels. What partnerships would you develop? How would you administer the survey?

5. What power (if any) does the government have to influence factors that impact overweight in children?

6. Discuss how the media may promote overweight in children and how it may be used to prevent this problem.

7. What should the public health nutritionist consider when he or she plans or implements overweight-in-children prevention interventions for families in clinic settings or special programs?

8. List ways a public health nutritionist can measure the success of an intervention related to preventing overweight in children. Provide an example of one of them.

Resources

Professional Organizations

American Academy of Pediatricians
http://www.aap.org
http://www.pediatrics.org

American Dietetic Association
http://www.eatright.org

American Medical Association
http://ama-assn.org

American Nurse Association
http://www.ana.org

American Psychological Association
http://www.apa.org

American Public Health Association
http://www.apha.org

Society of Nutrition Education
http://www.sne.org

Statistical or Surveillance Systems

Behavioral Risk Factor Surveillance System (BRFSS)
http://www.cdc.gov/brfss

Combined Health Information Database
http://chid.nih.gov

Kaiser Family Foundation's state health facts online
http://www.statehealthfacts.kff.org

Maternal and Child Health Bureau
http://www.mchdata.net

National Center for Health Statistics
http://www.cdc.gov/nchs

Pediatric and Pregnancy Nutrition Surveillance System
http://www.cdc.gov/pednss/

Statistical Abstract of the United States: 2004–2005
http://www.census.gov/statab/www

Statistics Related to Overweight or Obesity
http://www.niddk.nih.gov/statistics/index.htm

Youth Risk Behavior Surveillance System (YRBSS)
http://www.cdc.gov/HealthyYouth/yrbs/index.htm

Policy and Environmental Interventions

Center for Nutrition Policy and Promotion
http://www.usda.gov/cnpp

Center for Science in the Public Interest School Nutrition Policy
http://www.cspinet.org/nutritionpolicy

The Community Tool Box
http://ctb.ku.edu

Model School Wellness Policies
http://www.schoolwellnesspolicies.org

National Association of State Boards of Education: Fit, Healthy and
Ready to Learn: A School Health Policy Guide

http://www.nasbe.org/HealthySchools/fithealthy.html

National Recreation and Park Association
http://www.nrpa.org

Nutrition

Center for Science in the Public Interest Nutrition Policy
Project: School Foods Tool Kit. A Guide to Improving School
Foods and Beverages
http://www.cspinet.org/schoolfood

Children's Healthcare of Atlanta
http://www.choa.org

Dietary Guidelines for Americans
http://www.nal.usda.gov/fnic/dga

MyPyramid Plan
http://www.mypyramid.gov

Breast-feeding

Baby Friendly Hospital Initiative
http://www.babyfriendlyusa.org

Blueprint for Breastfeeding
HHS Blueprint for Action on Breastfeeding. DHHS Office
of Women's Health, 2000
http://www.cdc.gov/breastfeeding/report-blueprint.htm

Fruits and Vegetables

5 A Day
http://www.5aday.com
Junior Master Gardner Program
http://jmgkids.com

Dairy

1% or Less Campaign-School Kit
http://www.cspinet.org/nutrition/schoolkit.html

3-A-Day
http://www.3aday.org

Dairy Council
http://www.nationaldairycouncil.org

Exercise

Hearts N' Parks Program
http://www.nhlbi.nih.gov/health/prof/heart/obesity/
    hrt_n_pk/index.htm

National Association for Sport and Physical Education
http://www.aahperd.org/naspe

National Recreation and Park Association
http://www.nrpa.org

PE4life
http://www.pe4Life.com

The President's Council on Physical Fitness and Sports
http://www.fitness.gov

Take 10!
http://www.take10.net

Media

Centers for Disease Control and Prevention, Youth Media Campaign
http://www.cdc.gov/youthcampaign

TV Turnoff Network
http://www.tvturnoff.org

School Resources

Action for Healthy Kids
http://www.actionforhealthykids.org

The Center for Health and Healthcare in Schools: School
   Health Issues
http://www.healthinschools.org/sh/obesity.asp

National Association of State Boards of Education-Healthy Schools
http://www.nasbe.org/HealthySchools/States/state_Policy.html

Planet Health
http://www.hsph.harvard.edu/prc/proj_planet.html

School Health Index
http://apps.nccd.cdc.gov/shi

SPARK Program
http://www.sparkpe.org

Team Nutrition
http://www.fns.usda.gov/tn

Community Resources

Active Community Environments Initiative
http://www.cdc.gov/nccdphp/dnpa/aces.htm

Association for Community Health Improvement
http://www.communityhlth.org

Community Service Block Grant
http://www.acf.hhs.gov/programs/ocs/csbg/index/htm

North Carolina Prevention Partners
http://www.ncpreventionpartners.org

Task Force on Community Preventive Services
http://www.thecommunityguide.org

Other Resources

American Public Health Association Food and Nutrition Section:
Childhood Overweight
http://www.aphafoodandnutrition.org/overwt.html

Bright Futures
http://www.brightfutures.org

Center for Science in the Public Interest
http://www.cspinet.org

Centers for Disease Control and Prevention
http://www.cdc.gov

Centers for Disease Control and Prevention Evaluation and
Working Group
http://www.cdc.gov/eval/index.htm

Cooperative State Research, Education, and Extension Service
http://www.csrees.usda.gov

GrantsNet: Federal Grant Information
http://www.hhs.gov/grantsnet/

Healthy People 2010
http://www.healthypeople.gov

Institute of Medicine: Focus on Childhood Obesity
http://iom.edu/focuson.asp?id=22593

Maternal and Child Health Bureau
http://www.mchb.hrsa.gov

National Institute of Health
http://health.nih.gov

U.S. Department of Health and Human Services
http://www.hhs.gov

YMCA of the USA
http://www.ymca.org

References

1. Committee for the Study of the Future of Public Health Division of
   Healthcare Services. Institute of Medicine. *The Future of Public Health.*
   Washington, DC: National Academy Press; 1988.
2. Centers for Disease Control and Prevention. Use and Interpretation of
   the CDC Growth Charts. Available at: http://www.cdc.gov/nccdphp/
   dnpa/growthcharts/00binaries/growthchart.pdf. Accessed July 12, 2004.

3. Serdula MK, Ivery D, Coates RJ, Freedman DS, Williamson DF, Byers T. Do obese children become obese adults? A review of literature. *Preventive Medicine.* 1993;22:167–177.

4. Freedman DS, Khan LK, Dietz WH, Srinivasan SR, Berenson GS. Relationship of childhood obesity to coronary heart disease risk factors in adulthood: The Bogalusa Heart Study. *Pediatrics.* 2001;108:712–718.

5. Ellis KJ, Abrams SA, Wong WW. Monitoring childhood obesity: assessment of weight/height2 index. *Am J Epidemiol.* 1999;150:939–946.

6. Taylor RW, Jones IE, Williams SM, Goulding A. Body fat percentages measured by dual-energy X-ray absorptiometry corresponding to recently recommended body mass index cutoffs for overweight and obesity in children and adolescents aged 3–18 y. *Am J Clin Nutr.* 2002; 76:1416–1421.

7. National Center for Health Statistics. Prevalence of Overweight and Obesity among Adults: United States, 1999–2002. Available at: http://www.cdc.gov/nchs/products/pubs/pubd/hestats/obese/obse99.htm. Accessed March 15, 2005.

8. Ogden CL, Flegal KM, Carroll MD, Johnson CL. Prevalence and trends in overweight among US children and adolescents, 1999–2000. *JAMA.* 2002;288:1728-1732.

9. Freedman DS, Khan LK, Dietz WH, Srinivasan SR, Berenson GS. Relationship of childhood obesity to coronary heart disease risk factors in adulthood: The Bogalusa Heart Study. *Pediatrics.* 2001;108:712–718.

10. Hill JO, Wyatt HR, Reed GW, Peters JC. Obesity and the environment: where do we go from here? *Science.* 2003;299:853–855.

11. Berenson GS. Childhood risk factors predict adult risk associated with subclinical cardiovascular disease: The Bogalusa Heart Study. *Am J Cardiol.* 2002;90(suppl):3L-7L.

12. Hassink S. Problems in childhood obesity. *Prim Care Office Prac.* 2003;30:357–374.

13. Raman RP. Obesity and health risks. *J Amer Coll Nutr.* 2002;21(2):134S–139S.

14. Erickson SJ, Robinson TN, Haydel KF, Killen JD. Are overweight children unhappy? *Arch Pediatr Adolesc Med.* 2000;154:931–935.

15. Hill JO, Trowbridge FL. Childhood obesity: future directions and research priorities. *Pediatrics.* 1998;101(suppl):570–574.

16. Nelson JA, Chiasson MA, Ford V. Overweight children in a New York City WIC population. *Am J Public Health.* 2004 Mar;94(3):458–462.

17. Strauss RS, Pollack HA. Epidemic increase in overweight children, 1986-1998. *JAMA.* 2001;286:2845-2848.

18. Wang G, Dietz WH. Economic burden of obesity in youths aged 6 to 17 years: 197–999. *Pediatrics.* 2002;109(5). Available at: http://www.pediatric.aapublications.org/cgi/content/full/109/5/e81. Accessed March 27, 2005.

19. Editorial. Who pays in the obesity war? *Lancet.* 2004;363(9406):339.

20. Mokdad AH, Marks JS, Stroup DF, Gerberding JL. Actual causes of death in the United States. 2000. *JAMA.* 2004;291(10):1263–1264.

21. Dietz WH. Overweight in childhood and adolescence. NEJM. 2004;350(9):855–857.

22. Booth SL, Sallis JF, Ritenbaugh C, et al. (Working Group II). Environmental and societal factors affect food choice and physical activity: rationale, influences, and leverage points. *Nutrition Reviews.* 2001; 59(3, part 2): S21–S39.

23. O'Keefe JH, Cordain L. Cardiovascular disease resulting from a diet and lifestyle at odds with our paleolithic genome: how to become a 21st century hunter-gatherer. *Mayo Clin Proc.* 2004;79:101–108.

24. Simopoulos AP. The importance of the ratio of omega-6/omega-3 fatty acids. *Biomed Pharmacother.* 2002;56(8):365–379.

25. Briefel RR, Johnson CL. Secular trends in dietary intake in the United States. *Annu Rev of Nutr.* 2004;24:401–431.

26. Simopoulos AP. Evolutionary aspects of omega-3 fatty acids in the food supply. *Prostaglandins Leukot Essent Fatty Acids.* 1999;60:421–429.

27. Conner WE. Importance of n-3 fatty acids in health and disease. *Am J Clin Nutr.* 2000;71:171S-175S.

28. Bowman SA, Gortmaker SL, Ebbeling CB, Pereira MA, Ludwig DS. Effects of fast-food consumption on energy intake and diet quality among children in a national household survey. *Pediatrics.* 2004;113:112–118.

29. American Dietetic Association. The role of dietetics professionals in health promotion and disease prevention. *J Am Diet Assoc.* 2002;102:1680–1687.

30. Nicklas TA, Baranowski T, Cullen KW, Berenson G. Eating patterns, dietary quality, and obesity. *J Amer Coll Nutr.* 2001;20:599–608.

31. Kurzweil P. Taking the fat out of food. *FDA Consumer Magazine.* 1996 Jul-Aug.; 30 (6). http://www.fda.gov/fdac/696_toc.html. Accessed March 27, 2005.

32. Munoz KA, Krebs-Smith SM, Ballard-Barbash R, Cleveland LE. Food intakes of U.S. children and adolescents compared with recommendations. *Pediatrics.* 1997;100:323–329.

33. McBean LD, Miller GD. Enhancing the nutrition of America's youth. *J Amer Coll Nutr.* 1999;18(6):563–571.

34. Warren JM, Henry CJ, Simonite V. Low glycemic index breakfasts and reduced food intake in preadolescent children. *Pediatrics.* 2003 Nov; 112(5): e414.

35. Roberts SB. High-glycemic index foods, hunger and obesity: is there a connection? *Nutr Rev.* 2000 Jun;163–169.

36. Augustin LS, Franceschi S, Jenkins DJA, Kendall CWC, La Vecchia C. Glycemic index in chronic disease: a review. *Eur J Clin Nutr.* 2002;56:1049–1071.

37. Paeratakul S, Ferdinand DP, Champaqgne CM, Ryan DH, Bray GA. Fast-food consumption among U.S. adults and children: Dietary and nutrient intake profile. *J Am Diet Assoc.* 2003;103:1332–1338.

38. Harnack L, Stang J, Story M. Soft drink consumption among U.S. children and adolescents: nutritional consequences. *J Am Diet Assoc.* 1999;99:436–441.

39. Ludwig DS, Peterson KE, Gortmaker SL. Relation between consumption of sugar-sweetened drinks and childhood obesity: a prospective, observational analysis. *Lancet.* 2001;357:505–508.

40. Johnson SL. Improving preschoolers' self-regulation of energy intake. *Pediatrics.* 2000 Dec;106(6):1429–1435.

41. Birch LL, Fischer JO. Development of eating behaviors among children and adolescents. *Pediatrics.* 1998;101:539–547.

42. Allison DB, Faith MS. Genetic and environmental influences on human body weight: implications for the behavior therapist. *Nutr Today.* 2000;35(1):18–21.

43. Fisher JO, Birch LL. Restricting access to palatable foods affects children's behavioral response, food selection, and intake. *Am J Clin Nutr.* 1999;69:1264–1272.

44. Johnson SL, Birch LL. Parents' adiposity and children's eating style. *Pediatrics.* 1994;94:653–661.

45. Satter E. *How to Get Kids to Eat...But Not Too Much.* Palo Alto, Calif: Bull Publishing; 1987.

46. Satter E. *Secrets of Feeding a Healthy Family.* Madison, Wis: Kelcy Press; 1999.

47. Satter E. *Child of Mine: Feeding with Love and Good Sense.* Palo Alto, Calif: Bull Publishing; 2000.

48. Drewnowski A, Specter SE. Poverty and obesity: the role of energy density and energy costs. *Am J Clin Nutr.* 2004;79:6–16.

49. Alaimo K, Olson CM, Frongillo, Jr. EA. Low family income and food insufficiency in relation to overweight in U.S. children. Is there a paradox? *Arch Pediatr Adolsc Med.* 2001;155:1161–1167.

50. Jones SJ, Jahns L, Laraia BA, Haughton B. Lower risk of overweight in school-aged food insure girls who participate in food assistance. *Arch Pediatr Adolesc Med.* 2003;157:780–784.

51. Gibson D. Long-term food stamp program participation is differently related to overweight in young girls and boys. *J Nutr.* 2004;34:372–379.

52. Armstrong J, Reilly JJ. Breastfeeding and lowering risk of childhood obesity. Child Health Information Team. *Lancet.* 2002 Jun 8;359(9322):2003–2004.

53. Dietz WH. Breastfeeding may help prevent overweight children. *JAMA.* 2001;285(19):2506–2507.

54. Frumkin H. Urban sprawl and public health. *Public Health Reports.* 2002;117:201–217.

55. Burgenson CR, Wechsler H, Brener ND, Young JC, Spain CG. Physical education and activity: results from the School Health Policies and Programs Study 2000. *J Sch Health.* 2001;71:279–293.

56. Andersen RE, Crespo CJ, Bartlett SJ, Cheskin LJ, Pratt M. Relationship of physical activity and television watching with body weight and level of fatness among children: results from the Third National Health and Nutrition Examination Survey. *JAMA.* 1998;279:938–942.

57. Gortmaker SL, Must A, Sobol AM, Peterson K, Colditz GA, Dietz WH. Television viewing as a cause of increasing obesity among children in the United States, 198–990. *Arch Pediatr Adolesc Med.* 1996;150:356–362.

58. Dowda M, Ainsworth BE, Addy CL, Saunders R, Riner W. Environmental influences, physical activity, and weight status in 8- to 16-year-olds. *Arch Pediatr Adolesc Med.* 2001;155:711–717.

59. Kaiser Family Foundation. Kids & media @ the new millennium: a Kaiser Family Foundation report. Available at: http://www.kff.org. Accessed May 10, 2004.

60. Robinson TN, Hammer LD, Killen JD, Kraemer HC, Wilson DM, Hayward C, Taylor CB. Does television viewing increase obesity and reduce physical activity? Cross-sectional and longitudinal analyses among adolescent girls. *Pediatrics.* 1993;91:273–280.

61. Crawford P, Gosliner W, Anderson C, Strode P, Becerra-Jones Y, Samuels S, Carrol A, Ritchie LD. Counseling Latina mothers of preschool children about weight issues: suggestions for a new framework. *J Am Diet Assoc.* 2004;104:387–394.

62. Borzekowski DLG, Robinson TN. The 30-second effect: an experiment revealing the impact of television commercials on food preferences of preschoolers. *J Am Diet Assoc.* 2001;101:42–46.

63. Steinback KS. The importance of physical activity in the prevention of overweight and obesity in childhood: a review and an option. *Obes Rev.* 2001;2:117–130.

64. Antipatis VJ, Kumanyika S, Jeffery RW, Morabia A, Ritenbaugh C. Confidence of health professionals in public health approaches to obesity prevention. *Int J Obes Relat Metab Disord.* 1999;23:1004–1006.

65. Hill JO, Melanson EL, Wyatt HT. Dietary fat intake and regulation of energy balance: implications for obesity. *J Nutr.* 2000;130:284S–288S.

66. Jefferry RW. Public health strategies for obesity treatment and prevention. *Am J Health Behavior.* 2001;125(3):252–259.

67. Schmitz MK, Jeffery RW. Public health interventions for the prevention and treatment of obesity. *Med Clin North Am.* 2000;84:491–512.

68. Ariza AJ, Greenberg RS, Unger R. Overweight children: management approaches in young children. *Pediatr Ann.* 2004;33:33–38.

69. Copperman N, Jacobson MS. Childhood obesity: interventions for the prevention and treatment of pediatrics overweight. *Pediatric Perspectives Newsletter.* Mead Johnson and Company. 2004. Available at: http://www.meadjohnson.com/newsletterimages/0300cpp/0300c2.html. Accessed March 15, 2005.

70. Fox KR. Childhood obesity and the role of physical activity. *JR Soc Health.* 2004;124:34–39.

71. U.S. Department of Health and Human Services. *Healthy People 2010.* 2nd ed. With Understanding and Improving Health and Objectives for Improving Health. 2 vols. Washington, D.C.: U.S. Government Printing Office; November 2000.

72. Mullis RM. Entrepreneur in action. In: Boyle MA, Morris DH, eds., *Community Nutrition in Action: An Entrepreneurial Approach.* St. Paul, Minn: West Publishing;1994:434.

73. Temple SP. Professional focus. In: Boyle MA, Morris DH, eds. *Community Nutrition in Action: An Entrepreneurial Approach.* St. Paul, Minn: West Publishing;1994:324.

74. University of Kansas. Community Tool Box. Available at: http://ctb.ku.edu/index.jsp. Accessed March 15, 2005.

75. Centers for Disease Control and Prevention, National Center for Chronic Disease. Prevention and Health Promotion. School Health Index for Physical Activity, Healthy Eating and Tobacco-Free Lifestyle, 2002. Available at http://apps.nccdcdc.gov/shi. Accessed March 23, 2005.

76. Bogden JF. *Fit, Healthy, and Ready to Learn: A School Health Policy Guide, Part I: Physical Activity, Healthy Eating and Tobacco-Use Prevention.* Alexandria, Va: National Association of State Boards of Education; 2000.

77. Alfano CM, Klesges RC, Murray DM, Beech BM, McClanahan BS. History of sport participation in relation to obesity and related health behaviors in women. *Preventive Medicine.* 2002;34:82–89.

78. Centers for Disease Control and Prevention. Framework for program evaluation in public health. *MMWR.* 1999;48(No. RR-11):1–40.

79. Kettner PM, Moroney RM, Martin LL. *Designing and Managing Programs: An Effective-Based Approach.* Newbury Park, Calif: Sage Publications; 1990.

80. National Center for Chronic Disease Prevention and Health Promotion. 2005 State and Local Youth Risk Behavioral Survey. Available at: http://www.cdc.gov/HealthyYouth/yrbs/pdfs/2005highschoolquestionaire.pdf. Accessed March 15, 2005.

81. Position of the American Dietetic Association, Society for Nutrition Education, and the American School Food Service Association. Nutrition services: an essential component of comprehensive school health programs. *J Amer Diet Assoc.* 2003;103(4):505–514.

82. Centers for Disease Control and Prevention. Resource Guide for Nutrition and Physical Activity Interventions to Prevent Obesity and Other Chronic Diseases, 2003. Available at http://www.cdc.gov/nccdphp/dnpa/obesityprevention.htm. Accessed March 15, 2005.

83. Centers for Disease Control and Prevention. KidsWalk-to-School. Nutrition and Physical Activity. Available at http://www.cdc.gov/nccdphp/dnpa/kidswalk/index.htm. Accessed March 15, 2005.

84. TV Turnoff Network. Available at: http://www.tvturnoff.org. Accessed March 15, 2005.

85. Balaban G, Silva GAP. Protective effect of breastfeeding against childhood obesity. *J Pediatr (Rio J).* 2004;80:7–16.

86. Gillman MW, Rifas-Shiman SL, Camargo CA, Berkey CS, Frazier L, Rockett HRH. Risk of overweight among adolescents who were breast-fed as infants. JAMA. 2001;285:2461–2467.

87. Hediger ML, Overpeck MD, Kuczmarski RJ, Ruan J. Association between infant breastfeeding and overweight in young children. *JAMA.* 2001;285:2453–2460.

88. Armstrong J, Reilly JJ, Team CHI. Breastfeeding and lowering the risk of childhood obesity. *Lancet.* 2002;359:200–004.

89. Toschike AM, Vignerova J, Lhotska L, Osancova K, Koletzko B, von Kries R. Overweight and obesity in 6-to-14-year-old Czech children in 1991: protective effect of breastfeeding. J *Pediatr* 2002;141:764–769.

90. von Kries R, Koletzko B, Sauerwald T, et al. Breastfeeding and obesity: cross sectional study. *BMJ.* 1999;319:147–150.

91. Zive MM, McKay H, Frank-Spohrer GC, Broyles SL, Nelson JA, Nader PR. Infant-feeding practices and adiposity in 4-y-old Anglo and Mexican-Americans. *Am J Clin Nutr.* 1992;55:1104–1108.

92. O'Callaghan MJ, Williams GM, Andersen MJ, Bor W, Najman JM. Prediction of obesity in children at 5 years: a cohort study. *J Pediatr Child Health.* 1997;33:311–316.

93. Wadsworth M, Marshall S, Hardy R, Paul A. Breastfeeding and obesity. Relation may be accounted for by social factors. *BMJ.* 1999;319:1576.

94. American Academy of Pediatrics. Breastfeeding and the Use of Human Milk. Available at: http://www.aap.org/policy/re9729.html. Accessed March 15, 2005.

95. Butt N, Cobb K, Dwyer J, Graney L, Heird W, Rickard K. The start healthy feeding guidelines for infants and toddlers. *J Am Diet Assoc.* 2004;104:442–454.

96. American Dietetic Association. Dietary guidance for healthy children ages 2 to 11 years. *J Am Diet Assoc.* 2004;104:66–67.

97. Buechner J. *Stress-Free Feeding Curriculum and Video.* Atlanta, Ga: Children's Healthcare of Atlanta; 2001.

98. Epstein LH, Gordy CC, Raynor HA, Beddome M, Kilanowski CK, Paluch R. Increasing fruit and vegetable intake and decreasing fat and sugar intake in families at risk for childhood obesity. *Obesity Research.* 2001;9:171–178.

99. Rolls BJ, Ello-Martin JA, Tohill BC. What can intervention studies tell us about the relationship between fruit and vegetable consumption and weight management. *Nutrition Reviews.* 2004;62:1–17.

100. Agras WS, Hammer LD, Kraemer HC. Risk factors for overweight children. *J Pediatr.* 2004;145(1):20–25.

101. Strauss RS, Knight J. Influence of the home environment on the development of obesity in children. *Pediatrics.* 1999 June;103(6). Available at. http://www.pediatrics.org/cgi/content/full/103/6/e85. Accessed March 15, 2005.

102. Mokdad AH, Marks JS, Stroup DF. Correction: Actual Causes of Death in the United States, 2000. *JAMA.* 2005 Jan 19; 293(3): 292–294.

CHAPTER 6

INTERVENING TO CHANGE THE PUBLIC'S EATING BEHAVIOR

Yeemay Su Miller, MS, RD

Reader Objectives

After studying this chapter and reflecting on the contents, you should be able to:

1. Describe the social, economic, and environmental factors that influence eating behavior.
2. Discuss short-term and long-term intervention strategies for improving dietary behavior.
3. Compare and contrast individualized interventions versus community or population-wide interventions.
4. Understand the advantages of using an ecological model as the approach for planning effective dietary behavior change strategies.

The field and science of nutrition seem to be constantly changing. This keeps the work interesting for the nutrition professional, but for the average person nutrition can be quite confusing. It is no wonder that many people tend to just follow the most current diet trend or, alternatively, abstain from following any dietary recommendations. These latter individuals figure the advice will change soon anyway. Even when people are motivated to make positive changes in their eating habits, the environment in which they live, work, or attend school makes continuing healthy behaviors difficult. This is why an ecological approach to intervening in eating behaviors will make the strongest impact in causing and sustaining positive change. Furthermore, we must enlist and intervene in all sectors of society—individuals, families, schools, communities, employers, healthcare providers, mass media, and government. When all these players in all the various settings work together, favorable health outcomes can be achieved.

> **Ecological approach**—A framework that identifies multiple levels of influence (or factors) in the design, implementation, and evaluation of health promotion programs.[1]

Current Eating Trends

In the past two decades, we have seen an increase in nutritional labeling information on packaged foods, greater availability of healthy choices, and more organic foods in the marketplace and in some restaurants. The average daily consumption of vegetables, fruits, and grain products also increased during the 1990s.[2] The percentage of energy consumption from saturated fat over the last 30 years has declined; however, the total amount of fat in grams increased between 1981 and 2000.[3,4] Additionally, Americans are actually eating on average 250–300 calories more per day, much of it from carbohydrates, especially refined sugars.[3,5] Data from the National Health and Nutrition Examination Survey (NHANES) for 1971–2000 indicate similar trends in intake. According to the U.S. Department of Agriculture (USDA) survey data for 1977–1996, factors contributing to the increase in energy intake in the United States include consumption of food away from home; increased calorie consumption from salty snacks, soft drinks, and pizza[4]; and larger portion sizes.[5,6]

The increase in portion sizes for restaurant and processed foods and beverages has occurred concurrently with increases in the prevalence of obesity. The average fast food burger, which weighed approximately 1 ounce in 1957, weighs up to 6 ounces now; the typical serving of soda, which was 8 fluid ounces in 1957, is now 32 to 64 fluid ounces; and the average theater serving of popcorn, which was 3 cups in 1957, is now 16 cups.[7]

> Remember that for adults, overweight is a BMI of 25–29.9 and obesity is a BMI > 30.

In the 1990s, dietary fat was deemed the "enemy;" hence, the food industry responded with a reduced-fat or fat-free version of nearly every packaged food available in the market, from cheese to crackers, pepperoni, and ice cream. Although these foods are lower in fat, they are not necessarily any lower in energy density than their full-fat counterparts. This fact contributes to Americans' confusion about healthy food options. A further result of America's dietary and body fat phobia and dieting practices is that many individuals, unfortunately, found themselves heavier than before and with an unfavorable blood lipid profile. More specifically, people developed higher triglyceride levels (also known more recently as triacylglycerol) and decreased their levels of high density lipids (HDLs).[8-10] The reason for this may be because when individuals deliberately avoid dietary fat, the result is a much higher intake of carbohydrates. However, this increase in carbohydrate consumption is not from healthful fruits, vegetables, and whole grains, but primarily from sugars and processed "white flour" carbohydrates.

Now the pendulum on diet composition has swung in the other direction. Many dieters are shunning carbohydrate-containing foods in favor of foods high in protein and fat, such as cheese, bacon, and all types of meats. A typical meal of a person on a "low-carb" diet might be a cheeseburger with lettuce and tomato without the bun, or eating the cheese and sauce from a pizza, but not the crust. Many Americans have forgone fat gram counting in favor of carbohydrate counting, and the food industry is again catering to this diet trend. Supermarkets and some restaurant chains now sell "low-carb" milk,

> **Blood lipid profile**—A group of blood tests that are often ordered to determine risk of coronary heart disease. The lipid profile includes total cholesterol, HDLs, LDLs, and triglycerides.
>
> **Triglycerides**—These store energy, which is housed in fatty tissue and is gradually released between meals to meet the body's needs. High levels of triglycerides in the blood may be associated with coronary artery disease.

bread, pasta, and cereals. Restaurants offering low-carb meals have opened to the delight of many dieters. Many similar restaurants may follow suit if the popularity of this diet fad continues.

The average American purchases and consumes between 40% and 50% of meals and snacks away from home.[11] These foods tend to be higher in calories and fat, lower in fiber, and larger in portion sizes than what would be eaten at home. In addition, snacks are occupying a bigger proportion of the average American diet. In 1977, snacks comprised 11.3% of the total caloric intake; and in 1996, 17.7% of total calories were obtained from snacks.[11] This is a 60% increase during the span of 18 years. Snacks are now a booming segment of sales in the food industry, which parallels the snacking habits of Americans.

Eating is a normative, acceptable behavior in almost any setting, such as in the car, at meetings, at your desk at work, and in theatres and sporting events. Thus, eating and drinking on-the-go is also a normal everyday occurrence for commuters and multi-taskers with packed schedules. In contrast, ordering food or coffee to go in some countries is an unknown concept. As an example, cars in Japan do not have drink holders. Many of us have forgone the pleasurable, slower pace needed to truly enjoy a meal. Eating too fast is a habit many individuals admit to, which contributes to overeating. Of interest is a transcontinental study, conducted in 2003, comparing the amount of time spent eating in a McDonald's in Paris and one in Philadelphia.[12] Given that portion sizes are bigger in the United States compared to other countries, one might expect meals to take longer to eat. However, in Philadelphia, people on average finished their meals in 14.4 minutes, compared to 22.2 minutes in Paris.

Hectic schedules and less time for food shopping, preparation, and cooking at home has moved convenience to the top of the list that dictates food choice. "Our nation is a car culture," which led to the birth of drive-in restaurant chains, says Eric Schlosser in his book *Fast Food Nation*. "People are so lazy they don't even want to get out of them to eat!" said Jesse G. Kirby, the founder of an early drive-in restaurant chain.[13] However, the way our physical environment has been designed—evolving into suburban sprawl or car-centric cities throughout the United States—has made it unrealistic or unsafe to shop, run errands, or just go out on foot or by bike. The good news is that the city environment is beginning to change, as the Centers for Disease Control and Prevention (CDC) and other government agencies are recognizing the need to enlist city planners, architects, researchers, and transportation engineers to re-design cities and make them pedestrian-centered.[14,15]

Since the American lifestyle will likely not change in the immediate future, more options for healthy, convenient eating are needed. Some examples include low-fat prepared foods in supermarkets, an increased number and variety of restaurants that serve "lighter fare," the display of nutrition facts on menus, and drive-through "fast food" type establishments serving predominantly healthy choices. However, an essential factor for individuals is motivation to eat better and to become educated on the benefits of doing so.

Obesity in America

Two-thirds of American adults are overweight, and 50% of those overweight are considered to be obese. Obesity is an epidemic and one of the most complex public health issues that we have yet to fully understand, treat, and prevent. It will soon surpass smoking (if it hasn't already) as the strongest risk factor contributing to the top major causes of death in our country. What we do know is that nothing short of intense efforts from all sectors of society will make a difference in curbing this tidal wave of weight upon the health of Americans. According to a study of national costs attributed to both overweight and obesity, medical expenses accounted for 9.1% of total U.S. medical expenditures in 1998, and may have reached as high as $78.5 billion ($92.6 billion in 2002 dollars).[16]

The increasing prevalence of obesity has greatly increased the risk of chronic diseases for all age segments. Children and adolescents are presently showing the greatest increase, which is a sobering issue that has made some public health officials fear and predict that this present generation of children may be the first to live shorter life spans than their parents. Thus, the rationale exists behind the increase in interventions and social marketing programs specifically targeting youth.

This chapter strives to present some strategies and interventions that have shown promise in improving the nutritional health of adults and children. (See Chapter 5 for nutritional interventions for children.) An improvement in Americans' nutritional habits should help rein in the rise in obesity and the insurmountable healthcare costs the nation faces.

Dieting

Despite the billions of dollars that Americans continue to spend yearly on diets and weight loss drugs, products, and programs, the prevalence of obesity continues to increase at alarming rates. Clearly, dieting alone is not the answer, and actually may be causing additional harm, as well as further weight gain.

For now, diets and dieting books have moved away from counting calories as the method of controlling food intake to manage weight. Instead, the focus is on consuming directed proportions of macro-nutrients (fat, protein, and carbohydrates). Other diets promote eating disproportional and high amounts of fat and protein while keeping the carbohydrate amount quite low, at the expense of forgoing the known beneficial, cancer-preventive food groups of vegetables, fruits, and whole grains.[17] Many individuals desperately want to lose weight, and even those educated in the areas of nutrition and health will follow a diet that promises quick weight loss at the expense of health, nutrition, and even life. This is a major challenge for nutritionists, who attempt to educate the public on the harm of fad diets only to be ignored by the determined dieter.

For the obese patient and/or chronic dieter, nutritionists, behavioral therapists, physicians, and other health professionals who have influence over a patient's eating habits have a responsibility to educate the public about diets that do not work in the long term. When an individual goes "on a diet," the person often may successfully lose weight regardless of the type of diet. However, being *on a diet* implies that you will at some point in time come *off the diet*, which just leads to weight regain because no permanent dietary changes have been made. Only when an individual is ready and willing to make permanent, lifelong changes is he or she able to lose weight and keep it off. Helping an individual make a few small lasting changes in his or her eating behavior is an important goal, as opposed to facilitating many major changes for immediate, quick weight loss.

Trans-Fat

The public has become increasingly aware of the harm that trans-fatty acids (TFAs) can do to health, and this issue has become of great concern to many. Unfortunately, the amount of TFAs in North Americans' diets has increased markedly during the past decade. This increase can wreak havoc on individuals' blood lipid profile and thereby increase the risk of heart disease. We now know that trans-fat is more harmful in the diet than saturated fat in raising the

> **Low density lipoproteins (LDLs)—** Protein molecules that carry cholesterol in the blood and around the body for use by various cells.
>
> **High density lipoproteins (HDLs)—** Protein molecules that carry cholesterol back from tissues or organs to the liver, where cholesterol will be degraded or recycled.
>
> **Lipoprotein (a)—** A cholesterol-rich particle found in human plasma that combines structural elements from the lipoprotein and blood clotting systems and that is associated with premature coronary heart disease and stroke.

risk of developing cardiovascular disease. Although it is clear that saturated fat can raise low density lipoproteins (LDLs) in the blood, trans-fat can raise LDLs and also decreased high density lipoproteins (HDLs). In addition, TFAs, but not saturated fatty acids, tend to increase the levels of the highly atherogenic lipoprotein known as lipoprotein (a).[18]

Fortunately, the government, via the Food and Drug Administration (FDA), has responded by requiring that food manufacturers of packaged goods list the trans-fat content on the nutrition facts label starting by 2006. This should enable the average consumer to more easily choose among the plethora of packaged foods and select the more healthful option by a quick glance at the nutrition facts label, instead of a longer screening of all the ingredients. Some manufacturers have already begun labeling their products with their trans-fat content. This is a wise marketing ploy that appeals to the health-conscious consumer, especially if the product is made trans-fat free, as some spreadable butter companies and snack food manufacturers have already done.

Sadly, individuals who frequent fast food establishments would likely have a high trans-fat intake because partially hydrogenated oils are used for cooking and frying all of the fare. When Dr. Walter Willett, Chairman of the Nutrition Department of the Harvard School of Public Health, was asked, "What specific public health intervention do you think would make the greatest impact in helping people actually eat healthier?" He replied, "Although no single intervention will solve all our nutritional problems, a ban on the use of partially hydrogenated fats would have an enormous impact, in part because the whole population would benefit almost immediately."[19]

Until TFAs are completely eliminated from use in foods, education, public pressure, and consumer demand for the use of healthy oils by food manufacturers and restaurants remain as important strategies to advocate for our health.

Changing Eating Behavior

Current public health efforts tend to focus on reducing the prevalence of specific diseases, such as cardiovascular disease or cancer, by reducing blood cholesterol levels or improving screening practices. However, these efforts need to be balanced by addressing basic behavioral and social influences on food choice that may cause or prevent disease. To elucidate, we know that individuals who consume a diet rich in vegetables, fruits, and whole grains may reduce their risk of developing cardiovascular disease and certain cancers.[16] Unfortunately, among certain ethnic and socioeconomic groups, significant variations and disparities in disease exist. This can be partly due to minimized access to healthy foods, less offerings of good supermarkets, and, therefore, decreased variety of fresh, affordable produce and low-fat products in their community.[20] In addition, these communities often have many fast food establishments and small grocery stores that sell high-fat, energy-dense foods. Furthermore, high neighborhood crime rates discourage outdoor activities and limit safe places for walking and bicycling. Even when individuals are given specific dietary advice and physical activity encouragement and are motivated to make changes, the current environment may make follow-through difficult because of substantial barriers to establishing a healthy lifestyle.

The Institute of Medicine (IOM) stated, "Interventions must recognize that people live in social, political, and economic systems that shape behaviors and access to the resources they need to maintain good health."[21] Therefore, even if individual behavior changes are made, this alone is not likely to result in improved health and quality of life without an environment that enables sustenance of those changes. Persons with higher levels of education and socioeconomic status continue to be linked with better health, and are more likely to adopt more healthful behaviors.[22,23]

Making recommended dietary changes can cost more money and may require more knowledge, skill, time, or effort to prepare food. Therefore, understanding psychosocial and environmental influences on food choice and consumption is essential to creating nutrition programs, designing educational messages, and disseminating dietary recommendations that realistically help consumers make healthier dietary changes. According to a report from the IOM, *Promoting Health: Intervention Strategies from Social and Behavioral Research*, "The key to helping people enjoy longer, healthier lives is to understand how to promote behavioral change and create healthier environments."[24] However, some of the most meaningful changes that will have the greatest impact on the public's eating behavior will likely be the most difficult to achieve.

This chapter strives to communicate effective nutrition interventions ranging from individual behavior change strategies to the complex, long-term, costlier, difficult process of affecting policy and greater societal changes. A multilevel approach will have the greatest, most sustaining effect on improving the population's eating behavior. Therefore, using a social ecological model as the theoretical framework from which one plans, creates, researches, applies, and evaluates nutrition interventions would be most effective. The Healthy People 2010 goals are based on a multilevel approach to achieving those goals, as well as the IOM's recent report

The social ecological model—
An approach in which interventions address not only individual intentions and skills, but also the social and physical environmental context of a desired behavior, considering as well all social networks and organizations that share that environment, which will have the most potential for population-wide impact.[27]

on promoting healthy behavior.[25] The social ecological perspective, as it has evolved in behavioral sciences and public health, focuses on the nature of people's transactions with their physical and sociocultural surroundings.[26] (See Figure 6-1.)

Media is a principal source of information and influence on food and nutrition for many.[28] The leverage, or power, of media is its ability to persuade; alter norms, thinking, and behavior; and thereby prompt particular ways of eating.[29] Through experience, we have come to view mass media as a powerful way to promote the consumption of many unhealthy, processed food products. However, mass media can also positively encourage a significant proportion of people to alter their dietary habits. This was exhibited by a simple "1% or less" campaign in Wheeling, West Virginia, which used paid advertising and public relations to encourage members of one community to switch from whole or 2% milk to 1% or fat-free milk.[30] The effectiveness of the campaign was evident by

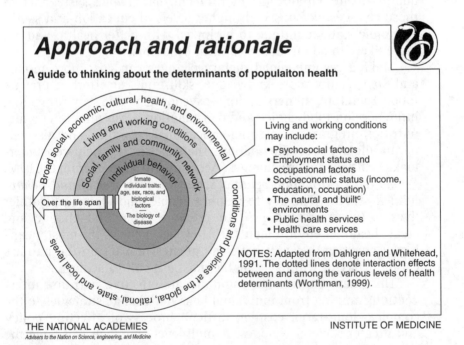

FIGURE 6-1 A useful framework for designing effective nutrition interventions. *Source:* Reprinted from *The Future of the Public's Health in the 21st Century.* ©2002 by the National Academy of Sciences. Courtesy of the National Academies Press, Washington, D.C.

a 17% increase in low-fat milk sales one month after the campaign; this increase was maintained at the 6-month follow-up. Pre- and post-telephone surveys revealed that 34.1% of high-fat milk drinkers had switched to low-fat milk in the intervention community compared to 3.6% in the control community (p < 0.0001).

This mass-media-based "1% or less" milk campaign was replicated by the California Adolescent Nutrition and Fitness Program in Spanish to reach predominantly Latino American communities in Santa Paula (in 1999) and East Los Angeles (in 2000).[31] Campaign elements included paid radio and print ads, point-of-purchase advertising, milk taste tests, community presentations, public relations, and a school-based program. After the 6-week campaign, sales of 1% and fat-free milk rose 60% in Santa Paula. A 6-month follow-up survey of retailers found that a large portion (25%) of this growth in sales was maintained.

The Food Industry

In 1988, the World Health Organization (WHO) recommended that sugars should account for no more than 10% of daily energy intake.[32] This recommendation has not received universal acceptance, especially from the food industry. This is no surprise given that the industry's most lucrative products are processed foods, laden with sugar and/or salt, that are calorically dense. This explains why new products like these enter the marketplace almost daily. Given the plethora of choices, selecting a granola bar or snack cracker makes food shopping a much lengthier, more complicated process. A large array of choices can also contribute to overeating. When presented with more variety, individuals eat more. When food options are more monotonous, individuals tend to eat less. Reducing easy access to energy-dense foods could help limit the opportunities for overeating.[33]

The food industry is colossal and can exert powerful influence on government policy via lobbying techniques.[34] Although the food industry may be an important factor contributing to the poor nutritional habits of consumers, industry must be enlisted now as part of the solution. In the past, industry has been a key player in curing and preventing nutritional deficiencies by vitamin and mineral fortification of foods.[34] Remember also that the food industry is quite responsive to consumer and market demands; therefore, as more grass-roots and consumer groups call for healthier food choices as a top priority, the industry can and will respond.

Schools

Schools are practical, ideal places to reach thousands of children to educate them about healthy eating behaviors. Scientific consensus panel reports have consistently recommended that children and adolescents eat at least five servings of fruit and vegetables daily and participate in daily physical activity to reduce the risk of chronic disease and premature death; however, youth are not meeting policy standards for these health behaviors.[25] Children should be a major focus of intervention efforts because many of the risk factors observed in adults can be detected in childhood, such as high blood pressure and cholesterol, as well as being overweight. There is considerable evidence that middle school years and adolescence are critical periods for influencing eating behavior, as more food choices are being made independently from parents as children grow older. For example, fruit consumption decreased by 41% between grades 3 and 8 in one cohort study.[35] In a longitudinal study following adolescents from 6th through 12th grade, researchers found that healthful and unhealthful behaviors that emerged by 6th grade continued throughout high school.[36] This is evidence for promoting healthful habits to children early during middle school and elementary school.

The National Heart, Lung, and Blood Institute (NHLBI) sponsored one of the largest school-based health promotion trials, the Child and Adolescent Trial for Cardiovascular Health (CATCH), which was implemented in 96 public elementary schools from 1991 to 1995.[37] This study was designed to decrease cardiovascular risk factors in children through interventions implemented in the classroom, during physical education class, and in the cafeteria via the school food service. The most significant results were decreases in total fat and saturated fat consumption, as well as increases in physical activity in the children who received the interventions in comparison to the control schools. Five years after the intervention, follow-up studies were conducted and showed that it is possible to maintain and sustain environmental changes to promote healthy behaviors.[38,39] This is encouraging news because many positive health behavior changes seen immediately post-intervention have not always been sustained long term (2+ years). Two of the most important factors in the viability and sustainability of the CATCH intervention in the schools were staff training and a more open and supportive school climate for the health promotion program.[40,41]

Health behavior theories and the literature dictate that the most potent interventions in schools are those that have comprehensive and multiple components. The critical components to changing fruit and vegetable consumption in young children include environmental changes, classroom curriculum, parental involvement, and partnerships with local produce companies. Although limited resources in some states and school districts preclude making multilevel changes, simple environmental changes can be adopted by schools almost immediately. For example, students who received the school-based intervention called Cafeteria Power Plus significantly increased their fruit intake.[42] As part of the intervention, the food service staff were encouraged to increase the choices and appeal of the fruits and vegetables offered in the lunch line and snack cart. The staff also verbally encouraged the students to eat fruits and vegetables by making positive comments when students went through the line.

Schools are an efficient, practical place to influence children's eating habits, because one or two meals and many snacks per week are consumed there. In addition to government programs that were created to provide healthful nutrition, such as the National School Lunch Program and the School Breakfast Program, many schools today offer a greater variety of eating options and opportunities. Unfortunately, aspects of the school environments can overshadow and diminish the benefits these programs were designed to provide. Examples include:

- poor quality and unpalatable food served in the cafeteria (i.e., many greasy, high-fat items and lack of healthy options)
- à la carte programs
- snack bars/carts and vending machines that serve non-nutritious foods
- short lunch periods
- in some cases, students' freedom to leave the premises to buy food elsewhere

Overall, few foods in this environment are low fat; quality fruits and vegetables are rare, and fruit juice is a less prevalent offering than carbonated or sweetened beverages.[43-47] Focus groups and interviews conducted with students, faculty, and staff in two New England middle schools revealed that lack of healthy options and poor quality food were the top barriers to eating healthier. Students stated that if the cafeteria offered fruits and vegetables in greater quantity and quality, they would choose to eat them instead of the less nutritious entrees or snack foods.[47]

Other in-depth focus groups conducted with schoolchildren in grades 2 through 11, randomly selected from 34 schools in Australia, elucidated the major perceived benefits and barriers to healthful eating and physical activity.[48] The most important benefits voiced by the children were the ability to think better, improved physical performance, increased energy, and mentally feeling better about oneself. The main barriers to eating healthy were convenience of less healthful alternatives, taste, peer pressure, lack of parental and school support, and few good role models. To overcome these barriers, the students in grades 5 through 11 suggested strategies that included:

- Parental support (availability of healthier foods at home)
- Planning to eat healthier by carrying nutritious foods to school
- Not taking money to school
- Reducing the availability of "junk food" at home, at school, and in the community

The core of the matter is that if non-nutritious foods and snacks are not available in schools, then students cannot purchase and eat them. Unfortunately, profits from the sale of snack foods, soda, and other sugar-sweetened beverages are used to fund scholarships and school events. Administrators admit to the challenge of relinquishing this kind of funding, especially because of the large sums of money distributed by soft drink companies, known as pouring rights contracts.[34] In exchange for this money (which can total millions of dollars over time), schools formally agree to stock their vending machines only with that particular company's beverages and use its brand exclusively at all games and school-sponsored events. School administrators will need opposing pressure from parents and state legislatures, and also encouragement, to be creative in finding alternative funding sources for student programs that do not compromise students' health. Instead, these vending machines could and should be stocked with healthy options, such as 100% fruit juice, bottled water, flavored seltzer, low-fat and non-fat milk and yogurt, baked pita and potato chips, fresh fruit, low-fat granola bars, nuts, and trail mix.

A one-year nutrition education program in schools in England with the simple message "ditch the fizz" was effective in reducing soda intake in children ages 7 to 11.[49] The intervention classrooms received a one-hour session each school term for 12 months that educated the children on the benefits of decreased sugar consumption from soda, such as improving overall well-being and dental health. The children completed diaries at the beginning and end of the trial, reporting on drinks consumed over 3 days. Consumption of carbonated drinks dropped by an average of 0.6 glasses over 3 days among the intervention children, but increased by 0.2 glasses among the children not receiving the educational session. The intervention group dropped 0.2% in prevalence of overweight compared to the control classrooms, where the percentage of overweight and obese children increased by 7.5%. This English trial has important implications because it reiterates what other research has shown—that there is an association between consumption of sugar-sweetened drinks and obesity in children.[50-52]

The American Academy of Pediatrics (AAP) Committee on School Health has recently published a statement to inform pediatricians, other healthcare professionals, parents, superintendents, and school board members about the nutritional concerns and health implications of soft drinks in schools:

> Potential health problems associated with a high intake of sweetened drinks include: 1) overweight or obesity due to excess calories; 2) displacement of milk consumption, resulting in calcium deficiency with a resultant risk of osteoporosis and fractures; and 3) dental caries and potential enamel erosion. A clearly defined, district-wide policy that restricts the sale of soft drinks will safeguard against health problems as a result of over-consumption of these nonnutritive, highly caloric beverages.[53]

The AAP appears to be speaking out against the pouring rights contracts between schools and the beverage companies. The good news is that school districts in Los Angeles, Philadelphia, San Francisco, Chicago, and New York City, as well as numerous smaller districts, are leading the way by taking steps to ban the sale of soft drinks during the school day. California and Texas have issued statewide bans on soft-drink sales in elementary and middle schools. Texas, New York City, and Los Angeles have actually taken the next important step by restricting the sale of potato chips, candy, and other junk food.[54]

Peer health education programs are also important in schools because the ability to tap into social networks and cliques can increase the adoption of behavior changes, which may not otherwise occur from pure teacher-led instruction. Adolescence is a time of autonomy, but also social conformity to peers. This can be advantageous if healthy norms and strategic changes can be inoculated into the group via the influential leaders of the cliques and social networks. A multicomponent, school-based intervention with a peer leader component conducted in 2002 showed the largest increase in fruit and vegetable consumption, as well as increased consumption of lower fat foods, compared to students who were exposed to classroom and environmental changes only.[55] However, a recent randomized controlled trial conducted in middle schools using a socioecological model (environmental changes) to improve nutrition and physical activity resulted in significant change in physical activity for the boys. The girls in this study did not show a change in physical activity habits.[56] Furthermore, the interventions did not help decrease dietary fat intake in these school children. More research with rigorous evaluation methods is needed to reveal why particular interventions may be effective in some schools and, perhaps, not in others.

In conclusion, because school-aged children and adolescents spend much of their day in schools and eat numerous meals, snacks, and beverages there, offering healthy food choices is the socially responsible thing to do. (Refer back to Chapter 1 on ethical responsibilities in public health.) In addition to providing a healthier food environment, students will be enabled to eat more nutritiously if: 1) access to "junk food" is limited; 2) healthy behavior is the group norm in the school environment; 3) peer leaders and others model nutritious choices; 4) the cafeteria offers appealing vegetables and fruits; and 5) cafeteria staff provide verbal encouragement to eat fruits and vegetables. (For more about obesity in childhood, please see Chapter 5.)

Organizational and Worksite Interventions

A review of 47 studies of worksite health promotion programs that addressed multiple risk factors revealed that almost all provided health education to their employees.[57] A smaller number of the programs (25%) implemented modifications in organizational policy or the work environment to facilitate employee behavior changes. But, imparting knowledge and skills for new health behaviors is not enough; targeting and intercepting workplace norms and eating environments is necessary to support change. Some examples of physical and environmental modifications include policies restricting or banning smoking on the premises, on-site exercise and kitchen facilities, as well as offering healthier fare in the cafeteria and vending machines. We have learned from existing studies that greater effort is needed to modify social factors and physical settings of the worksites. Also, having an understanding of the organizational climate and culture (e.g., attitudes, beliefs, needs, and resources of the members), including the organization's receptivity to health innovation, is important to create effective behavioral change interventions.[58]

Conducting solid formative research in the organization will elucidate perceptions and barriers to change. In addition, having all the relevant stakeholders and key figures participate in planning and conducting the health-promoting activities will help facilitate and maintain success in the organization. Management plays the important role of creating a work culture. For example, the management can provide eating norms in which employees can take a reasonable amount of time to eat a healthy lunch, as opposed to a work environment where individuals are expected to just "work through lunch" or eat at their desk. Employees, equipped with the knowledge and skills in a supportive environment with healthy norms, are much more likely to move into or remain in action and maintenance stages of change.[59,60]

Employees at their worksites are a captive audience and are ideal for intervention delivery. In particular, high traffic areas, such as the cafeteria and break rooms, are strategic places to deliver brief education. Some examples of low-intensity work-based nutrition interventions that have shown at least short-term beneficial results, such as a reduction in blood cholesterol levels,[61] include:

- Computer programs that appraise individual health risk
- Group education sessions
- Interactive activities with food sampling and recipes
- Contests (e.g., winners are individuals who exercise three times a week for one month or eat five fruits and vegetables per day for a month)
- Simple finger-prick blood glucose and cholesterol screenings accompanied by a dietitian to provide brief counseling, referrals, and follow-up plans[62]
- Printed information and materials for employees to take home

Having a personally tailored behavioral component (such as personalized education and/or a follow-up phone call) has been shown to promote continued employee participation in follow-up health screening compliance.[63]

Although implementation of nutrition activities has often been successful initially in numerous worksites, these health-promoting activities have generally not been sustainable 2 years post-intervention.[64] Upper management should increase their efforts in building capacity for sustaining health-enhancing activities in the organization that will facilitate increased commitment and follow-through by employees.

Family and Friends

The important influence of supportive family relationships and other social ties for good health is widely accepted in the scientific community.[65, 66] Family members and family dynamics are interconnected and mutually influential. Whether we realize or are conscious of this, family and friends influence our consumption of certain foods by modeling healthy or unhealthy choices by peer pressure (e.g., "You have to have some apple pie, I made it especially for you."). Parents or caregivers initially play the most influential role in a young child's development of eating preferences, habits, or patterns. Parenting and feeding styles will either foster or limit a child's ability to regulate their caloric intake by altering their responsiveness to internal or external cues of hunger and satiety.[67, 68] According to both Golan and Birch,[69,70] parents play a key role in preventing or treating overweight/obesity in their children. More specifically, parents who are overweight and are struggling to adopt healthier eating habits for themselves, or who are concerned about their children's risk for overweight, may adopt controlling or restrictive child-feeding practices in an attempt to prevent obesity in their children. This type of eating environment, which is inadvertently created by caring parents who only want the best for their children, may create or exacerbate an unhealthy eating pattern or genetic predisposition already present in their children.

In a longitudinal study, Caucasian girls, ages 5 to 9, with mothers that used restrictive feeding practices, ate in the absence of hunger.[71] These girls were less able to regulate their appetite and hunger needs by internal mechanisms. This point is particularly important given the rising rate of overweight and obese children and the importance of intervening to prevent parents from using restrictive feeding practices. Instead, parents need education on efficacious methods to promote healthier eating habits and physical activity with their overweight children.

How can parents foster the development of self-regulation in children? The development of self-regulation is grounded in a child's feelings of competence, autonomy, and connectedness.[72] When parents provide structure and guidelines for meals, as well as the reasons behind the guidelines, this motivates compliance and internalization for children. In addition, when parents support autonomy in their children and provide a warm, positive connection with them, this motivates compliance and affirms competence.[72]

Families are imbedded in a greater ecology, and therefore are subject to outside influences. Environments provide increased opportunities and resources, thus placing constraints on parental choices.[72] An important public health goal is to identify families that are at greater risk for poorer eating habits, such as those with limited income, high levels of stress, parents with obesity, or a single working parent, and provide a family-focused intervention relevant to their circumstances. This would be an opportunity to provide social support and/or education, enabling the provision of healthy meals in the home. Acquiring an understanding of parents' beliefs and their hierarchy of goals is necessary in order to impact or change parenting practices. A review of "parent education" literature reveals these three important principles for educating parents:

1. Information must be relevant to their life and family circumstances (e.g., both parents work full-time; therefore, home-cooked meals are not always realistic).
2. Information should come from a trusted source.
3. Information must be usable and accessible.[73, 74]

The advice parents receive from professionals must be practical, meaning that parents need to know not only what to do, but also how to do it within the constraints of their present circumstances. The modality of the education provided must also match the parents' learning style.[72] Printed materials can be helpful to some, but a video (available in different languages) can be a better method if there is a language barrier or literacy issues.

Interventions should take advantage of and build upon the momentum created by family transitions and changes, such as a couple expecting their first baby. Pediatric healthcare providers could begin disseminating advice to new parents during infancy on how to create a child who is a "healthy eater." This would give parents the opportunity and time it takes to begin the challenging process of altering suboptimal eating habits and replacing them with more healthful patterns. The result would be a home environment more conducive to healthy eating being the norm, since parental modeling of good habits is most influential in forming a child's eating pattern. How and where does a child initially learn about healthy foods and patterns of eating? Primarily, via exposure to foods from parents or caregivers. Parents also need to understand the detriments of coercive feeding practices and be given alternatives to restricting food and pressuring children to eat. Helpful practical advice for parents could include:

- How to promote acceptance of new foods by children, which entails offering the food repeatedly (10 different instances has been suggested)[75]

- Providing parents with easy-to-use, healthy recipes and tips on simple, quick, and inexpensive meals
- Recommendations on proper portion sizes from each food group
- How to avoid food struggles with picky eaters

Feeding children healthily and handling picky eaters can be two of the more stressful or frustrating aspects of child rearing. Picky eaters (those resistant to eating many familiar foods) and children with neophobia (reluctance to try new foods) are two different and distinct consumption behaviors. It is no surprise that vegetables are the one food group children are less apt to consume in adequate amounts, compared to children with neither pickiness nor neophobia. Given that vegetable intake among children is well below recommended levels in the United States, finding effective means to increase vegetable intake among children is important and needed.

One encouraging research study involving 192 seven-year-old girls and their parents revealed predictors of pickiness in girls, which are primarily environmental or experiential factors subject to change,[76] and not a genetically linked or normal trait of children as some may believe. Picky girls had mothers who:

- Perceived their family to have little time to eat healthful foods
- Had less variety in their vegetable intake
- Breastfed for fewer than 6 months

One explanation for this last finding is that breastfed children are exposed early in life to a diversity of flavors via breast milk (if the mother consumed a variety of foods in her diet).[76] These findings reveal important ways for dietitians, nutritionists, and other healthcare practitioners to intervene and prevent pickiness in children. Education should include encouraging:

- Longer duration of breastfeeding
- Parental modeling of eating a greater variety of vegetables
- The use of simple methods and time-saving preparation techniques for vegetables

For adolescents, the strongest correlation for vegetable and fruit intake are home availability of these foods and taste preferences for them.[77] However, this study found that even if taste preferences for fruits and vegetables was low among these adolescents, if fruits and vegetables were available, intake increased nevertheless. Parents, therefore, need to be encouraged to purchase produce regularly and have fruits and vegetables available in the home and offered at all meals as much as possible.

An example of a family nutrition intervention program includes "The High 5 Low Fat" nutrition intervention as part of the Parents as Teachers Program, which targets African American parents.[78]

Trained African American parents act as role models and disseminate the information via personal visits, group sessions, and newsletters to other parents. This intervention has been shown to improve the intake of fruits and vegetables, as well as lower overall dietary fat for parents receiving the intervention.

Another example of the importance of family support in promoting better health was shown in a study conducted with individuals with diabetes in a Diné (Navajo) Native American population. Individuals with active family nutritional support showed greater control in HgA(1c) (an indicator of longer term blood glucose control) and total cholesterol and triglyceride levels, compared to individuals with less family involvement.[79] The type of support these individuals received and reported included a family member helping with shopping and cooking healthy meals, or family members who would eat low-fat, low-sugar foods with them. These persons with diabetes and this type of family support demonstrated and improved self-care behavior.

In addition, a family-focused component that was added to a worksite intervention showed that consumption of fruits and vegetables was directly associated with level of household support for healthy eating.[80] Worksite interventions, with a component involving family members, has proven more effective than targeting the worksite alone.[80–82]

We need to recognize and acquire a better understanding of the influential role and burden that society must share in helping prevent obesity and promote opportunities and easier access to healthy food choices for children and adults. "Children are most vulnerable to the persuasive appeals by food marketers which can hook them with brand new processed products that enter the market daily."[83] Strong public policies and regulations should be created to limit advertising of non-nutritious foods to children. There will be more to follow on this issue in Chapters 7 and 8.

Community Interventions

A community can be any grouping of individuals who have a shared sense of identity or a common thread that draws all of them together. Therefore, a community can be a geographic area of persons, but is not necessarily limited to this.[21] Examples of communities can be a certain ethnic group; a professional group, such as small business owners; or a group of individuals who are all cancer survivors. The collective strength of a community to promote its own health is beyond the ability of any single person to control or change. That is what differentiates the effectiveness of community intervention from individual behavior change. Even individuals with few social ties, but who reside in socially cohesive communities, do not appear to suffer the same adverse health consequences as do socially isolated people living in less cohesive communities.[84, 85]

Valuable lessons have been learned from various community change interventions. They include the importance of the following: [86]

- Engaging the community, rather than an outside organizer or researcher, to define needs and priorities
- Identifying and building upon the strengths, assets, and resources of the community's members
- Being flexible and tailoring the change strategies to each particular community's context and milieu
- Building long-term sustainability of programs and identifying diversified sources of funding

Several community-based studies have shown that it is possible to change consumers' overall fat intake, without deliberate education on limiting fat intake, by increasing the availability and decreasing the cost of healthful products.[68] However, in some large, extensive community studies where this was done, no significant changes in dietary habits were observed. This suggests that perhaps more focused studies within high-risk subgroups, such as minority and low-literacy populations, may be more fruitful. In fact, a number of public health agencies and their academic, managed care, community health center, and other community partners have begun to implement smaller-scale cardiovascular disease prevention projects. A good example was the 15 WISEWOMAN projects, funded by the CDC, which targeted low-income, predominantly ethnic minority women screened by the Breast and Cervical Cancer Early Detection Program. The WISEWOMAN project successfully implemented screenings for high blood pressure, blood glucose, and total cholesterol in conjunction with cancer screenings the women were already receiving. This program was deemed successful in reaching underserved women, developing a more comprehensive women's health model, strengthening linkages to primary health care, experimenting with innovative behavioral interventions, and tapping into women's roles as social support providers and family/community gatekeepers.[87]

Churches and Places of Worship

Despite continued efforts to reduce health disparities among diverse populations in the United States, certain ethnic groups are faced with higher disease risk and death rates. African Americans continue to be disproportionately affected by all causes of disease compared to other groups. Greater effort is needed to reach this segment of the population with prevention strategies. Unfortunately, African Americans are more likely to be distrustful of investigators given negative historical events (e.g., the Tuskegee Institute) and sub-par medical access and care they tend to receive. The church, therefore, has become an ideal channel and setting for reaching members of this community with health education, given the high regard and level of trust members have for their pastors. For many African American families, life centers on the church and its activities, and therefore the church exerts a high degree of influence.[88]

Several interventions conducted in churches have shown clinically meaningful decreases in disease risk outcomes, such as body weight, blood pressure, and waist circumference.[89-91] Some of the specific successful behavioral and dietary outcomes these programs have achieved include decreased fat and sodium intake; increased fruit, vegetable, and fiber intake; and increased physical activity. One example of this type of intervention is the PRAISE! (Partnership to Reach African Americans to Increase Smart Eating) project, which was conducted in 60 churches in 8 North Carolina counties and that used a community-based participatory research (CBPR) approach.[92] The CBPR approach views community participants as partners in the research process, rather than just subjects upon whom research is conducted. At least one randomized clinical trial so far has found that research designed with a CBPR approach is associated with high levels of trust and a perceived benefit of satisfaction with the research process.[93]

Meals, coffee, and refreshments are common accompaniments to fellowship in church social gatherings and meetings. These gatherings afford an opportune setting for dietary intervention, such as offering lower fat dishes and recipes and incorporating more vegetables and fruits. This is one reason the National Institute of Health (NIH) has created a program titled, "Body & Soul: A Celebration of Healthy Eating and Living."[94] This program helps empower church members to be more physically active and to eat five to nine servings of fruits and vegetables every day for better health. The combined elements of this program include pastoral leadership, health education, an environment in church that supports healthy eating, and peer counseling.

Reaching Older Adults

Innovative and effective health promotion interventions targeted at older adults, within a public health framework, are becoming increasingly important as the U.S. population ages. The benefits of healthier lifestyles for older adults include increased functional ability, delaying the onset of disease, and an improved quality of life, which are important goals in program planning for this population.[95]

Specific nutritional goals for elders should include increasing the intake of vegetables, fruits, and calcium-rich foods, just like most segments of the population.[96] Some may think that interventions targeted toward adults over age 55 seem to have a limited effect, given the difficulty of changing nearly a lifetime of eating habits and behaviors. However, a review of the literature published from 1990 to 2003 regarding nutrition interventions targeting older adults revealed many positive outcomes. Features of the most effective nutrition programs included using the appropriate behavior change theory; limiting the education to one or two key messages; providing hands-on activities, incentives, and access to health professionals; reinforcing and personalizing the health messages; and a social environment that supports healthy behavior.[97]

An example of a community intervention targeting older adults was a creative partnership established among Tri-Parish Nursing Ministries, The Arthritis Foundation, Missouri Extension Services, and the Saint Louis County Department of Health.[98] The goal was to promote the quality of life for older adults through physical activity and health education messages. Twenty-nine participants met twice a week in a local church to exercise for one hour with a trainer from PACE (People with Arthritis Can Exercise). The participants received 30 minutes of nutrition education from a Saint Louis County registered dietitian using the Missouri Extension's Health for Everybody program. The participation rate for the program was 62% at the end of 6 weeks. The mean age of participants was 74 years. All participants reported favorably, indicating that they enjoyed sessions and "learned something new." Unfortunately, the reasons why some participants dropped out are unknown. Feedback also revealed that participants even asked for more ways to exercise outside of class. Providing older adults with encouragement, a place to exercise, and an opportunity to learn healthy eating tips could potentially make a significant difference in improving quality of life for this segment of the population.

Individual and Group Counseling

Until greater social change occurs and the long-term solution to improve our nation's nutrition and health is realized, nutritionists and other health educators play an important role in helping individuals manage better within our current "toxic food environment," as some have termed it.[34] Educating individuals and equipping people with tools and strategies is critical to resist or combat the powerful "eat more" marketing messages that we are constantly bombarded with by the food and restaurant industries.[34]

Brief counseling that incorporates principles of motivational interviewing and patient-centered behavioral change strategies have shown promise in medical settings.[99] For example, a randomized study of 206 adult patients with type 2 diabetes combined patient-centered self-management with interactive computer technology to improve dietary behaviors and decrease serum cholesterol levels.[99] This study integrated feasible, appealing behavioral interventions into the clinic flow of a primary care office. The intervention involved a sequence of the following: a 15-minute touch-screen computer assessment, which helped subjects identify dietary goals and barriers to accomplishing these goals; immediate scoring and two tailored feedback/goal printouts summarizing the information (one for the patient and one for the physician); a 20-second motivational message emphasizing the importance of the goal the patient had selected; a 15–20 minute meeting with a health educator to review the patient's goal and collaboratively develop barriers-based problem-solving strategies; and lastly, two brief follow-up phone calls from the health educator to check on progress. This sequence was repeated at a regular 3-month follow-up visit. The intervention group showed greater improvements in total and saturated dietary fat intake, as well as serum cholesterol levels, compared to the control group. Additionally, results were maintained at 12-month follow-up and the intervention proved to be cost-effective.

> **Motivational interviewing—**
> A directive, client-centered counseling style for eliciting behavior change by helping clients to explore and resolve ambivalence. Compared with nondirective counseling, it is more focused and goal-directed. Motivation to change is elicited from the client and not imposed by the counselor.[100]

Outside the medical setting, motivational interviewing (MI) techniques, which have traditionally been used for counseling patients with addictive behaviors, are showing promise in community settings with counselors via telephone to improve eating behaviors and increase physical activity.[101]

The U.S. Preventive Services Task Force (USPSTF) has extensively reviewed the literature between 1966 and December 2001 regarding the effectiveness of counseling to promote a healthy diet among patients in primary care settings.[102] They found that dietary counseling produces modest changes in self-reported consumption of saturated fat, fruits and vegetables, and possibly dietary fiber. More intensive interventions were more likely to produce greater changes than brief interventions, but may be more difficult to apply in typical primary care visits. Interventions using interactive health communications, including computer-generated telephone or mail messages, can also produce moderate dietary changes.

Since that extensive review by the USPSTF, two additional studies on counseling to produce dietary change have been published, which are consistent with the review's conclusion. The results showed increases in the consumption of fruits and vegetables, as well as a decrease in dietary fat intake. Between the two studies, patients exhibited significant improvements following either two 45-minute counseling sessions, including computer interaction,[103] or two 15-minute individual counseling sessions by research nurses.[104]

The Role of Government

Individual counseling in a healthcare setting and public health interventions in a variety of settings play significant roles in bringing preventative nutrition to the forefront. However, those methods as presently implemented are still limited in their effectiveness. In contrast, laws and regulations have proven to play a decisive and more effective role in advancing the public's health. Public health's contribution is particularly evident in the prevention and control of communicable diseases and in the realm of injury prevention, which were the leading causes of death at the beginning of the 20th century. Today, chronic disease is the leading cause of death and disability, but unfortunately we have no systematically developed frameworks for applying law toward preventive efforts.[105] Our strength in protecting the public has still primarily been in our means of responding to acute threats such as the SARS (Severe Acute Respiratory Syndrome) outbreak or, perhaps, terrorism since the attack on September 11, 2001. It is imperative for this country to move from a palliative medical model to one that is prevention-based if we are to make noticeable improvements in Americans' quality of life and control rising healthcare costs. In the relatively few instances where the role of law has been fully applied to the prevention and control of chronic diseases and their risk factors (e.g., tobacco control and smoking prevention), there has been a noteworthy impact on public health, such as a major decrease in smoking rates across the country for most segments of the population.

We have reached a point in healthcare history where we need to fully explore and create comprehensive legal frameworks for preventing and controlling the growing epidemics of obesity, heart disease, stroke, diabetes, and other chronic diseases and their related major risk factors.[106] "These frameworks will be a crucial addition to the tools available to the public health workforce, especially state and local health department program managers, as well as state and national policy makers. They also can assist program managers' interaction with city mayors, legislators, governors, and other policy makers."[106] Legal steps or laws may take the form of constitutional provisions, statutory enactments, regulations, ordinances, government-initiated litigation, court rulings, or policies adopted by public-sector bodies, such as schools and zoning boards. For example, we have seen bans on the sale of sodas and junk foods adopted by certain California schools and zoning boards, as mentioned earlier in this chapter.

Law can also include policies or treaties adopted by international bodies, such as the International Code of Marketing of Breast-Milk Substitutes ("The Code") passed in 1981 by the World Health Organization (WHO). It states that governments should provide information about the superiority of breast-feeding. The Code also outlines measures that would control use of inappropriate marketing practices that can undermine "a mother's ability to breast-feed her baby."[107] The enactment of this code was necessary in an effort to mitigate the aggressive marketing of infant formula by companies in developing countries, where infant mortality rates increased when mothers were disingenuously persuaded to formula-feed instead of breast-feed. The United States did not sign this

International Code until 1994, which was mostly due to the strength and extensive lobbying power of U.S. formula companies.

In 1995, the AAP issued a statement regarding the food industry's marketing effects on children: "Advertising directed at children is inherently deceptive and exploits children less than eight years of age." This strong statement should have set in motion the steps necessary by the federal government to ban junk food advertisements directed at children. The reason these measures have not been taken is again likely due to the strong lobbying powers of the food industry. However, it is time Congress did the ethically responsible thing to protect the most vulnerable, impressionable segment of the population, the children, for the future health of the nation. Norway, Sweden, Australia, Italy, and New Zealand have either banned advertising directed at children altogether or have legislative guidelines restricting it.[54]

Anti-junk food ads that promote healthy eating, via a government-sponsored public service campaign, could be another important strategy to combat the tens of thousands of commercials that the average child sees each year, enticing them to consume high-fat, high-sugar products that are continually being churned out in the marketplace.

Some select laws that have proven effective at promoting better health and preventing disease and injury include those listed in Table 6-1.[105]

TABLE 6-1   Selected Laws for the Prevention of Chronic Diseases and Injuries*

Law	Public Health Issue Addressed	Effectiveness	How It Works
Smoking bans or restrictions	Exposure to environmental tobacco smoke	Strong evidence	Requires behavioral change to change the environment
Tobacco excise taxes	Tobacco initiation and use	Strong evidence	Incurs a financial disincentive to invoke behavior change
Required coverage of cessation services costs	Tobacco use	Sufficient evidence	Requires organizational change that promotes behavioral change
Zoning and land use requirements	Physical inactivity	Review in progress	Requires environmental change to facilitate behavioral change
Child safety seat use laws	Unintentional injuries of children	Strong evidence	Directly requires behavioral change

Law	Public Health Issue Addressed	Effectiveness	How It Works
Safety belt use laws	Unintentional injuries of older children, adolescents, and adults	Strong evidence	Directly requires behavioral change
Blood alcohol concentration limit of 0.08% for operators of motor vehicles	Unintentional injuries of older children, adolescents, and adults	Strong evidence	Primarily provides powerful psychological deterrent to invoke behavioral change; also provides disincentive to invoke behavioral change through fines and other penalties
Sobriety checkpoints for motor vehicle operators	Unintentional injuries of older children, adolescents, and adults	Strong evidence	Provides psychological deterrent to invoke behavioral change
Fluoridation of community water supplies	Dental caries	Strong evidence	Directly changes the physical environment, requiring no action on the part of the target population
Food fortification	Nutritional deficiencies	Strong evidence	Directly changes the physical environment, requiring no action on the part of the target population

*Laws used to denote restrictions, bans, regulations, ordinances, or public policies, as well as legislation.

Source: Reprinted with permission from Mensah GA, Goodman RA, Zaza S, et al. Law as a tool for preventing chronic diseases: Expanding the spectrum of effective public health strategies. *Preventing Chronic Disease,* Jan 2004. Available at: http://www.cdc.gov/pcd/issues/2004/jan/03_0033.htm. Accessed March 18, 2005.

Price Adjustments, Taxation, and Subsidies

Many factors influence our food choices; however, the top four considerations of why we eat what we do are taste, convenience, cost, and nutritional value.[108] Studies reveal that simply lowering the price of healthier foods, including fruits, vegetables, and salad bars in cafeterias, as well as healthy snacks in vending machines in schools and worksites, has proven to be a highly effective method to increase the sales of these items. At minimum, this change in cost can positively change the proportion of sales of healthier choices versus less nutritious ones.[109-111] Price reductions of healthier foods in cafeterias or vending machines in 12 worksites and 12 secondary schools led to increased sales volume, which provided a constant level of profit, indicating a win-win situation for both consumers and food companies. This type of pricing strategy was pilot-tested in a midwestern suburban high school cafeteria during an entire school year.[112] Seven foods were targeted during the intervention: three popular higher fat foods (french fries, cookies, and cheese sauce) and four lower fat foods (fresh fruit, low-fat cookies, low-fat chips, and cereal bars). Prices ranged from $0.35 to $1.00. Prices on the higher fat foods were raised by approximately 10% and prices on the lower fat foods were reduced by approximately 25% for the school year. Sales data collected from school food services showed the revenue from the seven foods were within 5% of revenues estimated for usual price conditions. Therefore, students purchased based on price, which included more lower fat foods at lower prices, as revenue remained relatively unchanged.

In addition, French's study[111] in 2003 examined the impact of a 50% price reduction on fresh fruit and baby carrots in two secondary school cafeterias. Compared with usual price conditions, price reductions resulted in a four-fold increase in fresh fruit sales and a two-fold increase in baby carrot sales. These studies demonstrate the efficacy of price reductions in increasing purchases of more healthful foods in community-based settings, such as worksites and schools.

Paralleling the anti-smoking campaign, taxation on non-nutritious food and soda has been proposed as perhaps the most efficacious method to limit unhealthy food purchases and encourage better choices.[113-115] This strategy was originally suggested in the WHO's 1988 *Healthy Public Policy Report*, which stated, "Taxation and subsidies should discriminate in favor of easy access for all to healthy food and improved diet."[116] In other words, taxations on unhealthy food could and should be used to subsidize fruits, vegetables, and whole grains.

Implementation of a minimal tax (one or two cents) has already begun in at least 18 states and in some major U.S. cities on items such as soda, gum, candy, and other snack foods.[54,115] Revenue generated from these nominal taxes has totaled $1.5 billion in just one year.[54] This money could be used for health promotion programs as well as subsidies for produce companies. However, there are dissenters who believe that these types of economic or governmental measures are "food policing."[117] The question becomes, "How do we determine what foods are clearly 'unhealthy,' and therefore should be subject to taxation?" The United States faces the arduous task of creating and passing legislation for food and health polices that protect the health of Americans.

Another idea parallel to the well-known anti-smoking campaign, in addition to taxation of unhealthy food, is the banning of junk food commercials and advertisements to children, just as the federal government banned cigarette ads from television in 1971.[54] Food advertising to children has infiltrated every aspect of a child's life—in school, on the World Wide Web, at sports arenas, and on television. Children are now exposed to 40,000 TV ads a year, up from 20,000 in the 1970s, according to a report by the Henry J. Kaiser Family Foundation."[118]

Social Marketing

As discussed more thoroughly in Chapter 26, social marketing is a powerful tool for reaching an enormous number of people via a well-designed campaign. To improve personal and social welfare, social marketing campaigns apply commercial marketing strategies to influence the voluntary behavior of target audiences.[119] The three main attributes of a successful social marketing campaign are the following:

1. Its primary goal is to influence the voluntary behavior of target market members.
2. It offers benefits for changing behavior and reduced barriers to perform the behavior.
3. It primarily benefits members of the target audience, or society at large, rather than the organization that initiated it.[119]

This is what makes social marketing distinctly different from commercial marketing.

The VERB Campaign

VERB is a multiethnic media campaign sponsored by the CDC whose goal is to increase and maintain physical activity among tweens, that is, children aged 9 to 13 years.[120] It is an excellent example of successful social marketing that is reaching youth and changing behavior. Parents and other sources of influence on tweens (such as teachers, youth program leaders, and coaches) arc the secondary audiences of the VERB initiative. VERB is not an acronym, but simply a word that indicates action: "It's what you do."

VERB has successfully applied sophisticated commercial marketing techniques to address the public health problem of the sedentary lifestyles of American children. The social marketing principles address product, price, place, and promotion. Additionally, this initiative has been successful because it is quite focused and consumer-centric, and is designed specifically for and by kids of a specific age range.[121] Having an adequate budget to carry the message into all media that children use is necessary to "break through the clutter" of messages competing for their attention. VERB spent a total of $125 million in one year, which predominantly went to paid advertising on television stations most watched by tweens. VERB's financial resources are a major factor contributing to the campaign's success; unfortunately, many other well-designed campaigns often do not have this funding.

The VERB campaign strives for high brand awareness and affinity among tweens. The theory is that when tweens bond positively with VERB, they will be more receptive to messages about physical activity. Then many, if not most, will take the next step and be active. In the first year of VERB (launched in June 2002), marketing efforts were dedicated to creating and introducing the VERB brand to tweens. As a previously nonexistent brand, VERB initially had no value to tweens. VERB has now been successfully "sold" to tweens as "their brand for having fun," since the campaign associates itself with popular kids brands, athletes, celebrities, and activities and products that are appealing, fun, and motivating. When asked about VERB, the majority of children familiar with it respond with, "It's cool."[121]

More than 450 partners are involved in this initiative to promote more physical activity in children. As the VERB brand continues to be promoted and spreads throughout the country, eventually it should become a well-established, popular brand. A social marketing program that models VERB strategies to promote healthier eating should be the next campaign initiated in the effort toward obesity prevention.

Powerful Bones, Powerful Girls

Another initiative to note is the National Bone Health Campaign (NBHC): Powerful Bones, Powerful Girls. This initiative is a multiyear campaign to promote optimal bone health in girls aged 9–12, and thus reduce their risk of osteoporosis later in life.[122] The goal is to educate and encourage girls to establish lifelong healthy habits, especially increased calcium consumption and weight-bearing physical activity to build and maintain strong bones.

The following are some features of Powerful Bones, Powerful Girls that have contributed to its success in reaching its target audience:

- Paid print and radio advertising for girls and parents
- Participation in the Radio Disney Live World Tour 2001
- An award-winning website for girls—this girl-friendly website helps girls understand how weight-bearing physical activity and calcium can be a fun and important part of everyday life. The site's key features include interactive games and quizzes, recipes for tasty foods with calcium, and ideas to help girls get plenty of weight-bearing physical activity.
- A downloadable calendar—this free calendar for girls and parents allows girls to track their calcium intake and physical activity, with their parents' input

- Collaboration with the Girl Scouts of the USA, Girls Inc., and the National Association of School Nurses

Fuel Up/Lift Off! LA/Sabor y Energia!

A Los Angeles County Department of Health Services social marketing campaign, *Fuel Up/Lift Off! LA/Sabor y Energia!* is targeted at obesity control in predominantly African American and Latino American communities.[123-125] Primary interventions include demonstrations and training in strategies to integrate physical activity and healthy food choices into routine business activities. Examples include incorporating activity breaks with music into lengthy meetings, offering healthy food choices when refreshments are served, and hosting walking meetings. A randomized, controlled trial tested the feasibility of including physical activity breaks as a part of lengthy meetings. The trial demonstrated success in the feasibility of engaging more than 90% of a sample of predominantly middle-aged and older women in 10 minutes of moderate physical activity, regardless of their fitness level or overweight status. It is worth noting that 10 minutes of activity is one-third of the federally recommended daily allowance of physical activity. Therefore, if these women could add another 20 minutes of walking (for example, after work) on a daily basis, then they would be reaching the recommended goal of 30 minutes per day of physical activity to achieve better health and prevent many chronic diseases.[126-128]

Health Communication Technology

Printed educational materials and face-to-face communication are two basic and simple methods to increase knowledge and understanding of health risks and how to make healthful behavior changes. However, these two traditional methods for health education are now supplemented by or even being replaced by DVD, CD-ROM, the Internet, e-mail, wireless communication options such as cellular telephones, handheld computers, and instant messaging. Newer technologies have opened up an unprecedented range of options for communicating and facilitating health behavior change strategies.[129] Advancements in computer software have simplified the process of producing personalized printouts tailored to an individual's needs or stage of change. The question of whether tailored or general printed materials are more effective has no definitive conclusion as of yet. Research thus far shows mixed results, with some studies finding tailored material to be more effective than non-tailored and other research showing that either type has equal effects on changing behavior.[129-131]

For those seeking a program for weight loss, individuals are able to enroll and participate in one without even leaving home or having face-to-face contact with anyone. A copious number of Internet programs can provide sound nutrition and exercise advice from qualified fitness professionals and registered dietitians. The top-rated sites may include these features:

- Personal nutrition, exercise, and behavioral assessments
- Customized meal planning tools, healthy recipes, online food journal, and exercise logs
- Scientifically sound, up-to-date nutrition information and weight loss tips
- Personalized exercise plan appropriately matched to ability, interest, and fitness level
- Information addressing emotional and behavioral issues (such as stress) related to food, along with coping strategies and support
- An online "community" and chat rooms to motivate and provide support on a regular basis

Nine studies examining the effectiveness of online support groups for weight loss have shown mixed, but mostly nonsignificant, results. The results of one particular study suggest that Internet support does not appear to be as effective as minimal or frequent intensive in-person therapist support for facilitating the long-term maintenance of weight loss.[132]

Thousands of electronic health-related peer-to-peer support groups in the form of mailing lists, chat rooms, and discussion forums are available on the Internet. Internet access has created opportunities to access health information on any topic and has led some to self-diagnosis. This can be either a favorable or an unfortunate phenomenon, depending on whether the individual is then prompted to seek qualified medical advice in person. Numerous online support groups exist that serve as important social networks, especially for people with stigmatizing diseases such as AIDS, alcoholism, and certain cancers.[133] For individuals suffering from chronic pain, rare diseases, or conditions for which modern medicine has no effective remedy, and/or for those who are socially isolated with no family, these virtual friends and support groups can be life-giving. The primary medium for virtual communities today is the Internet in the form of e-mailing lists, newsgroups, listservs or discussion forums, Web-based discussion forums, and live chat rooms. As of April 2004, Yahoo! groups listed almost 70,000 electronic support groups in the health and wellness section. Anecdotal evidence shows that electronic peer-to-peer self-help groups might be beneficial social support interventions.

In contrast, a systematic review of studies examining the beneficial health effects of online peer-to-peer interaction failed to find robust evidence on the health benefits of virtual communities and

> **Listservs**—Contact with a specific group or organization through regular e-mail broadcasts.

peer-to-peer online support.[133] In 31 studies, investigators evaluated complex interventions, combining, for example, educational or cognitive behavior therapy components with peer-to-peer communications. Integrative approaches like this make it challenging to draw conclusions on the effectiveness of pure electronic peer-to-peer interactions used daily by millions of people participating in Internet discussion groups or listservs. However, this study did not find any harm or negative health effects on participants who engaged regularly in virtual communities.[123]

The use of nutrition education CD-ROM programs for particular populations, such as those receiving food assistance programs, is increasing and showing promising results. One randomized study with Women, Infants and Children's (WIC) program participants in North Carolina employed an interactive CD-ROM program consisting of a targeted video soap opera, dietary assessment, and individually tailored diet feedback with strategies for making changes.[134] After receiving the intervention just once, participants significantly increased their self-efficacy and scored higher on low-fat eating and infant-feeding knowledge as compared to controls. It remains to be tested whether repeated use of this program can be instrumental in impacting behavior change for these participants.

Another CD-ROM program, titled *Little by Little*, was created and tested with a low-income population of women in California with the aim to increase fruit and vegetable consumption and decrease fat intake.[135] This CD-ROM intervention program includes a brief assessment of fruit and vegetable intake, as well as messages and tips on how to increase it. This tool proved effective in improving fruit and vegetable intake, as well as advancing participants through the study's Stage of Readiness for Change continuum, as compared with the control group. This *Little by Little* CD-ROM could prove quite useful in increasing fruit and vegetable intake of clients in public health and clinical settings.

Additional Favorable Health Effects

The numerous goal-specific interventions discussed in this chapter can also have reverberating positive health benefits that are not captured only because a particular outcome was not measured or being studied. As one example, the goal of a British school-centered intervention was to slow the rise in obesity in children by decreasing soft drink consumption.[42] However, given the significant inverse relationship between soft drink consumption and bone mineral density,[136] as well the strong association between carbonated drink consumption and bone fractures,[137] interventions that decrease soda consumption in children could, in turn, improve bone health in young girls and lower their subsequent risk of osteoporosis.

Conclusion

As time passes, we will continue to learn and improve upon current strategies for intervening in dietary behaviors. At present, however, the most effective interventions are likely based on the social ecological theory. This theoretical model utilizes a multi-level approach, while altering the environment where individuals reside or work to be more conducive to and supportive of healthy eating. While recognizing the continued importance of intervening at all levels of society (from individual to population-wide), we must focus more attention and utilize the power and influence of media and governmental policy for effective and enduring change. Better health and quality of life can be achieved for every individual when all sectors of society work together in minimizing barriers to health and capitalizing on each other's strengths.

Issues for Discussion

1. Even when the study results of nutrition interventions appear efficacious, how strongly should we consider that self-reports of dietary intake are often wrought with random errors and recall bias, especially when revealing such personal behavior as eating?

2. Individuals who agree to participate and are captured in health interventions tend to be Caucasian, educated, English-speaking, and more health conscious.[138] How do we better engage marginalized individuals who need health-promoting interventions the most?

3. How transferable and practical do you feel these research intervention strategies are to implement in your own school, home, or work setting?

References

1. McLeroy KR, Bibeau D, Steckler A, Glanz K. An ecological perspective on health promotion programs. *Health Education Quarterly.* 1988;15:351–377.

2. Ory MG, Jordan PJ, Bazzarre T. The Behavior Change Consortium: setting the stage for a new century of health behavior-change research. *Health Educ Research.* 2002;17(5):500–511.

3. Kennedy ET, Bowman SA, et al. Dietary fat intake in the US population. *J Am Coll Nutr.* 1999;130:284S–288S.

4. Centers for Disease Control and Prevention. Trends in intake of energy and macronutrients—United States, 1981–2000. *MMWR Weekly.* 2004, Feb 6;53(01):80–82. Available at http://www.cdc.gov/mmwr/preview/mmwrhtml/mm5304a3.htm. Accessed March 18, 2005.

5. Nielsen SJ, Siega-Riz AM, Popkin BM. Trends in energy intake in US between 1977 and 1996: similar shifts seen across age groups. *Obes Res.* 2002;10:370–378.

6. Nielsen SJ, Popkin BM. Patterns and trends in food portion sizes, 1977–1998. *JAMA.* 2003;289:450–453.

7. Nicklas TA, Baranowski T, Cullen KW, Berenson G. Eating patterns, dietary quality, and obesity. *J Am Coll Nutr.* 2001;20:599–608.

8. Kris-Etherton PM, Binkoski AE, Zhao G, et al. Dietary fat: assessing the evidence in support of a moderate-fat diet; the benchmark based on lipoprotein metabolism. *Proc Nutr Soc.* 2002 May;61.

9. Sacks FM, Katan M. Randomized clinical trials on the effects of dietary fat and carbohydrate on plasma lipoproteins and cardiovascular disease. Review. *Am J Med.* 2002;30(113 Suppl 9B):13S-24S.

10. Hu FB, Willett WC. Optimal diets for prevention of coronary heart disease. Review. *JAMA.* 2002;288(20):2569–2578.

11. Food Marketing Institute. 1998 news publication, "Facts and Figures." Available online at www.fmi.org. Accessed on February 23, 2004.

12. Guggenbühl N. Obesity: it's super-size mania. *Belgian Journal of Health and Food.* 2003 Sept;60:9–10.

13. Schlosser E. *Fast Food Nation: The Dark Side of the All-American Meal.* New York: Houghton Mifflin; 2001: 17.

14. Frumkin H. Urban sprawl and public health. *Public Health Reports.* 2002 May–June;117:201–217.

15. Jackson RJ, ed. *American Journal of Public Health* (entire publication). 2003 Sept 1;93(9).

16. Finkelstein EA, Fiebelkorn IC, Wang G. National medical spending attributable to overweight and obesity: how much and who's paying? *Health Affairs.* 2003;W3;219–226.

17. Milner JA, McDonald SS, Anderson DE, Greenwald P. Molecular targets for nutrients involved with cancer prevention. *Nutr Cancer.* 2001;41:1–16.

18. Stender S, Dyerberg J, Holmer G, Ovesen L, Sandstrom B. The influence of trans fatty acids on health: a report from the Danish Nutrition Council. *Clin Sci* (Lond). 1995 Apr;88(4):375–392.

19. Walter Willett, personal communication via email on July 20, 2004.

20. Sloane D, Diamant A, Lewis L, et al. Improving the nutritional resource environment for healthy living through community-based participatory research. *J Gen Intern Med.* 2003;18:568–575.

21. Institute of Medicine. *Health and Behavior.* Washington, D.C.: National Academy Press; 2001.

22. Kaplan GA, Keil JE. Socioeconomic factors and cardiovascular disease: a review of the literature. *Circulation.* 1993;88:1973–1998.

23. Syme S, Berkman L. Social class, susceptibility, and sickness. *Am J of Epidemiology.* 1976;104:1–8.

24. Institute of Medicine, Smedley BD, Syme SL, eds. *Promoting Health: Intervention Strategies from Social and Behavioral Research report.* Washington, D.C.: National Academy Press; 2000.

25. U.S. Department of Health and Human Services. *Healthy People 2010.* Washington, D.C.: Department of Health and Human Services; 2000.

26. Stokols D. Establishing and maintaining healthy environments: toward a social ecology of health promotion. *Am Psychol.* 1992;47:6–22.

27. Stokols D. Translating social ecological theory into guidelines for community health promotion. *Am J Health Prom.* 1996;10(4):282–298.

28. Euromonitor International. *Making sense of global markets: beer in the USA.* Pub ID: EP971616. March 1, 2004.

29. Nestle M, Wing R, Birch L, et al. Behavioral and social influences on food choice. *Nutrition Reviews.* 1998;56(II):S50-S74.

30. Reger B, Wootan MG, Booth-Butterfield S. Using mass media to promote healthy eating: a community-based demonstration project. *Prev Med.* 1999;29(5):414–421.

31. Yancey AK, Kumanyika SK, Ponce NA, et al. Population-based interventions engaging communities of color in healthy eating and active living: a review. *Preventing Chronic Disease* 2004 Jan. Available at: http://www.cdc.gov/pcd/issues/2004/jan/03_0012.htm. Retrieved March 18, 2005.

32. World Health Organization Regional Office for Europe. *The Adelaide Recommendations: Healthy Public Policy.* Geneva, Switzerland: WHO; 1988.

33. Goldfield GS, Epstein LH. Can fruits and vegetables and activities substitute for snack foods? *Health Psychol.* 2002 May;21(3):299–303.

34. Nestle M. *Food Politics: How the Food Industry Influences Nutrition and Health.* Berkeley: University of California Press; 2002.

35. Tillotson JE. Pandemic obesity: is it time for change in economic and development policies affecting the food industry? *Nutrition Today.* 2003;38(6):242–246.

36. Lytle LA, Seifert S, Greenstein J, McGovern P. How do children's eating patterns and food choices change over time? Results from a cohort study. *Am J Health Prom.* 2000;14:222–228.

37. Kelder SH, Perry CL, Klepp KI, Lytle LL. Longitudinal tracking of adolescent smoking, physical activity, and food choice behaviors. *Am J Public Health.* 1994;84(7):1121–1126.

38. Perry CL, Stone EJ, Parcel GS, et al. School-based cardiovascular health promotion: the child and adolescent trial for cardiovascular health (CATCH). *J Sch Health.* 1990;60(8):406–413.

39. Hoelscher DM, Feldman HA, Johnson CC, et al. School-based health education programs can be maintained over time: results from the CATCH institutionalization study. *Prev Med.* 2004;38(5):594–606.

40. Osganian SK, Hoelscher DM, Zive M, Mitchell PD, Snyder P, Webber LS. Maintenance of effects of the eat smart school food service program: results from the CATCH-ON study. *Health Educ Behav.* 2003;30(4):418–433.

41. Parcel GS, Perry CL, Kelder SH, et al. School climate and the institutionalization of the CATCH program. *Health Educ Behav.* 2003;30(4):489–502.

42. Perry CL, Bishop DB, Taylor GL, et al. A randomized school trial of environmental strategies to encourage fruit and vegetable consumption among children. *Health Educ & Behav.* 2004;31(1):65–76.

43. American Food Service Association. *School Food Service and Nutrition Operations Study.* Alexandria, Va: American Food Service Association; 1999.

44. Story M, Hayes J, Kalina B. Availability of foods in high schools: is there cause for concern? *J Am Diet Assoc.* 1996;96:123–126.

45. Harnack L, Snyder P, Story M, Holliday R, Lytle L, Neumark-Sztainer D. Availability of a la carte food items in junior and senior high schools. *J Am Diet Assoc.* 2000;100:701–703.

46. Kubik, MY, Lytle LA, Hannan PJ, Perry CL, Story, M. The association of the school food environment with dietary behaviors of young adolescents. *Am J Public Health.* 2003;93(7):1168–1173.

47. Bauer KW, Yang YW, Austin SB. "How can we stay healthy when you're throwing all of this in front of us?" Findings from focus groups and interviews in middle schools on environmental influences on nutrition and physical activity. *Health Educ & Behav.* 2004;31(1):34–46.

48. O'Dea JA. Why do kids eat healthful food? Perceived benefits of and barriers to healthful eating and physical activity among children and adolescents. *J Am Diet Assoc.* 2003;103:497–500.

49. James J, Thomas P, Cavan D, Kerr D. Preventing childhood obesity by reducing consumption of carbonated drinks: cluster randomized controlled trial. Br Med J. 2004;328(7450):1237. Available at: www.bmj.com.

50. Ludwig DS, Peterson KE, Gortmaker SL. Relation between consumption of sugar-sweetened drinks and childhood obesity: a prospective, observational analysis. *Lancet.* 2001;357(9255):505–508.

51. Gillis LJ, Bar-Or O. Food away from home, sugar-sweetened drink consumption and juvenile obesity. *J Am Coll Nutr.* 2003;22(6):539–545.

52. Bellisle F, Rolland-Cachera MF. How sugar-containing drinks might increase adiposity in children. *Lancet.* 2001;357(9255):505–508.

53. American Academy of Pediatrics Committee on School Health. Soft drinks in schools. *Pediatrics.* 2004;113(1 Pt 1):152–154.

54. *Time.* Special issue: overcoming obesity in America; June 7, 2004.

55. Birnbaum AS, Lytle LA, Story M, Perry CL, Murray DM. Are differences in exposure to a multicomponent school-based intervention associated with varying dietary outcomes in adolescents? *Health Educ & Behav.* 2002;29(4):427–443.

56. Sallis JF, McKenzie TL, Conway TL, et al. Environmental interventions for eating and physical activity: a randomized controlled trial in middle schools. *Am J Prev Med.* 2003;24(3):209–217.

57. Heaney CA, Goetzal RZ. A review of health-related outcomes of multicomponent worksite health promotion programs. *Am J Health Prom.* 1997;11:290–308.

58. Emmons KM, Thompson B, McLerran D, et al. The relationship between organizational characteristics and the adoption of workplace smoking policies. *Health Educ Behav.* 2000;27(4):483–501.

59. Biener L, Glanz K, McLerran D, et al. Impact of the Working Well Trial on the worksite smoking and nutrition environment. *Health Educ & Behav.* 1999;26(4):478–494.

60. Kristal AR, Glanz K, Tilley BC, Li S. Mediating factors in dietary change: understanding the impact of a worksite nutrition intervention. *Health Educ & Behav.* 27(1):112–125.

61. Glanz K, Sorensen G, Farmer A. The health impact of worksite nutrition and cholesterol intervention programs. *Am J Health Promot.* 1996;10(6):453–470.

62. Karlehagen S, Ohlson CG. Primary prevention of cardiovascular disease by an occupational health service. *Prev Med.* 2003;37(3):219–225.

63. Tilley BC, Vernon SW, Myers R, et al. The Next Step Trial: impact of a worksite colorectal cancer screening promotion program. *Prev Med.* 1999;28(3):276–283.

64. Patterson, RE, Kristal AR, Biener L, et al. Durability and diffusion of the nutrition intervention in the Working Well Trial. *Prev Med.* 1998;27(5 Pt 1):668–673.

65. House JS, Landis KR, Umberson D. Social relationships and health. *Science.* 1988;241:540–545.

66. Uchino BN, Cacioppo JT, Kiecolt-Glaser JK. The relationship between social support and psychological processes: a review with emphasis on underlying mechanisms and implications for health. *Psych Bull.* 1996;119:488–531.

67. McCaffree J. Childhood eating patterns: the roles parents play. *J Am Diet Assoc.* 2003;103(12):1587.

68. Nestle M, Wing R, Birch L, et al. Behavioral and social influences on food choice. *Nutrition Reviews.* 1998;56(5):S50–S74.

69. Birch LL, Davison KK. Family environmental factors influencing the developing behavioral controls of food intake and childhood overweight. *Pediatr Clin North Am.* 2001;48(4):893–907.

70. Golan M, Crow S. Parents are key players in the prevention and treatment of weight-related problems. *Nutr Rev.* 2004;62(1):39–50.

71. Birch LL, Fisher JO, Davison KK. Learning to overeat: maternal use of restrictive feeding practices promotes girls' eating in the absence of hunger. *Am J Clin Nutr.* 2003;78(2):215–220.

72. McHale SM. Family dynamics: Challenges and opportunities for preventing childhood obesity. Workshop presentation, December 9, 2003. The Prevention of Childhood Obesity: Understanding the Influences of Marketing, Media, and Family Dynamics. Available at www.IOM.edu. Accessed on June 19, 2004.

73. Grusec JE, Goodnow JJ, Kuczynski L. New directions in analyses of parenting contributions to children's acquisition of values. *Child Dev.* 2000;71(1):205–211.

74. Dunst CJ, Trivette CM. Empowerment, effective help-giving practices and family-centered care. *Pediatr Nurs.* 1996 Jul-Aug;22(4):334–337, 343.

75. Birch LL. Development of food acceptance patterns in the first years of life. *Proc Nutr Soc.* 1998;57(4):617–624.

76. Galloway AT, Lee Y, Birch LL. Predictors and consequences of food neophobia and pickiness in young girls. *J Am Diet Assoc.* 2003;103(6):692–698.

77. Neumark-Sztainer D, Wall M, Perry C, Story M. Correlates of fruit and vegetable intake among adolescents. Findings from Project EAT. *Prev Med.* 2003;37(3):198–208.

78. Haire-Joshu D, Brownson RC, Nanney MS, et al. Improving dietary behavior in African Americans: the Parents As Teachers High 5, Low Fat Program. *Prev Med.* 2003;36(6):684–691.

79. Epple C, Wright AL, Joish VN, Bauer M. The role of active family nutritional support in Navajos' type 2 diabetes metabolic control. *Diabetes Care.* 2003;26(10):2829–2834.

80. Sorensen G, Hunt MK, Cohen N, et al. Worksite and family education for dietary change: the Treatwell 5-a-Day program. *Health Educ Res.* 1998;13(4):577–591.

81. Sorensen G, Stoddard A, Peterson K, et al. Increasing fruit and vegetable consumption through worksites and families in the Treatwell 5-a-Day study. *Am J Public Health.* 1999;89(1):54–60.

82. Macario E, Sorensen G. Spousal similarities in fruit and vegetable consumption. *Am J Health Prom.* 1998;12(6):369–377.

83. Schwartz, MB, Puhl R. Childhood obesity: a societal problem to solve. *Obesity Reviews.* 2003;4(1):57–71.

84. Seeman T, Berkman L, Kohout F, LaCroix A, Glynn R, Blazer D. Intercommunity variation in the association between social ties and mortality in the elderly: a comparative analysis of three communities. *Ann of Epidem.* 1993;3:325–335.

85. Kawachi I, Berkman L. Social cohesion, social capital and health. In: Berkman L, Kawachi I, eds. *Social Epidemiology.* New York: Oxford University Press; 2000.

86. Minkler M, Wallerstein N. Improving health through community organization and community building. In: Glanz K, Lewis FM, Rimer BK, eds. *Health Behavior and Health Education: Theory, Research, and Practice.* 2nd ed. San Francisco: Jossey-Bass; 1997: 241–269.

87. Viadro CI, Farris RP, Will JC. The WISEWOMAN projects: lessons learned from three states. *J Womens Health (Larchmt).* 2004;13(5): 529–538.

88. Yanek LR, Becker DM, Moy TF, Gittelsohn J, Koffman DM. Project Joy: faith based cardiovascular health promotion for African American women. *Public Health Rep.* 2001;116(Suppl 1):68–81.

89. Demark-Wahnefried W, McClelland JW, Jackson B, et al. Partnering with African American churches to achieve better health: lessons learned during the Black Churches United for Better Health 5 a Day project. *J Cancer Educ.* 2000;15(3):164–167.

90. Campbell MK, Motsinger BM, Ingram A, et al. The North Carolina Black Churches United for Better Health Project: intervention and process evaluation. *Health Educ Behav.* 2000;27(2):241–253.

91. Resnicow K, Jackson A, Braithwaite R, et al. Healthy Body/Healthy Spirit: a church-based nutrition and physical activity intervention. *Health Educ Res.* 2002;17(5):562–573.

92. Ammerman A, Corbie-Smith G, St. George DMM, Washington C, Weathers B, Jackson-Christian B. Research expectations among African American church leaders in the PRAISE! Project: A randomized trial guided by community-based participatory research. *Am J Public Health.* 2003;93(10):1720–1727.

93. Corbie-Smith G, Ammerman AS, Katz ML, et al. Trust, benefit, satisfaction, and burden: a randomized controlled trial to reduce cancer risk through African-American churches. *J Gen Intern Med.* 2003;18(7):531–541.

94. National Cancer Institute of the NIH. Eat 5 to 9 A Day for Better Health: Body and Soul: A Celebration of Healthy Eating and Living Program. Available at http://5aday.nci.nih.gov/bodyandsoul. Accessed on April 18, 2004.

95. Clark PG, Nigg CR, Greene G, Riebe D, Saunders SD, Study of Exercise and Nutrition in Older Rhode Islanders Project Team. The Study of Exercise and Nutrition in Older Rhode Islanders (SENIOR): translating theory into research. *Health Educ Res.* 2002;17(5):552–561.

96. Bernstein A., Nelson ME, Tucker KL, et al. A home-based nutrition intervention to increase consumption of fruits, vegetables, and calcium-rich foods in community dwelling elders. *J Am Diet Assoc.* 2002 Oct;102(10):1421–1427.

97. International Longevity Center, USA, Ltd. Maintaining healthy lifestyles: a lifetime of choices. Workshop Report. December 1999. Available at www.ilcusa.org. Accessed January 11, 2004.

98. Chapel DL, McCulla MM, Reinsch B, Warren C. Moving right along: a creative partnership to engage older adults in physical activity and nutrition programs. Abstract. *Preventing Chronic Disease.* 2004 Apr. Available at: http://www.cdc.gov/pcd/issues/2004/apr/03_0034d.htm. Accessed March 18, 2005.

99. Glasgow RE, La Chance PA, Toobert DJ, Brown J, Hampson SE, Riddle MC. Long term effects and costs of a brief behavioral dietary intervention for patients with diabetes delivered from the medical office. *Patient Educ and Couns.* 1997;32:175–184.

100. Rollnick S, Miller WR. What is motivational interviewing? *Behav and Cog Psychoth.* 1995;23:325–334.

101. Resnicow K, Jackson A, Wang T, et al. A motivational interviewing intervention to increase fruit and vegetable intake through black churches: results of the Eat for Life trial. *Am J Public Health.* 2001;91(10):1686–1693.

102. Pignone MP, Ammerman A, Fernandez L, et al. Counseling to promote a healthy diet in adults: a summary of the evidence for the U.S. Preventive Services Task Force. *Am J Prev Med.* 2003;24:75–92.

103. Stevens VJ, Glasgow RE, Toobert DJ, Karanja N, Smith KS. One-year results from a brief, computer-assisted intervention to decrease consumption of fat and increase consumption of fruits and vegetables. *Prev Med.* 2003;36:594–600.

104. Steptoe A, Perkins-Porras L, McKay C, Rink E, Hilton S, Cappuccio FP. Behavioural counselling to increase consumption of fruit and vegetables in low income adults: randomised trial. *BMJ.* 2003;326:855–860.

105. Mensah GA, Goodman RA, Zaza S, et al. Law as a tool for preventing chronic diseases: expanding the spectrum of effective public health strategies. *Preventing Chronic Disease.* 2004 Jan. Available at: http://www.cdc.gov/pcd/issues/2004/jan/03_0033.htm. Retrieved March 18, 2005.

106. Gostin LO. Public law in a new century. 1. Law as a tool to advance the community's health. *J Am Med Assoc.* 2000;83L:2837–2841.

107. Institute of Medicine. *The Future of Public Health.* Washington, D.C.: National Academy Press; 1988.

108. Glanz K, Basil M, Maibach E, Goldberg J, Snyder D. Why Americans eat what they do: taste, nutrition, cost, convenience, and weight control concerns as influences on food consumption. *J Am Diet Assoc.* 1998;98:1118–1126.

109. Jeffery RW, French SA, Raether C, et al. An environmental intervention to increase fruit and salad purchases in a cafeteria. *Prev Med.* 1994;23:788–792.

110. French SA, Jeffery RW, Story M, Hannan P, Snyder P. A pricing strategy to promote low-fat snack choices through vending machines. *Am J Public Health.* 1997;87: 849–851.

111. French SA. Pricing effects on food choices. *Journal of Nutr.* 2003; 133(3):841S-843S.

112. Hannan P, French SA, Story M, Fulkerson JA. A pricing strategy to promote purchase of lower fat foods in a high school cafeteria: acceptability and sensitivity analysis. *Am J Health Promot.* 2002;17:1-6.

113. Temple NJ, Balay-Karperien AL. Nutrition in cancer prevention: an integrated approach. Review. *J Am Coll Nutr.* 2002;21(2):79-83.

114. Jacobson MF, Brownell KD. Small taxes on soft drinks and snack foods to promote health. *Am J Public Health.* 2000;90(6):854-857.

115. Wilson N, Mansoor O. Getting the fat tax on the table. *N Z Med J.* 2000;27;113(1120):451.

116. World Health Organization. *Technical Report Series. Diet nutrition and the Prevention of Chronic Diseases.* Geneva, Switzerland: WHO; 2003: 916.

117. Byers T. Reflections on the war on cancer. *J Amer Coll Nutr.* 2002;21(2): 77-78.

118. American Dietetic Association. Position paper: total diet approach to communicating food and nutrition information. *J Am Diet Assoc.* 2002;102:100.

119. Glanz K, Lewis FM, Rimer BK, eds. *Health Behavior and Health Education: Theory, Research, and Practice.* 3rd ed. San Francisco: Jossey-Bass.

120. CDC. VERB: It's What You Do. Available at www.cdc.gov/youthcampaign. Accessed on March 18, 2005.

121. Rosenthal E. Marketing and Media Influences. Workshop presentation. December 9, 2003. The Prevention of Childhood Obesity: Understanding the Influences of Marketing, Media, and Family Dynamics. Available at www.IOM.edu. Accessed on June 19, 2004.

122. CDC.Powerful Bones. Powerful Girls. Available at: http://www.cdc.gov/powerfulbones/index_content.html. Accessed on March 18, 2005.

123. Sloane DC, Diamant AL, Lewis LB, et al. Improving the nutritional resource environment for healthy living through community-based participatory research. *J Gen Intern Med.* 2003;18(7):568-575.

124. Kumanyika S. Obesity treatment in minorities. In: Wadden TA, Stunkard AJ, eds. *Obesity: Theory and Therapy.* 3rd ed. New York: Guilford Publications; 2002: xiii, 377.

125. Yancey AK, Miles OL, McCarthy WJ, et al. Differential response to targeted recruitment strategies to fitness promotion research by African-American women of varying body mass index. *Ethn Dis.* 2001; 11(1): 115-123.

126. The National Cancer Institute. Eat 5 to 9 a Day for Better Health. Available at http://www.5aday.gov. Accessed March 18, 2005.

127. Foerster SB, Kizer KW, Disogra LK, Bal DG, Krieg BF, Bunch KL. California's "5 A Day-For Better Health!" campaign: an innovative population-based effort to effect large-scale dietary change. *Am J Prev Med.* 1995;11(2):124-131.

128. National Cancer Institute. *5-A-Day for Better Health Program.* NIH publication 01-5019; September 2001.

129. Brinberg D, Axelson ML, Price S. Changing food knowledge, food choice, and dietary fiber consumption by using tailored messages. *Appetite*. 2000;35:35–43.

130. Brug J, Steenhuis I, van Assema P, de Vries H. The impact of a computer-tailored nutrition intervention. *Prev Med*. 1996;25:236–242.

131. Campbell MK, DeVellis BM, Strecher VJ, et al. Improving dietary behavior: the effectiveness of tailored messages in primary care settings. *Am J Public Health*. 1994;84:783–787.

132. Harvey-Berino J, Pintauro S, Buzzell P, et al. Does using the internet facilitate the maintenance of weight loss? *Int J Obes Relat Metab Disord*. 2002;26:1254–1260.

133. Eysenbach G, Powell J, Englesakis M, Rizo C, Stern A. Health related virtual communities and electronic support groups: systematic review of the effects of online peer to peer interactions. *BMJ*. 2004 May 15;328(7449):1166.

134. Campbell MK, Carbone E, Honess-Morreale L, Heisler-Mackinnon J, Demissie S, Farrell D. Randomized trial of a tailored nutrition education CD-ROM program for women receiving food assistance. *J Nutr Educ Behav*. 2004;36(2):58–66.

135. Block G, Wakimoto P, Metz D, et al. A randomized trial of the Little by Little CD-ROM: demonstrated effectiveness in increasing fruit and vegetable intake in a low-income population. *Preventing Chronic Disease*. 2004 Jul. Available at: http://www.cdc.gov/pcd/issues/2004/jul/04_0016.htm. Retrieved March 18, 2005.

136. McGartland C, Robson PJ, Murray L, et al. Carbonated soft drink consumption and bone mineral density in adolescence: the Northern Ireland Young Hearts project. *J Bone Miner Res*. 2003 Sep;18(9):1563–1569.

137. Wyshak G. Teenaged girls, carbonated beverage consumption, and bone fractures. *Arch Pediatr Adolesc Med*. 2000 Jun;154(6):610–613.

138. Bull SS, Gillette C, Glasgow RE, Estabrooks P. Work site health promotion research: To what extent can we generalize the results and what is needed to translate research to practice? *Health Educ & Behav*. 2003;30(5):537–549.

PART III

SHAPING THE POLICIES THAT AFFECT THE PUBLIC'S HEALTH

Chapter 7   Creating Public Policy
Bruce Rengers, PhD, RD

Chapter 8   Advocating and Influencing Health and Nutrition Policies
Bruce Rengers, PhD, RD

Chapter 9   The Role of the United States Department of Agriculture (USDA) in Public Health Nutrition
Beverly J. McCabe-Sellers, PhD, RD
Margaret L. Bogle, PhD, RD

In Part III, we shift gears to investigate how science and needs assessment translate into public policy. It is through governmental policy that public health nutritionists are directed to educate and serve the public. Chapters 7 and 8 describe how nutrition policy is created, advocated for, and influenced by the public, health practitioners, lobbyists, and legislators. These chapters should highlight the need for dietitians and nutritionists to get involved in advocating for and influencing the passing of important nutrition policy. Chapter 9 demonstrates how the USDA acts on nutrition policy once it is made, and illustrates the complexity of that role in fulfilling the challenges of public health nutrition.

CHAPTER 7

CREATING PUBLIC POLICY

Bruce Rengers, PhD, RD

Reader Objectives

After studying this chapter and reflecting on the contents, you should be able to:

1. Define public policy.
2. Discuss some of the characteristics of public policy and why it is important.
3. Describe the conflicting aspects of public policy.
4. Discuss the evolution of nutrition policy in the United States.
5. Identify the steps involved in the creation of public policy.
6. Delineate the steps by which legislation is created in Congress.
7. Describe the role various levels of government play in creating public health policy.

Defining Public Policy

To accomplish something in an organized and efficient manner you must have a goal and a plan of action. This is the reason for having policy. Policy is "a course of action or principle adopted or proposed by a government, party, business, or individual".[1] Most policies consist of two parts.[2] The first is a statement or goal of what is to be accomplished, and the second is a set of practical rules, guidelines, programs, or regulations to accomplish the stated goal.

This chapter is about public policy, specifically public health policy as it relates to nutrition. Policy is labeled "public policy" when it is created by government. Government is, after all, according to Abraham Lincoln on November 19, 1863 in the Gettysburg Address, ". . . of the people, by the people, for the people. . . ." Public policy is created at all levels of government. It is how government functions. The government creates policies to regulate its own actions and to govern the actions of citizens and other entities under its control. Ultimately, what a government *does* is a reflection of its public policy. Some would say that what government does *is* public policy, regardless of what may be written or stated.[2]

Public policy may be created by the legislative, executive, or judicial branch of government.[3] Generally, policy is created by legislation that is introduced and passed by the legislative branch.[2] This legislation or policy is then translated into a set of practical rules by the executive branch to accomplish the intent of the legislation. Policy may, however, also be informal, indirect, and even unwritten. For example, a governing political party may have a philosophical belief of government involvement in environmental regulation. This philosophy becomes the government's guiding public policy.[4] Special interest groups, organizations, and certain individuals may also play an important role in determining public policy.

> A special interest group or organization may convince policy makers to create or avoid legislation that would affect their interests.[3,4]

Government policy is reflected as much in what government won't do as in what it will do.[2] Not all policies are created to accomplish a goal. Many unwritten and informal policies are more about what government will not be involved in. If the government identifies a problem, such as advertising directed at children, and then takes no action to regulate such advertising, this is a reflection of government policy. The decision to not become involved may be based on philosophies of downsizing government, reducing spending, increasing freedom, responding to special interest groups, or even a distrust of the evidence that says such advertising may be harmful. Because these philosophies direct the actions of the government, they become part of public policy.

Characteristics of Public Policy

Policy is generally created in response to a problem.[2,3] In an ideal world, policy would be created from objective assessments to identify potential problems and then prevent them. This, however, is rarely how public policy is created. Government officials generally create policy in response to emerging or existing problems that are important to the public, special interest groups, or professional or scientific groups. These emerging problems may be real or only perceived problems.[3] Sometimes popular belief or philosophies may result in identification of a concept as a problem or as a cause of a problem, when in fact there is little factual evidence to support the belief. It has been stated that more public policies fail from working to solve a perceived problem that is not real than from creating the wrong plan to solve a real problem.[3,5] Many policy issues are emotional, and solutions are created based on philosophical beliefs rather than actual understanding of the facts.[6]

Public policy is often controversial. It generally results in some form of control that limits the freedoms of some or all so that the majority may benefit.[7] There are those who feel government should limit its role and allow society to function with minimal interference.[2] Under this philosophy of limited involvement, economics and the free market create an environment where individuals have responsibility for their own actions and situations.

This is in contrast to a social justice philosophy, which acknowledges that society may share in the responsibility for a person's health.[2] Although it may be true that a person who overeats is responsible for his or her diet, there may also be societal factors that strongly influence a person's diet. For example, a person working for

> As an example of minimal government interference, one viewpoint could be that an obese person is obese because he or she chooses to overeat, and it is the individual's responsibility to eat less. An obese person is, therefore, responsible for the consequences of overeating. No action is required by the government.

low wages in a decaying neighborhood without grocery stores or public transportation may have few options other than to buy high-calorie prepared foods from a local convenience store. Public policy may be needed to alter those conditions in order for a person to have a reasonable ability to choose a healthy diet and lifestyle. Some argue that it is the role of government to create conditions that make healthy choices easier and unhealthy choices harder.[2,8] The mission of public health is to assure conditions in which people can be healthy.[9] To assure these conditions requires policies that do result in government intervention. The decision to limit personal choices and freedoms cannot be taken for granted, however, and the benefit from such public policies must be balanced against economic costs and losses of individual freedom.[7]

In the United States, we are conflicted with these two philosophies of public policy. For example, we want the government to ensure that our food supply is healthful, yet we also want the personal freedom to purchase unhealthful food. We want the government to guard us against becoming obese, yet we also want the freedom to make dietary and lifestyle choices that will lead to obesity. We want it both ways—freedom to make harmful choices, yet protection from harm when we do make those choices.

While many argue for less government, public policy is necessary in a complex society,[10] especially to safeguard health. To use a simple example, in a nation with little population and only a few cars, no significant public policy may be necessary with respect to automobiles. In a nation with millions of automobiles crowded into a dense area, public policies are needed with respect to driving, parking, passenger safety, road building and maintenance, car manufacturing, auto emissions, and even car disposal.

The same idea can easily be applied to other health issues in a society. For example, as societies become larger it becomes more important that a family not dump its sewage and other waste into the local water supply used by many others. Or, as our food supply changes and we become removed from production, policies are needed to ensure an adequate and safe food supply. Obviously, in a democratic society there must be a balance between the need to create a healthier society and the need to maintain personal freedoms.[7]

As a result of a need for public policy in a complex society, public policy touches almost every aspect of our lives.[2] One only need visit the government documents section of a library or peruse the *Code of Federal Regulations* to see that there are numerous public policies that affect our daily lives. Public policy is a reality. Life in a complex society without policies would be difficult and disorderly. Policy development for community living is a universal requirement.[10]

> The *Code of Federal Regulations* (CFR) is the codification of the general and permanent rules published in the *Federal Register* by the executive departments and agencies of the federal government. It is divided into 50 titles that represent broad areas subject to federal regulation.

U.S. Public Health Policy

Government has many reasons to be interested in the health of its citizens. A democratic government is elected by its citizens, and therefore has an interest in the welfare of the citizens who have created it.[11] Beyond the needs of individual health, the collective health of a country's citizens is vital to a country's economic health and independence as a nation. Health is a social as well as individual responsibility.[9]

The mission of public health, as stated by the Institute of Medicine (IOM) in its report *The Future of Public Health*, is "fulfilling society's interest in assuring conditions in which people can be healthy."[9] Many of the major improvements in the health of the American people have come about because of changes in public health policy. By one estimate, 25 of the last 30 years added to the U.S. life expectancy rate have been a result of changes brought about by public health policy.[12]

In its review of the U.S. public health system, the IOM noted that the United States has generally come to take the successes of public health for granted and that the nation has lost sight of its public health goals.[9] To date, the nation lacks a comprehensive public health policy.[11] Instead, the IOM[11] described a situation where public health policy tends to be antiquated, inconsistent, redundant, and at times ambiguous. Despite greater knowledge about health and the factors that affect health, technical knowledge plays a smaller role today in creating public policy than it did in the past.[9] Health policy is determined more by crises, hot issues, and the concerns of organized interest groups than careful analysis of objective data and technical knowledge about health.[9]

The IOM gave many reasons for the disarray of the U.S. public health system and challenged public health officials and policy makers to refocus on the three essential functions of public health: assessment, policy development, and assurance.[9] Although the responsibilities for public health are spread throughout the Federal Government, the Department of Health and Human Services (DHHS) is generally considered the principle agency of the federal public health infrastructure. It is also the principal contact for other federal agencies, as well as state and local agencies, with respect to public health issues.[11] Policy development is a critical function of DHHS in maintaining public health.[11] The U.S. Department of Agriculture (USDA), however, was designated as the lead for nutrition policy by the 1977 Farm Bill. Most federal nutrition programs are administered by USDA at the federal level.[2]

Nutrition Policy: A Brief History

As with the national health policy in general, there is no single or unifying public policy that guides the activities of government agencies with respect to nutrition in the United States.[2] Nutrition policy is fragmented amongst numerous laws, agencies, programs, and branches of the government.[2] Nutrition policy is often conflicting and inconsistent. Much of it is antiquated, having been created in the past when different nutritional problems affected the public.[2]

At the beginning of the twentieth century, little was known about nutrition. The main nutritional concerns of most people and the government were related to getting enough food to eat and avoiding foods that would make people sick. Early nutrition policy was, therefore, primarily agricultural policy. The government created policies to provide the population with a consistent and plentiful food supply at low cost. Since getting adequate calories was a major concern, emphasis was placed on providing foods that were a dense source of calories. These agricultural policies of the past had a major impact on shaping food supply that continues to this day.[2]

With the discovery of vitamins in the early part of the twentieth century, nutrition experts began to create guidelines encouraging people to eat certain groups of foods. In 1917, the USDA created the *Five Food Groups* to encourage people to eat food that provided all of the then-known nutrients. This guide was modified over time into a variety of forms to ensure that people were getting *adequate* diets. It wouldn't be until much later that nutrition guidelines from the government would start mentioning, moderating, or limiting intakes of certain types of foods, such as those high in fat or sodium. During the first half of the twentieth century, other nutrition policies were enacted, including fortification of salt with iodine, food distribution programs to feed children and other hungry people during the depression of the 1930s, the first Nationwide Food Consumption Survey, and establishment of the National School Lunch

Program. In 1941, the first set of "Recommended Dietary Allowances" was published, making recommendations for levels of
certain nutrients in the diet. The emphasis was still about getting an
adequate diet.

During the 1960s, the attention of the public health community
started to change from an emphasis on infectious diseases to one on
chronic diseases. Many accomplishments had been made in controlling communicable disease, and chronic diseases had become
the main causes of death in the United States. Public interest in nutrition and its effects on long-term health was also heightened by
the publication of books in the popular press by Adelle Davis,
Rachel Carson, and others, which stirred interest and controversy in
the long-term effects of food, food additives, and nutrients on
health. Continued interest in ensuring that people got enough food
led to the establishment of the Food Stamp Program, School Breakfast Program, and the Special Supplemental Food Program for
Women, Infants and Children (WIC) during the 1960s and 1970s.

In 1977, the Senate Select Committee on Nutrition and Human
Needs issued the first edition of the *Dietary Goals for the United
States*. It was one of the first governmental attempts at making nutritional recommendations, based on theories about the effects of
diet on chronic disease.[2] This started a change in diet recommendations that addressed moderation of certain foods and making
choices between foods within a food group.[2] The focus of recommendations and policy was changing from just getting an adequate
diet to making qualitative choices related to diet. Moderation and
choosing one type of food over another because of its effects on
chronic disease became important.

Since the *Dietary Goals for the United States* were released,
many government documents have been created that make recommendations about diet with respect to chronic diseases. The *Surgeon
General's Report on Nutrition and Health* presented the first comprehensive review of the scientific evidence associating diet with
chronic disease.[13] *Nutrition and Your Health: Dietary Guidelines for
Americans*, created by DHHS and USDA and jointly published every
5 years since 1980, recommended dietary changes to help people
avoid certain chronic diseases. The Dietary Guidelines were intended to be the foundation of all federal nutrition policies and programs and a vehicle for the government to speak with one voice on
nutrition and health.[14] Unfortunately, many federal and food programs are not compliant with the Dietary Guidelines. Government
policies still promote foods high in components such as saturated
fat and sodium that are overconsumed by the public.

The *Healthy People* initiative led by the DHHS Office of Disease
Prevention and Health Promotion has become the latest model for
policy development, including nutrition policy. *Healthy People 2010*
was developed by DHHS with input from all its operating divisions,
state and local government partners, more than 350 national mem-

bership organizations, nongovernmental organizations, corporate sponsors, and public input. It was a cooperative effort of government and nongovernment entities to create policy goals for the United States. *Healthy People 2010* contains a number of goals related to nutrition and is used by many public health agencies in creating nutrition policies. It has been suggested that *Healthy People 2010* may be DHHS's most effective nonlegislative policy vehicle for improving public health.[11]

Nutrition Policy: Goals and Methods

If the goal of public health policy is "fulfilling society's interest in assuring conditions in which people can be healthy,"[9] then nutrition policy would have the goal of assuring conditions in which people can be healthy through diet. There are two general ways that are used to try to influence what people eat: through education and through modification of the food supply.[2] In a very simplistic example, if a group of people were found to have a nutritional problem with inadequate amounts of vitamin A in the diet, the approach would be to teach them about the need for and sources of vitamin A *and* assure that they have a culturally acceptable, inexpensive, and appealing source of vitamin A available. (Another approach to finding a culturally acceptable and appealing source of vitamin A would be to create a new source for the vitamin through fortification of food, as has been done with some nutrients in the United States. This approach only works, however, when the lacking substances are known nutrients that can be easily added to common foods that are readily available.)

The problem becomes more complicated when the major nutritional problems being encountered are ones of excess, as with calories, sodium, and certain types of fat, or when whole food groups need to be increased, such as with fruits and vegetables. How does government create policies to discourage the consumption of certain foods and encourage the consumption of others?

The preferred policy method by many is education—educating the public on which foods should be consumed and which foods should be avoided or eaten in moderation.[2] This may be accomplished through consumer education campaigns, food assistance programs, and official documents of the government giving dietary advice, such as the Dietary Guidelines. Using education to influence food choices is a less powerful way to influence dietary behavior than actually trying to modify the food supply. Many prefer education, however, because it has less of an effect on personal freedom (you can still choose to eat junk food all day long), and it has less impact on the economic conditions of those producing and selling the foods to be avoided. Education may also be about prohibiting claims that provide false information or unfairly influence certain segments of the population. For example, it may be desirable to restrict unsubstantiated claims for foods and nutrients or to limit advertising of certain foods to children.

A more powerful way to influence dietary choices is through modifying the food supply.[2] Foods that are healthful should be more readily available and less expensive than those that would be considered less healthful or that are currently eaten in excess. Some have argued that the current obesity epidemic is due to a toxic environment where the wrong types of foods are readily available in supersized amounts.[15] Portion sizes of foods in restaurants have increased, the number of convenience foods has multiplied, and vending machines make low-nutrient foods readily available almost everywhere. Changes in the food supply, coupled with education, is generally considered a more successful strategy for dietary change.[2]

Government policies have a great impact on what foods are available to the public and at what price. Many of the current food policies come from a time when providing adequate food at a cheap price was the goal of U.S. agricultural and nutrition policy. The conditions and health issues that existed when those policies were created are not the same as exist now. From a nutrition policy point of view, these policies need to be reevaluated to create food policies that support the production, marketing, and low price of foods that are associated with a healthier diet. This is not a readily acceptable option to many, however, because it means dramatic changes in economic realities for those whose livelihoods depend on current government food and agricultural policy.

Beyond agricultural policy, there are ways to control the food supply that have been tried or suggested. Some of these suggestions include altering school lunch menus to meet the Dietary Guidelines, offering low cost or free fruits and vegetables to schools, adding fruits and vegetables and limiting the fat content in WIC food packages, limiting vending machines and pouring rights for soft drinks in schools, taxing empty-calorie foods, and removing candy from the checkout stands of supermarkets. Another way the government attempts to modify the food supply, at least for a select part of the population, is through redistribution. The government purchases foods for those who lack resources to purchase healthy or adequate amounts of food. Food Stamps, WIC, and commodities programs are examples of these types of programs. Nutrition policy is also required for nutrition monitoring and surveillance, research, food assistance, licensure, and food safety and quality.[11]

Policy Formulation

Policy formation is a complex, dynamic, and sometimes difficult process.[3] In an ideal world, nutrition policy would be formed using an accurate assessment of a community and its nutritional needs, the latest scientific information about nutrition, information about effective strategies, and community values. Policy would be evaluated on a regular basis and revised as needed, and would be created proactively to prevent, as well as, to solve problems. Nutrition policy would be integrated with other public policies, and all public policies would be supportive of the same goals. This is rarely the way public policy is created, however.

Public policy is created in a political environment.[2,7] Although public health officials prefer to look at problems and solutions in an objective manner, valuing technical expertise and scientific data, most policy makers work in a political environment where public values, popular opinions, and organized special interest groups have considerable influence.[9] There are many players in the public policy development process, and some are considered more important than others.[3] There are special interest groups, congressional committees and subcommittees, agencies of the executive branch of government, professional organizations, political parties, private and nonprofit organizations, economic and religious groups, individuals, and the media. Each of these has its own perspectives and philosophies that influence what is perceived as problems and what solutions should be created to solve problems. Scientific evidence may or may not coincide with the views of these groups. In the political process, all views become important, and public health officials must work to put forward solutions to problems that are objective and consistent with scientific observations. To many politicians, the opinion of public health officials may be just another opinion, and not necessarily an important, informed opinion.

Policy is generally created to solve a specific problem, often an emerging problem that has generated public concern.[2,3] As stated earlier in this chapter, the problem may be real or it may simply be something that is perceived to be a problem. The more severe the problem is perceived to be and the more public interest the problem generates, the more likely it will result in new policy.[4]

Most policies are created in an incremental fashion.[2,4] Public officials prefer incrementalism because it allows them to draw on past experience, work within an existing framework, and avoid major changes that could create large unforeseen problems and political fallout.[2,4] On the other hand, incrementalism stifles innovation and may add to the complexity of existing policy. If multiple small changes are made to a policy to solve immediate problems, sometimes the overall integrity of the original policy starts to break down. This is often observed in federal food programs, where incremental policy changes continue to add policy requirements without making changes to the overall program to accommodate these changes.

> **Incrementalism**—Policy making in small steps, rather than with large comprehensive reforms.

Once policies are created there is a reluctance to change them, especially as they become accepted practice. Old policies that become ineffective because the conditions for which they were created have changed often stay in force because of resistance to change.[16] Changing old policies is especially difficult when economic interests are dependent on the old policy. As noted by the IOM and others, much of U.S. public health policy was created at a time when conditions were quite different from what they are today.[2,9]

Most political scientists identify at least four steps for creating public policy[4]:

1. Agenda setting
2. Policy formulation
3. Policy implementation
4. Policy evaluation

Agenda Setting

The first step in creating new policy is to identify the problem to be solved, create broad goals to resolve the problem, and then position the issue on the policy maker's agenda. There are a number of potential problems that may make it difficult or impossible to move beyond this step in policy creation.

As stated, the first issue is identifying the real problem. This may be easier than it sounds. For example, one of the goals of *Healthy People 2010* is to increase breast-feeding rates. There are many theories about why women are unable or reluctant to breast-feed their infants for 6 months or a year, but which of these theories may be the real reason(s) and, therefore, most important for policy development? Changes to which of them would have the greatest impact on breast-feeding rates? Public opinion, people's belief structures, and special interest groups may be passionate about their views on what prevents breast-feeding rates from increasing, but the real reasons may not be readily apparent. Creating policy to solve the wrong problem would have limited impact on breast-feeding rates.

Once problems have been identified and policy goals set, then public health officials need to create a plan to get their recommended policy on the policy maker's agenda. Although the value of creating a policy to deal with a nutrition issue may be obvious to public health officials, it may not be to policy makers. In addition, getting a policy issue on the political agenda may be difficult and time-consuming. In general, policy issues are more likely to get on the political agenda when a great number of people believe the problem is real, and when people believe the consequences of the problem are likely to be severe, immediate, and to affect them personally.[4]

Even when a problem is perceived by many people to be a threat, it still may not get on the political agenda. Policymakers must believe that the problem is something that warrants government intervention.[2,4] There must also be room on the political agenda, and the issue must have enough priority over other issues. In a year when there are many significant problems facing policy makers, even an important issue may not make the political agenda.[4] Special interest groups that are opposed to a policy may also have enough clout to prevent a worthy policy issue from making the political agenda.[4]

Policy Formulation

Once an agenda has been set and a public health problem is placed on that agenda, the next step is formulation of an actual policy to address the issue. Alternative proposals are created. Information is collected about each of the proposals, and then a case is made for the proposal that seems to be the best solution for the problem.

Policy formation is about compromising and bargaining. Generally, one solution to a problem will not be accepted and championed to succeed without substantial changes and compromises. More likely, many different solutions and versions will be presented and debated. The solution that is eventually successful will often be modified before it reaches its final form. These modifications may weaken or strengthen the policy. Modifications are generally based on the ideologies and interests of various players in the political process, who have an interest in the outcome and effects of the proposal.

Policy Implementation

After a new policy has been created, it must be implemented. New policies are rarely written with adequate detail to allow their implementation.[4] The policy must be interpreted with the rules and regulations written to spell out how a policy will be implemented. Responsibility and financial resources must be assigned so that the policy may be implemented.

It may be tempting to believe that once a law has been passed public health officials should feel confident that the policy is now in place and will be effective. The implementation phase is very critical for the success of public policy.[4] Sometimes laws are passed establishing a new policy, but no funding is given for implementation, or those who write the rules and regulations do so in such a way as to make the policy weak or ineffective.[4] How a policy is implemented is critical to its success and must be guided by those who have the knowledge and expertise to create rules to make the policy successful.

Policy Evaluation

The final stage in policy development is policy evaluation. Despite the best efforts of everyone involved in policy development, new policies are rarely perfect. Once a policy has been implemented, it needs to be evaluated for success. If the policy is successful, it should be evaluated to see how it can be changed to make it more successful. Few policies retain the same level of value, simply because the environment and conditions for which they were created change with time. Policies need to be continuously evaluated so that they may be modified or discontinued as times change, because situations are complex and information is rarely complete.

Policy Creation at the Federal Level

The Federal Government was created to have a separation of powers. There are three branches of the federal government, each with its own responsibility and power. The legislative branch (Congress) is responsible for creating laws, the executive branch (the president) for enforcing laws, and the judicial branch (the courts) for interpreting laws.[11]

In the United States, most public policy is created by legislation.[2] Congress has the authority to pass laws that initiate, modify, and authorize, and appropriate funding for all programs and services is administered by the federal government. The legislative process is started when a member of Congress introduces a bill for consideration. If the bill is introduced in the Senate, it is given a designation starting with *S*, followed by an identifying number; if the bill is introduced in the House of Representatives, it is given a designation starting with *H.R.*, followed by an identifying number. The leadership of the Senate or House then assigns the bill to a subcommittee or committee that will consider the bill. Because of the numerous bills that are introduced to Congress each year, many die from neglect in subcommittees and committees.[17]

Congressional committees have considerable power in determining what will move forward to possibly become law and what will be tabled.[3,17] If the bill is of interest to the members of the assigned committee, is of sufficient priority, and the political climate is right, the committee may hold hearings on the bill. The committee may decide to amend the bill by adding or deleting parts. The clean bill (amended version) is voted on and is "reported out" either to a committee if it was in a subcommittee, or to the entire Senate or House if the bill was in a committee. If the bill was started in the Senate, it will be debated by the Senate, possibly amended, and then voted on. The bill would then go to a committee in the House for consideration. The House committee would then consider the bill, possibly amend it, and send it to the House for amendments and a vote. To save time, versions of the same bill may be introduced into both the Senate and House at the same time. These are referred to as companion bills.

If a bill is successfully voted on and passed by both the Senate and the House, the bill is sent to a conference committee made up of members of both the Senate and House. This committee attempts to resolve any differences between the two versions of the bill. The conference version of a bill must be sent back to both the Senate and House for a final vote before the bill is sent to the President.

The President has three choices when receiving a bill: First, he may sign the bill within 10 days and it becomes law. Second, he may veto the bill and send it back to Congress. This effectively kills the bill unless two-thirds of the members of both the Senate and House vote in favor of the bill to override the veto. Third, the President may do nothing with the bill when it is received.

If the President does nothing with the bill after it has been sent to him by Congress, there are two possibilities. If Congress is in session, the bill will become law in 10 days (excluding Sundays) even without the President's signature. If Congress is not in session, the bill does not become law. This is known as a "pocket veto."

Although most public policy in the United States is created by legislation through Congress, the other two branches of government can and do also create public policy.[18] Legislation passed by Congress must be turned into practical rules and regulations so that they may be carried out.[17] This is the duty of federal employees in the executive branch of government. The rules and regulations created to implement policy will have a great impact on whether the original intent of a policy can be accomplished. These employees have considerable policymaking power, because they create the rules and regulations.

The executive branch of government also is responsible for the enforcement of legislation. Decisions about how forcefully or even whether to enforce legislation have significant impact on policy. Public policy is what government actually does or does not do. If enforcement is lax, then the intended outcome of legislation or policy will be lost.

The agenda of a U.S. president and his political party can have significant impact on how legislation is turned into practical policies and how they are enforced and funded. Members of the executive branch of government, including the president, have a significant role in advocating for budget allocations, enforcing policy, and acting as advisors to members of Congress on technical issues.

The president may also create public policy through an executive memorandum. President Clinton did this when leaving office by making an Executive Order that the WIC program would screen children under age 2 for immunizations.

The judicial branch of the federal government makes public policy through court decisions that decide the intent and meaning of laws, whether a public health agency is operating within its scope of legislative authority, and whether public health statutes and regulations are constitutionally permissible.[11] The U.S. Supreme Court has made many decisions of importance to public health, including upholding the power of the government to protect the public's health.[11]

Policy Development at All Levels of Government: Federal, State, and Local

Policy development is important at all levels of government in order for public health agencies to fulfill their role in assuring health.[9] Each level of government has its own unique contributions to make in policy development and in providing public health services. From a historical and constitutional perspective, states have the primary responsible for the health of citizens of the United States.[9] Local governments, in turn, receive their authority from state governments. The federal government has, over time, developed a larger role in the promotion of health and now has many technical and leadership roles that influence state and local health policies.

It is important that all levels of government work together in creating effective health and nutrition policy.[11] By the very nature of having so many divisions of government, policies can become fragmented, overlapping, redundant, and at times contradictory. To deliver a convincing policy message in an organized and efficient way, all levels of government must work together.

Health problems, including nutritional problems, are seldom confined to one set of boundaries in the United States. For example, obesity may be more prevalent in some parts of the nation, but overall it is a problem in all parts of the nation. Food is grown in various parts of the country, but is then distributed to the entire country. Most processed foods are universally distributed across the nation. Television advertising and the lifestyle effects of television are universal throughout the United States. Food franchises, food labeling, and the effects of federal nutrition programs are nearly the same everywhere in the nation. The factors that improve or detract from our nutritional health are generally widespread, and not confined to a single state, county, or city. To make changes in policy that affect nutritional health requires a concerted policy effort by all levels of government giving a unified message.

Role of the Federal Government in Policy Development

The federal government plays a vital role in health and nutrition policy development. Many nutrition problems, such as obesity, increased prevalence of certain cancers, and heart disease, are problems that face the entire nation, and they are affected by behaviors and conditions that exist throughout the country. These problems require national policy attention, as well as state and local attention, if they are to be solved.

The federal government's policies affect the nutritional health of U.S. citizens in several ways.[9,11]

1. Federal policies greatly affect the food supply in the United States, including the quantity, types, and pricing of available

foods. Since the food supply affects nutritional health, any changes in agricultural policy would need to come from the federal level.

2. Since most food production, processing, packaging, labeling, and marketing are done at the national level, federal policies are necessary to bring about any changes.

3. The major food and nutrition programs in the United States are all administered and funded by the federal government. These programs impact a significant portion of the public. The policies of these programs determine what foods are given and what nutritional information is provided. For most states, the majority of the nutritionists and dietitians working in public health are employed by these programs. For some states, these programs constitute almost their entire public nutrition policy. Because federal programs, such as WIC, purchase such large quantities of foods such as cereals and infant formulas, program regulations affect manufacturing and marketing practices of the foods to the entire population.

4. The federal government plays an important role in assessing nutritional health of the population of the United States. The National Health and Nutrition Examination Survey, Behavioral Risk Factor Surveillance System, and other surveys give the nutrition public health community the nutritional data upon which to base policy decisions.

5. The federal government has built up a resource of scientific and technical assistance that may be used by states to identify nutrition and health issues and to help create effective policies for solving the problems.

6. Since most nutritional problems are national, the federal government must play a role in policy leadership to identify, monitor, and resolve nutritional issues.

7. The federal government has the technical and financial resources for research to understand and solve nutrition problems.

8. Finally, the federal government has financial resources to assist states with public policies to solve public health nutrition problems. A good example of this is the money states are receiving from the CDC to create policies and programs to prevent obesity.

Role of Public Agencies in Policy Development

In the context of this chapter, agencies are governmental units that oversee nutrition programs. These agencies can exist at all levels of government, from the federal to the local level. At the federal level, the USDA is the agency that has been given the primary responsibility for nutrition programs and policy. Nutrition programs such as Food Stamps, the Commodity Supplemental Food Program, WIC, and the National School Lunch Program are administered at the federal level by the USDA. Operation of these programs is delegated to state agencies, which in many cases then delegate the programs to local agencies where services are actually provided.

Nutrition programs are created through legislation that is written with broad goals and a basic design for a program. It is the responsibility of agencies to translate these broad goals and designs into practical rules and regulations that allow for the actual operation of programs. This arrangement permits legislatures to create broad policies to accomplish goals, and then allows agency staff to use their expertise to create the rules that provide for actual delivery of services. Agency staff have more expertise in nutrition and in techniques to improve nutrition behavior than legislative staff, so this is a good arrangement.[2] Agency staff can work out details in programs that allow them to be effective and to work in an efficient manner.

Agency staff have great influence on public policy because they write rules and regulations for programs. If rules and regulations are written poorly, then programs will be ineffective and the goals of legislated policy will not be achieved. If the rules and regulations are well written, then the program may have great success. Whatever the intent by legislators, the end result depends in great measure on those designing the details of the programs.[4]

Agency staff are also responsible for enforcement, interpretation, and prioritization of rules and regulations. This also can have a significant impact on policy. Most government programs have large numbers of rules with many details. It is virtually impossible to follow all rules to the letter. Which rules agency staff decide to focus their energy on or to enforce will substantially impact public policy by what the program accomplishes.

Agency staff also have a role in advising policymakers at various levels of government. Agency staff can make recommendations for legislation and budgets. Since many agency staff are experts in their subject areas, such as nutrition, they can advise policymakers about proposed policies and proposed budgets, and can recommend new policies. For example, if agency staff monitoring health statistics find that fruit and vegetable consumption in school-age children is lacking, they can make recommendations for legislation to encourage fruit and vegetable consumption. Likewise, if a legislator decides that a new program is needed to address obesity, agency staff can help develop the legislation and make recommendations for how the legislation is written, methods for decreasing obesity, and how much money should be allocated. Agency staff often make recommendations for policy when new legislation is being created and when programs are being reauthorized by Congress.

Role of State Government in Policy Development

State governments are responsible for the health of their citizens.[9] This responsibility was given to the states by the U.S. Constitution. States may delegate some of this responsibility to local governments, but the ultimate responsibility rests with the states.[9,18] Since the 1960s, the federal government has been playing a larger role, providing resources and expertise to help state governments fulfill their responsibility for the health of their citizens.[11] Because states have the ultimate responsibility for their citizens' health, however, they must be involved in the process of policy development related to health issues.

In its report, *Future of Public Health*, the IOM remarked that states must be the central force in public health.[9] States have a responsibility to collect and analyze information on the health of their citizens, to set policies and standards, to carry out national and state mandates, and to respond to health issues. The IOM recommended that each state have a health council that reports on health issues in the state and makes policy recommendations to the governor and legislature for policy development.

Policy does not just happen, and legislatures are generally not looking for new public health policies to create. Because many states do not have a single lead nutritionist responsible for policy development, it is the responsibility of all nutrition professionals in a state to assess their state's nutritional health and determine what legislation is needed. This includes nutritionists at the state-agency level and their professional associations. Nutritionists also need to monitor all legislative activities for policy changes that could affect the nutrition of the public.

State personnel are sometimes restricted in their government positions from advocating for legislation, at least while functioning as a government employee. Local dietetic associations and nutrition alliances, such as anti-hunger groups or nutrition networks, may be effective in proposing and advocating for nutrition policy changes.

State governments offer an advantage in policy development in that most state legislators are more accessible than are federal legislators. Legislators may be more responsive to small groups of advocates. Nutritionists at the state level have been successful at getting legislation introduced and passed regarding licensure of dietitians, pro-breast-feeding policies, issues affecting school nutrition, and reimbursement for certain types of nutrition counseling.

Role of Local Government in Policy Development

Local governments vary considerably in their form and configuration, as well as how they deal with health issues. There are a great many units of local government with a wide range of structures, functions, and size.[9] Some local governments are larger than some state governments, and some are so small that they have few resources and staff for health functions.

Local government is where nutrition services occur. State governments often delegate portions of their responsibility for health to local government units because it is local governments that are able to actually provide health services. Many nutrition programs, while administered at the state level, provide services through units of local governments.

Policy development needs to occur at the local level, as at all levels of government.[9] Local governments may be the most accessible of all when trying to create policy. One passionate nutritionist with good organizational and people skills can do great things with respect to nutrition policy while working with the school board, local health department, physicians, and city government. It may be possible to get legislation created and passed around nutrition education or vending machines in the school, breast-feeding issues, or senior nutrition programs. Policies created at the local level can become models and open doors to getting similar policies passed at the state level. Of course, it is always important that local policies target goals similar to national nutrition policies.

Much like agency personnel, local nutrition professionals have a great impact on actual nutrition policy as it is administered. A nutritionist working for a federal nutrition program at the local level can determine how well that program functions and interacts with other health programs. A local nutritionist working for WIC, who reaches out to the community and builds a quality WIC program, helps create effective nutrition policy. Likewise, a nutritionist who works to build coalitions with Head Start, preschools, day-care programs, nurse partnerships, and other programs can create an environment where nutrition issues are addressed and the nutritional health of the community benefits. A nutritionist in the same community who creates barriers to WIC services and builds walls with other programs will have the opposite effect on nutrition in the community.

Leadership Roles for Nutritionists

The purpose of public health policy is to create conditions in which people can be healthy. Public policy should create conditions where it is easier to be healthy and harder to make decisions that contribute to a person being less healthy. Policy makers at all levels of government are responsible for policy development.

Members of The American Dietetic Association can sign up to be a member of a listserv called "On the Pulse" to receive nutrition policy updates. To do this, go to http://www.eatright.org/Member/83_11027.cfm.

Good nutrition policy does not just happen. Policy development is a long, complex process, affected by many players and filled with compromises. There is no nutrition czar in the United

States to watch out for needed nutrition policy legislation. It is the role of every nutritionist to be involved and to work for good nutrition policy. Nutritionists need to be informed and work together to bring about changes for better nutrition. This is especially true as the United States faces one of its most challenging nutritional epidemics, that of obesity.

Issues for Discussion

1. Why is public policy important? Please discuss public policy in relation to obesity.
2. Nutritional concerns have changed significantly since the beginning of the twentieth century. Yet nutrition policy remains conflicting, inconsistent, and fragmented among numerous laws, agencies, programs, and branches of government. Please discuss how nutrition policy could be improved in the United States.
3. Public policy is created in a political setting. Please explain who you think the best group or groups are to create public policy. Why?

References

1. *The New Oxford Dictionary of English*. (1998). Oxford: Oxford University Press.
2. Sims, L. (1998). *The politics of fat: Food and nutrition in America*. Armonk, NY: M.E. Sharp.
3. Block, L. E. (2001). Health policy through the looking glass. In Harrington, Charlene & Estes, Carroll L. (eds.), *Health policy: Crisis and reform in the U.S. health care delivery system*, 3rd ed., 258–369. Sudbury, MA: Jones and Bartlett.
4. Anderson, G., & Hussey, P. S. (2001). Influencing government policy: A framework. In Pencheon, David, Guest, Charles, Melzer, David, & Muir Gray, J. A. (eds.), *Oxford handbook of public health practice*. Oxford: Oxford University Press,146–154.
5. Ackoff, R. L. (1974). *Redesigning the future: A systems approach to societal problems*. New York: Wiley.
6. Pencheon, D.; Guest, C. Melzer, D. & Muir Gray, J. A. (2001). Introduction. In *Oxford Handbook of Public Health Practice*. Oxford: Oxford University Press, 126–127.
7. Gostin, L. (2000). Public health law in a new century: Part III: Public health regulation: A systematic evaluation, *JAMA, 283*, 3118–3122.
8. Milio, N. (1976). A framework for prevention: Changing health-damaging to health-generating life patterns. *American Journal of Public Health*, 66, 435–439.
9. Institute of Medicine, Committee for the Study of the Future of Public Health. (1988). *The future of public health*. Washington, DC: National Academy Press.

10. Foege, W. (2001). Leadership and policy development. In Rowitz, Louis (ed.), *Public health leadership: Putting principles into practice.* Gaithersburg, MD: Aspen,126–147.

11. Institute of Medicine, Committee on Assuring the Health of the Public in the 21st Century. (2002). *The future of the public's health in the 21st century.* Washington, DC: National Academy Press.

12. Bunker, J. P., Frazier, H. S., & Mosteller, F. (1994). Improving health: Measuring effects of medical care. *Milbank Quarterly*, 72, 225–258.

13. McGinnis, J. M. & Nestle, M. (1989). The surgeon general's report on nutrition and health: Policy implications and implementation strategies. *American Journal of Clinical Nutrition*, 49, 23–28.

14. McMurray, K. Y. (2003). Setting dietary guidelines: The U.S. process. *Journal of the American Dietetic Association*, 103(12), S10–S16.

15. Murray, B. (2001). Fast-food culture serves up supersize Americans. *Monitor on Psychology*, 32(11).

16. Koh, Y. M. (2001). Shaping your organization's policy. In Pencheon, David; Guest, Charles; Melzer, David; & Muir Gray, J. A. (eds.), *Oxford handbook of public health practice.* Oxford: Oxford University Press, 128–135.

17. Hart, S. & Jackson, N. (2001). Primer on policy: The legislative process at the federal level. In Harrington, Charlene & Estes, Carroll J. (eds.), *Health policy: Crisis and reform in the U.S. health care delivery system*, 3rd ed., 370–372. Sudbury, MA: Jones and Bartlett.

18. Mensah, G. A.; Goodman, R. A.; Zara, S. Moulton, A. D.; Kocher, P. L.; Dietz, W. H. et al. (April 2004). Law as a Tool for Preventing Chronic Diseases: Expanding the Spectrum of Public Health Strategies [Part 2], Preventing Chronic Disease. Available at: http://www.cdc.gov/pcd/issues/2004/apr/04_0009.htm.

CHAPTER 8

ADVOCATING AND INFLUENCING HEALTH AND NUTRITION POLICIES

Bruce Rengers, PhD, RD

Reader Objectives

After studying this chapter and reflecting on the contents, you should be able to:

1. Describe the importance of being an advocate for public health policy.
2. Justify the role of politics in policy development.
3. Identify factors that influence policy development.
4. Delineate methods to build support for new policies.
5. Discuss the importance of building an infrastructure of support for policy development.
6. Name some individual skills needed for being an effective public health advocate.

The Importance of Being an Advocate for Public Health and Nutrition

Advocacy is the act of supporting or promoting a cause. Public health and nutrition professionals *must* advocate for nutrition policy. Nutrition policy does not just happen. We tend to take for granted nutrition policies from the past and to allow market forces and special interest groups to determine nutrition policies for the future. For nutrition and public health professionals, it is a primary responsibility to advocate for effective public policies that will improve the nutritional health of people in the United States.[1]

Public policy is how government creates conditions to maintain or improve the health of its citizens. Every aspect of our lives is influenced by public policy, including what we eat and our nutritional health.[2] Government has an interest in keeping its citizens healthy. Using public policy, government can have a powerful effect on a nation's health. Keeping citizens healthy results in a more productive society, lower healthcare costs, and an improved general well-being of society.

Good policy development is a result of a careful assessment of problems, objective knowledge about problems, establishment of priorities based on data, and allocation of resources for maximum benefit.[3] It is tempting to think that public health policy in the United States is generally created in this manner; however, this is often not the case. Policy development in the United States has been described as "complex, dynamic, confusing, and at times mysterious."[4] Development of public policy has been driven by crises, hot issues, and the concerns of well-organized interests.[5] As a result of this undisciplined and subjective process, public health policy in the United States has been described as outdated, fragmented, conflicted, and ineffective,[3] and the U.S. public health infrastructure as being in disarray.[5]

Policy development is one of the core functions of public health.[5] Leaders of public health have a responsibility to develop sound policy[6] and to use every opportunity to influence policy to improve the health of citizens.[1] Public policy is the primary tool public health officials have to maintain and improve the public health. If public health officials do not lead in policy development, then policy development will be dominated by well-organized special interest groups, motivated by profit,[7] and by those with agendas unfounded in science. The net effect will be ineffective policy, a waste of resources, and detrimental effects on the public's health. Because of a lack of effective leadership and support, current public health policy lags behind scientific knowledge and consumer concerns.[2]

Leadership and advocacy in nutrition policy development is the responsibility of all nutritionists.[8,9] Although those employed in leadership roles in public health nutrition have specialized roles for leading in policy development, it is the responsibility of all nutritionists to advocate for effective nutrition policy. Marianne Smith Edge, former president of The American Dietetic Association (ADA), noted that gains in policy and advocacy for nutrition issues have been the result of many individuals and their willingness to get involved.[8] ADA's State Issues Task Force recommended that all ADA members be trained in leadership and policy development.[9]

It takes many people working together to influence the political process for effective policy change. The Institute of Medicine (IOM)[5] noted that one of the difficulties of policy development in public health has been public health officials trying to work in isolation, without a broad base of support. Public health officials must learn to work in a political environment, using the political process to accomplish their goals.

Politics in Policy Development

Most public policy in the United States is created by legislation through passage of laws.[2] This process involves politicians and the political process. Many people view politics with cynicism, as something that is undesirable. Yet politics is a highly necessary way to bring about change.[10] Politics is the use of power to shape policy and accomplish goals.[10] Science and logic may help to identify a public health problem, but it is generally emotion and power in the political process that determine what will be done about a problem.[11]

The IOM[5] noted that many public health officials view politics as a contamination of the policy development process. Substantial tension between professional expertise and politics has been observed throughout the U.S. public health system.[5] Public health officials are accustomed to using professional judgment, technical expertise, and scientific information to identify and solve problems.[5] This is how public health officials have been trained. It is a central tenet of their professional ethic to use objective, scientific information to solve problems.[5] Public policy, however, is developed in a political atmosphere that is anything but objective and rational. This dichotomy of perspective has led to isolation and difficulty in creating new health policy. The IOM and others[5,9] strongly recommend that public health professionals learn how to use the political process to accomplish needed goals. This includes developing political skills and a broad base of support to use in the political process.

Influencing Legislation

The first step in creating new public policy is to get the proposed policy on the agenda of lawmakers. This may be the most difficult part of the policy-making process.[2] Legislators have many issues and many individuals and interest groups vying to capture their attention. Organized interest groups whose purpose is to create legislation have proliferated.[2] In a given year, far more bills are proposed than can possibly be turned into policies.[2] Also, health issues must compete with policy issues unrelated to health, as well with other health issues.[12]

> Read more about nutrition policy, terms, and procedures at these sites: http://www.loc.gov and http://thomas.loc.gov.

To create new federal policy, a sponsor or sponsors must be found to introduce a bill to the House of Representatives or Senate. If the bill is introduced, it is then assigned to a committee or subcommittee that has responsibility for food and nutrition issues. Committees and subcommittees are the "gatekeepers" for legislation, and they determine which bills will get testimony and which will pass on to the full House or Senate. Many bills die in committees because they are of low priority in a packed agenda. Policymakers can concentrate on only a few new policies during a legislative session.[12]

A number of factors help determine which bills are likely to get put on the policy agenda and successfully move on to become law.[12] Bills are more likely to be successful at being placed on the policy agenda if:

- A greater number of people perceive the policy issue to be a problem.
- The problem is perceived to have greater severity.
- The problem is more immediate and novel.
- More people are affected by the problem personally.
- The political atmosphere is supportive of the policy.
- The policy is appealing the public.

In democracies, public opinion and special interest groups have a substantial impact on whether a bill for new policy will be put on the legislative agenda.[11] It is, therefore, important for public health officials to know how to influence public opinion and to obtain the support of organized interest groups. Working effectively with the media to form public opinion is an important relationship and skill to cultivate.[12]

Public support alone will not always be enough to get a bill on the policy agenda.[12] The policy in question must be one that members of Congress consider appropriate for government action. For example, with respect to obesity, many legislators do not feel it is the government's role to discourage certain types of foods through taxation. In their view, people should be able to make choices about food without government interference. If this is the prevailing political view, then it is unlikely that such a policy would ever be placed on the policy agenda for consideration.

Well-organized and financed special interest groups can also sway policymakers away from following public opinion in some situations. This is especially true when the policy only affects a small number of people, large economic interests are involved, or the issue is very technical in nature.[12] Even if public opinion can get legislation passed, influential interest groups can have substantial impact on the fine print of legislation that substantially changes the actual intent or effectiveness of a new policy.[2]

Once a proposed policy is on the policymaker's agenda, continued support is needed until it is passed as law. Compromising, bargaining, expert testimony, and guidance of the bill through the legislative process are all required. There is potential at every step of policy development for something to go wrong and for the policy to be derailed.[12] The process of creating public policy rarely allows the original policy, as it was introduced, to remain unmodified. Public health officials must be willing to compromise and bargain to create a policy with the greatest public and political acceptance.[12] Compromising, however, must be balanced with a need to maintain at least some of the original intent of the policy.

Building Support for New Policies

The Policy

The first step in building support for a new policy is to create a defensible, sound policy.[6,13] Health policies must be based on accurate and complete scientific information. Cause and distribution of the health issue need to be known, as well as effective strategies for intervention.[5] Public health leaders must know the scientific literature and be able to present a strong case in favor of the policy. Is there sufficient scientific information to justify the policy? Sometimes, complete information is not available when creating policy. The potential risk of creating policy with inadequate information needs to be weighed against the need for the policy.[13]

Public health leaders must also be able to assess the feasibility of the new policy, the costs and benefits of having the policy, the costs and benefits of *not* having the policy, and the compatibility of the policy with public values.[5,14] The human rights burden, the effects of the new policy on personal freedoms, fairness of cost distribution, and reasonableness between means and end must also be considered.[15] It is the responsibility of the policy developer to justify the costs and burdens of new policy against its benefits.[15]

Public Opinion

Public policy tends to follow public opinion.[12] It is, therefore, very important to build public support for new policies. This can be done through the media, public officials, celebrities, and public awareness campaigns.[12] Public opinion can also be developed by building coalitions or alliances, citizen participation in policy development, communication with the public at large, and communication with elected officials.[5] The IOM noted that the public health system in the United States tends to be isolated and recommended that public health officials work at building a broad base of support.[5]

To be effective in building public support, public health officials need to cultivate a relationship with the public through regular communication, not just when policy issues are being discussed. Public health officials need to build ongoing credibility and a positive relationship with the public. The community, as well as elected officials, must see public health personnel as technical experts and as advocates for the community and supportive of community values.[5] Both technical knowledge and public values determine how public health is practiced.[5] Rather than having a paternalistic approach to communication, public health needs to encourage debate[11] and empower communities to create solutions to their own health issues.[6]

Timing of Policy Proposals

A new policy may not become part of the political agenda even when it is well supported. Timing is critical.[12] Policy agendas may be filled with other issues that are considered higher priorities. Reintroduction of the health policy in a different legislative session, when fewer priority items are on the agenda, may increase the likelihood of getting on the political agenda.

It is also important to judge the political climate when introducing new policy. What is the prevailing philosophy concerning the health issue and proposed solution? Who in the legislative committee will be in favor or strongly opposed to the new policy? If the political climate is not supportive, it may be impossible to get the new policy on the legislative agenda. Waiting another year until the players or climate changes may be the best option.

Sometimes it takes multiple tries to get a new policy on the legislative agenda. Once on the agenda, it may also take multiple tries to get the legislation passed. Repeated attempts help gather support and decrease opposition in many cases. Policy may also need to be created incrementally or in small steps over time.[2,12] To get legislation for dietetic licensure in one state, the sponsors of the legislation had to agree to exempt dietitians employed in certain practice settings. This wasn't the intent of the original policy, but it allowed a licensure bill to become law. In the following years, the legislation was amended to include some of the dietitians originally excluded. Through incremental change over time, the original intent of the policy was eventually accomplished.

Lobbying

Lobbying is the process of trying to influence the members of a legislature.[16] Lobbying is an art, not a science.[16] It can be done by professional lobbyists or it can be done by individuals or groups trying to advance their cause. By one estimate, there are close to 20,000 professional lobbyists in Washington, D.C.,[17] which makes for a lot of people trying to influence policymakers' decisions.

Lobbyists serve several functions in their roles. They attempt to educate legislators on issues important to their cause, stimulate public debate on issues, and encourage participation in the political process while trying to gather public support for their legislative issues.[2] "Lobby" has also come to have a negative connotation, referring to pressure groups that run sophisticated campaigns to influence legislators by a variety of persuasive methods.[16]

Public health professionals, health professionals, and consumer advocate groups have taken up lobbying as a way to influence legislation on public policy. Some have been reasonably successful.[16] In general, public health lobbyists are fewer in number and far less well-financed than those from economic interests. It is a challenge to overcome the influence of lobbyists from well-funded groups that may not favor certain policy changes important for health.

Government programs are generally prohibited from lobbying, as are government employees in many circumstances. Because government programs need the benefits of lobbying, they sometimes form private groups that will lobby for them. For example, many state and local WIC programs are members of the National WIC Association (NWA). NWA is a private, nonprofit organization that advocates for WIC and issues related to the WIC program. NWA provides information to legislators, makes recommendations on funding and policy changes related to WIC, and works to build community support for the program.

Groups That Are Part of the Political Process

Political Action Committees (PACs)

PACs are organized for the purpose of raising and spending money to elect or defeat political candidates.[17] Most PACs have specific legislative agendas and work to elect political candidates sympathetic to their cause. Health-related groups have created PACs so that their members can contribute money to help elect candidates that support their issues. As an example, The American Dietetic Association has an active PAC.

Coalitions

A coalition is a group of people and organizations that have come together to influence outcomes related to a specific problem.[6] For example, a coalition of interested citizens and health groups may come together to find ways to reduce the increasing prevalence of obesity in a community. Many communities have nutrition or hunger coalitions to solve nutrition and hunger issues.

Coalitions can be an excellent way for public health officials to design and propose new public health policies. They bring together community and health-related groups, as well as public and private organizations for public health issues. Building coalitions for policy development in public health was one of the recommendations made by the IOM to allow for more community involvement in public health.[5]

Alliances

Alliances are groups of healthcare and public health organizations that combine forces to address public health issues in a specific geographic area.[6] Alliances can also bring together public and private groups to work on a common issue. Coalitions and alliances allow for synergism in solving problems. Collectively, the group can do more than all of the partners separately.

Professional Organizations

Organizations of health professionals, such as The American Dietetic Association (ADA), the Society for Nutrition Education (SNE), or the American Public Health Association (APHA), have a strong role in advocating for public health issues. These organizations can create policy statements that support legislation. They can hire lobbyists, and they have the ability to mobilize members to lobby legislators on specific legislation. They can be technical resources when legislation is being created and provide expert testimony. Belonging to a professional organization that advocates for nutrition and public health is an important responsibility every nutritionist has to the nation's health.[9]

Health Advocacy Organizations

Health advocacy organizations generally focus on a specific health issue. They help advocate for public health in the same way as professional organizations. For example, The American Diabetes Association would be active in advocating for health issues related to diabetes. They can be an important partner in an alliance or coalition working for public policy change.

Consumer Advocacy Groups

Consumer advocacy groups can have a very powerful influence on legislatures. The American Association of Retired People (AARP) is one of the largest advocacy groups in the United States, and as such has tremendous influence with legislatures. It represents a very large and growing block of voting citizens.

The Center for Science in the Public Interest (CSPI) is another consumer advocacy group that has had considerable impact on nutrition policy in the United States. CSPI's goals include providing useful, objective information to the public and policymakers on food and nutrition; representing citizens' interests before government units; and ensuring that science and technology are used for the public good. CSPI has brought significant attention to nutrition issues, especially in controversial areas, through use of the media.

Political Parties

Political parties have a major role in determining public policy.[12] This is be done by formal party manifestos prior to elections,[1] or in an informal way through the philosophical beliefs under which the political parties operate. A political party that is supportive of health policy can be indispensable in helping to draft health legislation and to get it on the policy agenda. A political party opposed to health legislation can be a formidable hurdle.

National Academy of Sciences (NAS)/Institute of Medicine (IOM)

The National Academy of Sciences is a private, nonprofit society that was given a charter by Congress in 1863. NAS has a mandate to advise the federal government on scientific and technical matters. The Institute of Medicine is part of the NAS and conducts policy studies on health issues. Congress often refers health issues to the IOM when a nonpartisan, impartial review and recommendation is needed. Documents from the IOM are invaluable in advocating for change in public health and nutrition policy.

Media

The media helps shape the public's view of reality and can have strong effects on public opinion.[12] Anyone who has ever worked with the media is aware of how important it is to develop a positive and mutually beneficial relationship with the media. How the media "frames" an issue can make a major difference in whether the public will support or reject proposed policy. The media needs news stories of interest to entice the public, and public health officials need the media to educate the public. Public health officials must become dependable sources of accurate information for the media so that the media may frame them as knowledgeable experts when health issues arise.

The Importance of Building an Infrastructure of Support

To be able to build an ongoing base of support, it is necessary to cultivate relationships with the public and politicians; in essence, to create an infrastructure of support. Policy development should be an ongoing process to improve the health of the community, rather than a crisis-driven necessity when health issues arise. For public health officials to be effective advocates for policy change, they need to have the support of the community, other health professionals, and politicians. The IOM has made several recommendations for building a base of political support[5]:

- Public health officials should develop relationships with legislatures and other public officials and educate them on public health issues.
- Public health agencies should train staff in community relations and citizen participation.
- Public health agencies should develop relationships with physicians and other private sector representatives, including professional societies and academic medical centers.
- Public health agencies should seek stronger relationships and common goals with other professional and citizen groups involved with health issues.
- Agencies should undertake education of the public on health issues.
- Agencies should review the quality of contacts between employees and clients to ensure the public is treated with cordiality and respect.

The IOM noted that these relationships need to be cultivated and fostered on an ongoing basis.[5] Building these relationships is part of the political process necessary to accomplish goals. It has been suggested that political skills must be consistently used in order to maintain them.[7]

Advocacy Activities and Skills for Individuals

Individuals may be the most important advocates for public health and nutrition. All of the organizations and groups listed previously are made up of collections of individuals. It is the actions of those individuals that make groups effective.[8] Margaret Mead made the statement, "A small group of thoughtful people could change the world. Indeed, it is the only thing that ever has." It is important to not feel powerless when confronting major health or nutrition problems. Passionate, persistent individuals have made remarkable differences in the face of poor odds.

There are many ways that an individual can advocate for nutrition policy, either as a private individual or as a professional. The following suggestions apply to individuals advocating on their own or as part of groups made up of individuals:

- Know your elected officials. Read about their voting records, and get to know their philosophies and voting records related to health issues. Attend town hall meetings and make your opinions heard. Some professional associations, such as state affiliates of the ADA, have legislative luncheons where you can meet your elected officials. Attend these luncheons and talk to your elected officials. Be assertive, but polite, friendly, and tactful. Write letters, email, and telephone your elected officials telling them your views on public health and nutrition issues. Even when it is unlikely that the official will be swayed to change his or her mind on an issue, it is still good to let him or her know your views. It may soften his or her opposition.
- Vote in elections to influence who will represent your views in government.
- Be informed about the issues, current legislation, your community, and the arguments of those opposed to your views.
- Join a professional association or advocacy group(s) that advocates for public health. Many voices are generally louder than one. Be active in the group and encourage policy involvement.
- Respect others and their points of view even when they are diametrically opposed to your own.
- Conflicts arise. Don't take them personally. Learn from your opponent's position; it may strengthen your own position. Accept that some people may reject you for your position on an issue.
- Write letters to the editor of the newspaper when you have a strong position on a health or nutrition issue.
- Be persistent. Learn from your own mistakes and move on with that knowledge to do a better job next time.

Writing for Advocacy

There are a number of situations where advocacy is best done in writing. These could include letters to the editor of a newspaper, letters to elected officials, and written testimony for policy change.

For most writing it is important to remember that no one has to read what you have written.[18] Unless your letter is well written and catches the reader's attention, it may be ignored. Think before you write and organize your thoughts. Make your position clear early in the letter and find a way to get your reader's attention. Focus on one or two ideas and be brief. Most people are not motivated to read long essays.

Collect key statistics, research the literature, and make sure you are knowledgeable about current events related to your topic before you start writing.[18] Make sure that you are able to back up every fact and assertion with documentation and evidence. Accuracy is very important.

Use small words and short sentences, and don't be offensive.[19] Write while the issue is still in the public's attention. After writing, let the letter wait for a few hours or overnight before sending it. Reread the letter to make sure it says what you really intended and in a way you intended. Remember that what you write may be read by many thousands of people and will be remembered into the future. It may be helpful to have someone else read your letter and give you feedback before mailing it.

The government often requests written comments on new policies and policy changes. These requests for comments are printed in the *Federal Register* for comment periods of 30 to 90 days. This is one of those unusual times when someone is required to read your letter and comments. Federal employees are required to read and compile all comments received during a comment period. These compiled comments are then used to support approval, change, or rejection of proposed policies. Most people don't make a habit of reading the *Federal Register*, but news reports will often comment on certain proposed changes related to food or nutrition. The *Federal Register* can be accessed online for easy reading at http://www.gpoaccess.gov/fr/index.html. Organized special interest groups will comment on proposed policy, so it is important that public health advocates also comment.

> ***Federal Register***—A daily publication that compiles every regulation, and change in regulation, proposed and enacted upon by any branch of the U.S. government.

Media

Most people do not like talking in front of a crowd or on television. Media, however, is a very important tool in advocacy. The media can help form public opinion by reporting on issues related to nutrition and public health. How media frames an issue will help determine public reaction.

Many organizations actively look for media exposure to build their credibility in the eyes of the public. For example, universities often want faculty to comment on public health issues related to their research. Public health departments may want staff to discuss health issues when public involvement is needed. Nutritionists can use the media to discuss current issues, build credibility, and educate the public on nutrition principles.

With the media, there is always a danger of being misquoted or quoted out of context. There is also the possibility of a reporter, with an agenda, making the interview negative and combative. You should receive training in media interviews to help avoid such situations, but it is equally important that health officials not shy away from media attention for fear of negative consequences.

Public Testimony

Legislatures and government agencies often require public hearings on proposed legislation before a formal vote is taken or major policy changes are made. For example, a committee of a state senate may hold public hearings on a farmer's market bill before taking a vote. Again, most people are not eager to speak in public, but this can be a very important way of advocating for good nutrition or public health policy. It is also an example where public and private partnerships are very important for advocacy. A state agency may propose new legislation to offer fresh fruit snacks in schools but be limited by its government association from testifying in favor of the legislation. The local dietetic association or health coalition can be very helpful advocates by rallying members to testify in favor of the legislation.

The Future of Public Health

The future of public health will be determined by those with the greatest influence on public policy development. It is critical that public health officials work to become effective advocates of public health. Good public policy does not happen on its own. Without effective leadership from public health officials, public health will be determined by those with the greatest economic interest or political need. Effective skills and strategies in policy development must be developed by public health professionals. These skills require development of a broad base of support in the community and credibility as technical experts. As individuals, those with concerns for public health must remember that it is the actions of many individuals that result in positive changes for public health. Each public health professional as an individual and as part of organized groups must advocate for optimal health for all.

Issues for Discussion

1. Briefly describe the steps required to create new public health policy.
2. Please describe examples of how the media has helped shape the public's view of reality on public health policy.
3. Building a base of public support is important to get a public health policy through the legislature. Please explain how to develop public support in respect to a policy on obesity.

References

1. Wall, P. (2001). Influencing government policy: A national review. In Pencheon, David; Guest, Charles; Melzer, David; & Muir Gray, J. A. (eds.), *Oxford handbook of public health practice*. Oxford: Oxford University Press, 156–161.
2. Sims, L. (1998). *The politics of fat: Food and nutrition in America*. Armonk, NY: M.E. Sharp.
3. Institute of Medicine, Committee on Assuring the Health of the Public in the 21st Century. (2002). *The future of the public's health in the 21st century*. Washington, DC: National Academy Press.
4. Block, L. E. (2001). Health policy through the looking glass. In Harrington, Charlene & Estes, Carroll L. (eds.), *Health policy: Crisis and reform in the U.S. healthcare delivery system*, 3rd ed. Sudbury, MA: Jones and Bartlett, 358–369.
5. Institute of Medicine, Committee for the Study of the Future of Public Health. (1988). *The future of public health*. Washington, DC: National Academy Press.
6. Foege, W. (2001). Leadership and policy development. In Rowitz, Louis, *Public health leadership: Putting principles into practice*. Gaithersburg, MD: Aspen, 126–142.
7. Dodd, C. J. (2001). Can meaningful health policy be developed in a political system? In Harrington, Charlene & Estes, Carroll L. (eds.), *Health policy: Crisis and reform in the U.S. healthcare delivery system*, 3rd ed. Sudbury, MA: Jones and Bartlett, 373–382.
8. Edge, M. S. (2004). Get involved and make a difference. *Journal of the American Dietetic Association*, 104(2), 159.
9. Ochs, M. & McKnight, P. (2003). Preliminary report of the State Issues Task Force: Trends affecting the dietetics profession. *Journal of the American Dietetic Association*, 103(12), 1595–1596.
10. Koh, Y. M. (2001). Shaping your organization's policy. In Pencheon, David; Guest, Charles; Melzer, David; & Muir Gray, J. A. (eds.), *Oxford handbook of public health practice*. Oxford: Oxford University Press, 128–134.
11. Pencheon, D.; Guest, C.; Melzer, D.; & Muir Gray, J. A. (eds.). (2001). Introduction. *Oxford handbook of public health practice*. Oxford: Oxford University Press, 126–127.

12. Anderson, G. & Hussey, P. S. (2001). Influencing government policy: A framework. In Pencheon, D.; Guest, C.; Melzer, D.; & Muir Gray, J. A. (eds.), *Oxford handbook of public health practice*. Oxford: Oxford University Press, 146–154.

13. Cooper, M. J. & Zlotkin, S. H. (2003). An evidence-based approach to the development of national dietary guidelines. *Journal of the American Dietetic Association*, 103(12), S28–S33.

14. Frommer, Michael; Leeder, Stephen; Rubin, George; & Tjhin, Michelle (2001). Translating goals and targets into public health action. In Pencheon, D.; Guest, C.; Melzer, D.; & Muir G., J. A. (eds.), *Oxford handbook of public health practice*. Oxford: Oxford University Press, 136–144.

15. Gostin, L. (2000). Public health law in a new century: Part III: Public health regulation: A systematic evaluation. *JAMA 283*, 3118–3122.

16. Muir Gray, J. A. (2001). The public health professional as political activist. In Pencheon, D.; Guest, C.; Melzer, D.; & Muir G., J. A. (eds.), *Oxford handbook of public health practice*. Oxford: Oxford University Press, 262–267.

17. Misiroglu, G. (2003). *The handy politics answer book*. Canton, MI: Visible Ink Press.

18. Jessop, E. (2001). Writing to effect change. In Pencheon, D.; Guest, C.; Melzer, D.; & Muir G., J. A. (eds.), *Oxford handbook of public health practice*. Oxford: Oxford University Press, 428–434.

CHAPTER 9

THE ROLE OF THE UNITED STATES DEPARTMENT OF AGRICULTURE (USDA) IN PUBLIC HEALTH NUTRITION

Beverly J. McCabe-Sellers, PhD, RD

Margaret L. Bogle, PhD, RD

Reader Objectives

After studying this chapter and reflecting on the contents, you should be able to:

1. List the major agencies within the USDA that contribute to the practice of public health nutrition.
2. Identify the primary USDA programs that provide food assistance and nutrition education.
3. Discuss the agencies whose roles are to provide research data to support human nutrition in public health.
4. Discuss the major vehicles by which USDA agencies contribute to nutrition policy and promotion of health.
5. Discuss the historical perspective of nutrition education within the USDA.

The United States Department of Agriculture is a large and complex federal organization with seven undersecretaries that administer a diverse set of agencies and programs. Since the 1994 reorganization of the federal government, three undersecretaries supervise agencies, centers, and services that impact on public health nutrition: 1) Food, Nutrition, and Consumer Services (FNCS); 2) Food Safety; and 3) Research, Education, and Economics (REE). These agencies will be discussed for their individual major roles but, in reality, a large amount of interdependence and collaboration are needed to achieve their mutual mission and their goals of meeting the food and nutritional needs of Americans.

Overview of Food, Nutrition, and Consumer Services (FNCS)

The FNCS has two major agencies: the Food and Nutrition Service (FNS) and the Center for Nutrition Policy and Promotion (CNPP). FNCS's stated mission is to:

> . . . ensure access to nutritious, healthful diets for all Americans. Through food assistance and nutrition education for consumers, FNCS encourages consumers to make healthful food choices. Rather than simply providing food, FNCS works to empower consumers with knowledge of the link between diet and health, providing dietary guidance based on research (Bost, 2004).

The Food and Nutrition Service (FNS)

The Food and Nutrition Service increases food security and reduces hunger in partnership with cooperating organizations by providing children and low-income people access to food, a healthy diet, and nutrition education in a manner that supports U.S. agriculture and inspires public action.

FNS administers some 15 domestic food service programs that serve about one in five Americans at some point during the year (Lin & Smallwood, 2003). The programs work individually and in concert to provide a nutrition safety net for children and low-income adults and are a major component of the federal safety net. Together these programs account for about half of total USDA outlays. A total of $23.3 billion was distributed during the first half of fiscal 2004 (October 1, 2003 to March 31, 2004), and by the end of 2004 the USDA was projected to exceed the record $41.8 billion spent on food assistance in fiscal 2003 (Oliveira, 2004). These expenditures are up again after a decline in the 1990s, largely due to a decline in participation in the Food Stamp Program (FSP) to a low of $16 billon (18.2 million people) in 1999 (Wilde et al., 2000). Five programs account for almost 95% of the USDA's food assistance expenditures. These are the Food Stamp Program, the National School Lunch Program, the Special Supplemental Nutrition Program for Women, Infants and Children (WIC), the School Breakfast Program, and the Child and Adult Care Food Program.

> Read more about each of the food assistance programs online at the USDA's Food and Nutrition Services website at http://www.fns.usda.gov/fns/.

The Food Stamp Program

Since 1980, the Food Stamp Program has been the largest federal food assistance program and a mainstay of the federal safety net (Gleason et al., 1998). The program's intent is to enable people with low income to obtain a nutritionally adequate diet through coupons or *Electronic Benefit Transfer (EBT)* payments. These coupons or payments allow for the purchase of food and nonalcoholic beverages in authorized stores. These stores are then reimbursed by the federal government for the full value of the food. States administer the program in accordance with federal regulations and share the administrative expenses with the federal government (Wilde et al., 2000).

To qualify for FSP benefits, a household without an aged or disabled member must have gross income less than 130% of the official poverty guidelines. The household's net income must fall below the poverty line and must meet asset limits. In determining the benefit level, FNS assumes that a household will contribute 30% of its countable income toward food purchases. In addition, the Thrifty Food Plan for a family of four is determined

> Current eligibility criteria also appear on the Food and Nutrition Service's website at http://www.fns.usda.gov.

by FNS to calculate the basic expenditure by which a family of four could purchase a nutritionally adequate diet with minimum costs (Wilde et al., 2000).

Most people who receive food stamps rely on the program for support over a relatively long period of time because of high re-entry rates (Gleason et al., 1998). Individuals' economic circumstances, such as employment status and income level, are an important determination of participation patterns. Single females with children, older people, and people with disabilities have longer periods of participation (Gleason et al., 1998). Although no significant increase in food insecurity and hunger occurred in the 1995–1999 time period for those participating in the FSP, food insecurity and hunger did increase significantly (from 19.6% to 23.9%) for those low-income families not receiving food stamps in this same period (Nord et al., 2002). (Read more about food insecurity in the United States in Chapter 17.)

A major goal of the Food Stamp Program is to protect against food insecurity and hunger. Olson et al. (2004) recently studied factors that protect against and contribute to food insecurity among 316 rural families with household incomes of less than 200% of the federal poverty level. Mothers who used more food and financial skills, such as budget making, meal preparation, and stretching groceries, were more likely to have food-secure households than those who used

> Read more about the federal poverty levels and their impact in Chapters 4 and 20.

fewer of these skills. Reports of depression and of difficulty paying for medical expenses were related to increased risks of food insecurity. This report reinforces the need for teaching financial management and food preparation and purchasing skills to low-income families. Training in these skills is currently being provided by the Expanded Food and Nutrition Education Program (EFNEP) administered through State Cooperative Services. The report also highlights how health disparities of rural populations contribute to greater food insecurity.

Special Supplemental Nutrition Program for Women, Infants and Children (WIC)

The WIC program, administered by the USDA's Food and Nutrition Service, was established as a pilot program in 1972 and made permanent in 1974 (Oliveira & Gundersen, 2000). The program is based on two premises: 1) inadequate nutritional patterns and health behaviors of low-income women and children mean they are more vulnerable to adverse health outcomes; and 2) food interventions during critical times of growth and development can help prevent future medical and developmental problems (Rush, 1986; Rush et al., 1988). Data from the 1994–1996 Continuing Survey of Food Intakes by Individuals (CSFII) suggest that WIC recipients have higher intakes of all nutrients than income-eligible nonparticipants (Rose et al., 1998). A secondary data analysis of the cross-sectional survey of preschoolers from the 1994–1996 and 1998 CSFII confirmed beneficial effects, especially for the targeted nutrients (Siega-Riz et al., 2004). A recent study in Idaho (Dundas & Cook, 2004) examined the impact of WIC on the eating behaviors of preschool children and found significant improvement in eating behavior after 6 months on the WIC program with improved overall Healthy Eating Index (HEI) scores including scores for vegetables, fruits, and meats.

The WIC program is a broad-based and comprehensive food and nutrition program providing three main benefits to participants: 1) supplemental foods, 2) nutrition education, and 3) referrals to healthcare and social service providers (Committee on Scientific Evaluation of WIC Nutrition Risk Criteria, 1996). The specific aims of the WIC program are to augment available health care in order to prevent nutrition-related health problems and to improve the health of participants. The program serves not only as a secondary prevention program by providing risk appraisal and risk reduction, but also as a tertiary prevention program by providing treatment or rehabilitation to those with a diagnosed health condition.

Supplemental Foods

WIC food supplements to pregnant women are designed to improve nutritional status during pregnancy, improve pregnancy outcomes, and promote a better nutritional status for mothers and infants. Supplements for lactating women are designed to provide special nutrients needed for lactation, improve lactation performance, and promote a better nutritional status for the mother and infant. WIC food supplements for postpartum mothers who are not breast-feeding are intended to improve nutritional status during the postpartum period to better meet the physical demands of postnatal care and improve nutritional status and health for any future pregnancy.

The general consensus that "WIC works" has been questioned because most WIC research studies fail to control for selection into the program. A recent paper (Bitler & Currie, 2005) evaluated the selection problem using data from the national Pregnancy Risk Assessment Monitoring System and found

> See http://www.cms.gov/Medicaid/ to learn about those who qualify. Also, see Chapter 4 to read about those at highest nutritional risk in the United States.

that relative to Medicaid mothers, all of whom are eligible for WIC, participation was associated with improved birth outcomes, even after controlling for multiple factors.

The reduction or prevention of iron deficiency anemia is a primary goal of WIC food supplements for infants and children. Other goals are to improve diets and to support physical growth and mental development. These goals are perhaps even more important than previously thought, because the cross-sectional National Health and Nutrition Examination Survey III (1988–1994) demonstrated an increased prevalence of iron deficiency among overweight children and highlighted the need to screen for iron deficiency in children (Nead et al., 2004). WIC participation has a significant positive effect on children's intakes of iron, folate, and vitamin B-6 (Oliveira & Chandran, 2005, Oliveira & Gundersen, 2000), even after controlling for self-selection bias (Heckman, 1979). Iron is one of five nutrients specifically targeted by the WIC program; the four other nutrients besides iron are protein, calcium, vitamins A and C (Oliveira & Chandran, 2005) A 1991 USDA study recommended that folate, B-6, and zinc should also be targeted (USDA, Food and Nutrition Service, 1991).

Nutrition Education

The WIC program also provides nutrition education to improve the nutritional status of participants. At least one-sixth of WIC administrative funds must be spent by local agencies on nutrition education and counseling. Local agencies also must offer at least two nutrition education sessions to each participating woman in each 6-month certification period. With increased recognition of the value of breast-feeding, specific programs and earmarked funds, such as for the purchase of lactation aids like breast pumps, are intended to foster successful breast-feeding.

Referrals for Healthcare

Referrals to healthcare providers are intended to promote good healthcare by increasing the use of prenatal and postpartum care, and by improving access to routine preventive services such as immunization, smoking cessation, and family planning. Social service referrals to substance abuse treatment, housing assistance, Medicaid, and food stamps assistance are intended to meet a full range of health and nutrition needs of low-income women and their children.

The Center for Nutrition Policy and Promotion (CNPP)

The second major agency within FNCS is the Center for Nutrition Policy and Promotion (CNPP). It was created on December 1, 1994, as the focal point within the USDA where scientific research is linked with the nutritional needs of the public. CNPP works to improve the health and well-being of Americans by developing and promoting dietary guidance that links scientific research to the nutrition needs of consumers. Center staff help to define and coordinate nutrition education policy within the USDA and translate nutrition research into information and materials for consumers, policymakers, and professionals in health, education, industry, and the media. A recent issue of the agency's publication, *Family Economics and Nutrition Review* (Hentges, 2004), illustrates some of the major projects of CNPP. The issue includes research reports on factors influencing children's consumption of meals served in the Summer Food Service Program (Cotugna & Vickery, 2004), factors affecting food security among first-time WIC participants (Herman et al., 2004), and contributors to food insecurity among rural families (Olson et al., 2004). Another article (Basiotis et al., 2004) addresses the HEI for 1999–2000 as a means of charting dietary patterns of Americans and another way of assessing the nutritional quality of U.S. diets.

The Healthy Eating Index (HEI)

The HEI was developed by CNPP to assess and monitor the quality of the U.S. diet (Basiotis et al., 2002; Kennedy et al., 1995; USDA CNPP, 1995). The Interactive Healthy Eating Index (IHEI) program is an online dietary assessment tool that allows a consumer to calculate his or her own HEI score for a given day or days and provides information on the individual's diet quality. The program links to related nutrition messages and nutrient information. The Physical Activity Tool is a recent addition to the IHEI that assesses an individual's physical activity status and provides energy expenditure information and educational messages. Thus, the IHEI enhances the link between good nutrition and the health benefits of regular physical activity.

> The Interactive Healthy Eating Index program is available online at http://209.48.219.53/.

Dietary Guidelines for Americans and MyPyramid (formerly called the Food Guide Pyramid)

In conjunction with the Department of Health and Human Services, CNPP participates in the review and update of the nutrition science underlying revisions of the Dietary Guidelines for Americans (DGA) (USDA CNPP, 1996; USDA & USHHS, 2000, 2005). See Table 9-1 for a summary of DGA activities. The process for updating the Dietary Guidelines includes an evidence-based review of the latest science, which results in recommendations of the Dietary Guidelines Advisory Committee (DGAC). The committee consists of leading health and nutrition experts from across the country (USDHHS & USDA, 2005; Hentges, 2004). The process is open, and minutes of meetings of the DGA Committee are posted online through a federal website (http://www.usda.gov/cnpp/dietary_guidelines.html). Written and oral public comments and feedback about the proposed guidelines are solicited through *Federal Register* notices. A new revision of the Dietary Guidelines for Americans was released in January 2005. This version is discussed in Chapter 2. A revision of the food guidance system, commonly known as the MyPyramid (formerly called the Food Guide Pyramid), has been carried out by CNPP in conjunction with the revision of the Dietary Guidelines and was released in April 2005.

CNPP also maintains and updates the Thrifty Food Plan, which serves as the nutritional basis for determination of benefits in the Food Stamp Program. A recent publication (Carlson et al., 2003) outlined three additional food plans that specify the type and quantity of foods that people could consume at home to have a nutritious diet at various cost levels. Each food plan has 12 market baskets, one for each of 12 age-gender groups. These plans were developed when the USDA's 1989–1991 CSFII and the Food Price Database were merged.

> All of CNPP's projects are available on their website: http://www.cnpp.usda.gov.

TABLE 9-1   Recent USDA Food Guides and Tools

Name	Year Established
Dietary Guidelines for Americans	1980
Dietary Guidelines for Americans, First Revision	1990
Food Pyramid—Visual Tool	
Dietary Guidelines for Americans, Second Revision	1995
Healthy Eating Index—Assessment Tool	
Dietary Guidelines for Americans, Third Revision	2000
Individual Healthy Eating Index— Online Consumer Tool	
Dietary Guidelines for Americans, Fourth Revision	2005
MyPyramid	2005

Source: Compiled by the authors

Overview of the Food Safety and Inspection Service (FSIS)

The FSIS is the public health agency within the USDA responsible for ensuring that the nation's commercial supply of meat, poultry, and egg products is safe, wholesome, and correctly labeled and packaged (USDA, FSIS, 2004). It provides both education and inspection services. The USDA is responsible for nutrition labeling and inspection of foods not covered by the Food and Drug Administration. Although not a direct research agency, research does play an important role in FSIS's ability to fulfill its public health mission and to guarantee that the foods it regulates continue to be safe. The agency funds research in food safety and food safety education at various universities and institutes around the country. FSIS is now an important element in homeland security. (Read more about food safety in Chapter 16 and homeland security in Chapter 18.)

Overview of Research, Education, and Economics (REE)

The USDA-REE agency was created to provide federal leadership in creating and disseminating knowledge spanning the biological, physical, and social sciences related to agricultural research, economic analysis, statistics, extension, and higher education (CSREES, 2004). Research, Education, and Economics has four major service areas: Agricultural Research Service (ARS); Cooperative State Research, Education, and Extension Service (CSREES); Economics Research Service (ERS); and National Agricultural Statistics Service (NASS). Congress created CSREES through the 1994 Department Reorganization Act, which combined the former Cooperative State Research Service (CSRS) and the former Extension Service (ES) into a single agency (CSREES).

Agricultural Research Service

In 2004, the Agricultural Research Service celebrated its 50th anniversary as the principal research arm of the USDA and of human nutrition research. ARS is organized into 22 national programs that coordinate, communicate, and empower more than 1,200 research projects carried out by the ARS. The vision statement and the mission statement of the Human Nutrition National Program are:

Vision:

Provide a nutritious food supply, promote nutritional health, and quality of life, reduce morbidity and mortality associated with chronic diseases influenced by dietary intake and develop sound dietary recommendations which can be used to establish more effective nutrition assistance programs.

Mission:

> . . . to conduct basic and applied research to identify and understand how nutrients and other bioactive food components affect health. The ultimate goal of the food-based agricultural research is to identify foods and diets, coupled with genetics and physical activity, that sustain and promote health throughout the life cycle. (www.ars.usda.gov/research/programs/programs.htm?NP_CODE-107)

Important programs that are closely related to ARS's role in public health nutrition include:

- National Agricultural Library (NAL)
- Eight research locations concentrating on human nutrition
- Food consumption surveys
- Food composition databases
- Food and nutrition research publications

National Agricultural Library

Beyond the traditional functions of a national library of agriculture, the NAL provides six online information centers, one of which is the Food and Nutrition Information Center (FNIC). Founded in 1971, FNIC's mission is to collect and disseminate information about food and human nutrition. In 1977, the Food and Agriculture Act (Farm Bill) established FNIC as a permanent entity within the

> See the National Agricultural Library online at www.nal.usda.gov.

National Agricultural Library. Five special projects have their own Websites accessible through www.nal.usda.gov/fnic/general/general.html:

1. *Child Care Nutrition Resource System (CCNRS):* Provides information to people working in the USDA's Child Nutrition Programs.
2. *Food Stamp Nutrition Connection:* A resource system for Food Stamp Program nutrition education providers.
3. *Healthy School Meals Resource System (HSMRS):* Provides information to people working in the USDA's Child Nutrition Program.
4. *International Bibliographic Information on Dietary Supplements (IBIDS):* Databases that provide access to bibliographic citations and abstracts from published, international, scientific literature on dietary supplements. The USDA and agencies from NIH are working collaboratively to establish a dietary supplement database.
5. *WIC Works Resource System:* Serves as an encompassing resource for WIC nutritionists and other WIC professionals nationwide.

National Programs in Human Nutrition

The mission of the National Programs in Human Nutrition is carried out in eight locations that serve as major centers for human nutrition research. Each location has special research interests and extensive collaborations and partnerships with universities.

1. Arkansas Children's Nutrition Center (Little Rock, AK, founded in 1995) has primary studies in brain development and function, dietary factors affecting development, and bone development.
2. Beltsville Human Nutrition Research Center (Beltsville, MD, founded in 1941) focuses on defining the role of food and its components in optimizing human health and reducing the risk of nutrition-related diseases. It also houses the Nutrient Data Laboratory and the Food Surveys Research Group, which have a long history of important contributions to public health nutrition research.
3. Children's Nutrition Research Center at Baylor College of Medicine (Houston, TX, founded in 1979) studies the role of maternal, infant, and child nutrition in optimal health, development, and growth, including childhood dietary habits.
4. Grand Forks Human Nutrition Research Center (Grand Forks, ND, founded in 1977) has long served as the world's leading research center in basic and applied mineral nutrition.
5. Western Human Nutrition Research Center (Davis, CA, founded in 1980) strives to improve health through the study of diet, genetics, and environmental interactions.
6. Jean Mayer Human Nutrition Research Center on Aging at Tufts University (Boston, MA, founded in 1980) was founded to study the relationship between nutrition and aging.
7. Lower Mississippi Delta Nutrition Intervention Research Initiative (NIRI) (Little Rock, AK, founded in 1995) is focused on community intervention research through community-based participatory research in rural communities in Arkansas, Louisiana, and Mississippi. The Delta NIRI was established by congressional mandate to improve health and well-being in the Lower Delta through research in nutrition and intervention methodology.
8. Plant, Soil, and Nutrition Laboratory at Cornell University (Ithaca, NY, founded in 1940) was established to study the influence of soils on nutritional quality of plant foods and has a proud history of outstanding research, including the award of a Nobel Prize to one of its scientists.

Food Surveys Research Group (FSRG)

Housed within the Beltsville Human Nutrition Research Center, the FSRG has conducted food surveys on Americans since the 1930s.

These surveys have summarized nutrient intakes and monitored trends in food intakes. The Continuing Survey of Food Intakes by Individuals (CSFII) was conducted by the USDA in 1977–1978, 1985–1986, 1989–1991, and 1994–1996 before becoming combined with the National Health and Nutrition Evaluation Survey (NHANES) in 2000 as the "What We Eat in America" dietary component of NHANES 2000. Combining the two surveys has allowed data to be collected on an annual basis, rather than sporadically depending on the availability of monies. The first data from the combined survey is available online.

The FSRG has continued to develop, evaluate, and create new dietary assessment tools. In previous CSFII surveys, the Multiple Pass Method was used with pencil and paper using a five-step system to obtain free-flowing recall, remember forgotten foods, assign eating occasion, obtain more details, and allow one last opportunity to recall foods. Over a 7-year period, the original method was transferred to a computer-assisted interviewing instrument. The Automated Multiple Pass Method (AMPM) is the cornerstone of a Dietary Intake Data System consisting of

> Join the Food Survey Research Group listserv at http://www.barc.usda.gov/bhnrc/foodsurvey/home.htm.

three computer systems and an extensive food and nutrient database (Bliss, 2004; Raper et al., 2004). The Food and Nutrient Database for Dietary Studies (FNDDS) includes food descriptions, food portions, and their weights and nutrients. A recently established listserv (Food Survey Research Group Listserv, 2004) provides alerts when new data or instruments become available.

Effective, efficient, and validated dietary methodology allows the collection of accurate information on what people eat in research studies and over time as free-living individuals. Study of specific nutrients requires accurate and available food composition data of each nutrient in a sufficient number of foods. For large surveys, the food composition data need to include all the foods that the participants are likely to be consuming. Thus, the nutrient databases need continuous updating as new food products come on the market, new food varieties are developed, and new technologies for nutrient analysis are developed. (Read more about food intake surveys in Chapter 3 and managing data in Chapter 20.)

Food Composition Databases

Food composition databases are planned and developed by the USDA Nutrient Data Laboratory (NDL), ARS, and Beltsville Agricultural Research Center (BARC) and are considered to be the authority of composition data on foods available in the United States. NDL develops methods to acquire, evaluate, compile, and disseminate composition data on available foods. Table 9-2 provides a selected list of datasets created and compiled into national databases. Two major databases have been the USDA Nutrient Database for Standard Reference (SR), now in its 17th release, and the Primary Data Set (PDS) for USDA Nationwide Food Surveys. These have served as the numerical foundation of essentially all public and private work in the field of nutrition. These data were originally published in the form of *Agriculture Handbook 8* (AH-8), which is no longer available in print form. In order to provide timely release of nutrient data, the database is available for download from the Internet to a hard drive, CD, or handheld personal digital assistant (PDA), or they can be purchased on CD.

The Standard Reference Database consists of 21 sections and 4 supplements that contain over 6,000 foods. SR data are also included in the Child Nutrition (CN) Database, which is maintained for the School Lunch Program and other child nutrition programs. In 2003, NDL released the USDA Database for the Flavonoid Content of Foods and the USDA Table of Nutrient Retention Factors Release, and in 2004 it released the USDA Database for the Choline Content of Common Foods and the USDA Database for Proanthocyanidin Content of Selected Foods.

> Visit the USDA databases at http://www.nal.usda.gov/fnic/foodcomp/Bulletins/timeline.htm.

TABLE 9-2   Selected Tables of Food Composition Published by the USDA, ARS Nutrient Data Laboratory

Year(s)	Food Component(s)	Medium
1927	Vitamin content of food	Print
1939	Thiamin added	Print
1942	Nutritive value of the national food supply	Print
1944–1952	Amino acid content of food	Print
1950	Agricultural Handbook No. 8 containing proximate composition, 3 minerals, and 5 vitamins in 750 foods	Print
1959	Fatty acids	Print
1961	Vitamin B_{12}	Print
1963	Cholesterol	Print
1966	Vitamin E	Print
1973	Pantothenic Acid, Vitamin B_6, Vitamin B_{12}	Print

Year(s)	Food Component(s)	Medium
1981–1988	Handbook No. 8 Series of Various Foods, Fatty Acids and Cholesterol, Stearic Acid, Total Fat, Omega-3 Fatty Acids and Other Fat Components, Fast Foods, Amino Acids in Fruits and Vegetables, Dietary Fiber	Print
1987, 1990	Sugar content of selected foods	Print
1983	Iron	Print
1990–1994	Vitamin K, vitamin D, selenium	Print
1995	Trans Fatty Acids	Print/Electronic
1996		Transition from print to electronic software to allow free and easy access to updates and new additions to Standard Reference database
1993, 1998	Carotenoids	Electronic
1998, 2000	Isoflavonoids (Iowa State University)	Electronic
2002		Download software to handheld personal digital assistant (PDA)
2003	Isoflavonoids Database	Electronic
2004	Choline, proanthocyanidin	Electronic

Note: Home and Garden Bulletin No. 72 was again released in print form due to popular demand. All other food composition publications are available either online or on CD.
Source: Compiled by the authors.

Underlying human nutrition research and, subsequently, public health nutrition policy making and practice are quality food composition data (Harrison, 2004). Public health applications include assessing food and nutrient availability and intakes in populations, evaluation of programs to protect and improve nutritional status, research on diet and disease interrelationships, health education and promotion activities, assessment of risk from food-borne contamination, and preserving information on traditional foods. None of these applications can occur without a national nutrient database. The development and maintenance of a high-quality nutrient database began and continues under the leadership of USDA research scientists.

The collaboration of the food industry with the USDA Nutrient Data Laboratory is an essential element in capturing the latest food products. It is expensive to develop high-quality food composition data and is usually affordable only by governments. Representative sampling of perishable foods across a country, standardized procedures, and up-to-date technology are required for a valid food composition database.

According to Burlingame (2004), five conventional criteria are critical to quality food composition databases. Quality first begins with a "sampling plan" that may require a year of planning and that specifies the number of samples at every stage including sample preparation, discrete sample analyses, replicates, and variability. "Representativeness" is the traditional term used to describe the suitability of data to be entered into a database. The third factor is "completeness," a term suggesting all foods and all food components for all user groups. In reality, certain foods or food components are missing from every database. Choices and priorities have to be made to achieve a comprehensive database for most user groups. The foods in industrialized countries undergo constant change with the continuing introduction of new processed foods, many of which may be gone within a year. Continued development of new food varieties with more disease resistance, higher yields, or richer nutrients (phytochemicals) also changes the food supply. The fourth quality factor is "harmonization" of databases, which attempts to achieve international standards for defining elements in databases. The final quality criterion is "documentation." Although detailed documentation cannot be published, database compilers have the responsibility to fully record details and have these readily available (Burlingame, 2004).

Applications of these databases have been enhanced and increased by the development of websites that allow ready and free downloading of new releases of the Standard Reference database onto computer hard drives and handheld computers. Anyone with access to a personal computer can find the 90+ nutrients or components of some 6,000 foods.

ARS Publications

A major movement to increase efficiency and ease dissemination of research findings in a timely manner has been the increasing publication of online materials for both lay and professional audiences. *Agricultural Research* is the ARS bimonthly magazine that highlights research activities by ARS scientists, including development of new and improved varieties of fruits and vegetables that will provide more protective factors, community intervention projects, improved control of pests in crops, new methodology to study human nutrition, improved water quality projects, and other diverse topics.

Quarterly newsletters such as *Nutrition and Your Child* and *Research Briefs* provide updates on research and services from ARS scientists.

Cooperative State Research, Education, and Extension Service (CSREES)

The unique mission of CSREES is to advance knowledge for agriculture, the environment, human health and well-being, and communities by supporting research, education, and extension programs in the land-grant university system and other partner organizations. Although not performing actual research, education, or extension, CSREES helps fund these activities at the state and local level and provides program leadership in these areas.

Eleven targeted areas of interest and the 59 resulting programs include 4 areas closely related to public health: Economics and Commerce; Families, Youth, and Communities; Food, Nutrition, and Health; and Natural Resources and Environment (CSREES, 2004). Knowledge is advanced through two key mechanisms: 1) national program leadership that helps states identify and meet research, extension, and educational priorities in areas of public concern; and 2) federal assistance that provides annual funding to land-grant universities and competitively grants funds to researchers at universities.

An extensive network of state, regional, and county extension offices in every U.S. state and territory has a focus on critical issues affecting people's daily lives and the nation's future. The aim is to empower people and communities to solve problems and improve their lives on the local level. An example of such programs is the USDA's 102-year-old youth development program called 4-H (Heart, Hand, Head, and Health).

> To read more about the emphasis areas of the CSREES, visit http://www.csrees.usda.gov/nea/food/food.html.

Food, Nutrition, and Health

The Food, Nutrition, and Health National emphasis area is committing increased dollars and resources to remedy the negative effects of poor dietary choices and unhealthy lifestyles, food-borne illnesses, and the potential for terrorist-related and other threats to the food supply. Not to be forgotten, however, is that millions of Americans struggle to obtain sufficient food, and U.S. food suppliers attempt to keep up with changing food trends. Program leadership and funding opportunities work to strengthen the nation's capacity to address important issues surrounding diet, health, food safety, food security, and food science and technology. Six major programs in this area are:

1. Food safety and biosecurity
2. Food sciences and technology
3. Health

4. Hunger and food security
5. Nutrition
6. Obesity and healthy weight

Food Safety

Food safety activities illustrate the wide diversity supported by CSREES. Food safety concerns cover a broad spectrum from on-farm production to post-harvest processing, distribution, food preparation, selection, and consumption. Consumer education strives to increase understanding of disease-causing microorganisms, their products, naturally occurring toxicants, and chemical contamination in meat, poultry, seafood, and fresh fruits and vegetables. Protecting the national food supply, which can be threatened by both incidental and deliberate contamination, is another focus for research, education, and extension programs. Development of new technology such as thermal processing, irradiation, hydrostatic processing, and ohmic processing are just a few examples of adding value in processing, packaging, marketing, and distributing of wholesome and safe food.

Food Security

"Food security" has been defined as:

> . . . having access, at all times, to enough food for an active, healthy life for all its household members . . . including availability of nutritionally adequate and safe foods and assured ability to acquire personally preferred foods in a socially acceptable way (Anderson, 1990).

CSREES engages in a variety of education and awareness activities to increase public knowledge about nutrition, food safety, and community food security, such as a grant program that funds private nonprofit organizations to address community food security issues, as well as collaborating through partnerships across the USDA.

Community-Based Nutrition Education

In partnership with the Cooperative Extension Systems, CSREES delivers community-based nutrition education programs designed to help individuals, families, and communities make informed choices about food and lifestyles that support health and economic and social well-being. Four broad program areas are the foundation of CSREES nutrition education programs: food security, food safety, dietary guidance, and health. The Expanded Food and Nutrition Education Program (EFNEP) helps low-income families improve their diets for better health, to increase physical activity, and to save money. The EFNEP program is offered to all limited resource families who are eligible for food stamps. *EFNEP Success*

Research the EFNEP online at http://www.csrees.usda.gov/ProgView.cfm?prnum=2300.

Stories evaluate how EFNEP benefits have helped low-income audiences achieve good nutrition through knowledge and behavior change, and *EFNEP Impact Reports* include data and evaluations on the various EFNEP components.

CSREES Partnerships

CSREES has a partnership with the National Cancer Institute and the Produce for a Better Health Foundation to develop and promote the 5 A Day for Better Health Program. Another USDA partnership is with the Department of Health and Human Service's *Healthy People 2010* to set and promote health goals for the United States. Other partnerships exist among CSREES and other USDA agencies.

Economic Research Service (ERS)

The ERS studies the economics of food, farming, natural resources, and rural America. For example, the agency provides analyses of the economic issues affecting the safety of the U.S. food supply, including estimating: 1) the cost of specific food-borne diseases ($6.9 billion in 2000 for five organisms), and 2) the costs and benefits of programs aimed at improving food safety, including conducting a nationally representative survey of meat and poultry plants on the costs of the Hazard Analysis Critical Control Plan (HACCP). Another food safety report (Ralston et al., 2002) examined changes in hamburger preparation behavior, the reasons for the changes, the medical costs saved as a result of the changes, and the implications for future food safety education. Other examples of economic analysis include the study of how economics influence eating choices, body weight outcomes (Mancino et al., 2004), and the economic assessment of costs and benefits of food labeling (Golan et al., 2001).

The Food Assistance and Nutrition Research Program

Although the ERS does not administer food assistance programs, it does administer the Food Assistance and Nutrition Research Program (FANRP), which was established by the U.S. Congress in 1998 to conduct research and evaluation on topics relevant to USDA food assistance programs including program outcomes, program operations and integrity, vulnerable populations, the relationship between food assistance programs and the general economy, and food security in the United States. An example of an FANRP evaluation is *The WIC Program: Background, Trends, and Issues*, Report Number FANRR27 (Oliveira et al., 2002). FANRP's research emphasis is on the role of USDA food assistance and nutrition programs in promoting a healthy, well-nourished population. FANRP conducts intramural research such as the WIC report by Oliveira et al. (2002) and also sponsors extramural research. Extramural funding efforts include: 1) support of improved nutrition data, for example, funding of an annual collection of national data on household food security; 2) the FANRP Competitive Grants and Cooperative Agreements, which support policy-relevant research on food assistance programs and nutrition issues; and 3) support for the Small Grants Program, which encourages research innovation and broader scholarly participation in food assistance and nutrition research. Information about these is available online at http://www.ers.usda.gov/Briefing/FoodNutritionAssistance/.

ERS Publications

ERS publishes reports and periodicals that address the economic analysis of the impact of food assistance programs. Twice a year, ERS publishes *The Food and Assistance Landscape*, which provides a brief overview of the USDA's domestic food assistance programs including program statistics, expenditures, participation levels, and related economic indicators such as unemployment rates, income growth, and food price inflation. Another series, titled *Issues in Food Assistance*, addresses a variety of topics including effects of legislative changes, social changes, and operational issues on the Food Stamp Program, food insecurity, and other aspects of the well-being

> Another series of online information covers WIC and child nutrition issues. Find it at http://www.ers.usda.gov/publications/fanrr34/.

of low-income households. A lay magazine, *Amber Waves*, covers a wide variety of ERS research topics including food assistance, nutrition, and food safety.

Recent ERS reports document the importance of USDA food assistance and nutrition programs. For example, the September 2004 issue of the Food Assistance Landscape documents that the programs served approximately 1 in 5 Americans in fiscal year 2003 at a cost of $41.6 billion. ERS reports examine our understanding of how well the programs operate as a "food safety net." A new four-volume series, *Effects of Food Assistance and Nutrition Programs on Nutrition and Health*, is a comprehensive review and synthesis of research on the impacts of USDA food assistance and nutrition programs on numerous important outcomes including food expenditures, household nutrient availability, dietary intake, nutritional status, food security, birth outcomes, breast-feeding behaviors, immunization rates, use and cost of healthcare services, and selected non-health outcomes, such as academic achievement, school performance (children), and social isolation (elderly).

ERS studies also examine issues related to participation decisions. For example, the Food Stamp Program Access Study was a national study of Food Stamp Program accessibility at the local office level, and described the nature and prevalence of local office practices hypothesized to influence participation; households' stated reasons for not participating or ending their participation; and characteristics, attitudes, and experiences associated with participation behavior. It then analyzed the association between local office practices and household participation behaviors (Bartlett et al., 2004). Results provide information to policy and program officials on how programs can become more effective and efficient.

History of Nutrition Education in the USDA

The USDA has a rich history of providing science-based nutrition information and education to the public (Kennedy, 1996). The Organic Act of 1862 directed the newly formed Department of Agriculture to "acquire and diffuse among the people of the United States useful information on subjects connected to agriculture and rural development" (Kennedy, 1996). In the 1930s, the USDA's focus was on providing "common-sense knowledge of nutrition," followed by the RDAs in the early 1940s, which emphasized maintaining health for the war effort. In the 1950s, nutrient adequacy was emphasized, and the USDA focused on providing the right kind of information for an adequate diet (Kennedy, 1996). In 1969 the White House Conference on Food, Nutrition, and Health was held, and the focus became linking nutrition education to the promotion of optimal health with food. The president of the American Dietetic Association testified in favor of the amendment of the Food Stamp Act in 1969 and the expansion and improvement of the National School Lunch Act in 1969 (Cassell, 1990).

In the 1970s, the Food and Agriculture Act of 1977 named the USDA as the "lead government agency for nutrition research, extension, and teaching" (Kennedy, 1996). A call for the development of more effective systems for delivering nutrition information to the public was linked to the growing evidence relating some food components to risks for chronic disease. Increased public interest in diet and disease risks led to the first set of USDA Dietary Guidelines for Americans. Table 9-3 outlines the USDA Nutrition Education Programs with Legislative Authorization that began in the 1970s: 1) Nutrition Education and Training Programs (NET); 2) WIC; and 3) EFNEP.

The 1980s brought increased interest in nutrition education research for the development of improved materials and methods to better inform the general public about good nutrition. Evaluation of nutrition education tools was increased to measure comprehension and perceived usefulness by the targeted audiences.

In the 1990s, a revised Dietary Guidelines for Americans was released. A greater coordination of nutrition education efforts and survey efforts was called for by the Nutrition Monitoring and Related Research Act (Interagency Board for Nutrition Monitoring and Related Research, 1992, 1995). The focus shifted from a simple nutrition information provision to promoting behavioral change and motivating consumers to adopt eating practices to promote optimal health. The latest revision of the Dietary Guidelines for Americans was released in 2005.

TABLE 9-3 USDA Nutrition Education Programs with Legislative Authorization

Program	Target Audience	Agency Responsible	State Collaborators	Delivery
Nutrition Education and Training Program (NET)	Children, all incomes	FCS	State education departments	Training of school food service and teachers, school nutrition education curricula, training for child care providers and parents
Special Supplemental Nutrition Program for Women, Infants and Children (WIC)	Low-income pregnant and breast-feeding women, infants, and children up to age 5	FCS	State health departments and WIC clinics	Individual counseling or group lessons along with WIC food package or vouchers for supplemental foods; two contacts per 6-month certification period
Expanded Food and Nutrition Education Program (EFNEP)	Limited-resource families with young children; low-income youth	CSREES	State land-grant universities; county cooperative extension offices	One-on-one home visits or group classes by trained paraprofessional aides; in-depth 6-month program

Source: Compiled by authors.

Nutrition, Agriculture, and Health of Americans

The health of rural populations is essential to the production and maintenance of an adequate and safe food supply. Thus, the USDA has long been committed to improving the nutritional health of Americans through a program of research and education to maintain a food supply of high nutritional quality and to encourage consumption of a healthful diet.

Nutrition is a bridge between agriculture and the health of American consumers in a two-way process. Science-based nutrition messages can motivate Americans to make healthful changes in their diets that will create new demands in the kinds and amounts of food people buy in the marketplace (Kennedy, 1996). Market responses to consumer demands can lead, in turn, to the creation of new products and other changes in the food system. Examples include the development of low-fat and reduced calorie foods, leaner meats, and calcium-enriched orange juice and other beverages (Kennedy, 1996). Well-targeted nutrition education and health promotion activities can encourage Americans to adopt new agricultural products into healthy eating habits and lead, over time, to positive health outcomes and reduced healthcare costs.

History of the USDA's Research Role in Public Health Nutrition

The founding of food and nutrition science policy was nurtured by the establishment of the Land-Grant College System by the Hatch Act of 1887, shortly after the creation of the Department of Agriculture in 1862 (DuPont, 1999). The first federal funding of human nutrition research occurred in 1893-1894. An early beneficiary of the USDA Land Grant program at the University of Connecticut at Storrs was Dr. Wilbur O. Atwater, whose *Atwater values* for carbohydrates, protein, and fat are among the first nutrition facts taught in introductory nutrition courses and are used on a daily basis by dietitians and nutritionists (DuPont, 1999). Dr. Atwater, credited as the father of American food science, was appointed the Director of the Office of Experiment Stations, which was funded by the USDA (McBride, 1993). The contributions of Atwater and other pioneers of the 19th century are the cornerstone of current nutrition science and policy. These principles of rigorous quantitative analysis, using appropriate standard reference materials, are still applied today in the USDA nutrient data laboratory in Beltsville and in collaborating universities' laboratories (Harnly et al., 2004; Holden et al., 2004; Teague et al., 2004).

The first tables of average nutrient values of foods were published in 1896 as *The Chemical Composition of American Food Materials*, USDA Bulletin 28 (DuPont, 1999). The third version, by Atwater and Bryant in 1906, included analysis of more than 4,000 food items and served as a standard reference for dietitians and nutritionists for more than four decades (Cassell, 1990). Table 9-1, provided earlier in the chapter, presents a summary of the Food Composition Tables published by the USDA. The Nutrient Data Laboratory and the Food Survey Group of the Agricultural Research Service continue collaboration to plan, develop, and monitor nutrient databanks and methodology that underlie all nutrition surveys and nutrition intervention research in the United States.

The 1994–1996 CSFII was the USDA's 10th survey since the 1930s, producing the nutrient intakes of a stratified representative sample of Americans and providing standards against which regional and local nutrition studies have been compared (Borrud, 1998).

With the merging of the CSFII Survey and the National Health and Nutrition Examination Survey in 1999, continuous monitoring of the health and nutrient intake of Americans is now being carried out with the nutrition methodology developed and tested by the Food Survey Research Group. This merger of the USDA and NIH in nutrition monitoring for better health and disease prevention in Americans is a model from which Americans may benefit enormously, as the combined expertise of these departments promotes improved nutrition and health and helps prevent disease. The USDA has focused largely on promotion of health through supporting food production, food technology, nutrition research, and nutrition education.

Issues for Discussion

1. Is a single pyramid the best graphic model to represent the 2005 Dietary Guidelines for Americans in its food and physical activity recommendations?
2. How does a nutritionist translate research findings from large national studies into effective interventions for individuals?
3. Should nutrition interventions such as "healthy weights" be implemented on a community level or an individual level?
4. What are factors impacting participation in food assistance programs such as WIC, the Food Stamps Program, and the School Lunch Program? Conversely, what impacts does participation in food assistance programs have on health?

References

Anderson, S.A. (1990). Core indicators of nutritional state for difficult to sample populations. *Journal of Nutrition*, 120, 1559–1600.

Bartlett, S., Burstewin, N., Hamilton, W., Kling, R., & Andrews, M. (2004). *Food Stamp Program access study: Final report*. (E-FAN-03-013-3) Alexandria, VA: Economic Research Service.

Basiotis P. P., Carlson, A., Gerrior, S. A., Juan, W. Y., & Lino, M. (2002). *The healthy eating index: 1999–2000*. (CNPP-12). Washington, DC: U.S. Department of Agriculture, Center for Nutrition Policy and Promotion.

Basiotis, P. P., Carlson, A., Gerrior S. A., WenYen, J., & Lino, M. (2004). The Healthy Eating Index, 1999–2000: Charting dietary patterns of Americans. *Family Economics Nutrition Review*, 16, 39–48.

Bell, L., Pachikara, S., Schreiber-Williams, S., & Gabor V. (2002). *Re-engineering the welfare system—A study of administrative changes to the food stamp program*. (Food Assistance and Nutrition Research Report Number 17). Washington, DC: USDA Economic Research Service.

Bitler, M. P. & Currie J. (2005). Does WIC work? The effects of WIC on pregnancy and birth outcomes. *Journal of Policy Analysis and Management*, 24, 73–91.

Bliss, R. M. (2004). Researchers produce innovations in dietary recall. *Agricultural Research*, 52, 10–12.

Borrud, Lori. (1998). What's on the CD-ROM...the 1994–96 Continuing Survey of Food Intakes by Individuals and Diet and Health Knowledge, USDA, ARS, BHNRC, Foods Survey Research Group. What We Eat in America Research Results Survey Conference, September 14–15, 1998, Washington, DC.

Bost, E. M. (2004). Welcome to Food, Nutrition, and Consumer Services. Retrieved November 21, 2004, from http://www.fns.usda.gov/fns.

Burlingaem, B. (2004). Fostering quality data in food composition databases: Visions for the future. *Journal of Food Composition and Analysis*, 17, 251–258.

Carlson, A., Linn, M., Gerrior, S. A., & Basiotis, P. P. (2003). *The low-cost, moderate-cost, and liberal food plans: 2003 administrative report.* (CNPP-13). Washington, DC: Center for Nutrition Policy and Promotion.

Cassell, Jo Anne. (1990). *Carry the flame: The history of the American Dietetic Association.* Chicago, IL: American Dietetic Association.

Cooperative State Research, Education and Extension Service. Retrieved May 20, 2004, from http://www.csrees.usda.gov/nea/food/food.html.

Cotugna, N. & Vickery, C. E. (2004). Children rate the Summer Food Service Program. *Family Economics Nutrition Review*, 16, 3–12.

Dundas, M. L. & Cook, K. (2004). Impact of the Special Supplemental Nutrition Program for Women, Infants and Children on the healthy eating behaviors of preschool children in eastern Idaho. Topics in Clinical Nutrition, 19, 273–279.

DuPont, J. (1999). The third century of nutrition research policy-shared responsibility. *Nutrition Today*, 34(6), 234–241.

Fischer, F. E. (1970). President's report to members. *Journal of the American Dietetic Association*, 57, 411–414.

Food Surveys Research Group. (2004). Food Surveys Research Group Listserv. Retrieved July 1, 2004, from http://www.barc.usda.gov/.

Gleason, P., Schochet, P., & Moffett, R. (1998). *The dynamics of food stamp program participation in the early 1990's.* (Report submitted to the U.S. Department of Agriculture, Food and Nutrition Service). Princeton, NJ: Mathematica Policy Research.

Golan, E., Kuchler, F., Mitchell L., Greene, C., & Jessup, A. (2001). Economics of food labeling. (Agricultural Economic Report No. AER793). Washington, DC: United States Department of Agriculture.

Harnly, J. M., Doherty, R. F., Beecher, G. R., Haytowitz, D. B., Gebhardt, S. E., & Holden, J. M. (2004). Analytical determination of flavonoids (S Aglycones) in foods. *Proceedings of the 28th National Nutrient Databank Conference: From Farm to Fork-Practical Applications for Food Composition Data.* June 23–26, 2004. Iowa City, IA: University of Iowa.

Harrison, G. G. (2004). Fostering data quality in food composition databases: Applications and implications for public health. *Journal of Food Composition and Analysis*, 17, 259–265.

Heckman, J. (1979). Sample selection bias as a specification error. *Econometrica*, 41, 1.

Hentges, E. J. (2004). Front and center: Making a difference with dietary guidance: From science to promotion. *Family Economics Nutrition Review*, 16, 1.

Herman, D. R., Harrison, G. G., Abdelmonem, A. A., & Jenks, E. (2004). The effect of the WIC program on food security status of pregnant, first-time participants. *Family Economics Nutrition Review*, 16, 21–29.

Holden, J. M., Andrews, K., Ahao, C., Picciano, M. F., Dwyer, J., Saidanha, L., et al. (2004). Development of the dietary supplement ingredient database, phase II progress. *Proceedings of the 28th National Nutrient Databank Conference, From farm to fork-practical applications for food composition data*. June 23–27. Iowa City, IA: University of Iowa.

Interagency Board for Nutrition Monitoring and Related Research. (1992). *Nutrition monitoring in the United States: The directory of federal and state nutrition monitoring activities, 1992*. (DHHS publication [PHS] 92-1255-1). Hyattsville, MD: Human Nutrition Information Services.

Interagency Board for Nutrition Monitoring and Related Research, Life Sciences Research Office, FASEB (1995). *Third report on nutrition monitoring in the United States: Executive summary*. Washington, DC: Government Printing Office.

Kennedy, E. (1996). *The state of nutrition education in USDA: A report to the Secretary by the State of Nutrition Education in USDA Working Group*. Washington, DC: USDA Center for Nutrition Policy and Promotion.

Kennedy, E. T., Ohis, J., Carlson, S., & Fleming, K. (1995). The Healthy Eating Index: Design and application. *Journal of the American Dietetic Association*, 95, 1103–1108.

Lin, B.-H. & Smallwood, D. (2003). Research designs for assessing the USDA's food assistance and nutrition programs outcomes: Part I: Evaluation of ongoing national programs. *Nutrition Today*, 38, 139–145.

McBride, J. (1993). Wilbur O. Atwater: Father of American nutrition science. *Agricultural Research, 41*: 5–11.

Mancino, L., Lin, B.-H., & Ballenger, N. (2004). The role of economics in eating choices and weight outcomes. (Agriculture Information Bulletin Number 791). Washington, DC: USDA, *Economic Research Service.*

Mantovani, R. E., Daft, L., Macaluse, T. F., & Hoffman, K. (1997). *Food retailers in the food stamp program: Characteristics and service to program participants*. Alexandria, VA: Office of Analysis and Evaluation, Food and Consumer Service, USDA.

Nead, K. G., Halterman, J. S., Kaczorowski, J. M., Aulinger, P., & Weitzman, M. (2004). Overweight children and adolescents: A risk group for iron deficiency. *Pediatrics*, 114, 104–108.

Nord, M., Andrews, M. A., & Carlson, S. (2002). *Household food insecurity in the United States, 2001* (Food Assistance and Nutrition Research Report No. 29). Washington, DC: Economic Research Service, U.S. Department of Agriculture.

Oliveira, V. (2004). *Food assistance landscape, September 2004*. (Food Assistance and Nutrition Research Report No. FANRR28-5). Alexandria, VA: Economic Research Service, United States Department of Agriculture. Available at: http://www.ers.usda.gov/publications/fanrr28-5f. Accessed November 21, 2004.

Oliveira, V. & Chandran, R. (2005). *Children's consumption of WIC approved foods.* (Food Assistance and Nutrition Report No. 44) Washington, DC: Economic Research Service, United States Department of Agriculture.

Oliveira, V. & Gundersen, C. (2000). *WIC and the nutrient intake of children.* (Food Assistance and Nutrition Research Report No. 5). Washington, DC: USDA Economic Research Service, 1–22.

Oliveira, V., Racine, E., Olmstead, J., & Ghelfi, I. (2002). *The WIC program: background, trends, and issues.* (Food Assistance and Nutrition Report No. FANRR27). Alexandria, VA: Economic Research Service, U.S. Department of Agriculture.

Olson, C. M., Anderson, K., Kiss, E., Lawrence, F. C., & Seiling, S. B. (2004). Factors protecting against and contributing to food insecurity among rural families. *Family Economics and Nutrition Reviews*, 16, 12–26.

Ralston, K., Brent, C. P., Starke, Y., Riggins, T., & Lin, C. T. J. (2002). *Consumer food safety behavior: A case study in hamburger cooking and ordering.* (ERS Agricultural Economic Report No. AER804). Washington DC: Economic Research Service, United States Department of Agriculture.

Raper, N., Perloff, B., Ingwersen, L., Stainfeldt, L., & Anand, J. (2004). An overview of USDA's Dietary Data System. *Journal of Food Composition Analysis*, 17, 545–555.

Rose, D., Habicht, J.-P., & Devaney, B. (1998). Household participation in the food stamp and WIC programs increase the nutrient intakes of preschool children. *Journal of Nutrition*, 128, 548–555.

Rush, D. (1986). *Evaluation of the Special Supplemental Food Program for Women, Infants, and Children (WIC).* Volume 1: Summary. Research Triangle Park, NC.

Rush, D., Sloan, N., Leighton. J., Alvir, J., & Horwitz, D. (1988). The national WIC evaluation: Evaluation of the special Supplement Food Program for Women, Infants, and Children. *American Journal of Clinical Nutrition*, 48, S389–S519.

Siega-Riz, A. M., Kranz, S., Blanchett, D., Haines, P. S., Gulkey, D. K., & Popkin, B. M. (2004). The effect of participation in the WIC program on preschoolers' diets. *Journal of Pediatrics*, 144, 229–234.

Teague, A. M., Sealey, W. M., McCabe-Sellers, B. J., & Mock, D. M. (2004). Biotin is stable in frozen foods. *FASEB Journal*, 18, A118.

United States Department of Agriculture, Agricultural Research Service. (2004). Vision and mission statements. Retrieved November 21, 2004, from http://www.ars.usda.gov/research/programs/programs.htm? NP_CODE_107.

United States Department of Agriculture, Center for Nutrition Policy and Promotion. (1995). *The Healthy Eating Index* (CNPP-1). Washington, DC: United States Government Printing Office.

United States Department of Agriculture, Center for Nutrition Policy and Promotion. (1996). *The Food Guide Pyramid.* (Home and Garden Bulletin Number 252) CNPP. Washington, DC: United States Department of Agriculture.

United States Department of Agriculture, Food and Nutrition Service. (November 1991). *Review of WIC food packages: Technical paper*, Economic Research Service. Washington, DC: United States Department of Agriculture.

United States Department of Agriculture, Food Safety and Inspection Service. (2004). Fulfilling the vision: Updates and initiatives in protecting public health. Retrieved November 21, 2004, from http://www.fsis.usda.gov/About_FSIS/Fulfilling_the_Vision/index.asp.

United States Department of Agriculture, National Agricultural Library (NAL). (2004). Online Information Centers. Retrieved November 21, 2004, from http://www.nal.usda.fnic/general/general.html.

United States Department of Agriculture and United States Department of Health and Human Services. (2000). *Nutrition and your health: Dietary guidelines for Americans* (5th ed.). (Home and Garden Bulletin No. 232). Washington, DC: U. S. Government Printing Office.

United States Department of Health and Human Services and the United States Department of Agriculture. *Dietary Guidelines for Americans 2005*. Washington, DC: U.S. Government Printing Office.

Wilde, P., Cook, P., Gundersen, C., Nord, M., & Tiehen, L. (2000). *The decline in food stamp program participation in the 1990's.* (Food Assistance and Nutrition Research Report No. 7). Washington, DC: USDA, Economic Research Service.

PART IV

PROMOTING THE PUBLIC'S NUTRITIONAL HEALTH

Part IV includes those chapters that illustrate the programs and services public health nutrition provides for different groups of Americans. Through needs assessment, scientific study, and policy, many groups have been identified as qualifying to receive public health nutrition. Chapter 10 discusses these programs and services, along with the challenges of serving children, adolescents, and women. In Chapters 11–15, the reader is then educated about the public health nutrition programs that affect adults, a special subset of adults—the baby boomers and the elderly. Each group has different needs and challenges, but all will need to be provided for by public health nutrition now and in the future.

CHAPTER 10

GROWING A HEALTHIER NATION: MATERNAL, INFANT, CHILD, AND ADOLESCENT NUTRITION

Shortie McKinney, PhD, RD, LDN, FADA

Beth Leonberg, MS, RD, CSP, FADA, LDN

Bonnie Spear, PhD, RD

Reader Objectives

After studying this chapter and reflecting on the contents, you should be able to:

1. Discuss the need for public health nutrition services for women, infants, children, and adolescents.
2. Identify the health maladies that can occur without public health nutrition services in these groups.
3. Describe the nutrient requirements for each group.
4. Forecast how adolescent mothers may fare in society without public health programs.
5. Clarify the reasons for supplying maternal, child, and adolescent public health nutrition programs.

Receiving adequate food and nutrition throughout the various stages of growth and development is crucial to lifelong health and optimal functioning. Numerous studies have documented the physiological and mental deficits that can occur when pregnant women, infants, and children are not provided with the nutritional resources and advice they need for optimal health. With medical interventions becoming more sophisticated than ever, society must find ways to support the provision of nutrition and health care to these vulnerable groups to minimize the strain on the already overburdened healthcare system. Numerous negative outcomes, such as preterm births, small-for-gestational-age infants, fetal alcohol syndrome, gestational diabetes, anemia, obesity, stunting, nutrient deficiencies, and eating disorders, can result when adequate food and nutrition are not provided during pregnancy and the early stages of life.

Pregnancy, infancy, childhood, and adolescence are all life stages in which nutrients are needed for the development of important body systems. In addition, the preconceptional period for women of childbearing age is a time when nutrition education can help promote an optimal environment for a healthy pregnancy.

Healthy People Objectives

The Healthy People (HP) 2010 objectives were established to promote improved health across the nation. Maternal and child health programs provide key interventions to help achieve these objectives. This chapter will review the important issues that public health professionals should consider. The importance of the mother and maternal–child programs is well recognized in the HP 2010 guidelines. Objective 16 of HP 2010 focuses on a variety of issues related to healthy pregnancies, infant birth rates, child growth and development, and preventable health consequences during development. Objective 18 focuses on food and nutrition goals. Most of the nutrition goals apply to mothers and children and their diets, and some objectives specifically address children's issues. Table 10-1 lists the HP 2010 objectives that relate to nutrition issues in pregnancy, lactation, infancy, childhood, and adolescence.

Table 10-1   HP 2010: Nutrition-Related Maternal–Child Health Objectives

Fetal, Infant, Child, and Adolescent Deaths

16-1.   Reduce fetal and infant deaths.

16-4.   Reduce maternal deaths.

16-5.   Reduce maternal illness and complications due to pregnancy.

Prenatal Care

16-6.   Increase the proportion of pregnant women who receive early and adequate prenatal care.

Risk Factors

16-10. Reduce low birth weight (LBW) and very low birth weight (VLBW).

16-11. Reduce preterm births.

16-12. Increase the proportion of mothers who achieve a recommended weight gain during their pregnancies.

Developmental Disabilities and Neural Tube Defects

16-14. Reduce the occurrence of developmental disabilities.

16-15. Reduce the occurrence of spina bifida and other neural tube defects (NTDs).

16-16. Increase the proportion of pregnancies begun with an optimum folic acid level.

Prenatal Substance Exposure

16-17. Increase abstinence from alcohol, cigarettes, and illicit drugs among pregnant women.

16-18. Reduce the occurrence of fetal alcohol syndrome (FAS).

Breastfeeding, Newborn Screening, and Service Systems

16-19. Increase the proportion of mothers who breast-feed their babies.

Weight Status and Growth

19-3. Reduce the proportion of children and adolescents who are overweight or obese.

19-4. Reduce growth retardation among low-income children under age 5 years.

Food and Nutrient Intake

19-5. Increase the proportion of persons aged 2 years and older who consume at least two daily servings of fruit.

19-6. Increase the proportion of persons aged 2 years and older who consume at least three daily servings of vegetables, with at least one-third of them being dark green or orange vegetables.

19-7. Increase the proportion of persons aged 2 years and older who consume at least six daily servings of grain products, with at least three being whole grains.

19-8. Increase the proportion of persons aged 2 years and older who consume less than 10 percent of calories from saturated fat.

19-9. Increase the proportion of persons aged 2 years and older who consume no more than 30 percent of calories from total fat.

19-10. Increase the proportion of persons aged 2 years and older who consume 2,400 mg or less of sodium daily.

19-11. Increase the proportion of persons aged 2 years and older who meet dietary recommendations for calcium.

Iron Deficiency and Anemia

19-12. Reduce iron deficiency among young children and females of childbearing age.

19-13. Reduce anemia among low-income pregnant females in their third trimester.

19-14. Reduce iron deficiency among pregnant females.

Schools, Worksites, and Nutrition Counseling

19-15. Increase the proportion of children and adolescents aged 6 to 19 years whose intake of meals and snacks at school contributes to good overall dietary quality.

Food Security

19-18. Increase food security among U.S. households, and in so doing reduce hunger.

As a result of the growing overweight/obesity epidemic, many of the HP 2000 nutrition objectives were not reached, and some categories moved even further away from the target goals. For example, the prevalence of overweight increased rather than decreased. The overall nutrition and overweight objective for 2010 is to ". . . reduce the proportion of children and adolescents who are overweight or obese" (Healthy People 2010, Goal 19-3). Eleven percent of children and adolescents were at or above the gender- and age-specific 95th percentile of the Body Mass Index (BMI) during baseline measurements between 1988 and 1994. The target percentage for overweight or obese children and adolescents in 2010 is 5%. The overweight/obesity epidemic is more prevalent among African Americans and Mexican Americans, and reaching this objective will be more challenging for these populations. The differential between the existing and targeted rates of overweight, as well as nutrient and food pattern goals, is substantial (Story, Neumark-Sztainer, French, 2002).

Maternal Health

The health of the mother is especially important to the health of the child. The nutritional status of the mother before she conceives establishes the quality of the environment in which the fetus will develop and is a key determinant in the life of the newborn. The mother's nutritional health also affects her ability to breast-feed the infant and provides postnatal nurturing. The interconceptional period before the woman becomes pregnant again is vital to the health of both the mother and the next baby she will conceive. If she becomes pregnant too soon or does not have sufficient food intake before she becomes pregnant, her limited body stores will put both the mother and the fetus at risk. Beyond pregnancy and infancy, the mother's health impacts her interactions with her family and her ongoing ability to feed her children and provide them with an optimal maternal-child experience as they move to adulthood. Health professionals who work with women of childbearing age have the potential to make significant impacts on the entire society by focusing on ways to improve the health of the mother.

Preconceptional Period

The preconceptional period is the time before a woman becomes pregnant. Women who are trying to become pregnant are more likely to be aware of their food intake and the importance of nutrition in relation to the success of their eventual pregnancy. But most women are pregnant for 6 to 8 weeks before they know it. This early pregnancy period is especially important in fetal development, and women who have health problems, nutritional deficiencies, or who consume alcohol or illicit drugs have a much higher risk of poor pregnancy outcomes. For this reason, health messages directed at women in the preconceptional period need to focus on information about the importance of a healthy diet before becoming pregnant so any future baby will be healthy. Women are most likely to receive this advice during visits to their gynecologist, family physician, or family planning clinic.

The primary nutrition messages for women in their childbearing years relate to weight management, nutritional intake, and alcohol intake. Women who are at extremes of either underweight or obese are at higher risk of delivering preterm or experiencing health problems during pregnancy. For this reason, as well as others, these women should be advised to maintain their weight in the normal range. With increasing numbers of women in the overweight and obese categories, this issue will take on more importance in relation to pregnancy and childbirth. Adequate nutritional intake in the preconceptional period is important to ensure that the woman enters pregnancy with fully replete body stores; this is especially important for women who are in the interconceptional period. Nutrient intake should be kept in the recommended range to avoid both deficiencies and excesses. Women should be evaluated for dietary practices that may put them at increased risk for either extreme. Alcohol intake during the first trimester is associated with higher rates of fetal alcohol syndrome. Because no level of alcohol has been identified as being safe, women should be advised to keep their alcohol intake levels low if they decide to drink alcohol during this time period. The following are guidelines for nutritional assessment and intervention for women in their childbearing years that should be conducted by the health professional:

1. Screen and assess women for preconceptional nutritional status. A self-administered questionnaire can be used to collect pertinent data, which is then reviewed by a healthcare professional. Criteria for referral to the dietitian can be established.
2. Nutrition information should be provided to all women. Women categorized as healthy and with no nutritional problems can be given a standard pamphlet to review. Women with low-risk problems can be counseled by the healthcare provider who is monitoring her care. Women identified as high risk should be referred to the dietitian for more intensive nutrition counseling.
3. Specific nutritional guidance should include:
   - Maintaining a healthy weight in the normal BMI range
   - Consuming a healthy diet that meets the Dietary Guidelines
   - Maintaining adequate intake of all nutrients, with special attention to iron, folic acid, calcium, vitamin C, vitamin D, and protein

- Stopping smoking due to its impact on infant development
- Avoiding alcohol
- Monitoring medical conditions, such as diabetes and hypertension

Prenatal Care

Once a woman learns she is pregnant, she needs to be evaluated and provided with appropriate guidance to assist her in staying healthy and delivering a healthy full-term baby. Nutritional assessment and advice, though similar to the preconceptional period, becomes more precise to the woman's particular status and needs.

Weight Gain

Prepregnancy weight, in conjunction with height, provides the baseline for determining weight gain ranges for the pregnant woman. Recommendations of the Institute of Medicine (IOM) of the National Academy of Sciences are based on the BMI of the woman when she became pregnant. Women are placed into one of four categories (underweight, normal weight, overweight, or obese) based on their BMI. Women in the normal weight category (BMI 19.8 to 26) should gain between 25 and 35 pounds during pregnancy. Underweight women (BMI < 19.8) should gain between 28 and 40 pounds. Overweight women (BMI > 26 to 29) should gain between 15 and 20 pounds. And, obese women (BMI > 29) should gain at least 15 pounds. If a woman is carrying twins, she should gain 35 to 45 pounds.

Once the woman has been placed into a weight category, her weight should be measured and plotted at each prenatal visit. Weight gain should be lowest during the first trimester (range 2 to 5 pounds). Weight gain higher than this indicates that too many calories are being consumed. During the second and third trimesters, most women should gain one pound per week, on average. Underweight women should gain slightly more (1.07 lb.) and overweight women should gain only two-thirds of a pound weekly. Maternal weight gain is an important factor in reducing the incidence of preterm delivery (Schieve et al., 1999).

Although excessive weight gain can be harmful, weight loss and dietary restrictions are not recommended. A woman may be advised to slow her rate of weight gain, but women should never be told to lose weight while pregnant.

Weight gain components include the fetus, fat stores, extracellular fluid, blood volume, uterus, amniotic fluid, placenta, and breast tissue (listed in order from highest to lowest weight for a term pregnancy). After delivery of a full-term infant weighing 7.5 to 8.5 pounds on average, most mothers will retain 10–20 pounds. By 6 weeks postpartum, most women are 5–10 pounds heavier than preconception levels (Gunderson et al., 2001). Some reports indicate that women who breast-feed are able to lose fat tissue more readily than women who formula-feed their infants (Kramer et al., 1993).

Appropriate strategies should be used to help mothers to lose the weight gain of pregnancy (Wosje & Kalkwarf, 2004). This weight retention contributes to the high nationwide obesity rates for women.

Nutrient Intake

In order to support the recommended level of weight gain, the pregnant woman needs to eat and drink wisely. Although health professionals know that pregnant women should not "eat for two," many women tend to eat more than advised. Review of food intake during pregnancy can help the pregnant woman eat the food she needs to maintain a healthy pregnancy and deliver a healthy baby, while ensuring that she does not consume more than she needs.

Calories

The Dietary Reference Intakes (DRIs) for pregnant women vary by trimester. The Estimated Energy Requirements (EER) for a woman in the first trimester is the same as a non-pregnant woman due to the low level of additional energy needed to sustain the pregnancy. A pregnant woman needs an additional 340 kcal/day in the second trimester and 452 kcal/day in the third trimester. These calorie goals may need to be adjusted for women who are in the underweight or overweight/obese weight categories.

These additional calories need to be used wisely to ensure that they are nutrient-rich foods that contribute to the other nutrients that need to be consumed in levels higher than for a non-pregnant woman. Recommended intake for nearly all nutrients is higher in pregnancy. Vitamin/mineral supplementation should be evaluated on an individual basis. Supplements cannot replace the combination of nutrients found in food. Some women tend to rely on the supplements and are less careful about their food intake. Nutrients that may require supplementation include iron, calcium, and folic acid. Additional nutrients may be indicated in some cases, such as an adolescent or a woman who is carrying multiple fetuses.

> Visit the DRIs online at http://www.nal.usda.gov/fnic/etext/000105.html to see the nutrition requirements of non-pregnant, pregnant, and lactating women.

Protein

Protein intake is especially important in pregnancy. Growth and development of the fetus, as well as the tissues to support the pregnancy, rely on adequate protein for tissue development. The DRI for protein in pregnancy is an additional 25 gm/day for all three trimesters. This level of additional protein is relatively easy for most women to consume. This is a key example of wise food selection. If one cup of non-fat milk is consumed, protein, calcium, vitamin D, and numerous other nutrients are significantly increased with only 100 kcal added to the diet. Dairy products are not appropriate for all women, however, particularly those who are lactose intolerant, but other solutions can be developed for them.

Smoking

Smoking cessation should be advocated as part of the nutrition education session. Smoking is totally contraindicated during pregnancy due to the profound impact it has on development of the fetus. Less oxygen is available to the fetus of a mother who smokes, so the baby is likely to be small for gestational age (SGA). SGA babies are at higher risk of complications of birth and to have higher rates of problems during the first year of life. Pregnant women who smoke need to be referred to an appropriate smoking cessation program if they are willing to try to stop smoking.

Alcohol

Alcohol abstinence is an essential element of pregnancy. Alcohol is a known teratogenic agent and is linked to fetal alcohol syndrome (FAS). Infants born with FAS exhibit numerous permanent developmental problems, including mental retardation. Infants who have been exposed to alcohol in utero may have fetal alcohol effects even if they are not diagnosed with FAS. Most pregnant women willingly abstain from alcohol to eliminate any risk of FAS.

Teratogenic—Causing birth defects.

Special Conditions

Adolescent Pregnancy

Recommended weight gains during pregnancy may be slightly higher for the teenager than for the adult. The current recommendation is that pregnant adolescents should gain weight within the upper range of that currently recommended for adults (i.e., 30 to 35 lb.) (Institute of Medicine, 1990). For adolescents with a below-normal pre-pregnancy weight, a 35- to 40-lb weight gain may be desirable (Institute of Medicine, 1990; Story & Stang, 2000).

Pregnant adolescents who are of young gynecologic age (the number of years between the onset of menses and the date of conception) or who are undernourished at the time of conception have the greatest nutritional needs. A young woman who conceives soon after her first menstrual period is at greatest physiologic risk. It was once thought that adolescents with advanced physiologic maturity had no more physical complications during pregnancy than adult women, but the Camden Study (Scholl, 1998) has shown that both these adolescents and their infants are at increased risk. This longitudinal study sought to explain why, with increasing maternal weight gains in adolescent mothers, the infant birth weights remained low. This increased risk of fetal growth restriction may be attributed to disruption in the fetal-placental blood flow and in the transmission of nutrients to the fetus as a result of the physiology associated with maternal growth.

Aside from the consequences to the outcome of pregnancy, adolescents who begin their childbearing early (while still growing themselves) may be at particular risk for overweight and obesity. The Camden Study (Hediger et al., 1998) has documented that the excessive accrual of subcutaneous fat stores at central body sites often, in later life, leads to the development of cardiovascular disease, non–insulin-dependent diabetes mellitus, and hypertension.

A clinically practical method of ensuring nutritional adequacy is to encourage the pregnant adolescent to gain the recommended amount of weight by consuming nutrient-rich foods. Most important, contact with health professionals during prenatal care provides the opportunity to teach adolescents about feeding themselves and their families (American Dietetic Association, 1994). Because of the economic instability of the pregnant adolescent, it is impossible to assume that she will have an adequate food supply. Health professionals can help provide access to and information about resources, such as food stamps, food banks, and the Women, Infants and Children (WIC) program.

Gestational Diabetes

Gestational diabetes is a form of diabetes that develops in some women when they become pregnant, but resolves once the pregnancy ends. Many of these women will go on to have type 2 diabetes later in life, particularly if they become obese. Gestational diabetes can have harmful effects on both the mother and the infant. The mother has an increased risk

> **Pre-eclampsia**—A hypertensive disorder of pregnancy that is characterized by the presence of protein in the urine and swelling, putting both mother and infant in danger.

of pre-eclampsia and delivering by Cesarean section. Infants born to women with all types of diabetes have a higher risk of becoming too large in utero (*macrosomia*—weighing more than 10 pounds). The infant also is at higher risk to be stillborn, to have hypoglycemia at birth, and to develop hypertension, diabetes, and obesity as an adult.

Women in moderate to high risk categories need to be screened for gestational diabetes using a glucose tolerance test. This is usually done by weeks 24–27 of pregnancy. Once diagnosed, an intervention plan is developed to bring the diabetes under control. Interventions generally start with diet and exercise and move to include medications as necessary to control blood glucose levels. Women with gestational diabetes need to be counseled and monitored by a dietitian (Kaiser & Allen, 2002).

Professional guidelines for nutritional assessment and intervention in pregnancy include:

1. Screen and assess the nutritional status of pregnant women. A self-administered questionnaire can be used to collect

pertinent data, which is then reviewed by a healthcare professional. Criteria for referral to the dietitian can be established.

2. Nutrition counseling should be provided to all pregnant women. Counseling strategies can be based on:
   - Women categorized as healthy and with no nutritional problems can be provided routine prenatal nutrition advice as part of their routine care.
   - Women with low-risk problems can be counseled by the healthcare provider who is monitoring her care using materials provided by the dietitian.
   - Women identified as high risk should be referred to the dietitian for more intensive nutrition counseling. High-risk women may include those who are not gaining sufficient weight; those who are gaining excessive amounts of weight; women with preexisting health conditions, such as diabetes, that require dietary intervention; and women who develop diseases requiring nutrition advice.

3. Specific nutritional guidance for women during pregnancy can include:
   - Maintaining a healthy weight gain as appropriate for her BMI category. Weight should be plotted at every prenatal visit to monitor growth.
   - Increasing calorie and protein intake during the second and third trimesters.
   - Consuming a healthy diet that meets the Dietary Guidelines. Emphasis should be placed on fruits and vegetables, whole grains, dairy products, and protein foods.
   - Maintaining adequate intake of all nutrients, with special attention to iron, folic acid, calcium, vitamin C, vitamin D, and protein. Supplements should be recommended if needed.
   - Maintaining physical activity as advised.
   - Consuming adequate amounts of fluid.
   - Stopping smoking due to its impact on infant development.
   - Abstaining from alcohol.
   - Learning about infant feeding methods; strong consideration should be given to breast-feeding with an emphasis on the benefits for both the mother and baby.
   - Monitoring medical conditions, such as diabetes and hypertension.
   - Providing nutrition intervention as needed.

Infancy

The first 12 months of a child's life are a critical period for establishing health and health-related habits. Key issues include the parent's decision to breast-feed or formula-feed; monitoring growth and development; introducing appropriate complementary foods when the infant is developmentally ready; and providing adequate amounts of key nutrients such as vitamin D, iron, and fluoride. This section will provide an overview of these key issues and describe several initiatives aimed at helping infants get a good start.

Breast-Feeding

Breast milk is the undisputed optimal food for both term and pre-term newborn infants (Lawrence & Lawrence, 1999). The unique characteristics of breast milk and breast-feeding confer many advantages, including health, nutritional, immunological, developmental, psychological, social, economic, and environmental benefits. The American Academy of Pediatrics (Breastfeeding Working Group, 1997), American Dietetic Association (ADA, 2001), and World Health Organization (WHO Expert Consultation, 2001) support exclusive breast-feeding of infants for the first 6 months. The AAP further recommends that breast-feeding be continued for the first 12 months and beyond for as long as it is mutually desired by the mother and toddler.

Although breast-feeding rates are on the rise in the United States, they remain below nationally established goals. In 2001, 69.5% of mothers initiated breast-feeding and 32.5% continued to breast-feed at 6 months (Ryan et al., 2002). The HP 2010 goals target 75% initiation of breast-feeding, with 50% continuing to breast-feed at 6 months, and 25% continuing to breast-feed at 12 months (U.S. Department of Health and Human Services, 2005). The rates of breast-feeding are different across demographic groups within the United States. Mothers who are less educated, single, young, have other children, work, or are African American or Hispanic American may be less likely to breast-feed. However, from 1993 to 1998, breast-feeding promotion was credited with significantly increasing the rates among vulnerable groups in 10 states from 57.0% to 67.5%. The groups most changed included low-income and African American women, participants in WIC, and mothers of infants admitted to the neonatal intensive care unit (Ahluwalia et al., 2003).

There are very few instances when breast milk and/or breast-feeding are not recommended (Kleinman, 2004). These include infants with galactosemia or certain other metabolic disorders, infants whose mothers abuse illegal drugs, or those mothers with certain other medical conditions, as recommended by the infant's pediatrician. In the United States, breast-feeding is not recommended for infants of mothers with human immunodeficiency virus (HIV).

Formula-Feeding

Infant formula is the appropriate food for infants who are weaned from the breast before 12 months and for infants who are not breast-fed. Infant formulas sold in the United States must meet safety and nutritional guidelines that are established and updated periodically by the U.S. Food and Drug Administration (Congressional Record, 1986; Life Sciences Research Office, 1998). The WHO *International Code of Marketing of Breast-Milk Substitutes* recommends that infant formulas should not be advertised or promoted to the general public and that manufacturers should not provide samples of products to pregnant women, mothers, or members of their family (WHO, 1981). In agreement, the AAP has stated their disapproval of direct advertising because it may negatively impact breast-feeding initiation or continuation (Kleinman, 2004).

Infant formulas are available as ready-to-feed liquid, or as concentrated liquid or powder to which water must be added. The majority of infant formulas are made from modified cow milk; however, soy-based and specialty formulas designed for medical conditions are also available. Cow milk–based infant formulas are available either as iron-fortified or low iron. Both the AAP and the Centers for Disease Control and Prevention (CDC) recommend that infants less than 12 months old be fed only iron-fortified infant formula (Committee on Nutrition, American Academy of Pediatrics, 1999; Centers for Disease Control and Prevention, 1998). Soy-based formulas are appropriate for infants with galactosemia, hereditary lactase deficiency, documented lactose intolerance following acute gastroenteritis, and for vegetarian infants. However, the routine use of soy-based formulas has not been demonstrated to be effective in preventing or managing colic, or in preventing the development of food allergies, and is not appropriate for pre-term infants weighing less than 1,800 grams (Committee on Nutrition, AAP, 1998). Infants who develop symptoms of food allergy may benefit from using a soy-based formula or a hypoallergenic formula in which the protein is partially or totally hydrolyzed (Committee on Nutrition, AAP, 2000).

In recent years, infant formula manufacturers have begun to examine the benefits of adding a variety of nutrients and biological factors to mimic the composition and quality of breast milk (Carver, 2003). These include long-chain polyunsaturated fatty acids, nucleotides, and prebiotics/probiotics. At this time, the benefits of these and other ingredients are still being studied.

Growth and Development

Infancy is a period of rapid growth and development. Most infants double their birth weight by the 6th month and triple it by the 12th month (Butte et al., 2000). However, there are normal differences in growth between healthy breast-fed and formula-fed infants during the first year of life. Breast-fed infants tend to gain weight more rapidly than formula-fed infants in the first 2 to 3 months, but less rapidly from 3 to 12 months (Story et al., 2002). These differences in weight gain and growth tend to disappear in the second year (Butte et al., 2000a).

Growth can best be assessed by plotting weight and length for age, and weight for length on an appropriate National Center for Health Statistics Growth Chart (as discussed in Chapter 3). These charts have been constructed using data from large population groups over time and are a way to assess an individual's growth against group norms. However, each infant will establish and follow his or her own growth curve.

Rapid development during the first year is responsible for the infant changing from a newborn that needs head support to feed and is capable of a simple suck-swallow-breathe pattern during feeding, to an older infant who can easily feed herself with her fingers and can

> You'll find The Start Healthy Feeding Plan at: http://www.gerber.com/feedingplan/.

drink from a cup. The Start Healthy Feeding Plan reflects a recent evaluation of many years of research and graphically represents the advancement of developmental and feeding skills throughout infancy (Butte et al., 2004).

Healthcare providers can monitor growth and development by comparing an infant's progress against these tools. Periodic visits allow the provider to establish a relationship with the infant and his caregivers, through which a dialogue can be held. At the appropriate times, questions about the child's development and feeding will provide the basis for anticipatory guidance or counseling to help provide a smooth transition between developmental stages as the child grows (Story et al., 2002).

Complementary Foods

Research has demonstrated that exclusive breast-feeding can meet the nutrient needs of infants through the first 6 months. Most infants are developmentally ready for the introduction of complementary foods and beverages by 4 to 6 months.

Solids

In the United States, an infant's first solid food is typically iron-fortified, single-ingredient (rice) infant cereal. Recent research has affirmed the importance of a good source of iron for breast-fed infants by 4 to 6 months in meeting daily requirements (Devaney et al., 2004). This can be provided by iron-fortified infant cereal and later by meats. Following cereal, single ingredient pureed fruits and vegetables are offered to the infant, with at least 2 to 4 days between introductions of each new food. Whether fruits or vegeta-

This chapter introduces the reader to the many public health nutrition issues of feeding infants and children. Additional training and research on the appropriate feeding practices of infants and children should be a part of the education of those healthcare providers counseling parents of young children.

bles should be offered first has long been a subject of debate, but a recent review of the literature indicates the order in which they are introduced isn't critical (Butte et al., 2004). It is well-established that it can take 10 to 15 exposures to a new food for it to be accepted by an infant or toddler, and parents should be encouraged to present the food repeatedly to encourage acceptance (Birch et al., 1998; Sullivan & Birch, 1990).

Juice

Juice manufacturers have successfully marketed 100% fruit juice as a healthy beverage. However, some fruit juices, such as prune, apple, and pear, contain a significant amount of sorbitol (a sugar alcohol) and proportionally more fructose than glucose. Infants can absorb only a portion of the sorbitol (as little as 10%) and fructose in these juices (Lifschitz, 2000). The unabsorbed carbohydrate is fermented in the lower intestine, causing diarrhea, abdominal pain, or bloating. These symptoms are commonly reported in infants and toddlers who drink excessive amounts of juice. The AAP has concluded that fruit juice offers no nutritional benefit for infants younger than 6 months and no benefit over whole fruits for infants older than 6 months. They recommend that juice not be introduced to infants before 6 months, should not be given in a bottle or easily transported covered cup, should not be given at nap- or bedtime, and should be limited to 4 to 6 ounces daily for infants and children up to 6 years old (Committee on Nutrition, 2001).

Key Nutrients

Vitamin D

Rickets is a disease of vitamin D and/or calcium deficiency, characterized in infants by poor bone growth leading to bowing of the legs or knock knees. Although the incidence of rickets in developed countries is very low, cases have continued to be reported regularly over the last 20 years. Most cases have occurred in breast-fed infants of dark-skinned mothers who had minimal exposure to sunlight (Kreiter et al., 2000; Pugliese et al., 1998; Welch et al., 2000) and in toddlers on vegetarian diets (Carvalho et al., 2001). Although rickets can be prevented by regular exposure to sunlight, increasing concern over the long-term affects of early sun exposure on the development of skin cancer have led to new recommendations for vitamin D supplementation of all infants. The AAP now recommends that all breast-fed infants receive 200 IU of vitamin D daily, unless they are weaned, to at least 500 ml per day of vitamin D–fortified formula or milk (AAP, 2003). They further recommend that formula-fed infants who consume less than 500 ml of formula daily receive 200 IU of vitamin D daily.

Iron

Iron deficiency anemia in infancy has been associated with significant developmental deficits, including language difficulties, poor motor skills and balance, and poor attention, responsiveness, and mood, which may be only partially reversible with subsequent supplementation (Nokes et al., 1998). Fetal iron stores are exhausted by 4 to 6 months of age, making it necessary that iron be supplied by the diet (Kleinman, 2004). This need corresponds well with the introduction of high-iron complementary foods, such as iron-fortified infant formula, iron-fortified infant cereals, and/or meats. The AAP recommends that full-term breast-fed infants need a supplemental source of iron beginning at 4 to 6 months and that only iron-fortified formula should be used for weaning or supplementing breast milk for infants up to 12 months (Committee on Nutrition, 1999; Kleinman, 2004). The immature gastrointestinal (GI) tract of infants is unable to digest and absorb cow milk during the first year, and its ingestion is responsible for GI blood loss leading to anemia (Ziegler et al., 1999). The AAP recommends the avoidance of regular cow, goat, or soy milk for the milk-based part of the diet before 12 months of age (Kleinman, 2004).

Fluoride

Exposure to appropriate levels of fluoride is effective in reducing the prevalence of dental caries. Most public water supplies are fluoridated to provide 0.7 ppm to 1.2 ppm of fluoride. The need for fluoride supplementation depends on the total amount of fluoride available to the infant from all sources, including infant formula, water, and commercial and home-prepared baby foods. Human milk contains little fluoride, even in areas with fluoridated water (Hale, 2004). The amount of fluoride in commercial concentrated or powdered infant formula depends on the amount of fluoride in the formula and in the water used for mixing. Infants fed formula made with fluoridated water may receive up to 1.0 mg/day of fluoride (Institute of Medicine, Food and Nutrition Board, 2004). Ready-to-feed infant formulas are manufactured with non-fluoridated water. The AAP, the American Academy of Pediatric Dentistry, and the CDC recommend no fluoride supplementation for infants less than 6 months old (American Academy of Pediatric Dentistry, 2003; CDC, 2001; Kleinman, 2004). For infants older than 6 months whose community drinking water contains < 0.3 ppm fluoride, they recommend supplementation of 0.25 mg sodium fluoride/day.

Guidelines for nutritional assessment and intervention in infancy are recommended in the following steps:

Birth to 6 months:

1. Breast-feed for the first 4–6 months. Supplement with iron and vitamin D.
2. If breast-feeding is not selected, provide a fortified infant formula that approximates breast milk. Ensure that the formula is prepared under sanitary conditions and according to directions.
3. Begin complementary foods when the infant is developmentally ready.
4. Measure length and weight growth status and plot on NCHS growth charts.

Six months to one year:

1. Continue breast milk or formula.
2. Continue to introduce foods as directed by pediatrician or dietitian.
3. Include infant in family meals.
4. Provide finger foods and child-sized utensils to encourage self-feeding.
5. Measure length and weight growth status and plot on NCHS growth charts.
6. Provide opportunities to develop physical abilities.
7. Refer to WIC when indicated.
8. Provide appropriate care for disease or other health conditions.

Childhood and Adolescence

Beyond infancy, children move through various stages of growth and development on their journey to becoming young adults. Each age level has different nutrient needs. Toddlers have a slower growth rate that continues through childhood until the growth spurt of adolescence starts. Children also move from being dependent on parents to provide healthy food choices to making all their own food choices when they are in late adolescence. An important role for parents and other caregivers is to provide a wide variety of healthy foods and let the children decide which foods and the amount to eat. Mealtime struggles can create an unpleasant environment for everyone and do little to encourage children to eat more foods.

Assessment of Growth

Growth assessment is the best way to determine if children are well nourished. When children are getting enough to eat and do not have health problems, they should be growing normally. Plotting height (or length for very young children) and weight on the NCHS standardized growth charts can help determine if a child's growth is appropriate.

The CDC/NCHS BMI tables are available at http://www.cdc.gov/growthcharts/.

Weight and height can be plotted on growth grids to determine whether individuals are maintaining their growth pattern or growth channel. The relationship between weight and height can be evaluated by using the CDC/NCHS BMI tables. Appropriate weights for height, according to age and sex, lie between the 10th and 85th percentiles, a range that allows for individual differences in body build (Story et al., 2000).

Use of BMI, which is highly correlated with body fatness, can also indicate weight status. BMI is calculated by dividing body weight (expressed in kilograms) by the square of height (in meters); that is, $BMI = kg/m^2$. Children with BMIs below the 5th percentile should be assessed for organic diseases or eating disorders. Children with BMIs between the 85th percentile and the 95th percentile are at risk for overweight, and a nutritional screening/assessment should be performed to determine health risk. Children with BMIs $\geq$ 95th percentile for age and gender are overweight and should have an in-depth medical assessment (Barlow & Dietz, 1998) that includes data on family history, blood pressure, total cholesterol level, any major change in BMI, and concern about weight (Dietz, 1998; Story et al., 2000).

A skinfold evaluation yields a further degree of precision. For example, a low skinfold measurement in an individual who is above the 85th percentile BMI indicates a state of being overweight, but not overfat. An assessment of muscle and arm circumference can confirm the muscular composition. However, a skinfold in the 90th percentile or greater with a BMI greater than the 95th percentile suggests overfat or truly overweight.

Excessive or less-than-normal growth can be detected by plotting height changes on the CDC growth charts. The major cause of short stature during adolescence is genetically late initiation of puberty, although other conditions, such as chronic disease or skeletal and chromosomal abnormalities, also can account for certain children being shorter than normal. Hormonal imbalances leading to abnormal growth are rare.

Nutrient Requirements

Energy

Energy requirements are designed to maintain health, promote optimal growth and maturation, and support a desirable level of physical activity. Children who limit energy intake or have food security issues that limit energy intake may limit ultimate adult growth. In 2002, the National Academy of Sciences released new guidelines for energy requirements (National Academy of Sciences, 2002). Estimated Energy Requirements (EER) are based on energy expenditure, requirements for growth, and level of physical activity. Variability in the EER exists for both males and females because of variations in growth rate and physical activity.

To derive the EER, the adolescent's gender, age, height, weight, and physical activity level (PAL) were utilized in calculations, with an average of 25 kcal/day added for energy deposition. In order to determine adequate energy (kcal) intake, an assessment of physical activity is required. The energy requirements allow for four levels of activity (sedentary, low active, active, and very active). This physical activity reflects the energy expended in activities beyond the activities of daily living. Activity levels are based on the equivalence shown in Table 10-2.

TABLE 10-2   Physical Activity Levels

Physical Activity Level Category	Walking Equivalence (at 2–4 mph)
Sedentary	No additional activity
Low Active	1.5–2.2 miles/day
Active	3.0–4.4 miles/day
Very Active	7.5–10.3 miles/day

Protein

Protein needs, like those for energy, correlate more closely with the growth pattern than with chronological age. The 2002 Dietary Reference Intakes for protein are based on the amount of protein needed for growth and positive nitrogen balance (National Academy of Sciences, 2002). The DRIs provide for both the Estimated Average Requirements (EAR) and the Recommended Dietary Allowances (RDA). The DRIs recommend using the EAR when assessing nutrient intakes of groups. The EAR provides for adequate intake of 50% of the population. The RDA is recommended for assessing the intake of an individual. Average intakes of protein for adolescents are well above the RDA for all age groups. In fact, when comparing protein intakes of adolescents from the United States with teens from other countries, studies show that U.S. adolescents have a much higher intake of protein. There is little evidence to show that insufficient protein intake is common in the adolescent population. However, if energy intake is inadequate for any reason (i.e., food security issues, chronic illness, or attempts to lose weight), dietary protein may be used to meet energy needs and will, therefore, be unavailable for synthesis of new tissue or for tissue repair. This may result in a state of insufficient protein, which will lead to a reduction in growth rate and a decrease in lean body mass. Current dieting patterns in some adolescent females can result in restricted calorie intakes that are potentially harmful, especially when protein sources are used to meet energy needs. However, excessive intakes of protein can also have an impact on nutritional status. For example, a high protein intake can interfere with calcium metabolism as well as increase fluid needs. These increased fluid needs may put adolescent athletes at high risk for dehydration.

Minerals and Vitamins

Micronutrients (vitamins and minerals) play an important role in the growth and health of adolescents. Inadequate fruit and vegetable consumption has been linked to certain types of cancer and other diseases. Because of the many health benefits associated with fruits and vegetables, national recommendations support increased consumption of these foods. The 2005 Dietary Guidelines, released January 12, 2005, recommend 2 cups of fruit and $2^{1}/_{2}$ cups of vegetables per day (U.S. DHHS/USDA, 2005). Unfortunately, surveys show that, for adolescents, there are significant gaps between actual intake and these recommendations. The 2003 Youth Risk Behavior Survey (YRBS) revealed that only 22.0% of all adolescents ate ≥ 5 servings of fruits/vegetables a day—20.3% of females and 23.6% of males (CDC, 2004).

Despite the low levels of fruits and vegetables, most children get sufficient amounts of vitamins and minerals until they reach adolescence, when requirements increase dramatically due to growth demands. Because of increased energy demands during this period, increased quantities of thiamine, riboflavin, and niacin are required for the release of energy from carbohydrates. With tissue synthesis, there is an increased demand for vitamin B_6, folic acid, and vitamin B_{12}. There is also an increased requirement for vitamin D (for rapid skeletal growth), and vitamins A, C, and E are needed for new cell growth. Although there are few reports of low serum vitamin C levels in teens, those who habitually avoid fruits and vegetables and those who smoke cigarettes may be at increased risk for deficiency.

Calcium

Because of accelerated muscular, skeletal, and endocrine development, calcium needs are greater during puberty and adolescence than in childhood or during the adult years. At the peak of the growth spurt, the daily deposition of calcium can be twice that of the average during the rest of the adolescent period. In fact, 45% of the skeletal mass is added during adolescence (Lytle, 2002).

Calcium requirements are expressed as Adequate Intakes (AIs). The AI is believed to cover needs of all individuals in a group, but lack of data or uncertainty in the data preclude specifying, with confidence, the percentage of persons covered by this intake (Institute of Medicine, 1997). This is especially true for adolescents. *The National Institutes of Health Consensus Development Conference Statement on Optimal Calcium Intake* (NIH, 1994) recommended

1,200 to 1,500 mg of calcium per day for adolescents aged 11 to 24 years. In its statement, the committee acknowledged that there appears to be a certain threshold level of dietary calcium that is necessary to allow growing adolescents to achieve their genetically predetermined peak bone mass. Dietary survey data indicate that adolescents, particularly females, are at greatest risk for inadequate calcium intake (Alaimo et al., 1994). Calcium intake tends to decline among females 10 to 17 years of age. Consumption surveys show an average intake for females to be 780 to 820 mg per day. In male adolescents, the average intake is 800 to 920 mg per day.

Several recent human and animal studies have suggested a specific role for calcium in modulating body fat. Zemel et al. (2003) demonstrated that increased dietary calcium inhibited adipocyte intracellular calcium, resulting in increased stimulation of lipolysis and inhibition of lipogenesis during energy restriction. National Health and Nutrition Examination Survey (NHANES) III data showed an inverse relationship between calcium and BMI. These data indicate that individuals with higher calcium intake had lower BMIs. More recently, Skinner et al. (2003) showed the same effect in children. In examining children ages 9–14, she found that those who consumed more calcium tended to weigh less and have lower body fat than those with low calcium consumption. In this study, the intake of calcium accounted for 4.5%–9.0% of the variance in body fat. Skinner suggested that children could reduce their body fat if they increased their calcium intake with one glass of skim milk or 8 oz of yogurt per day. Even the slightest decrease in body fat could help in preventing co-morbidities associated with overweight/obesity.

Iron

Iron is a key indicator nutrient throughout childhood and adolescence. Iron deficiency anemia is fairly common, with 4%–7% of children exhibiting low hemoglobin and hematocrit. During adolescence iron requirements are increased. Dallmon et al. (1989) noted that in boys there is a sharp increase in the requirements for iron from approximately 10 to 15 mg/day. This increase reflects not only the expanding blood volume, but also a rise in hemoglobin concentration that occurs with sexual maturation in males. After the growth spurt and sexual maturation, growth increases rapidly and so does the need for iron. In females, the growth spurt is not as great, but menstruation typically starts about one year after peak growth. The mean requirement for iron reaches a maximum of approximately 15 mg/day at peak growth, but settles to a mean of approximately 13–15 mg/day because of the need to replace menstrual iron losses.

In girls with marginal intakes, iron deficiency anemia may result from growth demands. Conversely, iron deficiency may be a limiting factor for growth during adolescence. Additionally, anemia in adolescence may impair the immune response. A study of Native American children aged 1–14 indicated that the cell-mediated immune response and the bactericidal capacity of leukocytes (in vitro methods) were significantly depressed in those with hemoglobin concentrations below 10 mg/day (Dallmon et al., 1989).

Reports from dietary surveys indicate that iron intakes of adolescents with normal dietary patterns were between 12.5 and 14.2 mg/day for females compared to between 13.6 and 18.0 mg/day for males. The average U.S. diet contains an estimated 6 mg iron/1,000 kcal (CDC, 1998). Adolescent females, who typically have lower caloric intakes than males, may have more difficulty in obtaining adequate levels of iron from their diets.

NHANES III found iron deficiency in 14.2% of the 15 to 18-year-old females and 12.1% of the 11 to 14-year-old males (Alaimo et al., 1994). Iron deficiency is prevalent in adolescents of both genders and in teens of all ethnicities and socioeconomic levels. In its recommendations to prevent and control iron deficiency in the United States, the CDC includes guidelines for prevention, screening, and treatment of iron deficiency anemia (CDC, 1998).

Nutrition Education

School settings are ideal for nutrition education. The majority of U.S. children between the ages of 5 and 17 are enrolled in school, and this provides a unique learning community through which children are able to participate in nutrition-based education. A familiar environment and the support of teachers and peers strengthens the impact of nutrition education. Programs are likely to be more widely accepted by the participants when they are culturally and socially sensitive. Multidimensional strategies including health/physical education, parental involvement, and food service involvement along with nutrition education helps to promote learning and behavior change. Children seem most interested in teaching methods that use discovery learning, student learning stations, cooperative groups, situation analysis, and cross-age and peer teaching. Extensive research on school-based methods to improve nutritional intake supports their continued use, but confirms that behavioral change is slow. Nutrition education needs to be part of the comprehensive school health education program to strengthen and advance positive food and nutrition messages.

Physical Activity

Physical Activity and Health: A Report of the Surgeon General is a comprehensive overview of research related to physical activity and health (CDC, 1996). The report: 1) summarizes the benefits of physical activity; 2) reinforces the importance of promoting physical activity; 3) states that many children and adolescents are at risk for health problems because of inactive lifestyles; and 4) states that everyone should participate in a moderate amount of physical activity (e.g., 15 minutes of running, 30 minutes of brisk walking, 45 minutes of playing volleyball) on

> Read more about *Physical Activity and Health: A Report of the Surgeon General* at: http:// www.cdc.gov/nccdphp/sgr/sgr.htm.

most, if not all, days of the week. The 2003 YRBS (CDC, 2004) indicated that 30% of teens did not participate in at least 20 minutes of vigorous physical activity at least three times a week. The rate of inactivity increased with each grade level, from 28.2% in 9th grade to 40.2% in 12th grade. This same pattern was seen with ethnicity (Caucasian 31%, African American 41.2%, Hispanic American 36.5%).

These findings are disturbing in view of the numerous health benefits that children and adolescents derive by being physically active on a regular basis. Physical activity can lead to improved body composition (e.g., increased lean muscle mass, reduced total body fat) and can help reduce other coronary heart disease (CHD) risk factors among adolescents. For example, increased physical activity levels can favorably alter blood lipid profiles in adolescents at high risk for CHD (e.g., children and adolescents who are obese or who have type 1 or 2 diabetes mellitus) and can reduce blood pressure, especially in adolescents whose blood pressure is elevated. Physical activity plays a substantial role in the development of bone mass during adolescence and can help maintain the structure and functional strength of bone throughout life (Patrick et al., 2001; Salis & Patrick, 1994).

Efforts to increase physical activity levels among children and adolescents have been most successful in school settings. However, little attention has been focused on promoting physical activity among children and adolescents in settings other than schools, including healthcare settings (i.e., health professionals counseling children and adolescents about physical activity during health supervision visits) (Corbin & Pangrazi, 1998).

Health professionals, families, peers, and communities can influence children's and adolescents' physical activity levels. Parents who participate in physical activity themselves and who support and encourage physical activity in their adolescents have a positive influence on adolescents' physical activity levels. In addition, older children and adolescents whose friends are physically active tend to be more physically active themselves.

Little is known about which factors motivate children and adolescents to become physically active, remain physically active, and increase their physical activity levels as they become older. In addition, it is not clear why these factors differ for females and males or for different racial and ethnic groups. However, it is clear that females are less likely than males to participate in vigorous physical activity, participate in strengthening or toning activities, or participate on sports teams. Strategies different from those used to promote physical activity in boys and male adolescents may be needed to promote physical activity in girls and female adolescents (Patrick et al., 2001). Strategies that take into account children's and adolescents' race or cultural background could also be beneficial. The Surgeon General's report recommends the following intervention strategies to promote physical activity in children and adolescents:

- Make physical activity enjoyable.
- Help adolescents succeed and increase their confidence in their ability to be physically active.
- Support adolescents' efforts to be physically active.
- Help adolescents learn about the benefits of physical activity and help them develop positive attitudes toward it.
- Help adolescents overcome barriers that keep them from being physically active.

Family Mealtime

Increasing emphasis is being placed on family mealtime because of its positive impact on food intake and child development. Project EAT surveyed middle school and high school students from ethnically and socioeconomically diverse communities (Eisenberg et al., 2004). Results show that almost one-third of participants reported only eating one to two meals with their family each week, or never eating family meals. Children eating more than three family meals per week were significantly less likely to skip breakfast and report poor consumption of fruits, vegetables, and dairy foods, compared to children

> Read more about Project EAT at http://www.epi.umn.edu/research/eat/.

eating less than three family meals per week. African Americans and Hispanic Americans were less likely to skip breakfast and report poor fruit consumption compared to Caucasian children. A higher frequency of family meals is associated with significantly lower odds of the following variables: cigarette, alcohol, and marijuana use; low grade point average; high depressive symptoms; and suicidal ideation. Family meal frequency had a strong positive association with intake of energy; percentage of calories from protein; calcium; iron; vitamins A, C, E, B_6; folate; and fiber (Story et al., 2002).

Another family meal study involved children of participants in the ongoing Nurses' Health Study II. Subjects who ate family dinner every day consumed an average of 0.8 more servings of fruits and vegetables than those who never ate family meals or did so only on some

> Read more about the Nurses' Health Study II at http://www.channing.harvard.edu/nhs/.

> Childhood overweight and obesity are critical public health threats, but are addressed in an earlier chapter. Please refer to Chapter 5 to learn about their cause and recommended treatments.

days. Additionally, consumption of fried food and soda was inversely associated with frequency of family meals. Participants who ate family meals more often reported slightly higher energy intakes and also higher intakes of several nutrients including fiber; calcium; folate; vitamins B_6, B_{12}, C, and E; and iron. In addition, they consumed less trans-fat and saturated fat as a percentage of energy intake (Gillman et al., 2000). Family mealtime may be a potentially protective factor in the lives of children for nearly all these variables.

School-Based Growth Screening

Until recently, most schools did not assess weight status using BMI. In many school districts, the school nurse measured height and weight and plotted them on a growth chart; however, no additional referral or reporting procedures were required.

In response to the increasing epidemic of childhood obesity across the nation, many state and local governments have implemented programs to measure children's growth and educate and inform parents about their child's weight status. These screening programs are designed to provide a mechanism by which parents of high-risk children are:

- Informed about their child's risk of overweight
- Educated on the risks of childhood overweight on health
- Referred for available community and school-based interventions

Screening programs provide an excellent way for parents and children to more easily access the needed resources to address childhood overweight in an effective manner and facilitate collaboration between school, family, primary care providers, and interested community partners. For example, the Pennsylvania Growth Screening Program requires that school nurses and/or teachers measure height and weight and calculate BMI, record these results in the child's school health record, plot results on the CDC growth charts, and inform parents of children who are at risk for overweight (85th to less than 95th percentile on the BMI-for-age chart) or who are overweight (above 95th percentile on the BMI-for-age chart). Results are submitted on an annual basis to the Division of School Health for surveillance and program planning purposes. This program will provide a comprehensive way to identify overweight children and those at risk for becoming overweight, and then link them with available interventions (PANA, 2004).

Early Childhood Specifics

After the rapid growth of infancy, the toddler and preschool child's growth slows. Toddlers (age 1–3) gain about half a pound a month and grow ¼ inch to ½ inch. Preschool children gain about 4–5 pounds and grow 2 inches per year. Children generally lose some of the body fat accumulated as an infant, their bodies elongate, and they begin to look more like children. All baby teeth should be in place by age 2. Brain development continues to be important, with brain growth 75% complete by age 2, and attaining adult size during the elementary school years.

Total energy needs continue to increase to support body maintenance and a slow rate of growth, but calories per kilogram declines until the growth spurt of adolescence. Along with the gradual increase in total calories, the need for protein, vitamins, and minerals also increases.

Eating Patterns

Young children develop lifelong eating patterns in response to the food environment in which they live. This is easily demonstrated by the diverse foods eaten by children of different cultures. Children learn to prefer the foods that they are exposed to at mealtimes. Parents and other adults have an important role to play as food and nutrition gatekeepers by ensuring that a wide variety of nutritious foods are served. Foods rejected by children should continue to be offered on other occasions. Children are naturally neophobic about new foods, and frequency of exposure to food promotes increased preference. Food choices of other children in the home or in childcare settings also influence what children like to eat. Children often go on food jags where they want to eat the same foods; fortunately, they generally don't last long enough to impact nutritional intake.

Young children respond well to small frequent meals; snacks contribute as much as 20% of daily calories. Portion sizes need to be kept in balance with the child's appetite. Children like foods with interesting shapes, colors, and contrasting temperatures. Foods that might cause choking if swallowed whole, such as grapes, popcorn, hard candy, and hot dogs, should be avoided. Parents and caregivers can help promote a healthy variety of food choices by maintaining a positive attitude towards food and minimizing mealtime conflicts (Nicklas & Johnson, 2004).

Guidelines for nutritional assessment and intervention in early childhood, ages 1–5, may include the following:

1. Screen and assess growth status and plot on NCHS growth charts.
2. Provide a wide variety of healthy foods with emphasis on nutritious choices such as whole grains, fruits, vegetables, dairy foods, and lean meats and protein alternatives.

3. Continue to serve new foods even if not initially preferred.

4. Avoid using food as a reward or punishment.

5. Provide opportunities for physical activity through active play.

6. Avoid low nutrient-dense foods as snack choices.

7. Evaluate nutrition services in childcare facilities to ensure standards are met.

8. Provide appropriate care for disease or other health conditions.

9. Teach children to wash their hands before eating.

Childcare Programs

Many parents work, which means that many children are in childcare programs during the preschool years. Generally, these programs provide some level of food service to the children they serve. The ADA position paper on childcare programs recommends that childcare menus provide one-third of a child's nutritional requirements in the meals and snacks provided (Briley & Roberts-Gray, 1999). Levels of fat, salt, and sugar should be maintained at modified levels. Childcare centers are advised to use the services of a dietitian in planning the menus and to include nutrition education in the classroom. Cleanliness in food production and service are important to minimize food-borne illness. The Child and Adult Care Food Program administered by the USDA provides assistance to childcare programs in setting food standards and gives financial support to provide nutritious foods for low-income children (Stang & Bayerl, 2003).

> Read more about The Child and Adult Care Food Program administered by the USDA at http://www.fns.usda.gov/cnd/care/cacfp/cacfphome.htm.

Lead Exposure

Concerns about lead in the environment have resulted in numerous bans on the use of lead in such things as gasoline and paint. Although these efforts have had a positive impact, the lingering lead in the environment continues to contribute to lead poisoning in young children. Many young children are exposed to lead in their homes. Lead is present in old paint and water pipes. Lead absorption is highest during stages of rapid growth such as early childhood. Lead intake is harmful to children because it contributes to iron deficiency and anemia. Low levels of lead toxicity can be difficult to diagnose because the symptoms, such as diarrhea, irritability, and fatigue, are nonspecific. Early identification is important due to the permanent damage that can occur, leading to nerve damage and mental retardation (Farley, 1998).

Food Allergies

Food allergies are caused when the body's immune system reacts to a whole food protein. Allergic responses can range from inflammation of the nasal passages to skin rashes to anaphylactic shock. Food allergies can be difficult to identify, particularly if the response is delayed. Non-allergenic adverse reactions to foods can be misidentified as food allergies. Most children outgrow food allergies. Foods likely to cause allergies include eggs, milk, fish, peanuts, and soybeans. Children with severe allergic reactions need to be evaluated by a physician and will require careful monitoring of their food intake.

School-Aged Child Specifics

By the time she enters school, a child should weigh twice as much as she did at age 1. During the elementary school years, children continue to grow at a steady rate, gaining approximately 2.5 inches per year and 5–7 pounds. Children's appetites will ebb and wane as their growth patterns change, with increased food intake during a growth spurt. Families continue to play an important role in food choices, but peer pressure and media influences begin to play a strong role in food decisions.

Children mature physically and mentally during this time span. They become progressively stronger and their motor coordination increases. Body image becomes important in relation to peers, as children don't want to be seen as different. Their independence grows and they learn how to make decisions for themselves. This can lead to conflicts over food choices and emotional struggles with parents.

School Meals

The USDA National School Lunch Program provides financial support to schools to provide nutritious lunches to low-income children. In addition, these programs mandate food and nutrition criteria for schools to use in planning school meals. The USDA allows for several methods for schools to meet the nutrient requirement for school lunches. The traditional meal planning approach includes five components; newer strategies include computerized nutrient analysis. Nutrition education displays are often provided in the school lunchroom. The USDA's Team Nutrition was established to provide resources and technical support to help schools improve healthy eating and physical activity patterns (Briggs et al., 2003).

The School Breakfast Program extends free nutritious food to the breakfast period. More schools in low-income neighborhoods should be encouraged to participate in this program. Many low-income children go to school hungry or eat low nutrient foods before starting school. A healthy breakfast has been shown to improve school performance.

> Read more about The School Lunch and Breakfast Programs administered by the USDA at http://www.fns.usda.gov/cnd/.

Guidelines for nutritional assessment and intervention in school-aged children, ages 6–10, should include:

1. Screen and assess growth status and plot on NCHS growth charts.
2. Children identified as at risk for overweight or who are overweight should be referred for further evaluation and possible treatment.
3. Provide a wide variety of healthy foods with emphasis on nutritious choices, such as whole grains, fruits, vegetables, dairy foods, and lean meats and protein alternatives.
4. Ensure that children eat breakfast before going to school.
5. Promote regular physical activity at school and at home.
6. Reduce sedentary activity with an emphasis on reduction of screen time.
7. Provide nutrition education in school.
8. Ensure regular meals and snacks.
9. Encourage reduced levels of low nutrient-dense beverages.
10. Support school lunch and breakfast programs.
11. Provide appropriate care for disease or other health conditions.

Food Advertising

Television and magazines probably have a greater influence on children's eating habits than any other form of mass media. It is estimated that, by the time the average child reaches the teen years, he or she has viewed 100,000 food commercials, most of them for products with high concentrations of fat and simple carbohydrates. More than 65% of food advertisements promote beverages (primarily alcohol) and sweets (Brown & Witherspoon, 1998; Story et al., 2002). Food advertisements use a variety of techniques to appeal to children such as cartoon characters, catchy songs, colorful images, and appealing colors and tastes. Many advertisers use prizes and other incentive items to encourage food purchases. Advertisements for low nutrient-dense foods, such as soda, candy, and snacks, have a dominant presence in the time slots in which children's programming is aired.

Recently, food manufacturers have been under tremendous pressure to modify their advertising to children. Some fast food outlets and food manufacturers have started to respond with plans to eliminate some advertising directed at children. Efforts such as these will help to improve the unhealthy food environment in children's television.

Adolescence Specifics

Adolescence is a time of dramatic change in the life of every human being. The relatively uniform growth of childhood is suddenly altered by an increase in the velocity of growth. This sudden spurt is also associated with hormonal, cognitive, and emotional changes. All of these changes create special nutritional needs. Adolescence is considered an especially nutritionally vulnerable period of life for several reasons. First is the greater demand for nutrients due to the dramatic increase in physical growth and development. Second is the change of lifestyle and food habits of adolescents that affect both nutrient intake and needs. Third are those adolescents with special nutrient needs, such as those who participate in sports, have a chronic illness, diet excessively, or who use alcohol or drugs (Spear, 1996).

Physiologic Changes

Puberty, the process of physically developing from a child to an adult, is initiated by physiological factors and includes maturation of the entire body. Adolescence is the only time following birth when the velocity of growth actually increases. The adolescent gains about 20% of adult height and 50% of adult weight during this period.

This growth continues throughout the approximately 5–7 years of pubertal development. A great percentage of this height will be gained during the 18- to 24-month period of the growth spurt. The growth spurt or peak height gain velocity occurs at different ages for different individuals, as does the initiation of puberty. In general, girls began the pubertal process approximately 2 years earlier than boys. Although growth slows following the achievement of sexual maturity, linear growth and weight acquisition continue into the late teens for females and early twenties for males. Most females gain no more than 1 to 2 inches following menarche, although girls who have early menarche tend to grow more after its onset than do those having later menarche.

In the process of total body maturation, the composition of the body changes. Prepubertal boys and girls tend to be similar, with body fatness averaging about 15% and 19%, respectively. Girls gain more fat than boys during puberty, and in adulthood they have about 22% to 26% body fat, compared with around 15% to 18% in males. During puberty, males gain twice as much lean tissue as do females.

Psychological Changes

Adolescence is a period of maturation for both mind and body. Along with the physical growth of puberty, emotional and intellectual development is rapid. Adolescents' capacity for abstract thinking, as opposed to the concrete thought patterns of childhood, enables them to grow cognitively during adolescence. Many of these tasks have implications for their nutritional well-being.

Cognitive and emotional development can be divided into early, middle, and late adolescence. Determining the adolescent's stage can be very helpful in providing nutritional counseling as well as in designing educational programs (Sigman-Grant, 2002). In *early adolescence*, the adolescent:

- Is preoccupied with body and body image
- Trusts and respects adults
- Is anxious about peer relationships
- Is ambivalent about autonomy

The nutritional implications are that adolescents in this stage are willing to do or try anything that will make them look better or improve their body image. However, adolescents at this stage want immediate results, so nutrition counseling should be geared to short-term goals and to addressing nutritional concerns that impact the teen's appearance, performance (e.g., dance, sports), or both.

A teen in *middle adolescence*:

- Is greatly influenced by his or her peer group
- Is mistrustful of adults
- Sees independence as being very important
- Experiences significant cognitive development

During this stage, the teen will listen to peers more than to parents or other adults. Teens are becoming more in charge of the foods they eat. The drive toward independence often results in temporary rejection of the family dietary patterns. At this age, adolescents often experiment with vegetarianism. Nutritional counseling should include making wise decisions when eating away from home.

The teen in *late adolescence*:

- Has established a body image
- Is oriented toward the future and is making plans
- Is increasingly independent
- Is more consistent in his or her values and beliefs
- Is developing intimacy and permanent relationships

By late adolescence, teens are thinking about the future and are interested in improving their overall health. Nutritional counseling during this stage can address long-term goals. Adolescents in this stage still want to make their own decisions, but are open to information provided by healthcare professionals. Nutritional counselors should not only present current recommendations, but also explain the rationale behind them.

As adolescents strive for independence, they often take risks. Many of these risks are important to becoming independent (e.g., trying out for a sports team, applying to college, dating), but many risk behaviors can be dangerous. Resnick et al. (1993) found that serious behaviors, termed *acting out behaviors*, can be grouped together and include the following: drug use, school absenteeism, and unintended injury risk, such as drinking and driving, not wearing seatbelts, and not using a bicycle helmet. The second group of serious behaviors, termed *quietly disturbed behaviors*, are of concern to nutritionists because these behaviors include the following: poor body image; disordered eating, including bingeing, bulimia, and chronic dieting; fear of loss of control over eating; emotional stress; and suicidal ideation.

Food Habits

Recommendations for fulfilling the nutritional needs of adolescents arise from a small research base. Often, the amounts recommended are extrapolated from studies in adults or children. Part of the difficulty lies in the fact that studies of requirements must consider not only age, but also stage of physical ma-

> Read more about the DRIs, RDAs, AIs, and ULs at http://www.fcs.uga.edu/pubs/PDF/FDNS-E-65.pdf.

turity. The DRIs, which include the RDAs, AIs, and Tolerable Upper Intake Levels (ULs) for adolescents, can be accessed online.

Adolescents search for identity, strive for independence and acceptance, and are concerned about appearance. Irregular meals, snacking, eating away from home, and following alternative dietary patterns characterize the food habits of adolescents. These habits are further influenced by family, peers, and the media.

Irregular Meals and Snacking

Meal patterns of adolescents are often chaotic. Teenagers miss an increasing number of meals at home as they get older. Breakfast and lunch are often the meals most frequently missed, but social and school activities may cause a teen to miss an evening meal as well. Female adolescents tend to miss more meals than their male counterparts (Story et al., 2002).

Although concern has been expressed about the habit of snacking, teenagers may obtain substantial nourishment from foods eaten outside traditional meals. Thus, the choice of foods is more important than the time or place of eating.

As a result of health and science education at school, most adolescents know what they should and should not eat (Story & Resnick, 1986; Story et al., 2002). However, overcoming barriers to act on that knowledge is the concern. Teens identify the biggest barrier as time. Teens perceive themselves as too busy to worry about food, nutrition, meal planning, or eating right. Additionally, adolescents tend to form different associations with healthy foods and junk foods. Adolescents form mainly negative associations with healthy foods, but positive associations with junk foods (Chapman & Maclean, 1993). In order for adolescents to change their eating habits to better behaviors, counseling must center on fitting proper nutrition into allowable time, making selection of healthy foods easier, and making healthy foods appealing to teens and their peers.

During the time of peak growth velocity, adolescents usually need to eat large amounts of food often. They are able to use foods with a high concentration of energy; however, they need to be increasingly careful of the amounts and frequency of eating when growth has slowed. Habits of overeating adopted during adolescence may ultimately contribute to a number to adult obesity and related diseases.

Fast Foods

The use of fast foods for meals or snacks is especially popular with busy adolescents. So-called fast foods include foods from vending machines, self-service restaurants, convenience groceries, and franchised food restaurants. Fast foods tend to be low in iron, calcium, riboflavin, and vitamin A, and there are few sources of folic acid. The vitamin C content of fast foods is also low unless fruit or fruit juice is consumed. Although most places offer a selection of healthy foods, many of the food items provide more than 50% of their calories from fat. Adolescents should be counseled on how to make wise and healthy choices when eating out in a restaurant.

Adolescents as Food Purchasers

For marketers, being a teenager is a matter of lifestyles and spending habits, not age. Marketing to teens has become a multi-billion-dollar business. It is estimated that the nation's approximately 23 million teens spend nearly $100 billion annually (Channel One, 2000). Teenagers spend $15 billion annually on fast food and other food and snacks. Teens not only spend money themselves, but also wield a tremendous influence over purchases made by their parents (Channel One, 2000).

Teens are frequent visitors to different stores. In a 30-day period, the top two types of stores teens visited were food stores, with more than 200 million visits to convenience stores and supermarkets. Teens eat in fast food restaurants often, with most visits occurring either immediately after school or at a weekday dinnertime.

Guidelines for nutritional assessment and intervention in adolescence may include:

1. Screen and assess growth status and plot on NCHS growth charts.
2. Adolescents identified as at risk for overweight or who are overweight should be referred for further evaluation and possible treatment.
3. Provide a wide variety of healthy foods with emphasis on nutritious choices such as whole grains, fruits, vegetables, dairy foods, and lean meats and protein alternatives.
4. Promote daily physical activity that fits with the adolescent's interests.
5. Reduce sedentary activity with an emphasis on reduction of screen time.
6. Provide nutrition education in school.
7. Ensure regular meals and snacks.

8. Encourage reduced levels of low nutrient-dense beverages and promote intake of milk and dairy foods.
9. Provide appropriate care for disease or other health conditions.

Situations with Special Needs

Vegetarian Eating Practices

Adolescents tend to be attracted to vegetarian eating practices, especially during middle or late adolescence, because of their concerns about animal welfare, ecology, the environment, or personal health. Additionally, concerns about body weight motivate some adolescents to adopt a vegetarian diet, since this a socially acceptable way to reduce dietary fat. Vegetarian eating is often seen in adolescents with anorexia nervosa, who adopt the diet in an attempt to hide their unnecessary restriction of food intake (Story et al., 2000).

Vegetarian diets are consistent with the Dietary Guidelines for Americans and can meet the DRIs/RDAs for nutrients. With planning, vegetarian diets can provide a variety of nutrient-dense foods that promote health, growth, and development. Diets need to be planned to provide adequate energy, protein, calcium, iron, zinc, and vitamins B_{12} and D. The bioavailability of calcium, iron, and zinc should also be ensured. When adolescents become vegetarians, parents are often concerned about the diet's nutritional adequacy, especially about meeting protein requirements. Parents need reassurance that a vegetarian diet can meet their adolescent's nutrition needs, and they should receive information on the principles of healthy vegetarian eating for adolescents. But both parents and adolescents should be informed that overly restricted or inappropriately selected vegetarian diets can result in significant malnutrition. Some vegetarian adolescents have suffered from a delayed growth spurt, iron-deficiency anemia, and vitamin B_{12} deficiency (Sanders, 1995; Story et al., 2000).

Eating Disorders

Eating disorders rank as the third most common chronic illness in adolescent females, with an incidence of up to 5%. The prevalence has increased dramatically over the past three decades (Kreipe, 2000; Spear & Stellefson-Myers, 2001). Large numbers of adolescents who have disordered eating do not meet the strict DSM-IV (AAP, 2000) criteria for either Anorexia Nervosa or Bulimia Nervosa, but can be classified as Eating Disorders Not Otherwise Specified (EDNOS). In one study (Bunnell et al., 1990), more than half of the adolescents evaluated for eating disorders had subclinical disease but suffered a similar degree of psychological distress as those who met strict diagnostic criteria. Diagnostic criteria for eating disorders such as DSM-IV may not be entirely applicable to adolescents. The wide variability in the rate, timing, and magnitude of both height and weight gain during normal puberty, the absence of menstrual periods in early puberty along with the unpredictability of menses soon after menarche, and the lack of abstract concepts limit the application of diagnostic criteria to adolescents (Spear, 2001; Kreipe, 2000).

Just as adolescents are at increased risk for developing eating disorders, they are also more vulnerable to the complications of these disorders. The impact of malnutrition on linear growth, brain development, and bone acquisition can be long-standing and irreversible. Yet, with early and aggressive treatment, there is also potential for a better outcome than in adults who have more long-standing disease (Golden, 1997).

Early identification of adolescents with disordered eating habits has been linked to improved long-term outcome, but this is difficult to accomplish. Often, parents will bring an affected teen in for another reason—gastrointestinal complaints, amenorrhea, or unexplained weight loss. A screening for disordered eating can easily be done, and this should include questions about fear of becoming fat, amount of dieting, use of laxatives, fasting or frequent meal skipping to lose weight, fear of certain foods (e.g., foods containing fat or sugar), vomiting, binging, and excessive exercise.

Because adolescence is the greatest period of risk for development of an eating disorder, efforts must be made to reduce the incidence of malnutrition, or at least provide early intervention to prevent its serious complications (Striegel-Moore, 1997).

Adolescence is one of the most challenging periods in human development. Because of the extent of the physical and psychological changes taking place, a number of important issues arise that influence the nutritional well-being of the teenager. Knowledge of the developmental processes is a prerequisite to understanding the nutritional aspects of this period of life. Understanding the nutritional and physical activity needs of adolescents will help nutrition professionals provide counseling and programs that can impact the future health of these individuals.

Public Health Initiatives

WIC

For more than 30 years, the Special Supplemental Nutrition Program for Women, Infants and Children (WIC) has provided supplemental foods and nutrition education to low-income women, infants, and children up to 5 years of age. The ultimate goal of WIC is to improve the nutritional status of low-income pregnant or lactating women, infants, and young children who have been identified as being at nutritional risk. The primary method of achieving that goal is through the provision of specific nutrient-dense foods paid for through WIC checks or vouchers and selected by eligible pregnant or lactating women and mothers/caregivers of eligible infants and children (USDA, FNS, 2003).

WIC is funded at the federal level by the U.S. Department of Agriculture, and is administered by states through public and private organizations, such as county and regional health departments. Breast-feeding promotion and support are central to the WIC program, and it has been credited with improving breast-feeding rates among vulnerable populations (Wright & Schanler, 2001). WIC participation includes regular nutrition risk screening, growth assessment, and counseling by healthcare providers. During the infant's first year, WIC supplemental food packages for breast-feeding mothers provide milk, iron-fortified breakfast cereals, 100% juice containing vitamin C, eggs, and either dried beans/peas or peanut butter. Mothers of exclusively breast-fed infants also receive cheese, tuna, and carrots. Breast-fed infants do not receive food packages until they are weaned. Food packages for infants who are weaned provide iron-fortified infant formula for the first 6 months with the addition of iron-fortified infant cereal and infant juices at 4 to 6 months.

WIC provides nutritional services to a very large proportion of the population. WIC benefits are received by 24% of children ages 1 to 4, 35% of all pregnant and postpartum women, and 50% of all infants in the United States (Fox et al., 2004). Food availability and food insecurity are problems for many WIC recipients, with approximately one-third of all WIC recipients on food stamps. Any barriers that decrease food resources for these individuals make them more vulnerable to food insecurity as well as nutritional risk (Conrey et al., 2003).

Numerous studies have been conducted to evaluate WIC. Many have focused on specific outcomes such as the incidence of low-birth-weight infants (Kowaleski-Jones & Duncan, 2002), nutritional assessment of pregnant women (Swensen et al., 2001), and the nutrient intakes of infants and young children (Ponza et al., 2004). Recently, some studies have investigated barriers to WIC usage. Woelfel et al. (2004) identified several key barriers to the use of WIC services. Their survey of over 3,000 WIC recipients rated 68 potential barriers to WIC use as measured by likelihood of not picking up WIC checks. Of greatest interest are the top 11 items that were identified by more than 20% of respondents. Based on these findings, dietitians and nutritionists who are involved with WIC programs, or who are interested in enhancing the success of WIC programs, can take specific steps to determine if these barriers exist in their local setting and decrease their incidence, if present. These barriers can be broken into three broad categories: office procedures, the WIC food package, and nutrition education.

Office Procedures

The office setting is a key area for change. The most frequently reported barrier (Rosenberg et al., 2003; Woelfel et al., 2004) relates to the long waiting times to receive WIC services. When combined with three related items from the top 11 (more than an hour to re-certify, overcrowded waiting rooms, and no activities for children), office procedures become a logical target for improvement. The image of unhappy, crying children waiting with their mothers in a cramped waiting room does not create a positive response. WIC providers can make the greatest impact on clients' use of WIC services by identifying reasons for long waiting times and improving contributing processes. Less wait time results in fewer clients and children in the waiting room. In addition, all WIC sites should provide enjoyable activities for infants and children. Creatively developed activities could become nutrition education opportunities for children and caregivers.

WIC Food Package

Dissatisfaction with the WIC food package has been recognized by many practitioners. The food package barriers include problems with the actual food items and purchasing issues. Mothers report that they do not receive enough formula and juice; this may indicate a need for improved education on appropriate amounts of formula and juice to feed children and a review of procedures for mixing formula. Excessive consumption of energy-dense beverages, such as juice, in early childhood could contribute to child obesity problems. Dissatisfaction with the types and amounts of foods included in the WIC package often come from ethnic subgroups who do not consume some WIC foods. Mothers also report difficulties in purchasing some foods due to problems with package size and store policies about WIC. If clients are having problems identifying the correct size cereal package to select or are uncertain about store policies, dietitians can design a learning activity that simulates the options available in the store (McKinney, 2004).

WIC Nutrition Education

To be effective, nutrition education must engage the client in the learning process in a meaningful way. Less than optimal nutrition education could result from a variety of reasons, ranging from staff training and available nutrition education materials to inappropriate techniques, as well as insufficient nutrition staff and requirements for time efficiency. Very often, the WIC nutritionist is an entry-level position for a nutritionist, dietitian, or other health professional or paraprofessional, and suffers from frequent turnover. These frontline nutrition educators need to be provided with the skills and resources to be most effective in making meaningful connections with their clients and to be a stimulating and vibrant part of the WIC experience. WIC nutritionists need to objectively evaluate the effectiveness of their customary nutrition education programs and involve clients in determining pros and cons of current practices and ways to improve.

Improvements in WIC office procedures, the WIC food package, and WIC nutrition education can have a significant impact on the nutritional status of WIC clients. The more barriers encountered by WIC recipients, the less likely they are to obtain the nutritious food needed to improve nutrition status. Most of these areas of barrier reduction are within the control or influence of dietitians. WIC nutrition practitioners can make the greatest impact by identifying and eliminating barriers in their locale (McKinney, 2004).

Bright Futures

Launched in 1990 by the Health Resources and Services Administration's Maternal and Child Health Bureau, Bright Futures is an initiative aimed at improving health promotion and preventive services for infants, children, and adolescents. Bright Futures has produced a series of guidelines and supportive materials for health supervision

> Read more about Bright Futures at http://www.brightfutures.org.

focused on the areas of oral health, nutrition, physical activity, and mental health. The nutrition guidelines include recommendations for nutrition supervision from infancy through adolescence, common nutrition issues and concerns, and nutrition tools (Story et al., 2002). In 2002, collaboration with the AAP led to the establishment of the Bright Futures Education Center and Pediatric Implementation Project, whose objective is to support the implementation of the guidelines.

Start Healthy, Stay Healthy

In 2002, the ADA began a partnership with Gerber Products Company to launch a research and education initiative focused on infant and toddler feeding. The Start Healthy Feeding Guidelines for Infants and Toddlers are based on existing recommendations of authoritative organizations, careful analysis of the feeding and nutrition literature, and evaluation of the nutrient needs of infants and toddlers (Butte et al., 2004). Its recommendations are grouped into five areas: nutrients and foods, infant

> Read more about Start Healthy, Stay Healthy at http://www.gerber.com/starthealthy.

and toddler development, healthy feeding relationships, safe feeding, and physical activity. These recommendations are being disseminated to healthcare professionals through professional publications and presentations and to parents through education materials. *Start Healthy, the Guide to Teaching Your Little One Good Eating Habits* delivers the following six messages:

1. Establish healthy eating habits right from the beginning—
   by breast-feeding.
2. Healthy eating starts with a positive parent-child partnership.
3. If he rejects a new food, try, try again!
4. Build your baby's taste buds with variety.
5. Five servings of fruits and vegetables a day are important.
6. The other side of the healthy habits equation: Activity!

Summary

Public health nutrition programs that provide services to women in the childbearing years, pregnant and lactating women, infants, children, and adolescents are vital to the health of the nation. Nutritionists, dietitians, and other health professionals have important roles to play in improving the health of the nation by ensuring that these vulnerable groups get the services they need to grow and develop to their full potential. Attainment of the Healthy People 2010 goals that relate to maternal, child, and adolescent issues can be used as an indicator of how successful public health programs are in providing the necessary services. Many of the programs mentioned in this chapter have websites that provide extensive information.

The stages of growth and development covered in this chapter are the most nutritionally challenging periods in human development. Knowledge of the developmental processes is a prerequisite to understanding the nutritional aspects of these life stages. Understanding these groups' nutritional and physical activity needs will help nutrition professionals provide counseling and programs that can impact the future health of these individuals and the nation.

Issues for Discussion

1. After reading the chapter's description of some of the problems with the WIC program, how would you plan to go about making changes?
2. After your plan is in place for changing WIC, strategize how you would institute the changes.
3. What types of problems might you expect from both staff and clients if you change public health programs?

Maternal Child Health Internet Resources

American Medical Association Adolescent Health Online — http://www.ama-assn.org/ama/pub/category/1947.html

Breastfeeding Legislative Updates — http://www.house.gov Search under *breastfeeding*

Breastfeeding Policy — http://www.aap.org/policy/re9729.html

Bright Future Lactation Resource Centre — http://www.bflrc.com

Bright Futures — http://mchb.hrsa.gov/programs/training/brightfutures.htm

Bureau of Maternal and Child Health Library — http://mchlibrary.info

CDC/NCHS BMI tables — http://www.cdc.gov/growthcharts/

Center for Health and Health Care in Schools — http://www.healthinschools.org

Coalition for a Healthy and Active America — http://www.chaausa.org

DHHS HRSA Maternal and Child Health Bureau — http://www.mchb.hrsa.gov

Dietary Guidelines, 2005 — http://www.health.gov/dietaryguidelines/dga2005

Food Allergy & Anaphylaxis Network — http://www.foodallergy.org

Healthy People 2010 — http://www.healthypeople.gov

Human Milk Banking Association of North America — http://www.hmbana.org

International Lactation Consultants Association — http://www.ilca.org

Kidnetic — http://www.kidnetic.com

Kids Count — http://www.kidscount.org

La Leche League — http://www.lalecheleague.org

National Academies Press, Dietary Reference Intakes — http://www.nap.edu

National Center for Education in Maternal and Child Health — http://www.ncemch.org

National Center for Health Statistics (source of growth charts) — http://www.cdc.gov/nchs/

National Early Childhood Technical Assistance Center	http://www.nectac.org.
Neonatology on the Web	http://www.neonatology.org
School Meals Programs	http://www.fns.usda.gov/cnd/
Start Healthy, Stay Healthy	http://www.gerber.com/content/usa/bin/pdf/ Feeding_Plan.pdf
Support Breastfeeding.com	http://www.supportbreastfeeding.com
Team Nutrition	http://www.fns.usda.gov/tn/
U.S. Breastfeeding Committee	http://www.usbreastfeeding.org
U.S. government's food and nutrition site	http://www.nutrition.gov
USDA Center for Nutrition Policy and Promotion	http://www.usda.gov/cnpp/
USDA Food and Nutrition Information Center	http://www.nal.usda.gov/fnic/
USDA Women, Infants and Children (WIC) Program	http://www.fns.usda.gov/wic/

References

Ahluwalia IB, Morrow B, Hsia J, Grummer-Strawn LM. Who is breastfeeding? Recent trends from the pregnancy risk assessment and monitoring system. *J Pediatrics*. 2003;142(5):486-491.

Alaimo K, et al. Dietary intake of vitamins, minerals and fiber of persons ages 2 months and over in the United States: Third National Health and Nutrition Examination Survey, Phase 1, 1988–91. *Advance Data from Vital and Health Statistics*, No. 258. Hyattsville, MD: National Center for Health Statistics; 1994.

Albertson AM, et al. Estimated dietary calcium intake and food sources for adolescent females 1980–92. *J Adol Health Care*. 1997;20:20.

American Academy of Pediatric Dentistry. Clinical guideline on fluoride therapy. *Pediatric Dentistry*. 2003;25(7):67-68.

American Academy of Pediatrics, Section on Breastfeeding and Committee on Nutrition. Prevention of rickets and vitamin D deficiency: new guidelines for vitamin D intake. Pediatrics. 2003;111(4):908-910.

American Dietetic Association. Position of the American Dietetic Association: Breaking the barriers to breastfeeding. J Am Dietet Assoc. 2001;101(10):1213-1220.

American Dietetic Association. Position on nutrition care for pregnant adolescents. *J Am Diet Assoc*. 1994;94:449.

American Psychiatric Association. Diagnostic and statistical manual of mental disorders. 4th ed., text rev. Washington, DC: APA Press; 2000.

Barlow SE, Dietz WH. Obesity evaluation and treatment: expert committee recommendations. *Pediatrics*. 1998;102(3):1-11.

Berenson GS, et al. Precursors of cardiovascular risk in young adults from a biracial (black-white) population: The Bogalusa Heart Study. In: Jacobson MS, Rees JM, Golden NH, Irwin CE, eds. *Adolescent Nutritional Disorders: Prevention and Treatment.* New York: The New York Academy of Science; 1998.

Birch LL, Gunder L, Grimm-Thomas K. Infants' consumption of a new food enhances acceptance of similar foods. *Appetite.* 1998;30:283–295.

Breastfeeding Working Group, American Academy of Pediatrics. Breastfeeding and the use of human milk. *Pediatrics.* 1997;100(6):1035–1039.

Briggs M, Safii S, Beall DL. Position of the American Dietetic Association, Society for Nutrition Education, and American School Food Service Association: Nutrition services: An essential component of comprehensive school health programs. *J Am Dietet Assoc.* 2003;103:505–514.

Briley ME, Roberts-Gray C. Position of the American Dietetic Association: Nutrition standards for child-care programs. *J Am Dietet Assoc.* 1999;99:981–988.

Brown JD, Witherspoon EM. The mass media and American adolescents' health. P*roceedings of the Health Futures of Youth! Pathways to Adolescent Health Conference.* Annapolis, MD; September 14, 1998.

Bunnell DW, Shenker IR, Nussbaum MP, Arden MR, Jacobson MS. Subclinical versus formal eating disorders: differentiating psychological features. *Int J Eating Disorder.* 1990;9:357–362.

Butte NF, Cobb K, Dwyer, J, Graney L, Heird WC, Rickard KA. The Start Healthy Feeding Guidelines for infants and toddlers. *J Am Dietet Assoc.* 2004:104:442–454.

Butte NF, Hopkinson JM, Wong WW, Smith EO, Ellis KJ. Body composition during the first 2 years of life: an updated reference. *Pediatric Research.* 2000a;47(5):578–585.

Butte NF, Wong WW, Hopkinson JM, Smith EO, Ellis KJ. Infant feeding mode affects early growth and body composition. *Pediatrics.* 2000b;106(6):1355–1366.

Carvalho NF, Kenney RD, Carrington PH, Hall DE. Severe nutritional deficiencies in toddlers resulting from health food milk alternatives. *Pediatrics.* 2001;107(4):e46.

Carver JD. Advances in nutritional modifications of infant formulas. *Am J Clin Nutrition.* 2003;77(suppl):1550S–1554S.

Centers for Disease Control and Prevention. Obesity Still on the Rise, New Data Show. National Center for Chronic Disease Prevention and Health Promotion, Division of Nutrition and Physical Activity Web site. Available at: http://www.cdc.gov. Accessed May 15, 2004.

Centers for Disease Control and Prevention. *Physical activity and health: A report of the Surgeon General.* Washington, DC: National Center for Chronic Disease Prevention and Health Promotion, President's Council on Physical Fitness and Sports; 1996.

Centers for Disease Control and Prevention. Recommendations to prevent and control iron deficiency in the United States. *MMWR.* 1998;47(No. RR-3).

Centers for Disease Control and Prevention. Recommendations for using fluoride to prevent and control dental caries in the United States. *MMWR.* 2001;50(RR-14).

Centers for Disease Control and Prevention. Youth risk surveillance—United States 2003. *MMWR*. 2004;53(SS-2):1–29.

Channel One Network. *Teen fact book*. New York: Channel One Network; 2000.

Chapman G, Maclean H. "Junk food" and "healthy food": meanings of food in adolescent women's culture. *J Nutr Educ*. 1993;25:108.

Christoffel KK, Ariza A. The epidemiology of overweight in children: relevance for clinical care. *Pediatrics*. 1998;101:103.

Committee on Nutrition, American Academy of Pediatrics. Soy protein-based formulas: recommendations for use in infant feeding. *Pediatrics*. 1998;101(1):148–153.

Committee on Nutrition, American Academy of Pediatrics. Iron fortification of infant formulas. *Pediatrics*. 1999;104(1):119–123.

Committee on Nutrition, American Academy of Pediatrics. Hypoallergenic infant formulas. *Pediatrics*. 2000;106(2):346–349.

Committee on Nutrition, American Academy of Pediatrics. The use and misuse of fruit juice in pediatrics. *Pediatrics*. 2001;107(5):1210–1213.

Congressional Record. 99th Congress 2nd Session, Senate S 14042–14047. Washington, DC: U.S. Government Printing Office; 1986:132(130).

Conrey EJ, Frongillo EA, Dollahite JS, Griffin MR. Integrated program enhancements increased utilization of farmers market nutrition program. *J Nutr*. 2003;133(6):1841–1844.

Corbin CB, Pangrazi RP. *Physical activity for children: A statement of guidelines*. Reston, VA: National Association for Sport and Physical Education; 1998.

Dallmon, PR. Iron deficiency: does it matter? *J Intern Med*. 1989; 226:367–372.

Devaney B, Ziegler P, Pac S, Karwe V, Barr SI. Nutrient intakes of infants and toddlers. *J Am Dietet Assoc*. 2004;104(1):S14–S21.

Dietz WH. Use of the body mass index (BMI) as a measure of overweight in children and adolescents. *J Pediatrics*. 1998;132:191–193.

Eisenberg ME, Olson RE, Neumark-Sztainer D, Story M, Bearinger LH. Correlations between family meals and psychsocial well-being among adolescents. *Archives of Pediatrics and Adolescent Medicine*. 2004;158:792–796.

Farley, D. Dangers of lead still linger. *FDA Consumer*. 1998, Jan/Feb:16–21.

Fox HB, McManus MA, Schmidt HJ. *WIC reauthorization: opportunities for improving the nutritional status of women, infants, and children*. Washington, DC: National Health Policy Forum; 2004.

Freedman DS, Khan LK, Dietz WH, Srinivasan SR, Berenson GS. Relationship of childhood obesity to coronary heart disease risk factors in adulthood: the Bogalusa heart study. *Pediatrics*. 2001;108(3):712–718.

Freedman DS, Khan LK, Serdula, MK, Dietz WH, Srinivasan SR, Berenson GS. The relationship of childhood BMI to adult adiposity: the Bogalusa heart study. *Pediatrics*. 2005;115(1):22–27.

Gillman MW, Rifas-Shiman SL, Frazier AL, Rockett HR, Camargo CA Jr., Field AE, Berkey CS, Colditz GA. Family dinner and diet quality among older children and adolescents. *Archives of Family Medicine*. 2000;9(3):235–240.

Golden NH. The adolescent: vulnerable to develop an eating disorder and at high risk for long-term sequelae. *Annals of the New York Academy of Sciences.* 1997; 817:94–97.

Golden NH. Osteoporosis prevention: a pediatric challenge. *Arch Pediatr Adolesc Med.* 2000;154:542–543.

Greger N, Edwin CM. Obesity: a pediatric epidemic. *Ped Annals.* 2001;30(1):694–700.

Gunderson EP, Abrams B, Selvin S. Does the pattern of postpartum weight change differ according to pregravid body size? *Intl J Obesity.* 2001;25:853–862.

Hale TW. *Medications and mothers' milk,* 11th ed. Amarillo, TX: Pharmasoft Publishing; 2004.

Hediger ML, et al. Implications of the Camden Study of Adolescent Pregnancy: Interactions among maternal growth, nutrition status, and body composition. In: Jacobson MS, Rees JM, Golden NH, Irwin CE, eds, *Adolescent Nutritional Disorders: Prevention and Treatment.* New York: The New York Academy of Science; 1998.

Institute of Medicine, Committee on Nutrition Status During Pregnancy and Lactation. *Nutrition during pregnancy, Pt. 1. Weight gain.* Washington, DC: National Academy Press; 1990.

Institute of Medicine, Food and Nutrition Board. *Dietary Reference Intakes for calcium, phosphorus, magnesium, vitamin D, and fluoride.* Washington, DC: National Academy Press; 1997.

Institute of Medicine. *Childhood obesity.* Washington, DC: National Academy Press; 2004.

Jacobson MF. *Liquid candy: How soft drinks are harming Americans' health.* Washington, DC: Center for Science in the Public Interest; 1998: 1–13.

Kaiser LL, Allen L. Position of the American Dietetic Association: Nutrition and lifestyle for a healthy pregnancy outcome. *J Am Dietet Assoc.* 2002;102:1479–1490.

Kleinman RE, ed. *Pediatric nutrition handbook,* 5th ed. Elk Grove Village, IL: American Academy of Pediatrics; 2004. Breastfeeding: 55–78. Formula Feeding of Term Infants: 87–95, Iron Deficiency: 299–312. Nutrition and Oral Health: 789–800.

Kowaleski-Jones L, Duncan GJ. Effects of participation in the WIC program on birthweight: evidence from the National Longitudinal Survey of Youth. *Am J Pub Health.* 2002;92(5):799–804.

Kramer FM, Stunkard AJ, Marshall KA, McKinney S, Liebschutz J. Breastfeeding reduces maternal lower body-fat. *J Am Dietet Assoc.* 1993;93(4):429–433.

Kreipe RE, Birndorf DO. Eating disorders in adolescents and young adults. *Medical Clinics of North America.* 2000;84(4):1027–1049.

Kreiter SR, Schwartz RP, Kirkman HN, Charlton PA, Calikoglu AS, Davenport ML. Nutritional rickets in African American breast-fed infants. *J Pediatrics.* 2000;137(2):153–157.

Lawrence RA, Lawrence RM. *Breastfeeding: a guide for the medical profession,* 5th ed. St. Louis, MO: Mosby, Inc: 1999.

Life Sciences Research Office, Food and Drug Administration. Assessment of nutrient requirements for infant formulas. *J Nutrition. 1998*;128:11S.

Lifschitz CH. Carbohydrate absorption from fruit juices in infants. *Pediatrics*. 2000;105(1):e04.

Lytle L. Nutritional issues for adolescents. *J Am Dietet Assoc*. 2002;102: S8–S12.

Marshall WA, Tanner JM. Variations in the pattern of pubertal changes in boys. *Arch Dis Child*. 1970;45:13.

McKinney, S. Steps to improving WIC usage: office procedures, food package, and nutrition education. *J Am Dietet Assoc*. 2004;93:743–745.

Must A, et al. Long-term morbidity and mortality of overweight adolescents. *N Engl J Med*. 1992;327:1350.

National Academy of Sciences. *Recommended dietary allowances*, Washington, DC: National Academy Press; 2002.

National Cholesterol Education Program (NCEP). *Report of the expert panel on blood cholesterol levels in children and adolescents*. NIH Publication No. 91–2732. Washington, DC: National Heart, Lung and Blood Institute, Public Health Service; September 1991.

Nicklas TA, et al. School-based programs for health-risk reduction. In: Jacobson MS, Rees JM, Golden NH, Irwin CE, eds. *Adolescent Nutritional Disorders: Prevention and Treatment*. New York: The New York Academy of Science; 1998.

Nicklas TA, Johnson R. Position of the American Dietetic Association: Dietary guidance for healthy children ages 2 to 11 years. *J Am Dietet Assoc*. 2004;104:660–677.

NIH Consensus Conference. Optimal calcium intake. NIH consensus development panel on optimal calcium intake. *JAMA*. 1994;272: 1942–1948.

Nokes C, van den Bosch C, Bundy DA. *The effects of iron deficiency and anemia on mental and motor performance, education achievement, and behavior in children: a report of the International Nutritional Anemia Consultative Group*. Washington, DC: ILSI Press; 1998.

Ogden CL, Flegal KM, Carroll MD, Johnson CL. Prevalence and trends in overweight among U.S. children and adolescents, 1999–2000. *JAMA*. 2002;288:1728–1732.

Patrick K, Spear B, Holt, Sofka D, eds. *Bright futures in practice: physical activity*. Arlington, VA: National Center for Education in Maternal and Child Health; 2001.

Pennsylvania Nutrition and Activity (PANA). *Pennsylvania growth screening process*. Harrisburg, PA; 2004.

Ponza M, Devaney B, Ziegler P, Reidy K, Squatrito C. Nutrient intakes and food choices of infants and toddlers participating in WIC. *J Am Dietet Assoc*. 2004;104S:S71–S79.

Pugliese MT, Blumberg DL, Hludzinski J, Kay S. Nutritional rickets in suburbia. *J Amer Coll Nutr*. 1998;17(6):637–641.

Resnick MD, et al. Health and risk behaviors of urban adolescent males involved in pregnancy. Families in Society: *J Contemporary Human Services*. 1993;74:366.

Rosenberg TJ, Alperen JK, Chiasson MA. Why do WIC participants fail to pick up their checks? An urban study in the wake of welfare reform. *Am J Pub Health*. 2003;93(3):477–481.

Ryan AS, Wenjun Z, Acosta A. Breastfeeding continues to increase into the new millennium. *Pediatrics*. 2002;110(6):1103–1109.

Sallis JF, Patrick K. Physical activity guidelines for adolescents: consensus statement. *Pediatric Exercise Science.* 1994;6(4):302–314.

Sanders T. Vegetarian diets and children. *Pediatric Clinics of North America.* 1995;42(4):955–965.

Schieve LA, Cogswell ME, Scanlon KS. Maternal weight gain and preterm delivery: differential effects by body mass index. *Epidemiology.* 1999;10:141–147.

Scholl TO, et al. Maternal growth and fetal growth: pregnancy course and outcome in the Camden Study. In: Jacobson MS, Rees JM, Golden NH, Irwin CE, eds. *Adolescent Nutritional Disorders: Prevention and Treatment.* New York: The New York Academy of Science; 1998.

Sigman-Grant M. Strategies for counseling adolescents. *J Am Dietet Assoc.* 2002;102:S32–S39.

Skinner JD, Bounds W, Carruth BR, Zeigler P. Longitudinal calcium intake is negatively related to children's body fat indexes. *J Am Dietet Assoc.* 2003;103:1626–1631.

Spear BA. Adolescent growth and development. In: Rickets VI, ed. *Adolescent Nutrition: Assessment and Management.* New York: Chapman and Hall; 1996:3–24.

Spear BA, Stellefson-Myers E. Position of the American Dietetic Association: Nutrition intervention in the treatment of anorexia nervosa, bulimia nervosa, and eating disorders not otherwise specified (EDNOS). *J Am Dietet Assoc.* 2001;101(7):810–819.

Stang J, Bayerl C. Position of the American Dietetic Association: Child and adolescent food and nutrition programs. *J Am Dietet Assoc.* 2003:103:887–893.

Steen SN. Timely statement of the American Dietetic Association: Nutrition guidance for adolescent athletes in organized sports. *J Am Dietet Assoc.* 1996;96:610.

Story M, Holt K, Sofka D, eds. *Bright futures in practice: nutrition.* Arlington, VA: National Center for Education in Maternal and Child Health; 2000.

Story M, Holt K, Sofka D, eds. *Bright futures in practice: nutrition,* 2nd ed. Arlington, VA: National Center for Education in Maternal and Child Health; 2002.

Story M, Neumark-Sztainer D, French S. Individual and environmental influences on adolescent eating behaviors. *J Am Dietet Assoc.* 2002;102:s40–s51.

Story M, Resnick MD. Adolescents' views on food and nutrition. *J Nutr Educ.* 1986;18:188.

Story M, Stang J. *Nutrition and the pregnant adolescent.* Minneapolis, MN: Center for Leadership Education and Training in Maternal and Child Health, University of Minnesota; 2000.

Striegel-Moore R. Risk factors for eating disorders. In: Jacobson MS, Rees JM, Golden N, Irwin C, eds. *Adolescent Nutritional Disorders: Prevention and Treatment.* New York: Annals of the New York Academy of Sciences; 1997:98–109.

Suitor CW, Bailey LB. Dietary folate equivalents: interpretation and application. *J Am Dietet Assoc.* 2000;100:88–94.

Sullivan SA, Birch LL. Pass the sugar, pass the salt: experience dictates preference. *Developmental Psychology.* 1990;26(4):546–551.

Swensen AR, Harnack LJ, Ross JA. Nutritional assessment of pregnant women enrolled in the Special Supplemental Program for Women, Infants, and Children (WIC). *J Am Dietet Assoc.* 2001;101(8):903–908.

Troiano RP, et al. Overweight prevalence and trends for children and adolescents. The National Health and Nutrition Examination Surveys, 1963–1991. *Arch Pediatr Adolesc Med.* 1995;149:1085.

Troiano RP, Flegal KM. Overweight children and adolescents: description, epidemiology and demographics. *Pediatr.* 1998;101(suppl):497.

U.S. Department of Agriculture, Food and Nutrition Services. Special Supplemental Nutrition Program for Women, Infants and Children. *Federal Register:* 7 CFR Part 246. Washington, DC: National Archives and Records Administration; January 1, 2003.

U.S. Department of Health and Human Services. Healthy People 2010. Available at: http://www.healthypeople.gov. Accessed January 17, 2005.

U.S. Department of Health and Human Services and U.S. Department of Agriculture. U.*S. Dietary Guidelines for Americans, 2005,* 6th ed. Washington, DC: Government Printing Office; January 2005.

Welch TR, Bergstrom WH, Tsang RC. Vitamin D-deficient rickets: the reemergence of a once-conquered disease. *J Pediatrics.* 2000;137(2):143–145.

Whitaker RC, Wright JA, Pepe MS, Seidel KD, Dietz WH. Predicting obesity in young adulthood from childhood and prenatal obesity. *New Engl J Med.* 1997;337:869–873.

Williams CL, et al. Management of childhood obesity in pediatric practice. In: Jacobson MS, Rees JM, Golden NH, Irwin CE, eds. *Adolescent Nutritional Disorders: Prevention and Treatment.* New York: The New York Academy of Science; 1998:225–240.

Woelfel ML, AbuSabha R, Pruzek RM, Stratton H, Chen SG, Edmunds LS. Barriers to use of WIC services. *J Am Dietet Assoc.* 2004;738–743.

World Health Organization. *International code of marketing of breast-milk substitutes.* Geneva, Switzerland: World Health Organization; 1981.

World Health Organization (WHO). Physical status: the use and interpretation of anthropometry. Report of a WHO Expert Committee. *WHO Tech Rep Ser.* 1995;854:1–452.

World Health Organization (WHO) Expert Consultation. The Optimal Duration of Exclusive Breastfeeding. 2001. Available at: http://www.who.int. Accessed January 18, 2005

Wosje KS, Kalkwarf HJ. Lactation, weaning and calcium supplementation: effects on body composition in postpartum women. *Am J Clin Nutr.* 2004;80:423–429.

Wright AL, Schanler RJ. The resurgence of breastfeeding at the end of the second millennium. *J Nutrition. 2001;*131:421S–425S.

Wyshak G. Teenage girls, carbohydrate beverage consumption and bone fractures. *Arch pediat adolesc med.* 2000;154:610–613.

Yates AM, et al. Dietary Reference Intakes: the new basis for recommendations for calcium and related nutrients, B vitamins and choline. *J Am Dietet Assoc.* 1998;98:699.

Zemel MB. Role of dietary calcium and dairy produce in modulating adiposity. Lipids. 2003;38:139–146.

Ziegler EE, Jiang T, Romero E, Vinco A, Frantz JA, Nelson SE. Cow's milk and intestinal blood loss in late infancy. *J Pediatrics.* 1999;135(6): 720–726.

THE IMPORTANCE OF PUBLIC HEALTH NUTRITION PROGRAMS IN PREVENTING DISEASE AND PROMOTING ADULT HEALTH

Judith Sharlin, PhD, RD

Reader Objectives

After studying this chapter and reflecting on the contents, you should be able to:

1. Identify the primary causes of death and disability in adults in the United States.
2. Describe primary, secondary, and tertiary levels of health prevention and health promotion and their relationship to nutrition program planning.
3. Identify risk factors for chronic diseases and their implication for nutrition.
4. Describe the dietary risk factors associated with the leading chronic diseases.
5. Discuss the common features of the dietary guidelines issued by the major U.S. health organizations.
6. Compare different dietary interventions a public health nutritionist or dietitian offers to the community, family, or an individual at risk.
7. Recognize the mission and role of public health nutrition in preventing disease and promoting adult health.
8. Name some of the public health nutrition programs that exist today for maintaining adult health.

Preventing Disease and Promoting Health

Growing scientific evidence reveals that nutrition or dietary intake in adults contributes significantly to preventing illnesses and premature deaths in the United States.[1] Life expectancy has increased

dramatically over the past 100 years, and today the average life expectancy is 77 years.[2] Health and nutrition programs for adults aim
at prevention, as well as improving quality of life. However, chronic
diseases account for 7 out of every 10 deaths in the United States.[3]
The increasing cost of crisis medical care and the growing economic
burden provide a cost-effective incentive for individuals and our
nation to prevent chronic disease. Chronic diseases cost the United
States 75% of the $1 trillion spent on healthcare annually.[3] In spite
of this, only 3% of the total annual healthcare expenditures in our
nation were spent on prevention.[4] Nutrition interventions and policies target the factors related to adult health, and aim to prevent
chronic diseases that are the leading causes of death and disability.

Chronic Diseases: The Leading Causes of Death and Disability

In order to successfully create programs to promote health,
longevity, and the quality of life, we must examine the leading
causes of death and disability. Data from the National Center for
Health Statistics (NCHS) show that chronic diseases are the leading
causes of death and disability (Table 11-1).[5] Cardiovascular diseases
and cancer account for more than half of all deaths in the United
States.[3] More than 60% of chronic disease mortality can be attributed to lifestyle factors, such as diet, which can be modified.[6] A recent report on the health status of U.S. adults emphasized that
increasing numbers of people still smoke, are physically inactive,
and are overweight.[7] Researchers noted recently that about half of
the deaths among U.S. adults in 2000 could have been prevented.[8]
These findings revealed that 400,000 deaths occur each year due to
poor diet and physical inactivity.[8] (This number was found to be
20% less in a subsequent study.)[9] It appears that the increasing trend
of overweight and obesity will likely overtake tobacco as the leading preventable cause of mortality in the United States.[8] Although
mortality rates from heart disease, stroke, and cancer have declined,
behavioral changes have led to an increased prevalence of obesity
and diabetes.[10,11] Dietary factors are now associated with 4 of the 10
leading causes of death: coronary heart disease (CHD), some types
of cancer, stroke, and type 2 diabetes.[12] The Surgeon General's report in 1988 confirmed these findings: "For two out of three adult
Americans who do not smoke and do not drink excessively, one personal choice seems to influence long-term health prospects more
than any other, what we eat."[13]

TABLE 11-1   Deaths and Percentage of Total Deaths for the 10 Leading Causes of Death: United States, 2001–2002

Causes of death and year	Rank[1]	2001		2002	
		Deaths	Percent of total deaths	Deaths	Percent of total deaths
All causes		2,416,425	100.0	2,403,351	100.0
Diseases of the heart (I00–I09, I11, I13, I20–I51)	1	700,142	29.0	710,760	29.8
Malignant neoplasms (C00–C97)	2	553,768	22.9	553,091	23.0
Cerebrovascular diseases (I60–I69)	3	163,538	6.8	167,661	7.0
Chronic lower respiratory diseases (J40–J47)	4	123,013	5.1	122,009	5.1
Accidents (unintentional injuries) (V01–X59, Y85–Y86)	5	101,537	4.2	97,900	4.1
Diabetes mellitus (E10–E14)	6	71,372	3.0	69,301	2.9
Influenza and pneumonia (J10–J18)	7	62,034	2.6	65,313	2.7
Alzheimer's disease (G30)	8	53,862	2.2	49,558	2.1
Nephritis, nephrotic syndrome and nephrosis (N00-N07, N17–N19, N25–N27)	9	39,480	1.6	37,251	1.5
Septicemia (A40–A41)	10	32,238	1.3	31,224	1.3

[1]Rank based on number of deaths

Source: From *National Vital Statistics Report,* vol. 52, no. 9. Nov. 7, 2003; in Deaths and Leading Causes for 2001.

Risk Factors and Chronic Disease

Chronic diseases, although prevalent and costly, are among the most preventable. Research has identified a Health Promotion and Preventive Action model (HPA) for risk factors.[14] In this model, risk factor identification, reduction, modification, and education are related to human health and developmental stages.[14] Risk factors can be defined as those specific characteristics associated with an increased chance of developing a chronic disease. Risk factors that can be changed or modified, such as diet or physical activity, are under an individual's personal choices.[15] There are four types of risk factors:[2]

1. Biological factors such as an individual's genetic make-up, family history, age, or gender
2. Environmental conditions—social and physical environment
3. Access to quality healthcare
4. Individual behavior and lifestyle factors such as smoking, exercise, and good eating habits

Healthy People 2010 (HP 2010) provides the most recent guidelines and recommendations for specific health objectives and goals for the nation.[2] HP 2010 reveals that individual biological behaviors and environmental factors are responsible for approximately 70% of all premature deaths.[2] Biological factors such as age or gender are not modifiable. However, the leading causes of death are associated with dietary factors, which are modifiable. The determinants of health illustrate how individual biology and behaviors influence health through the individual's social and physical environments.[2] Finally, health can be improved through policies that provide access to health care and interventions with access to quality health care. Because the leading causes of illness and death in the United States, such as CHD, some types of cancer, stroke, type 2 diabetes, and atherosclerosis, are associated with dietary factors, we must address the concern that chronic diseases have resulted from dietary excesses and imbalance.[2] Furthermore, there is evidence that more intensive dietary counseling can lead to reduced intakes of dietary fat and cholesterol, and increased fiber, fruit, and vegetable consumption.[16]

> Healthy People 2010 outlines 28 focus areas that include risk factors for chronic diseases and addresses nutrition and overweight, physical activity, tobacco use, cancer, diabetes, cardiovascular disease, and access to quality healthcare.

Prevention Strategies

Health promotion and disease prevention provide complementary interventions to change health risk factors. Prevention efforts in public heath, community, and worksite settings are divided into three levels: primary prevention (health promotion), secondary prevention (risk appraisal and reduction), and tertiary prevention (treatment and rehabilitation).[17-19]

Primary Prevention (Health Promotion)

Primary prevention strategies, or health promotion, encourage health-enhancing behaviors by giving individuals, families, and communities ways to reduce risk factors associated with disease and injury.[19] Risk factors include environmental, economic, social, and biological aspects. Good examples of primary prevention strategies include nutrition and weight management classes in a community center for adults, environmental changes to provide nutritious choices in a school cafeteria vending machine, and local 5-A-Day for Better Health campaigns to increase the availability of fresh fruits and vegetables from farmers' markets.[19] Primary prevention strategies seek to expand the positive potential of health.[20]

A holistic approach, embracing individual lifestyle factors, the environment, and economic, social, and political factors, can help communities and private sector partners achieve health promotion and disease prevention goals. Providing information, available on food labels and through health messages to the public, is one effective method. These messages encourage consumers to apply the U.S. Dietary Guidelines, MyPyramid (formerly called the Food Guide Pyramid), Dietary Reference Intakes, and the Dietary Guidelines Alliance's through the It's All About You campaigns.[21-23] Voluntary community and health organizations, the federal government, worksite programs, and schools can reach consumers daily to promote nutrition interventions.

The media remains an effective means of communicating nutrition issues to the public.[24] Programs to promote physical activity and fitness, good nutrition, and smoking cessation must be broadly accessible. Worksite nutrition-centered health promotion and disease prevention programs provide opportunities to harness social support and influence.[25]

Motivations should be provided for food processors and vendors, restaurant chefs, and school and worksite cafeteria managers to prepare and serve foods lower in fat, calories, and sodium. Finally, legislation and regulations can be ratified to endorse more complete food and nutrition labeling. Food labels that provide short, unequivocal, positive messages aimed at a single behavior prove beneficial to consumers.[26]

Secondary Prevention (Risk Appraisal and Risk Reduction)

Secondary prevention includes risk appraisal and screening to emphasize early detection and diagnosis of disease.[14,18,19] Secondary prevention begins at the point where the pathology of a disease may occur. It encompasses diagnostic services that include screening, surveillance, and clinical examinations.[14] Screening strategies include follow-up education, counseling, and health referral. One model for secondary prevention involving screening is a cholesterol screening program for early detection of cardiovascular problems, such as elevated blood pressure, elevated blood cholesterol, and high glucose levels.[28] For people with an elevated blood cholesterol level, this means introducing "therapeutic lifestyle changes" such as reducing total and saturated fat in the diet, increasing physical activity, and reducing or maintaining a healthy weight. If this is not effective, or if low density lipoprotein levels are abnormally high, drug therapy can be recommended by the physician.

Strategies in secondary prevention are aimed at self-care for people with chronic diseases. An example of a secondary prevention program involving self-care would be an educational and awareness program to teach a woman with a history of gestational diabetes how to control her weight through diet and exercise.[18,19]

Tertiary Prevention (Treatment and Rehabilitation)

Tertiary prevention involves treatment and rehabilitation, and is defined as the reduction in the amount of disability caused by a disease to achieve the highest level of function.[27] Tertiary factors include diabetes, kidney disease, and angina. The goal of treatment and rehabilitation is the prevention of further disability and any secondary conditions that might result from the initial health problem.

Examples of tertiary prevention programs include medical nutrition therapy (MNT) for people suffering from kidney disease, nutrition education about vitamin and mineral supplementation and feeding strategies to prevent further complications of wasting from HIV/AIDS, and cardiac rehabilitation through diet, exercise, and stress management. The ultimate goal of tertiary prevention is, through rehabilitation, to restore the individual to an "optimal" level of functioning, given the constraints of the disease.[19]

Implications of the Prevention Levels

The prevention levels are useful concepts to help set objectives for public health programs concerned with adult health in communities, worksites, and other settings. Recent findings underscore the need to emphasize population-based prevention programs.[15, 29] As discussed earlier, research points to a holistic approach that aims at health, as well as prevention, when using the level concept for public health programs. This approach is embraced in HP 2010 in terms of the nutrition and health objectives.[2] For each goal, the holistic approach involving individual lifestyle factors, environmental factors, social and political issues, and access to quality healthcare is addressed.

Public health endeavors focus on primary or secondary prevention. It is important to choose the appropriate prevention level when planning a public health program. This is illustrated with two different approaches for handling CHD risk factors: one intended to reduce the prevalence of high blood pressure and one to reduce obesity levels.

Almost all Americans have had their blood pressure measured sometime in their lives. Ninety percent of Americans had their blood pressure measured in the past 2 years and could state whether it was normal or abnormally high.[30] Over 90% of Americans are aware of the relationship between hypertension and stroke and hypertension and heart disease.[31] Almost 70% of people with hypertension know about high blood pressure, yet the same percentage (70%) do not have their blood pressure under control (less than 140/90 mm Hg).[32] Recent findings show that systolic (higher number) blood pressure is a more important predictor of heart disease than diastolic blood pressure, especially in the elderly.[33] In addition, ethnic disparities exist for prevalence rates of high blood pressure, and African Americans in the United States have a greater prevalence of high blood pressure than do Caucasians.[32] These data suggest that in order to reduce mortality from hypertension, secondary prevention strategies should be directed toward persons with hypertension (especially those with elevated systolic pressures), African Americans, and the elderly. This would be more effective than primary prevention strategies aimed at increasing public awareness.

In contrast, many Americans are just beginning to be aware of the growing obesity epidemic and the significance of elevated Body Mass Index (BMI) (30 and above) for the risk of death and illness.[3] Americans understand the viability of lowering this risk factor associated with many chronic diseases. Extensive data exist to substantiate that making lifestyle changes such as engaging in regular physical activity and healthy eating could, at the very least, halt the continued growth of the obesity epidemic.[3] Given the dramatic increases in overweight and obese U.S. adults between 1976–1980 and 1999–2000,[3] population-based efforts could be more efficient at reducing the obesity epidemic than efforts to identify those individuals at risk.

One primary prevention effort is called *America on the Move*,[34] a national initiative dedicated to helping individuals and communities become more physically active and to eat more healthfully. The program creates and supports an "integrated grassroots network" at the state level to build communities that support individual behavior changes. In addition, America on the Move involves public and private partnerships at the national, state, and local levels. It publicizes small behavioral changes, such as cutting 100 calories a day and taking 2,000 steps daily.

Health promotion and chronic disease prevention programs should focus on coalition building (as previously discussed at length in Chapter 5) between community-based nutrition and health professionals, government, local businesses, health agencies, and insurers.[19] In this rapidly changing healthcare environment, continued training and research in public health program development is crucial to provide evidence of the efficacy of health prevention and promotion.

All levels of prevention should be addressed when devising strategies for dietary behavior changes for chronic disease prevention. However, for some diseases, the nutrition strategy may prove similar at each prevention level. Weight reduction, for example, may prevent the onset of hypertension or be part of the treatment for type 2 diabetes. In the case of other diseases, such as cancer, nutrition strategies might vary with the prevention level.

Dietary Guidelines for Disease Prevention

Various health organizations and government agencies have issued dietary guidelines and recommendations based on current scientific evidence. In 1989, the National Research Council published its report, *Diet and Health: Implications for Reducing Chronic Disease Risk*, providing evidence for the relationship between all major chronic conditions and diet.[3] More recently, HP 2010 set forth a comprehensive health promotion and disease prevention program for the nation. HP 2010's comprehensive health agenda has two overarching goals: 1) to increase the quality and years of a

> Visit www.health.gov for more information about the National Research Council's report, *Diet and Health: Implications for Reducing Chronic Disease Risk.*

healthy life, and 2) to eliminate health disparities.[2] These goals embrace the dietary recommendations set forth by several government and health organizations.[35]

In 2001, the U.S. Dietary Guidelines were assessed in terms of surveillance and research needs, especially related to risk for chronic diseases, such as cancer.[36] In the same year, the revised Dietary Guidelines of the American Heart Association (AHA) gave greater emphasis to the diet as a whole and, specifically, to certain protective foods for chronic disease risk prevention.[37] Recent scientifically based dietary guidelines from the American Cancer Society and the American Institute for Cancer Research reinforce these guidelines and further emphasize eating foods from plant sources.[38] More recent dietary recommendations for women issued by the American Dietetic Association reiterated these health-promoting dietary guidelines.[39] In addition, the Alternate Healthy Eating Index (AHEI) was developed to target food choices and nutrient intake associated with chronic disease risk.[83]

> **U.S. Dietary Guidelines—**
> www.health.gov/dietaryguidelines/
>
> **Dietary Guidelines of the American Heart Association—**
> www.americanheart.org/
> presenter.jhtml?identifier=1466
>
> **American Cancer Society—**
> www.cancer.org
>
> **American Institute for Cancer Research—**www.aicr.org
>
> **America Dietetic Association—**
> www.eatright.org
>
> **Alternate Healthy Eating Index—**
> www.hsph.harvard.edu/
> nutritionsource/pyramids.html
>
> **American Diabetes Association—**
> www.diabetes.org
>
> **North American Association for the Study of Obesity—**www.naaso.org

The dietary guidelines from these major health organizations agree in their basic message. The American Institute for Cancer Research stated: "Our research has shown that a diet that prevents cancer can also prevent other chronic diseases . . . the United States Department of Agriculture (USDA) and other major health organizations are now largely in agreement about specific dietary guidelines that protect overall health."[40]

The American Heart Association, the American Cancer Society, the American Diabetes Association, the American Institute of Cancer Research, and the North American Association for the Study of Obesity concur with the new dietary recommendations.[40] In July 2004, the American Cancer Society, the American Diabetes Association, and the American Heart Association collaborated to work on health promotion and disease prevention.[41] In their collaborative efforts, these organizations are making unified health statements concerning the prevention of heart disease, cancer, diabetes, and related risk factors. Furthermore, all of these organizations agree on the following dietary patterns, which may help reduce the risk of chronic diseases:[40,41]

- Consume a diet that emphasizes whole grains and legumes, vegetables, and fruits.
- Decrease saturated fat and dietary cholesterol; limit red meat and full-fat dairy products.
- Limit intake of foods and beverages high in added sugars.
- Limit overall intake of calories and engage in regular physical activity to maintain a healthy body weight.

Despite the evidence of the importance of diet to health, vegetable and fruit consumption among adults continues to be below recommended amounts: Less than 25% of U.S. adults consume five servings a day.[42] According to the U.S. Department of Agriculture's 1994–1996 Continuing Survey of Food Intakes by Individuals and the Food Guide Pyramid, only 3% of individuals meet four of the five recommendations for the intake of grains, fruits, vegetables, dairy products, and meats.[49]

The 2005 Dietary Guidelines for Americans (6th edition) were released in January 2005 by the Department of Health and Human Services (HHS) and the USDA. In the past, a diet low in fat was recommended, but in 2000, this recommendation was changed to a diet "moderate" in total fat, and specifically low in saturated fat and cholesterol. The dietary guidelines have consistently encouraged the consumption of complex carbohydrates and fiber by eating more fruits, vegetables, and whole grains. In 2000, the guidelines separated the recommendations for eating fruits and vegetables and eating whole grains. The issue of safe foods was added. The two separate guidelines—"aiming for a healthy weight" and "increasing physical activity"—also were added in 2000.

In revising the Dietary Guidelines and MyPyramid (formerly called the Food Guide Pyramid) for 2005, the following revisions have been proposed:[43]

- Balancing calories from foods and beverages according to the amount of calories expended and using MyPyramid to determine appropriate caloric requirements based on age and physical activity levels.
- Select nutritional goals for food intake patterns, such as the USDA Food Guide or DASH eating plan.
- Propose food intake patterns for educating the American public about healthful eating patterns, such as consuming

more fruits and vegetables, whole grains, and fat-free or low-fat milk.

- Use "cups" and "ounces" instead of "servings" in educational materials.
- Select appropriate illustrations of food patterns for consumer materials.

(See Chapter 2 for more information on these revisions.)

In summary, diverse health organizations stress the similarities in the dietary recommendations for reducing disease risk. These recommendations are to eat less saturated fat and cholesterol (limit red meat and full-fat dairy products); increase consumption of fruits, vegetables, whole grains, and legumes; limit added sugar and sodium; drink alcohol in moderation; and increase physical activity. By using clear terms, public health nutrition and dietetic professionals can make the nutrition message easier for the public to understand, value, and implement.

Diet and Health: Nutrition Strategies and Risk Factors

Nutrition strategies are essential in the prevention and management of several chronic diseases and their risk factors. When developing a public health program, risk factor assessment needs to be addressed. The following criteria can be assessed:

- The risk factor must have a strong association with the development of a chronic disease (e.g., obesity and heart disease).
- The risk factor must affect a significant number of people.
- The risk factor must be modifiable, so it can be reduced or changed.
- The risk factor must have a modification that, when changed or reduced, results in decreased mortality.

Because many risk factors can be modified by healthy lifestyle changes, early recognition of the risk factors for chronic disease prevention is critical. Figure 11-1 outlines general prevention guidelines for average-risk adults endorsed by the American Cancer Society, American Diabetes Association, and American Heart Association. The guidelines present screening recommendations for disease prevention and health promotion related to risk factors, and general nutrition and physical activity recommendations.

Obesity

Obesity has reached epidemic proportions in the United States. In 1999–2000, nearly 65% of adults were overweight or obese.[3,41]

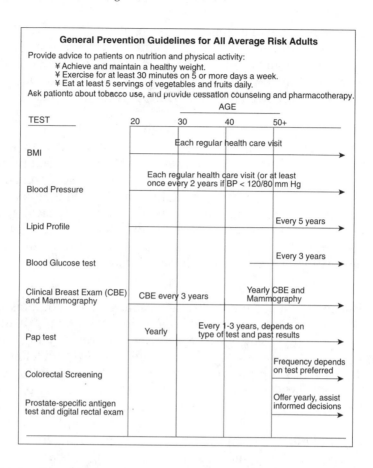

General Prevention Guidelines for All Average Risk Adults

Provide advice to patients on nutrition and physical activity:
¥ Achieve and maintain a healthy weight.
¥ Exercise for at least 30 minutes on 5 or more days a week.
¥ Eat at least 5 servings of vegetables and fruits daily.
Ask patients about tobacco use, and provide cessation counseling and pharmacotherapy.

TEST	AGE 20	30	40	50+
BMI	Each regular health care visit			
Blood Pressure	Each regular health care visit (or at least once every 2 years if BP < 120/80 mm Hg)			
Lipid Profile				Every 5 years
Blood Glucose test				Every 3 years
Clinical Breast Exam (CBE) and Mammography	CBE every 3 years		Yearly CBE and Mammography	
Pap test	Yearly	Every 1-3 years, depends on type of test and past results		
Colorectal Screening				Frequency depends on test preferred
Prostate-specific antigen test and digital rectal exam				Offer yearly, assist informed decisions

FIGURE 11-1   General Prevention Guidelines for All Average Risk Adults
Source: Reprinted with permission from the American Diabetes Association. Copyright © 2004 American Diabetes Association. From *Diabetes Care,* Vol. 27, 2004; 1812–1824.

Rates of overweight and obesity are steadily growing in our country. Nearly 55% of the U.S. adult population was overweight or obese in 1988–94, compared to 46% in 1976–80.[45] The National Institutes of Health (NIH) Expert Panel uses BMI for defining overweight and obesity.[44] The cut-off point for *overweight* is a BMI of 25 kg/m². *Obesity,* defined as having a BMI of 30 kg/m² or greater, has doubled among adults since 1980. Many diseases are associated with overweight and obesity, including CHD, stroke, high blood pressure, diabetes, arthritis-related disabilities, sleep apnea, gallbladder disease, and some cancers.[45]

The public health burden of overweight and obesity is overwhelming in terms of premature deaths and disability, lost productivity, and social stigmatization.[46] In 2000, the total cost of obesity was estimated at $117 billion.[3] Obesity rates are higher among certain population groups such as Hispanic Americans, African Americans, Native Americans, and Pacific Islander American women.[45]

Recent research has reported, however, that overweight has increased in *all* parts of the U.S. population.[47,48] The recent trend of overweight in the United States has become so severe that if it is not reversed in the next few years, poor diet and lack of physical exercise will likely become the leading preventable cause of mortality among adults.[8]

Many factors contribute to overweight and obesity. For each individual, metabolic and genetic factors, as well as behaviors affecting dietary intake and physical activity, contribute to being overweight. Cultural, environmental, and socioeconomic influences also play a role. Most overweight and obese individuals eat more calories from food than they expend through physical activity. As body weight increases, so does the prevalence of health risks in an individual. For this reason, encouraging obese individuals to adopt new eating and physical activity habits is of vital importance.

Weight Management

The goals and outcomes of weight management programs should be guided by an assessment of an individual's weight (BMI) and health. The National Heart, Lung, and Blood Institute (NHLBI) guidelines recommend intervention for people who are overweight and have two or more risk factors associated with their weight.[50]

Visit www.nhlbi.gov for more information about the National Heart, Lung, and Blood Institute's recommendations.

Furthermore, according to the position paper of the American Dietetic Association for weight management, assessment should incorporate the following areas:[51]

- *Anthropometrics:* The assessment of height, weight, BMI, and waist circumference (as waist measurement increases, so do health risks)
- *Medical causes:* Identifying potential causes, age of onset, obesity-associated complications, and severity of obesity
- *Psychological causes:* Eating disorders, possible psychological causes, and barriers to treatment
- *Nutritional causes:* Weight history, diet history, current eating patterns, nutritional intake, environmental factors, meals eaten away from home, exercise history, and motivation to change

For an individual, the goal of a weight management program should focus on the prevention of weight gain as well as weight loss. This recommendation encourages individuals to adopt healthier lifestyles, such as increasing physical activity and choosing less calorically dense foods. With this approach, weight loss will lead to reductions of health risks.[53] A weight loss of as little as 10% can improve health risks associated with overweight and obesity.[52]

For effective weight management programs, a multidisciplinary team should be involved, including a physician, a dietitian, an exercise physiologist, and a behavioral therapist. Healthcare professionals ought to be especially dedicated and sensitive to the needs of overweight and obese individuals. It is appropriate to discuss realistic goals of weight loss and maintenance so that shared responsibility for weight management can develop between the provider and individual. Goals might include the following:[51]

- Prevention or cessation of weight gain in an individual who is continuing to see an increase in his or her weight
- Progress in physical and emotional health
- Small, realistic weight losses achieved through sensible eating and exercise
- Improvements in eating, exercise, and any behaviors apart from weight loss

Establishing both short- and long-term treatment goals and documenting measures before implementing the weight management plan and after the individual has started on the plan are an important part of care. Positive behavior changes, other than absolute weight, should be rewarded, as these can be very motivating.

Physical activity is highly recommended as an essential part of a weight-management program. It is well established that to maintain weight loss, healthful dietary habits must be coupled with increased physical activity.[45] Physical activity contributes to weight loss not only by changing energy balance, but also by positively changing body composition by increasing lean body mass. Exercise decreases the risk of chronic disease and improves mood and quality of life. Many experts believe that physical inactivity is responsible for the increasing prevalence of overweight and obesity in the United States.[46] Combining weight loss with regular physical activity reduces one's risk for chronic diseases such as heart disease and diabetes by reducing both blood cholesterol and blood glucose levels.

The biggest challenge in weight management is to maintain a healthy weight once it is achieved. It is essential to include physical activity in weight-loss programs because regular physical activity is one of the best predictors of weight maintenance.[54] Unfortunately, studies show that within 5 years, a majority of people regain the weight they have lost.[55] The NIH recommends that both dietary and physical activity changes need to be continued indefinitely for weight loss to be maintained.[52] A comprehensive lifestyle program that focuses on nutrition, exercise, cognitive behavioral changes, and medical monitoring has been shown to be most effective for long-term success.[56]

Due to the increased prevalence in overweight and obesity in the United States, weight management becomes crucial for primary prevention of many chronic diseases. It is the foundation of secondary and tertiary prevention of hypertension, high blood cholesterol, diabetes, arthritis, and some cancers. It is important for healthcare providers to lobby for public health policies that endorse the treatment and management of weight, as discussed in Chapters 7 and 8. Also, clients must be informed of the known healthy and positive outcomes achieved through weight management programs.

Cardiovascular Disease

Cardiovascular disease is the nation's leading cause of death, accounting for more than 38% of all deaths in the United States. In 2001, more than 930,000 Americans died of cardiovascular disease.[57] Three modifiable health behaviors—poor nutrition, lack of physical activity, and smoking—contribute greatly to the burden of heart disease.

Cardiovascular diseases include diseases of the heart and blood vessels: CHD, stroke, and peripheral vascular diseases. CHD is the most common form of cardiovascular disease, and usually involves atherosclerosis and hypertension. Atherosclerosis is characterized by the build-up of plaques along the inner walls of the arteries, causing inadequate blood flow and leading to serious cardiovascular problems.

The consequences of cardiovascular disease are usually heart disease and stroke; these two diseases combined cause 1 death every 33 seconds.[3] About 61 million Americans live with the effects of heart disease and stroke. The annual cost of cardiovascular disease and stroke is estimated at $194 billion.[3] The death rate from cardiovascular disease fell by 17% in the last part of the 20th century; however, the number of deaths increased by 2.5% each year due to the growth and size of the population aged 65 years and older.[32] The decrease in the mortality rates due to cardiovascular disease is attributed to primary prevention (e.g., a decrease in dietary intake of saturated fat), secondary prevention (e.g., early detection and treatment of hypertension), and improved medical and surgical treatments.[57] In general, mortality and prevalence rates of cardiovascular disease could be improved by reducing the major risk factors: high blood pressure, high blood cholesterol, tobacco use, physical inactivity, and poor nutrition. Controlling one or more of these risk factors could have a major public health impact in our country.

Hypertension

High blood pressure or hypertension remains a "silent killer" in the United States, affecting about 50 million or 1 in 6 Americans.[58] High blood pressure is a major independent risk factor for cardiovascular disease. Hypertension increases the risk of heart attack, heart failure, stroke, and kidney disease.[59] This is significant because heart disease and stroke are, respectively, the first and third leading cause of death in the United States.[3]

In the latest classification of blood pressure for adults, normal blood pressure is considered to be < 120/80 mmHg and prehypertension is designated as 120–139 systolic or 80–89 mmHg diastolic pressure.[59] High blood pressure for adults is defined as a systolic pressure of 140 mmHg or higher, or a diastolic pressure of 90 mmHg or higher. A recent finding has determined that systolic blood pressure is a more important predictor of CHD in older adults than diastolic blood pressure.[60]

The number of people who were able to control their high blood pressure from lifestyle changes and the use of antihypertensive drugs rose from about 16% in 1971–1972 to about 65% in 1988–1994.[61] The age-adjusted death rate attributed to hypertension rose by about 36.4% over the past decade (data from 1991 to 2001), with the actual number of deaths increasing by 53%.[41] Twenty-five percent of people with hypertension are on medication but are inadequately controlled; only 34% are on medication and well controlled.[59,62] Significant disparities exist among persons diagnosed with hypertension; for example, African Americans have high blood pressure at an earlier age, and in general have higher blood pressures.[63] Thirty percent of Americans are unaware that they have hypertension.[62]

The latest guidelines for the treatment of hypertension are found in *The Seventh Report of the Joint National Committee on Prevention, Detection, Evaluation, and Treatment of High Blood Pressure.*[59] This report advocates major lifestyle modifications shown to lower blood pressure, enhance antihypertensive drug efficacy, and decrease cardiovascular risk.

> Visit www.nhlbi.nih.gov/guidelines/hypertension/ for more information about the *Seventh Report of the Joint National Committee on Prevention, Detection, Evaluation, and Treatment of High Blood Pressure.*

General lifestyle modifications include weight reduction for overweight or obese individuals (the goal is for a BMI of 18.5–24.9),[64,65] the adoption of the Dietary Approaches to Stop Hypertension (DASH) eating plan,[66] reducing sodium intake,[66] increasing physical activity,[67] and moderating alcohol consumption.[68,69] The DASH eating plan is a diet rich in calcium and potassium, consisting of fresh fruits, vegetables, and low-fat dairy products.[66,70] The DASH eating plan advocates a low sodium intake; intakes of 1,600 mg have been found to be as effective as single drug therapy in lowering blood pressure.[66] Other specific lifestyle modifications include reducing sodium to 2,400 mg a day, engaging in regular aerobic physical activity at least 30

> A usual food intake in the United States, complete with convenience and fast foods, may provide 10,000–20,000 mg of sodium per day.

minutes a day (most days of the week), and limiting alcohol consumption (2 drinks/day for men; 1 drink/day for women).[59] The report's guidelines recommend these lifestyle modifications for all individuals. For those people who have not achieved the goal blood pressure (< 140/90 mmHg), antihypertensive drugs, such as thiazide-type diuretics, may also be recommended.[71]

Cholesterol

High blood cholesterol is one of the major independent risk factors for heart disease and stroke.[3] Modifying this risk factor is effective in reducing cardiovascular disease mortality. Animal, epidemiologic, and metabolic research show that having elevated blood cholesterol levels is associated with cardiovascular disease. In spite of recommended dietary guidelines and medications available, over 50% of Americans have total blood cholesterol levels of 200 mg/dl or greater and almost 46% have an LDL cholesterol of 130 mg/dl or higher.[3]

Research from the 1980s showed that lowering high blood cholesterol significantly reduces the risk for heart attacks and reduces overall mortality rates. As a result, the National Cholesterol Education Program (NCEP) was launched in 1985.[72] Since its inception, the percentage of people who have had their cholesterol checked more than doubled, from 35% in 1983 to 75% in 1995.[73] Current guidelines recommend that all adults age 20 or older have their blood cholesterol levels checked every 5 years as a preventive measure.[63] Nevertheless, over 80% of Americans who have high blood cholesterol do not have it under control.

In terms of dietary trends and blood cholesterol levels, as dietary consumption of total fat, saturated fat, and cholesterol declined in the 1980s and 1990s, average blood cholesterol levels in adults declined from 213 mg/dl in 1978 to 203 mg/dl in 1991.[72] Research shows that as little as a 10% decrease in total cholesterol levels can reduce the incidence of CHD by almost 30%.[3]

In 2001, the NCEP released updated clinical guidelines in its report of the Expert Panel on the Detection, Evaluation and Treatment of High Blood Cholesterol in Adults, referred to as the Adult Treatment Panel (ATP) III.[74] This report updates the recommendations made in ATP II and I for people with high blood cholesterol levels, and reinforces findings from studies that confirm elevated LDL cholesterol to be a major cause of CHD. The guidelines in ATP III focus on LDL-lowering cholesterol strategies and on primary prevention in persons with multiple risk factors.[75] In 2004, an update was added to the NCEP guidelines on cholesterol management that advised physicians to consider new, more intensive medical treatments, such as statin drugs for people at high and moderately high risk for a heart attack.[76]

Statin drugs—These lower blood cholesterol by inhibiting HMG-CoA reductase (3-hydroxy-3-methylglutaryl coenzyme A reductase), a liver enzyme that is responsible for producing cholesterol.

The ATP III report recommends a complete lipoprotein profile that includes total cholesterol, LDL cholesterol, high density lipoprotein (HDL) cholesterol, and triglycerides as the preferred test rather than screening for total cholesterol and HDLs alone. For LDL-lowering therapy, a person's risk status needs to be assessed based on multiple risk factors including cigarette smoking, hypertension, low HDL, family history of premature CHD, and age. Diabetes is considered as a CHD equivalent in assessing a person's risk. In addition, the current guidelines use the Framingham scoring projections of 10-year absolute CHD risk to identify people who need more intensive therapy and those with multiple metabolic risk factors. NCEP[74] defines high-risk patients as those who have CHD, or diabetes, or multiple (two or more) risk factors, such as hypertension or smoking, which give them a greater than 20% chance of having a heart attack within 10 years. Very high-risk patients are those who have cardiovascular disease together with either multiple risk factors (especially diabetes), or badly controlled risk factors (e.g., smoking), or metabolic syndrome (a constellation of risk factors associated with obesity). For moderately high-risk and high-risk persons, the ATP III report and update recommend drug therapy in addition to therapeutic lifestyle changes (TLC), which include intensive use of nutrition, weight control, and physical activity.[74,76]

The specific parts of TLC include the following: reducing intakes of saturated fat to < 7% of total calories and decreasing cholesterol to < 200 mg per day. Total fat from calories can be in the 25%–35% range, as long as saturated and trans-fatty acids are kept low. Individuals are encouraged to use plant stanols and sterols in their diet (2g/day). Small amounts of plant sterols, or phytosterols, occur naturally in pine trees and foods like soybeans, nuts, grains, and oils. Increasing soluble fiber to 10–25 g/day is also recommended with weight reduction and increased physical activity. Since overweight and obesity are considered major underlying risk factors for CHD, weight reduction enhances LDL-lowering interventions.

In comparing the recommendations set forth in the ATP III report to the more recent updates, more intensive treatment options are delineated for very high-risk individuals. For high-risk patients, the goal in both reports remains an LDL level of less than 100 mg/dL; for very high-risk patients, a therapeutic option is to treat with statins to lower levels to < 70 mg/dL. The update lowers the threshold for drug therapy to an LDL of 100 mg/dL or higher, and recommends drug therapy for those high-risk people whose LDL is 100 to 129 mg/dL.

> The decision to go on drug therapy for high LDL levels is dependent on a multitude of risk factors and is decided between the physician and the patient.

In ATP III, for moderately high-risk persons, the LDL treatment goal is < 130 mg/dL and drug therapy is recommended if LDL levels are 130 mg/dL or higher. In the update, there is a therapeutic option to set the treatment goal at LDL < 100 mg/dL and to use statin drug therapy if LDL is 100–129 mg/dL to reach the goal. In the update, when LDL drug therapy is used, it is advised that enough medication be used to achieve at least a 30% to 40% reduction in LDL levels. In both reports, anyone with LDL above the goal is a candidate for TLC. In the update, any person at high or moderately high risk who has lifestyle-related risk factors should follow TLC, regardless of LDL level.[74,76]

As individuals learn about their risk factors and begin TLC, more registered dietitians and nutritionists will be asked to help people make necessary dietary changes. ATP III guidelines recommend that physicians refer individuals to dietitians for MNT.[74] At all stages in the model of TLC, the referral to a dietitian is recommended. This challenges public health providers to provide diet and exercise recommendations that will make a difference to those with elevated blood cholesterol levels. Nutritionists also need to consider prevailing eating and ethnic habits when counseling people to lower blood cholesterol levels. In terms of adhering to the ATP III protocol guidelines (and the update), patients and healthcare providers are key players in realizing the benefits of cholesterol-lowering and in attaining the highest possible levels of CHD risk reduction. Both screening for risk factors and compliance in adopting the lipid-lowering guidelines are essential; in reality, fewer than 50% of those persons eligible for meeting the criteria actually receive treatment.[74]

Physical Activity

Research demonstrates that virtually all individuals benefit from regular physical activity. Yet, more than 60% of American adults are not regularly physically active.[77] Twenty-five percent of all adults are not active at all. Inactivity increases with age and is more common among women than men. Also, those with lower incomes and less education exercise less than those with higher incomes or education.[77] Thus, physical inactivity is a prevalent risk in the United States. People who are sedentary are almost twice as likely to develop CHD as people who engage in regular physical activity.[75] The risk imposed by physical inactivity is almost as high as other well-known CHD risk factors, such as high blood cholesterol, high blood pressure, or smoking.[75,77] Even moderate physical activity produces significant health benefits, such as a decreased risk of CHD.[78] Research shows that moderate physical activity, such as walking 30 minutes a day/5 times a week, is more likely to be adopted and maintained than vigorous activity.[79]

There are many health benefits to be gained from regular physical activity. It enhances cardiovascular function, reduces very low density lipoprotein (VLDL) levels, raises HDL cholesterol, and can lower LDL cholesterol levels.[74] Physical activity lowers blood pressure and reduces insulin resistance. Overall, physical activity improves muscle function, cardiovascular function, and physical performance, and aids in weight management.[77] Nutritionists should become aware of the different types of physical activity, especially moderate levels of activity, that can lower an individual's risk for cardiovascular disease.

Smoking

Cigarette smoking is responsible for more than 440,000 deaths each year and is the single largest preventable cause of death and disease among U.S. adults.[80] Public health professionals, concerned about the risk factors for cardiovascular disease, need to discuss smoking with clients because it is a leading risk factor. Almost 20% of deaths from cardiovascular disease are attributed to smoking, including both active and second-hand smoke.[80] In 2003, an estimated 1.1 million Americans had a new or recurrent heart attack. Cigarette smoking was associated with sudden cardiac death in adult men and women.[80] Smoking-related CHD may also contribute to congestive heart failure, causing 4.6 million to suffer from this disease.[80] Smoking is also a major cause of stroke, which is the third leading cause of death in the United States. However, the risk of stroke decreases when an individual stops smoking.

Smoking cessation is also effective in preventing heart disease. In fact, after just one year of smoking abstinence, people who quit smoking have a 50% lower risk of death from CHD than those who continue to smoke.[81] Studies have shown that secondhand smoke exposure causes heart disease among adults, with an estimated 35,000 deaths each year.[80,82]

Smoking is a modifiable risk factor, and its modification is effective in preventing cardiovascular disease mortality. Smoking cessation is particularly important in people with other cardiovascular risk factors such as high blood pressure and elevated blood cholesterol, since these risk factors work synergistically. Cigarette smoking is also a risk factor for other leading causes of death and disability, including several kinds of cancer and chronic lung diseases.[80]

Trends

Progress has been made in decreasing mortality and risk factors for cardiovascular diseases. Between 1987 and 1996, the age-adjusted death rate for CHD declined by 22.2%, while deaths caused by stroke declined by 13.2%.[86] However, the HP 2010 objectives on CHD and stroke were not reached. Hypertension rates climbed from 11% to 29%. The prevalence of high blood cholesterol, however, declined from 26% to 19% between 1988 and 1994. There was a slight decline in smoking between 1995 and 1999/2000, yet deaths from smoking, poor diet, and physical inactivity still accounted for almost one-third of all deaths in the United States.[8]

Results from epidemiologic studies suggest that diets rich in fruits, vegetables, whole grains, and low-fat dairy foods are associated with a lower risk of mortality from many chronic diseases, including heart disease.[83] This nutritional pattern is supported by all of the major health organizations. Nevertheless, a large gap remains between recommended dietary patterns and what U.S. adults actually eat. Only about one-fourth of U.S. adults eat the recommended five or more servings of fruits and vegetables each day.[3] Recent research on frequency of fruit and vegetable consumption shows little change from 1994 to 2000.[84] Caloric intake from total fat declined from 36% to 34% from 1976 to 1994, but fell short of the target goal of 30% set by HP 2010.[63] According to data from the National Health and Nutrition Examination Surveys, decreases in calories from dietary fat and dietary cholesterol coincided with decreases in blood cholesterol levels.[85]

From 1950 to 1996, age-adjusted death rates from cardiovascular diseases declined 60%.[86] Although this is a positive trend, other health indicators have not improved significantly. Increasing prevalence rates in obesity and the continued high levels of blood pressure and stroke pose a continued public health challenge.[86]

Cancer

Cancer is an umbrella term used to describe a large group of diseases characterized by uncontrolled growth and spread of abnormal cells.[42] Cancer is the second leading cause of death in the United States, causing one in every five deaths. In 2004, an estimated 564,000 Americans died from this disease.[3] According to the American Cancer Society about one-third of cancer deaths are preventable, and are attributed to dietary factors, physical inactivity, overweight, or obesity.[42] For U.S. adults who don't smoke, dietary choices and physical activity are the most modifiable determinants of cancer risk. All cancers caused by cigarettes and the heavy use of alcohol could be prevented. The National Cancer Institute estimates that about 9.6 million Americans who had been diagnosed with cancer at some point in their life were alive in 2000.[42] This estimate includes people living with cancer and those who were cancer-free.[87] The 5-year relative survival rate for all cancers is 63%, or about 6 in 10 persons, which represents people who are living 5 years after diagnosis of cancer.[42]

Age-standardized death rates from all cancers decreased by 7.2% between 1991 and 2000.[87] Despite a decrease in the death rate from cancer, the total number of people who develop or die from cancer each year continues to increase because of our aging population.[96] The overall decrease in death rates from cancer is due to a decline in smoking and more effective detection and screening. The recent decrease in deaths from breast cancer in Caucasian females, for example, is due to a greater use of breast screening in regular medical care. Cancer death rates vary by gender, race, and ethnicity. For example, African Americans are more likely to die from cancer than are Caucasians.[88]

Although inherited genes play a significant role in cancer risk, they only explain part of all cancer incidences.[42] Most of the variation in cancer incidence cannot be explained by inherited factors. The predominant causes of cancer are external factors such as cigarette smoking, diet or nutrition, weight, and physical activity.[42,88] These factors act to modify the risk of cancer at all stages. It is estimated that more than 50% of all cancers could be prevented through dietary improvements, such as reducing total fat and increasing fruit and vegetable consumption, and smoking cessation.[80,89] Doll and Peto[90] estimated that about 10% to 70% of deaths from cancer were attributable to diet. However, recent evidence showing actual causes of death in the United States found that 14% of cancer deaths occurring in 1990 could be attributed to diet.[91] The science of nutrition and cancer is evolving, but still is not as developed as that of diet and cardiovascular disease. Many large-scale studies are currently underway to further elucidate the relationship between various nutrients and cancer.[91] Future research points to the areas of diet and gene interactions, and biomarkers for cancer that will further our understanding in this area.[92]

Current dietary recommendations are based on evidence from the American Cancer Society, the American Institute of Cancer Research/World Cancer Research Fund, and the Harvard Cancer Prevention Study.[42,93,94] In 2001, the American Cancer Society updated its guidelines on nutrition and physical activity after reviewing current scientific evidence.[95] In general, the current dietary guidelines support the existing 2005 Dietary Guidelines for Americans, and also encourage the consumption of plant-based diets, without relying on processed foods. The guidelines endorse eating a diet that promotes healthy weight control along with being physically active.[42,94] Specifically, nutrition and food scientists agree on the following recommendations to lower cancer risk:[42]

- Eat a plant-based diet that includes a wide variety of fruits, vegetables, whole grains, beans, and legumes. The recommendation is to choose whole grains over refined sources, and eat three to five servings of vegetables and two to four servings of fruits per day.
- Eat less fat from all food sources.
- Limit excess calories and maintain a healthful weight throughout life. Eat a sound diet and incorporate moderate or vigorous physical activity 5 days a week or more to further reduce risks of cancer.
- If you drink alcohol, do so in moderation.

Nutrition supplements are not universally recommended for cancer prevention. Instead, the cancer-prevention benefits of diet are considered among the best due to the interactions of many vitamins, minerals, and other plant-derived substances found naturally occurring in foods.[42,93] However, the possible benefits of supplemental folate, calcium, and selenium are noted.[42,95] By eating whole foods and following the cancer-prevention dietary recommendations along with physical activity, the protection of the body's cells may take place during the initiation, promotion, and progression stages of cancer. These food substances may repair damage that has already occurred in cells. Some literature sources state that individuals do not need to be concerned about the pesticide residues on fruits and vegetables, since the benefits of eating fruits and vegetables far outweigh any potential risk.[93] More long-term studies may help to state this definitively.

The study of diet and cancer prevention is relatively new. Dietitians and other public healthcare professionals need to stay abreast of these discoveries in order to give appropriate guidance to individuals at risk. The basis of MNT should include those recommendations set forth by the American Cancer Society and the World Cancer Research Fund/American Institute for Cancer Research.[42,93]

Diabetes

Diabetes is a serious, costly, and increasingly common chronic disease that poses a significant public health challenge. In 2001, diabetes was the sixth leading cause of death in the United States.[3] About 18 million Americans have diabetes, and over 5 million of these people are unaware that they have the disease.[3] Type 2 diabetes used to be called adult-onset diabetes and may account for about 90% to 95% of all diagnosed cases of diabetes.[97] By 2050, an estimated 29 million Americans are expected to have been diagnosed with diabetes. The increase in the number of cases has been particularly high within certain ethnic and racial groups in the United States.[98]

Medical complications of type 2 diabetes include heart disease, kidney failure, leg and foot amputations, and blindness. Each year about 12,000–24,000 people become blind because of diabetic eye disease.[3] The majority of the deaths caused by diabetes are due to diabetes-associated cardiovascular disease. The presence of diabetes in adults is associated with a two-to-four-fold increase in CHD compared to non-diabetic adults. Almost three-quarters of adults with diabetes have hypertension.[3] Diabetes is the cause of 44% of end-stage renal disease cases. Severe forms of nervous system damage occur in 60%–70% of diabetic adults. Approximately 60% of all non-traumatic amputations in the United States occur in people with diabetes.[99] Periodontal or gum disease is also more common among diabetics. As a result, diabetes is a costly disease, with the total attributable costs (direct and indirect) estimated at $132 billion annually.[99]

Type 2 diabetes is associated with the following factors:

- *Age*: Diabetes is most common in people over 60 years of age.[99]
- *Ethnicity*: Deaths from diabetes are twice as high for African Americans than for Caucasians; Native Americans, Hispanic Americans, and certain Pacific Islander American and Asian American populations also have higher rates.[98]
- *Genetics and family history*: Genetic markers that indicate a greater risk for type 2 diabetes have been identified.
- *Obesity*: The increased prevalence of obesity among adults is positively associated with the increased rates of diabetes.[100] Data from clinical trials strongly support the potential of moderate weight loss to reduce the risk of type 2 diabetes.[101]
- *History of gestational diabetes in women*: Gestational diabetes is a form of glucose intolerance that develops in some women during pregnancy. Obesity is associated with gestational diabetes. Women with a family history of gestational diabetes and Hispanic American and African American women are at an increased risk.[102]
- *Impaired glucose metabolism*: People with prediabetes, or who at increased risk of developing diabetes, have impaired fasting blood glucose. Research studies suggest that weight loss and increased physical activity among people with prediabetes may return glucose levels to normal and prevent the onset of diabetes.[98]
- *Physical inactivity*: If you are at higher risk and fairly inactive, or exercise fewer than three times a week, you are more likely to develop type 2 diabetes.

In the United States, recent lifestyle changes such as decreased physical activity and increased energy consumption, which contribute to the increased prevalence rates of obesity, are also strong risk factors for diabetes.[101] On the other hand, positive lifestyle changes such as diet, weight loss of 5%–7%, and moderate-intensity physical activity (e.g., walking 30 minutes a day) can delay the onset of diabetes. The Diabetes Prevention Program,[101] a major, large-scale study of over 3,000 people at high risk for developing diabetes, confirmed this, and found a 58% reduction in the development of diabetes over a 3-year period. The findings from this study, sponsored by the NIH, showed that exercise, a healthy diet, and weight loss can reduce the risk of developing diabetes by as much as 71% in high-risk individuals.[101]

MNT is an essential part of diabetes management for adults. Objectives for MNT include the following:[102]

- Attaining and maintaining optimal metabolic outcomes including normalizing blood glucose levels, maintaining a lipid profile that reduces vascular disease risk, and normalizing blood pressure levels

- Preventing, delaying, and treating the onset complications by modifying nutrient intake and lifestyle to prevent and treat obesity, cardiovascular disease, hypertension, and nephropathy
- Optimizing health through sensible food choices and physical activity
- Addressing personal and cultural preferences as well as lifestyle factors, including a person's willingness to change, when determining individual nutritional needs[102]

In terms of specific nutrients and dietary recommendations for type 2 diabetes, studies in healthy subjects and those at risk for type 2 diabetes support the importance of including foods containing complex carbohydrates in the diet, particularly those from whole grains, fruits, vegetables, and low-fat milk.[102] Reduced intake of total fat, especially saturated fat, may reduce the risk of diabetes.

In summary, lifestyle changes such as reduced energy intake, increased physical activity, and nutrition education (with the goal of promoting weight loss) represent essential aspects of type 2 diabetes management for adults. HP 2010[99] discusses the challenges of diabetes and the preventive interventions aimed at them: primary prevention, screening and early diagnosis, access, and quality of care. This includes secondary and tertiary prevention, such as glucose control and decreasing complications from diabetes.[99] As dietitians, public health professionals, and educators, many opportunities exist to contribute to the effective management of diabetes.

Osteoporosis

As one grows, bones develop and become larger, heavier, and denser. At approximately age 30 years peak bone mass is achieved in both men and women. After this time period, adults begin to lose bone mass, and this continues as they get older. Osteoporosis, or porous bone disease, develops when bone loss reaches the point of causing fractures under common, everyday stresses. Due to increased bone fragility, there is a greater susceptibility to fractures of the hip, spine, and wrist. Both men and women suffer from osteoporosis.

Osteoporosis currently affects 44 million Americans, or 55% of people aged 50 and older, 68% of women over 50 have the disease.[103,104] These rates correspond to one in two women and one in four men (aged 50 and older) who will experience an osteoporosis-related fracture in their lifetime.[103] Osteoporosis causes significant disability with important economic consequences, costing about $14 billion each year in direct expenditures (hospitals and nursing homes).[106] Of the 1.5 million fractures occurring each year due to osteoporosis, over 300,000 are hip fractures, 700,000 are vertebral fractures, and 250,000 are wrist fractures. Of the 300,000 annual hip fractures, 24% result in death following complications from the fracture.[104]

Osteoporosis is often called the "silent disease" because it can occur without any overt symptoms. The technical standard for measuring bone mineral density is dual-energy x-ray absorptiometry (DXA). A low bone mass density is a strong predictor of fracture risk.[104] Bone density tests can detect osteoporosis before a fracture occurs, and they can serve as a predictor for future fracture risks.

Your chances of developing osteoporosis are greatest if you are a Caucasian woman beyond menopause. Women have less bone tissue and lose bone more easily than men due to the hormonal changes involved in menopause. Those individuals who have a low dietary intake of calcium and vitamin D over a lifetime, who are physically inactive, who are cigarette smokers, who are excessive alcohol drinkers, who are thin and small-framed, and who have a family history of osteoporosis are at increased risk.[103,104] Additionally, Caucasians and Asian American women are at highest risk, whereas African American and Hispanic American women have lower risks.[104] Anorexia nervosa, the use of certain medications, and low testosterone levels in men are also risk factors for osteoporosis.

The five factors that can be modified to prevent osteoporosis are: 1) a diet rich in calcium and vitamin D; 2) weight-bearing exercise; 3) a healthy lifestyle that excludes smoking and excessive alcohol intake; 4) routine bone density measurements; and 5) the use of medication, when appropriate.[104]

Nutrition is an important modifiable risk factor in terms of both bone health and the prevention and treatment of osteoporosis. An adequate amount of calcium and vitamin D contributes significantly to bone health. Low calcium intakes are associated with low bone mass, rapid bone loss, and high fracture rates.[105] Bone is a living, growing tissue, and 99% of the body's calcium is found in bone. Throughout one's lifetime, bone formation and resorption occurs. This process, which is known as bone turnover, is responsive to dietary calcium regardless of age. Dietary calcium works to strengthen bone by suppressing bone resorption and parathyroid hormone.[105]

According to the NIH Consensus Statement on Osteoporosis,[106] calcium is the most important nutrient for the prevention of osteoporosis. In spite of this, actual calcium intakes for most of the U.S. population are considerably lower than the current Dietary Reference Intakes (DRI).[107] Many studies have shown that adult skeletal health is improved by increasing dairy foods or calcium intake in the diet.[108] The DASH diet, used to treat hypertension, is a low-fat diet, rich in calcium, that has been shown to reduce bone turnover and reduce the risk of osteoporosis.[66] Calcium requirements can be met with low-fat dairy products; however, low consumption of milk and other dairy products in the U.S. diet is mainly responsible for low calcium intakes among U.S. adults.[108] Other foods contain calcium, such as dark leafy greens, but these foods usually provide less calcium per serving than milk, and most Americans do not eat these vegetables often. For individuals who do not consume enough calcium in their diets, calcium supplements are recommended.

Vitamin D also plays an important role in calcium absorption and bone health. Vitamin D is a major determinant of intestinal calcium absorption. When skin is exposed to sunlight, the body synthesizes vitamin D. However, studies show decreased production of vitamin D in the elderly and individuals who are housebound, especially in the winter months.[103] Due to inadequate intake of vitamin D in a high proportion of older adults, the most recent DRI have increased the vitamin D requirements for people 50 years and older.[107] Low-fat and nonfat milk, excellent sources of calcium, are fortified with 100 IU of Vitamin D per serving.

> For those living in colder climates without much sunshine, vitamin D supplementation is suggested to accompany calcium intake.

In conclusion, osteoporosis is a serious public health disease and is largely preventable. Starting early in life, both females and males should be advised on how to incorporate sources of calcium into their diets. The use of low-fat and nonfat dairy foods should be recommended, and if persons can't consume dairy products, other food sources and calcium supplements are necessary. Adequate vitamin D intake needs to be addressed, as well. Public health nutritionists should encourage individuals to participate regularly in physical activity. Modifiable lifestyle factors should be discussed to promote bone health throughout life.

Acquired Immune Deficiency Syndrome (AIDS)

In 1981, a new infectious disease, AIDS, was first identified in the United States. A few years later, human immunodeficiency virus (HIV) was discovered, and this was identified as the viral agent that causes AIDS. HIV/AIDS has affected almost every ethnic, socioeconomic, and age group in the United States.[109]

AIDS, a deadly disease, is the end stage of HIV infection. The infection progresses to overwhelm the immune system and leaves individuals defenseless against numerous other infections and diseases. HIV is spread through direct contact with contaminated body fluids, sexual intercourse, direct blood contact, or from mother to infant. In 1996, death rates from AIDS in the United States declined for the first time.[109] Nevertheless, HIV/AIDS remains a significant cause of illness, disability, and death in the United States. According to the Centers for Disease Control and Prevention (CDC)[109] in 2002, the estimated number of diagnosed AIDS cases was about 890,000. Death rates have dropped dramatically in the United States due to the introduction of antiretroviral therapies.[109]

Health complications for people with HIV/AIDS are immune dysfunction and its associated complications, which include malnutrition and wasting. HIV targets the immune system, rendering an individual susceptible to infections and disease. The CDC defines the AIDS-related wasting syndrome as a 10% weight loss in a 6-month period accompanied by diarrhea or fever for more than 30 days.[110] Malnutrition and its complications can reduce one's tolerance to medications and other therapies. Malnutrition occurs in the form of tissue wasting, fat accumulation, increased lipid levels, and risk of other chronic disease. The American Dietetic Association's (ADA) Position Paper[111] strongly supports nutrition evaluation and MNT as parts of the ongoing health care of HIV-infected individuals. In terms of MNT, this includes early assessment and treatment of nutrient deficiencies, the maintenance and restoration of lean body mass, and continued support for performing daily activities and maintaining quality of life. According to the ADA, nutrition education and guidance should incorporate the following aspect:[111]

- Healthful eating principles
- Water and food safety issues
- Perinatal and breast-feeding issues
- Nutrition management for symptoms such as anorexia, swallowing problems, diarrhea, and so on
- Food-medicine interactions
- Psychosocial and economic issues
- Alternative feeding methods (supplementation, tube feeding, or parenteral nutrition)
- Additional therapies, including physical activity and disease management
- Guidelines for evaluating nutrition information, diet claims, and individual mineral and vitamin supplementation
- Strategies for treatment of altered fat metabolism

In addition, it is important for an HIV-infected individual to have adequate access to food, health care, and other support systems. The maintenance and restoration of nutrition stores are interrelated with recommended medical therapies; therefore, it is essential that a public health nutritionist be an active participant in the healthcare team to provide optimal MNT.

Issues for Discussion

1. What would you propose should be incorporated into public health programs that focus on nutrition as an important preventive factor in illness, disability, and death?

2. What advice would you give to the individual in the community with regard to preventing chronic disease risk factors such as obesity, physical inactivity, and smoking in order to reduce society's financial burden?

3. What proportion of public funds designated for nutrition services should be given for primary, secondary, and tertiary prevention versus acute medical care?

4. Programs such as for-profit weight loss centers are proliferating in this country. What are positive and negative aspects of this trend compared with public health weight management programs?

References

1. Frazao E. The high costs of poor eating patterns in the U.S. In: Frazao E., ed, *America's Eating Habits: Changes and Consequences.* Washington, DC: U.S. Department of Agriculture (USDA), Economic Research Service (ERS), AIB-750; 1999.

2. U.S. Department of Health and Human Services: *Healthy People 2010: understanding and improving health.* 2nd ed. Washington, DC: U.S. Government Printing Office; 2000.

3. National Center for Chronic Disease Prevention and Health Promotion. *The burden of chronic diseases and their risk factors.* Washington, DC: Department of Health and Human Services; 2004. Section 111: Risk Factors and Use of Preventive Services, US.

4. Centers for Disease Control and Prevention, National Center for Health Statistics. Effectiveness in disease and injury prevention; estimated national spending on prevention. U.S., 1988. *MMWR.* 1992; 41: 529–531.

5. Deaths: preliminary data for 2001. *National Vital Statistics Report.* March 14, 2003;51.

6. Krauss RM, Eckel RH, Howard B, et al. AHA dietary guidelines: revision 2000: a statement for healthcare professionals from the Nutrition Committee of the American Heart Association. *Circulation.* 2000; 102: 2284–2299.

7. National Center for Health Statistics. *Health, U.S., 2003*; U.S. Government Printing Office, Washington, DC, 2003.

8. Mokdad AH, Marks JS, Stroup DF, Gerberding JL. Actual causes of death in the U.S., 2000. *JAMA.* 2004;291:1238–1245.

9. Mokdad AH, Marks JS, Stroup DF, Gerberding JL. Correction: Actual causes of death in the U.S., 2000. *JAMA.* 2005; 293(3): 293–294.

10. Department of Health and Human Services, Centers for Disease Control and Prevention. *Health, U.S., 2002.* Rockville, Md: Department of Health and Human Services, Centers for Disease Control and Prevention; 2002. DHHS Publication No. 1232.

11. Koplan JP, Dietz WH. Caloric imbalance and public health policy. *JAMA.* 1999;282:1579–1581.

12. National Center for Health Statistics (NCHS). Report of the final mortality statistics,1995. Monthly Vital Statistics Report. 1997;5(11); Suppl. 2.

13. U.S. Department of Health and Human Services. The Surgeon General's report on nutrition and health. Washington, DC: U.S. DHHS; 1988. DHHS (PHS) Publication No. 88–50210.

14. Elo SL, Caltrop JB. Health promotive action and preventive action model (HPA model) for the classification of healthcare services in public health nursing. *Scand J Public Health.* 2002;30:200–208.

15. Wimbush FB, Peters RM. Identification of cardiovascular risk: use of a cardiovascular-specific genogram. *Public Health Nursing.* May/June 2000;17(3):148–154.

16. U.S. Preventive Services Task Force. *Guide to clinical preventive services.* 3rd ed. Washington, DC: U.S. Department of Health and Human Services; January 2003.

17. Kaufman M, ed. *Nutrition in public health: a handbook for developing programs and services.* Rockville, Md.: Aspen Publishers; 1990.

18. Shamansky SL, Clausen C. Levels of prevention: examination of the concept; *Nurs Outlook.* 1980;28:104–108.

19. Position of the American Dietetic Association: the role of nutrition in health promotion and disease prevention programs; *J Amer Diet Assoc.* 1998;98:205–208.

20. Brunner E, White I, Thorogood M, Bristow A, Curle D, Marmot M. Can dietary interventions change diet and cardiovascular risk factors? A meta-analysis of randomized controlled trials. *Am J Public Health.* 1997;87:1415–1422.

21. Dietary Guidelines Advisory Committee. *Report of the Dietary Guidelines Advisory Committee on the Dietary Guidelines for Americans, 2000.* Washington, DC: U.S. Department of Agriculture; 2000.

22. U.S. Departments of Agriculture and Health and Human Services. *The food guide pyramid.* Washington, DC: U.S. Departments of Agriculture, Health and Human Services; 1992. Home and Garden Bulletin, No. 249.

23. Dietary Guidelines Alliance. Do it yourself: crafting consumer tips. In: *Reaching consumers with meaningful health messages.* Washington, DC: Dietary Guidelines Alliance; 1996.

24. Position of the American Dietetic Association: nutrition education for the public. *J Amer Diet Assoc.* 1996;96:1183–1187.

25. American Dietetic Association and the Office of Disease Prevention and Health Promotion, Public Health Service, U.S. Department of Health and Human Services. *Worksite nutrition; a guide to planning, implementation, and evaluation.* 2nd ed. Chicago, Ill.: American Dietetic Association; 1993.

26. Goldberg JP. Nutrition and health communication: the message and the media over half a century. *Nutr Rev.* 1992;50:71–77.

27. Pender NJ. *Health promotion in nursing practice.* 3rd ed. Stamford, Conn.: Appelton-Lange; 1996.

28. Sharlin J, Posner BM, Gershoff S, Zeitlin M, Berger P. Nutrition and behavioral characteristics and determinants of cholesterol levels in men and women. *J Amer Diet Assoc.* 1992;92:434–440.

29. Resnicow K, Orlandi M, Vaccaro D, Wynder E. Implementation of a pilot school-site cholesterol reduction intervention. *J School Health.* 1989;59(2):74–78.

30. U.S. Department of Health and Human Services, Centers for Disease Control and Prevention, National Center for Health Statistics. National Health Interview Survey (NHIS). 2003. Available at: http://www.cdc.gov/nchs/. Accessed on May 26, 2004.

31. U.S. Department of Health and Human Services. National Heart, Lung, and Blood Institute (NHLBI). National High Blood Pressure Education Program. Available at: www.nhlbi.nih.gov/about/nhbpep. Accessed on May 26, 2004.

32. Centers for Disease Control and Prevention, National Center for Chronic Disease Prevention and Health Promotion, USDHHS. Preventing heart disease and stroke, addressing the nation's leading killers. *At-a-Glance Summary Tables*; The American Heart Association, 2004.

33. Kannel WB, Dawber TR, McGee DL. Perspectives of systolic hypertension, the Framingham Study. *Circulation*. 1980;61:1179–1182.

34. America on the Move. Available at: http://www.americaonthemove.org. Accessed on May 26, 2004.

35. National Academy of Sciences, National Research Council, Food and Nutrition Board. *Diet and health: implications for reducing chronic disease risk*. Washington, DC: National Academy Press; 1989.

36. The dietary guidelines: Surveillance issues and research needs. *J Nutrition, supplement: AICR 11th Annual Research Conference on Diet, Nutrition and Cancer*. 2001;131(2 3154S-3155S).

37. Kris-Etherton P, Daniels SR, Eckel RH, et al. Summary of the scientific conference on dietary fatty acids and cardiovascular health. Conference summary from the Nutrition Committee of the American Heart Association. *Circulation*. 2001;103:1034–1039.

38. American Institute of Cancer Research. Available at: http://www.aicr.org. Accessed on May 26, 2004.

39. Position of The American Dietetic Association and the Dietitians of Canada: nutrition and women's health. *J Amer Diet Assoc*. 2004;104(6);.984–1001.

40. American Heart Association. AHA Comment, May 31, 2004. Health agencies applaud HHS/USDA new dietary guidelines. Available at: http://www.americanheart.org. Accessed June 29, 2004.

41. Eyre H, Kahn R, Robertson RM. Preventing cancer, cardiovascular disease, and diabetes. *Diabetes Care*. 2004;27(7):1812–1824.

42. American Cancer Society. *Cancer prevention and early detection facts and figures 2004*. Atlanta, Ga: ACS; 2004.

43. U.S. Department of Agriculture. News release: scientific update of food guidance presented to the Dietary Guidelines Committee, January 28, 2004. Available at: http://www.usda.gov. Accessed June 29, 2004.

44. National Institutes of Health, National Heart, Lung, and Blood Institute. *Clinical guidelines on the identification, evaluation, and treatment of overweight and obesity in adults, 1998*. Washington, DC: U.S. DHHS, Public Health Service: xxiii.

45. U.S. Department of Health and Human Services. *Healthy People 2010: understanding and improving health*. 2nd ed. Washington, DC: U.S. Government Printing Office; 2000. 19: Nutrition and Overweight. 19-3-19-49

46. U.S. Department of Health and Human Services, Public Health Service, Office of the Surgeon General. *Surgeon General's call to action to prevent and decrease overweight and obesity*. Washington, DC: U.S. DHHS; 2001.

47. Mokdad AH, Bowman BA, Ford ES, Vinicor F, Macks JS, Koplan JC. The continuing epidemics of obesity and diabetes in the U.S. *JAMA*. 2001;286:1195–1200.

48. Flegal KM, Carroll MD, Ogden CL, Johnson CL. Prevalence and trends of obesity among U.S. adults, 1999–2000. *JAMA*. 2002;288:1723–1727.

49. U.S. Department of Agriculture. *USDA continuing survey of food intakes by individuals (CSFII), 1994–1996*. Washington, DC: USDA; 1998.

50. Kuczmarski RJ, Flegal KM. Criteria for definition of overweight in transition: background and recommendations for the U.S. *Am J Clin Nutr*. 2000;72(5):1074–1081.

51. Position of the American Dietetic Association: Weight management. *J Amer Diet Assoc*. 2002;102(8):1145–1155.

52. National Institutes of Health and National Heart, Lung, and Blood Institute. Clinical guidelines on the identification, evaluation, and treatment of overweight and obesity in adults—the evidence report. *Obesity Research*. 1998;6(2):1105.

53. Kassiger JP, Angell M. Losing weight—an ill-fated New Year's resolution. *N Eng J Med*. 1998;338:52–54.

54. Pavlou KN, Krey S, Stefee WO. Exercise as an adjunct to weight-loss and maintenance in moderately obese subjects. *Am J Clinc Nutr*. 1989;49:1115–1123.

55. NIH Technology Assessment Conference Panel. Methods for voluntary weight loss and control. Consensus development conference. March 30-April 1, 1992. *Annals of Internal Medicine*. 1993;119(7.2):764–770.

56. Jeffrey RW, Drewsiowski A, Epstein LH, et al. Long-term maintenance of weight-loss: current status. *Health Psych*. 2000;1 (supplement):5–16.

57. American Heart Association. *Heart disease and stroke statistics: 2004 update*. Dallas, TX. : American Heart Association; 2004.

58. Centers for Disease Control and Prevention. *Fact sheet: high blood pressure*. Hyattsville, MD: CDC; May 11, 2004.

59. U.S. Department of Health and Human Services, NIH, NHLBI, NHBPEP, JCN 7 Express. *The seventh report of the Joint National Committee on Prevention, Detection, Evaluation, and Treatment of High Blood Pressure*. Bethesda MD, National Institutes of Health. May 2003. NIH Pub. No. 03–5233.

60. Systolic Hypertension in the Elderly Program (SHEP) Cooperative Research Group. Prevention of stroke by antihypertensive drug treatment in older persons with isolated systolic hypertension. Final results of the SHEP. *JAMA*. 1991;265:3255–3264.

61. National Heart, Lung, and Blood Institute. *Morbidity and mortality: 1998 chartbook of cardiovascular, lung, and blood diseases*. Bethesda, MD: Public Health Service, National Institutes of Health, NHLBI; October 1998.

62. NHLBI. National High Blood Pressure Education Program, Program Description. Available at: www.nhlbi.nih.gov. Accessed May 19, 2004.

63. U.S. Department of Health and Human Services. *Healthy People 2010: understanding and improving health*. 2nd ed. Washington, DC: U.S. DHHS; 2000. 12-Heart Disease and Stroke12-3-12-33.

64. The Trials of Hypertension Prevention Collaborative Research Group. Effects of weight-loss and sodium reduction intervention on blood pressure and hypertension incidence in overweight people with high-normal blood pressure. The Trials of Hypertension Prevention, Phase 11. *Arch Intern Med*. 1997;157:657–667.

65. He J, Whelton PK, Appel LJ, Charleston J, Klag MJ. Long-term effects of weight-loss and dietary sodium restriction on incidence of hypertension. *Hypertension.* 2000;35:544–549.

66. Sacks FM, Syerkey LP, Vollmer WM, et al. Effects on blood pressure of reduced dietary sodium and Dietary Approaches to Stop Hypertension (DASH) diet. DASH-Sodium Collaborative Research Group. *N Engl J Med.* 2001;344:3–10.

67. Chobanian AV, Hill M. National Heart, Lung, and Blood Institute Workshop on Sodium and Blood Pressure: a critical review of current scientific evidence. *Hypertension.* 2000;35:858–863.

68. Whelton SP, Chin A, Xin X, He J. Effect of aerobic exercise on blood pressure: a meta-analysis of randomized, controlled trials. *Ann Intern Med.* 2002;136:493–503.

69. Xin X, He J, Frontini MG, et al. Effects of alcohol reduction on blood pressure. A meta-analysis of randomized controlled trials. *Hypertension.* 2001;38:1112–1117.

70. Vollmer WM, Sacks FM, Ard J, et al. Effects of diet and sodium intake on blood pressure. Subgroup analysis of the DASH-sodium trial. *Ann Intern Med.* 2001;135:1019–1028.

71. Psatsy BM, Smith NL, Siscovick DS, et al. Health outcomes associated with antihypertensive therapies used as first-line agents. A systematic review and meta-analysis. *JAMA.* 1997;277:739–745.

72. Cleeman JL, Lenfant C. The National Cholesterol Education Program: progress and prospects. *JAMA.* 1998;280:2099–2104.

73. National Heart, Lung, and Blood Institute. Consumer awareness surveys. Press conference. Bethesda, MD: NHLBI; December 4, 1995.

74. U.S. Department of Health and Human Services, NHLBI. *National Cholesterol Education Program, Third Report of the Expert Panel on the Detection, Evaluation, and Treatment of High Blood Cholesterol in Adults (Adult Treatment Panel III)* Bethesda, MD: National Institutes of Health. May 2001. NIH Pub. No. 01–367.

75. U.S. Department of Health and Human Services. *Healthy People 2010: understanding and improving health.* 2nd ed. Washington, DC: U.S. DHHS; 2000: 22-Physical activity and fitness. Bethesda, MD 22–3-22–36,

76. Grundy SM, Cleeman JI, Barrey Merz CN, et al. For the coordinating committee of the National Cholesterol Education Program. Implications of recent clinical trials for the National Cholesterol Education Program Adult Treatment Panel III Guidelines. *Circulation.* 2004;110:227–239.

77. U.S. Department of Health and Human Services. *Physical activity and health: a report of the Surgeon General, 1996.* Atlanta, Ga: Centers for Disease Control and Prevention, National Center for Chronic Disease Prevention and Health Promotion; 1996.

78. NIH Consensus Development Panel on Physical Activity and Cardiovascular Health. Physical activity and cardiovascular health. *JAMA.* 1996;276(3):241–246.

79. Pate RR, Pratt M, Blair SN, et al. Physical activity and public health: a recommendation from the Centers for Disease Control and Prevention and the American College of Sports Medicine. *JAMA.* 1995;273(5):402–407.

80. U.S. Department of Health and Human Services. *The health conse-quences of smoking: a report of the Surgeon General, 2004*. Atlanta, Ga: Centers for Disease Control and Prevention, National Center for Chronic Disease Prevention and Health Promotion, Office on Smoking and Health; 2004.

81. U.S. Department of Health and Human Services. *The health benefits of smoking cessation: a report of the Surgeon General, 1990*. Atlanta, Ga: U.S. DHHS, CDC, Center for Chronic Disease Prevention and Health Promotion, Office on Smoking and Health; 1990.

82. Glanz SA, Parmely WW. Passive smoking and heart disease: mechanism and risk. *JAMA*. 1995;272:1047–1053.

83. McCullough ML, Feskanich D, Stampfer MJ, et al. Diet quality and major chronic disease in men and women: moving toward improved dietary guidance. *Am J Clin Nutr*. 2002;76:1261–1271.

84. Serdula MK, Gillespie C, Kettel-Khan L. Farris R, Seymour J, Denny C. Trends in fruit and vegetable consumption among adults in the U.S.: Behavioral Risk Factor Surveillance System, 1994–2000. *Am J Publ Health*. 2004;94(6):1014–1018.

85. Ernst ND, Sempos ST, Briefel RR, Clark MB. Consistency between U.S. dietary fat intake and serum total cholesterol concentrations; the National Health and Nutrition Examination Surveys. *Am J Clin Nutr*. 1997;66:965S-972S.

86. Centers for Disease Control and Prevention. Decline in deaths from heart disease and stroke–United States, 1990–1999. *MMWR*. 1999;48:649–656.

87. Ries L, Eisner M, Kosary C, et al. SEER: *cancer statistics review, 1975–2000*. National Cancer Institute; 2003.

88. Key TJ, Allen NE, Spencer EA, Travis RC. The effect of diet on risk of cancer. *Lancet*. 2002;360:861–868.

89. Willett, W. Diet and nutrition. In: Schottenfield D., Frammeni, Jr. JF, eds. *Cancer Epidemiology and Prevention*. 2nd ed. New York: Oxford University Press; 1996: 438–461.

90. Doll R, Peto R. The causes of cancer: qualitative estimates of avoidable risks of cancer in the U.S. today. *J Natl Cancer Inst*. 1981;66:1191–1308.

91. McGinnis JM, Forge WH: Actual causes of death in the U.S. *JAMA*. 1993;270:2207–2212.

92. Mandelson MT, Oestreicher N, Porter PL, et al. Breast density as a predictor of mammographic detection: comparison of interval- and screen-detected cancers. *J Natl Canc Inst*. 2000;92:1081–1087.

93. American Institute of Cancer Research. Available at: www.aicr.org. Accessed July 8, 2004.

94. FANSA. Statement on Diet and Cancer Prevention in the U.S. Available at: www.eatright.org. Accessed July 7, 2004.

95. Byers T, Nestle M, McTiernan A, et al. American Cancer Society guidelines on nutrition and physical activity for cancer prevention: reducing the risk of cancer with healthy food choices and physical activity. *CA Cancer J Clin*. 2002;52:92–111.

96. Stewart SL, King JB, Thompson TD, Friedman C, Wingo P. Cancer mortality surveillance–U.S., 1990–2000. National Center for Chronic Disease Prevention and Health Promotion. *MMWR*. 2004;53(S503):1–108.

97. National Institutes of Health, National Institute of Diabetes and Digestive and Kidney Diseases. Diabetes Prevention Program. Available at: www.preventdiabetes.com. Accessed July 9, 2004.

98. Centers for Disease Control and Prevention. National diabetes fact sheet: general information and national estimates on diabetes in the U.S., 2003. Rev. ed. Atlanta, Ga.: U.S. Dept. of Health and Human Services, Centers for Disease Control and Prevention; 2004.

99. U.S. Department of Health and Human Services. *Healthy People 2010: understanding and improving health.* 2nd ed. Washington, DC: U.S. DHHS; 2000. 3-34–5-35.

100. Mokdad AH, Ford ES, Bowman BA, et al. Diabetes trends in the U.S.: 1990–1998. *Diabetes Care.* 2000;23:1278–1283.

101. Diabetes Prevention Program Research Group. Reduction in the incidence of type 2 diabetes with lifestyle intervention or metformin. *N Engl J Med.* 2003;346:393–403.

102. Franz MJ, Bantle JP, Beebe CA, et al. Nutrition principles and recommendations in diabetes. *Diabetes Care.* 2004;27:S36.

103. National Institutes of Health. Osteoporosis and Related Bone Diseases, National Resource Center, 2003. Available at: www.osteo.org. Accessed July 12, 2004.

104. National Osteoporosis Foundation. Osteoporosis, Disease Statistics, 2004. Available at: www.nof.org. Accessed July 12, 2004.

105. Heany RP. The importance of calcium intake for lifelong skeletal health. *Calcif Tissue Int.* 2002;70:70–73.

106. National Institutes of Health. Consensus Development Panel on osteoporosis. *JAMA.* 2001;285:785.

107. Standing Committee on the Scientific Evaluation of Dietary Reference Intakes. Food and Nutrition Board, Institutes of Medicine. *Dietary Reference Intakes for calcium, phosphorus, magnesium, vitamin D, and fluoride.* Washington, DC: National Academy Press; 1999.

108. The benefits of dairy foods in health promotion. *Dairy Council Digest.* 2004;75(3).

109. Centers for Disease Control and Prevention. HIV/AIDS Surveillance Report, CDC. Addendum. 2002;13(2).

110. U.S. Department of Health and Human Services. *Healthy People 2010: understanding and improving health.* 2nd ed. Washington, DC: U.S. DHHS; 2000. 13-3–13-27-HIV.

111. Position of the American Dietetic Association and Dietitians of Canada. Nutrition intervention in the care of persons with human immunodeficiency virus infection. *J Am Diet Assoc.* 2000;100:708–717.

CHAPTER 12

ASSURING NUTRITION FOR OLDER ADULTS

Joseph M. Carlin, MS, RD, LDN, FADA*

Reader Objectives

After studying this chapter and reflecting on the contents, you should be able to:

1. Describe how the number of older Americans is growing due to improvements in healthcare, including nutrition.
2. Discuss the degree to which older Americans suffered from food insecurity and hunger prior to the implementation of government-sponsored nutrition intervention programs.
3. Describe the factors that laid the groundwork for federally funded elderly nutrition programs.
4. Outline factors that promoted the success of the Older Americans Nutrition Program.
5. Learn the importance of evaluation as a critical step in planning nutrition interventions.
6. Suggest ideas that might influence better nutrition among the elderly in the future.

An Aging Population

The second half of the twentieth century was a time when Americans began to take notice of the growing sea of older people around them. While the total population of the United States grew from 150 million to 281 million from 1950 to 2000 (almost doubling in size), the population of those 65 and older grew more rapidly, increasing from 12 million to 35 million (an almost three-fold increase).[i] Even more impressive was the growth in the population over 75 years of age, which increased from 4 million to 17 million persons. This trend is expected to continue for the next 50 years, but at a slower rate.

During the first half of the twentieth century, improvements in the prevention and control of infectious diseases had a profound ef-

*Joseph M. Carlin, MS, MA, RD, LDN, FADA is a Regional Nutritionist with the U.S. Administration on Aging, Boston, Massachusetts. The views expressed in this paper are the author's and do not necessarily reflect those of the Administration on Aging.

fect on increasing life expectancy. After 1950 improvements in nutrition, housing, hygiene, and medical care contributed to a longer life span. Life expectancy at birth increased for men from 48 years in 1901 to 74 years of age in 2001; for women, the increases were even more impressive, increasing from 51 to almost 80 years of age.[ii] The life expectancy of those in other countries, particularly Japan, holds out hope that longevity can be increased even more in the United States.

One of the major reasons people are living longer is due to decreases in mortality due to heart disease, stroke, and unintentional injuries. Government statistics reveal that although heart disease is still the leading cause of death in the United States, the death rate from heart disease decreased 59% from 1950 to 2002. The death rate from stroke declined 69% during the same period. Both of these diseases are closely associated with high blood pressure, high cholesterol, lack of physical activity, and obesity. Health promotion initiatives, healthier lifestyles, and exercise programs offer the potential of increasing life expectancy.

The aging of the population has important consequences to the health and well-being of all Americans. Not only will it put increased demands upon the healthcare system, but at the community level there will be a similar demand for a full range of services, including nutrition services.

Prior to the 1970s, older Americans were more likely to be classified as living in poverty than any other age group. With the availability of inflation-adjusted government social insurance programs—Social Security, Supplemental Security Income, and nutrition intervention programs such as Food Stamps and the Elderly Nutrition Program—the poverty rate for older Americans declined rapidly from about 30% in 1970 to about 12% in 2000.

See www.nutrition.gov to search for the different nutrition programs provided by the U.S. government.

One method of assessing food and nutrition problems in the community is the concept of "food insecurity." Food insecurity is a term used to convey the idea that the "availability of nutritionally adequate and safe foods or the ability to acquire acceptable foods in socially acceptable ways is limited or uncertain."[iii] Among those who experience food insecurity can be people who suffer from true hunger, which is defined as the "uneasy or painful sensation caused by a lack of food."[iii] The ideal is to ensure that all older Americans are food secure, meaning that throughout the year they have "access, at all times, to enough food for an active, healthy life."[iv] A household food security study conducted by the U.S. Department of Agriculture in 2003 found that the prevalence rate for food insecurity in households with elderly persons was 1.7%. This

Read more about food insecurity in all ages of the U.S. population in Chapter 17.

increased to 2.1% for elderly persons living alone.[v] The idea of food insecurity, and the more precise definition of hunger, are major improvements over the vague and difficult-to-define term *malnutrition*—both under- and over-malnutrition—that was popular for most of the twentieth century.

Feeding America's Elderly

On March 27, 1972, Congress passed Public Law 92-258, adding a new Title VII to the Older Americans Act (OAA), establishing a permanent program to provide lifesaving meals to the elderly. Even though the new Elderly Nutrition Program (ENP) had bipartisan support in Congress, it was held hostage when the appropriation bill, which provided funding for the new ti-

> Read more about Public Law 92-258 and Title VII at:
> www.grantcommunity.com/cfdaprog/p93045.htm.

tle, was attached to the "Cease Fire in Cambodia Bombing Bill," and was repeatedly vetoed by the President. During the summer of 1973, the funds were finely released to the states. Almost overnight, thousands of community centers opened their doors to the elderly and began the process of delivering meals to older people's homes.

At that time, the law specified that meals were to be served in a congregate setting for socialization purposes and were to be delivered to the homes of those with serious mobility problems. The justification for this new program grew out of the social activism that paralleled America's soul searching during the 1960s, which was at the height of this country's involvement in the Vietnam War and the Civil Rights movement. Providing nutritious meals to America's elderly was viewed as one of the many corrective actions society needed to take to provide for a more just America. Ending the Vietnam War and providing justice for African Americans were similar goals. The elderly were not the only group in society to be singled out for nutrition intervention programs. Both the U.S. Department of Agriculture's Food Stamp and Commodity Foods Distribution programs were expanded and the Supplemental Nutrition Program for Women, Infants and Children (WIC) were initiated.

Following the implementation of these new nutrition intervention programs, the United States became acutely aware of its domestic hunger issues. The Food Stamp Program grew from a $288 million program, serving 2.8 million people, to a $6 billion program by 1978. Free or reduced price lunches for poor children grew from a $42 million program for 3 million children to a $1.2 billion program serving 12 million children. Child care and summer food service for children grew from a $3.2 million program serving 140,000 to a $250 million program serving 3 million children.[vi]

The idea that would eventually result in the federal government promoting and financing a nutrition program for the elderly started to take shape shortly after the Second World War. In 1954, a group of women in a Philadelphia neighborhood decided to pack sandwiches in brown paper bags and deliver them to elderly "shut-ins." Newspaper accounts of the efforts of these "angels" delivering "meals on wheels" captured the imagination of America. As the story was repeated across the nation in newspaper accounts, women in other communities began to copy the Philadelphia angels. A survey conducted at the request of the federal government in 1971 counted 311 of these "meals on wheels" programs. Some programs served as few as 10 people a day, while others served over 100. No one knows where the women got the original idea for this successful program. We know that in London during the Second World War, efforts were made by relief groups to deliver meals to older people trapped by the blitz. Some of these Philadelphia women may have heard about these British efforts from their soldier husbands stationed in London during the war.[vii]

Before these small efforts to deliver meals to the homebound were created, formal programs to protect the nutritional well-being of the elderly did not exist. It was believed at that time that the needs of older people were being met at home by their families. Forgotten were the tremendous sociological changes that had occurred during the twentieth century, particularly after World War II. Children were moving away from home to take jobs a considerable distance away from their parents and grandparents. Furthermore, many older people, particularly women, found themselves living alone after the premature death of a husband. With decreased economic resources to provide for their health and well-being, a large number of older people suffered from food insecurity. When faced with the decision of whether to spend their scarce resources on food, prescription drugs, rent, or utilities, they chose to pay the rent. As their numbers grew, their desperate situation could no longer be ignored. In retrospect, it would not be unreasonable to conclude that prior to the establishment of elderly nutrition programs, many older people suffered from high mortality and morbidity rates because of the lack of proper nutrition.

In the late 1960s, the health and nutrition-related problems of the elderly came to the attention of Congress, particularly the Senate Select Committee on Nutrition and Human Needs chaired by Senator George McGovern. This committee held some of the first hearings ever on the nutritional problems associated with aging in America. These hearings were just one of several defining events during the 1960s that focused attention on the nutritional needs of America's elderly. In 1968, Congress authorized President Johnson to fund several demonstration programs to investigate the extent of the problem and test methods for delivering nutritional resources to the elderly.

The idea for a federally supported nutrition program specifically targeting the elderly began taking root during the 1961 White House Conference on Aging. The deciding event during this turbulent period was the negative findings that came from the USDA's 1965 National Food Study on Food Consumption and Dietary Level. This study produced the shocking finding that as many as 6 to 8 million older persons might have deficient diets. These troubling statistics resulted in the creation of a task force on nutrition to develop both administrative and legislative recommendations for correcting the problem. This task force decided to spend $2 million yearly for 3 years on demonstrations and to collect data in a systematic way concerning the nutrition needs of the elderly. These early demonstration programs tested two potential models for providing meals to older people: home-delivered meals and meals provided in group settings, called congregate meals. The home-delivered meals model was clearly modeled after existing community meals on wheels programs. The congregate program took as its model programs operated in the Jewish settlement houses located in the lower east side of Manhattan. Two of the original 23 demonstration programs were located in Manhattan at the Henry Street Settlement House and the Hudson Guild-Fulton Senior Association.[viii]

By the time the White House Conference on Nutrition and Human Needs was held in 1969, the idea for a federally supported nutrition program for the elderly had the backing of federal policy makers. At the 1971 White House Conference on Aging, solid information from the many Title IV demonstration programs was available. By this time a set of shared principles about the urgent need to respond to the nutritional needs of the elderly existed within the professional nutrition community and among political leaders. These values were incorporated into the Older Americans Act and to this day continue to serve as the basic justification for Congress and the administration to continue to support the program. These fundamental principles, as written into the Older Americans Act, declare that:

> More information about the Older Americans Act is available at www.aoa.gov/about/legbudg/oaa/legbudg_oaa.asp.

> . . . the purpose of the new nutrition program is to meet the acute need for a national policy which: provides older Americans, particularly those with low incomes, with low cost, nutritionally sound meals served in strategically located centers such as schools, churches, community centers, senior citizen centers, and other public or private facilities where they can obtain other social and rehabilitative services. Besides promoting better health among the older segment of the population through improved nu-

trition, such a program is aimed at reducing the isolation of old age, offering older Americans the opportunity to live their remaining years in dignity.

When the above statement was written, it was not envisioned that home-delivered meals would be a major part of the program. In the beginning, federal regulations required that state plans ensure that nutrition programs "provide home-delivered meals where necessary and feasible to meet the needs of target group eligible individuals who are homebound."[ix] There was a perception, at least at the federal level, that private *Meals on Wheels* programs would continue to grow parallel with the OAA home-delivered meals component. Because of this perception, home-delivered meals were capped, and the total number of meals served that way could not exceed 10% of the total meals served in the state. It was assumed that independent *Meals on Wheels* providers had the capacity to expand and would want to remain independent of the federally funded programs.

This assumption was unfounded, and *Meals on Wheels* programs soon petitioned the states to be designated as the local service provider. They aggressively pursued federal funding to expand their programs. A few did remain independent, at least for a time, and continued to use the designation *Meals on Wheels* to distinguish themselves from the rapidly expanding federal home-delivered meals programs.

It soon became clear that the policy restricting home-delivered meals to 10% was unworkable. It was raised incrementally over the first couple of years by the Administration on Aging (AoA) until Congress intervened in 1978 to amend the OAA, eliminating Title VII. The new amendments created the nutrition program anew, providing separate funding for congregate and home-delivered meals.

That separation continues to be in effect, with home-delivered meals representing almost 60% of all meals served. Clearly, the United States' expanding population of very frail elderly homebound is vulnerable and at great nutritional risk. Today, home-delivered meals and *Meals on Wheels* are different names for the same program.

In their yearly budget requests to Congress, the AoA has put the following clear and convincing reasons forward as to why home-delivered meals should continue to exist and even expand.[x] A home-delivered meal:

- "[Is] the first in-home service that an older adult receives . . ."
- "Serves as a primary access point for all other in-home services."
- "Improves participant nutrient intake, decreases food insecurity, increases social interaction and decreases social isolation, contributing to improved quality of life."

- "Play[s] an important role in the treatment, management, and delay of chronic disease and disease-related disability."
- "Provides an essential service to many caregivers by helping them maintain their own health and continued functionality."
- "Assists in decreasing the risk of complications associated with acute and chronic disease and contribute to improvements in quality of life."

In summary, the home-delivered meal program "is a smart, cost-effective investment of public funds."

Factors That Promote Program Success

Over the past 30-plus years, the Elderly Nutrition Program, also called the Older Americans Nutrition Program, has been viewed as a resounding success for many reasons. First, it set out to do exactly what it was charged to accomplish and had a positive and lasting nutritional impact on those who participated in the program. Second, states, area agencies on aging, and local service providers did not rely solely upon federal funding to support the program. In addition to participant donations, service providers tapped into their state legislatures for additional funding and received financial support from cities and towns in which the programs operated. To supplement these funds, programs turned to fund-raising and the use of in-kind resources including facilities, and developed one of the most extensive and effective volunteer efforts in the country. In short, this program was made a success by the hundreds of thousands of volunteers who daily perform labor-intensive tasks, such as delivering hot meals to the homes of the isolated elderly.

> The Elderly Nutrition Program can be found on the AoA website at www.aoa.gov.

Another reason for the success of the program, which seldom gets full credit today, is the careful planning that went into its design and implementation. These carefully planned steps ensured the stability and longevity of the program. These steps can serve as a textbook case study of how to implement a complicated nutrition intervention program.

AoA put in place an administrative structure, detailed policies and procedures, and a training strategy that effectively ensured that all providers of this new and unproven program had the knowledge and skills to operate a successful program. Even before the first meals were served, AoA had authored a carefully thought-out set of regulations, policies, and a comprehensive training manual. That training manual was so comprehensive and carefully thought out that after 30 years, it is still in use and is affectionately referred to as the "Green Bible," because of its green vinyl cover.

Within AoA, a unit was created to oversee this new program, headed up by Donald Watkins, MD, an international authority in the area of nutritional gerontology. He had 3 experienced nutritionists on his immediate staff, plus 10 highly skilled nutritionists, one in each of AoA's 10 regional offices. This team of experienced nutritionists provided technical assistance to the states on issues of nutrition, nutrition education, food service management, and food safety.

AoA funded five training centers strategically located across the country to train state and local service providers. The first directors of these Elderly Nutrition Programs received a minimum of 80 hours of instruction on the nutritional needs of older people, food service operations, sanitation, and basic social gerontology concepts, in addition to accounting and fiscal management basics.

Behind the backbone of this strong administrative structure, training, and technical assistance was the law itself, which provided straightforward guidance to the states on how to implement this program. It was clear from the language in the law that Congress expected the meals to be nutritious. Each meal had to contain one-third of the Recommended Dietary Allowances (RDAs), a reasonable target, given that very little was known about the nutritional needs of older persons at that time. When the program was first created, there was a strong belief that meals should be hot at the time of service, a concession to those older people and professional nutritionists who wanted to set the quality bar as high as possible. Older people, consulted in the 1970s about the design of the program, had vivid memories of the depression and did not want to participate in a program that would be demeaning or humiliating. They did not want a meal that could in any way be interpreted as "being on the dole." They wanted to sit down to a "hot meal." This program was not to become a soup and sandwich program common during the depression!

Considerable thought was given to the delicate issue of how much participants should contribute to the cost of these meals. Some elderly people clearly had the resources to pay for these meals while others, just as clearly, did not. The solution to this dilemma was to install a donation system; participants could determine for themselves what they considered fair. Furthermore, this donation system was to be implemented in a way that protected the confidentiality and dignity of the participant. The decision not to charge older people for their meals has contributed in large measure to the success of the program. The need for humans to reciprocate in kind with a token of value is a concept that sets our species apart from other animals and has been part of our character throughout our evolutionary progress. In short, human adults feel a sense of anxiety, or at least a state of discomfort, when sharing food with others outside the family. Humans feel a natural tendency to reciprocate with something of equal value when offered food. This something of value can be money. Based upon present data, older people contributed at least $160 million yearly to the support of this program.

The genius of this program lies in part in the simplicity of the legislation and accompanying regulations, which advocate for the needs of the elderly while promoting objectives that respect older people's needs for independence.

Like any law, it was not designed without flaws. As originally written, only hot meals could be served, and each meal had to meet one-third of the RDAs. In 1978, the law was amended to permit other than hot meals to be served, but they still had to meet the strict one-third RDA requirement. In 1990, the law was amended again to permit programs to offer a two-meals-a-day program, as long as the two meals combined equaled two-thirds of the RDA. Similarly, if three meals were served, the combined meals had to equal 100% of the RDA. (Note that the RDAs have now been replaced with the Dietary Reference Intakes.) These two changes, although not minor, attest to how well the program was designed in the beginning. These examples also demonstrate three truths: First, it is difficult, if not impossible, to write a flawless law because all variables cannot be anticipated. Second, when writing legislation, extreme care needs to be taken; once something is put in the law, it might take years to make a correction. Third, all programs need to be monitored and periodically evaluated to ensure that the program is doing what it is supposed to do. Changing policy, procedures, or even the law may be necessary to put the program back on track. The simplicity of the nutrition provisions in the OAA has afforded both AoA and the states maximum flexibility on administering this program.

Meals are provided in a variety of settings, such as senior centers, senior housing facilities, schools, and church basements. Some meals are cooked on site; some are prepared in central commissaries and delivered to meal sites. In most cases meals are prepared under contract with large food service management companies. A growing number of service providers have turned to frozen pre-plated meals, not only for home-delivered meals, but also for congregate participants. Approximately 250 million meals are served yearly, with about 57% home-delivered and 43% congregate.

Evaluation

The question has to be asked: "Did the Elderly Nutrition Program accomplish what it set out to accomplish?" Between 1993 and 1995, AoA funded a nationwide evaluation of the Elderly Nutrition Program (ENP) as required under the Older Americans Act of 1965 when it was amended in 1992.[xi] The legislation specified 19 areas for evaluation, with emphasis on the following:

- ENP's effects on participants' nutrition and socialization, compared with a similar population that does not participate in congregate or home-delivered meals programs.
- Is the program targeted to those who need the services most?
- How efficiently and effectively are services administered and delivered?
- What funds are available, and how are they allocated to service providers?

Mathematica Policy Research, Inc. was the contractor for the evaluation. It found that both congregate and homebound ENP participants, when compared with the overall U.S. population 60 years of age and older, were: 1) older by 4 to 6 years; 2) more than two-thirds female (69%); 3) lived alone; and 4) were more likely to be impoverished.[xii]

For almost all of the nutrients studied, both congregate and home-delivered meals supplied well over a third of participants' daily intake. Many meals provided 40% to 50% of the RDAs. As to how the participants thought about the meals, about two-thirds of both congregate and home-delivered participants described themselves as being "very satisfied" with the taste of the food. The Mathematica team summed up their findings as follows:

> The ENP serves highly vulnerable people with characteristics that tend to put them at increased health and nutritional risk. ENP participants tend to be older, poorer, more likely to be members of racial or ethnic minorities, and more likely to live alone, compared with the overall population in the U.S. age 60 and older. Participants are also more likely to be in poor health, to have greater difficulty performing everyday tasks, and to have relatively high nutritional risk.[xiii]

The 1990s evaluation found that the program is serving the target population. This information is critical to the future of the program because it demonstrates that the ENP program is doing exactly what it set out to do. Programs that do what they are designed to do, and do it efficiently and effectively, are more likely to be successful in attracting future funding.

Because comprehensive evaluation research, such as that carried out by Mathematica, is expensive, AoA has used a number of tested performance measurement surveys to get a snapshot of how recipients of services rate the service, whether services are effectively targeted to vulnerable individuals, and whether services help older persons to maintain their independence and avoid premature institutionalization. AoA's 2003 *Annual Report*[xiv] shared with the aging network the results on this survey.

AoA found that home-delivered nutrition services "are effectively targeted to vulnerable populations." They found that 59% of respondents lived alone, 69% were 75 years of age or over, and 79%

had difficulty with at least one activity of daily living (ADL), such as eating.

One element, critical to the success of the home-delivered meals program, is how well the participants like their meals. If the meals are not consumed, or only half eaten, no benefit is derived. This can be observed directly at congregate sites, but direct observation of eating patterns in the home of participants is difficult. In addition, delivering hot and tasty meals to people's homes has always been a major logistical and quality challenge. In spite of all the difficulties in delivering these meals, 94% of respondents surveyed said that they liked the meal; 91% reported that meals almost always arrive when expected.

Since the early 1990s, nutrition programs have been using the Determine Your Nutritional Health[xv] checklist as a tool to see to what degree participants are at nutritional risk. The survey found that 73% of respondents were at high nutritional risk. This figure does not sound unrealistic when 62% of respondents are reporting that the typical home-delivered meal provides one-half or more of their daily food intake. Twenty-five percent of respondents said that they did not always have enough money or food stamps to buy food. Clearly, food insecurity is a major problem among this vulnerable population.

> Find the Determine Your Nutritional Health checklist at www.aafp.org/x16095.xml.

When congregate meal participants were surveyed, 64% were 75 years or older and 56% lived alone. As for the quality of the meals, 92% of respondents said they were satisfied with the taste of the food, and 97% were satisfied with the temperature of the food.

When the congregate meals program was designed in the early 1970s, socialization opportunities for participants was one of the primary goals. The importance of socialization as a health factor was highlighted in a major study published in *Science*. The authors, after examining the literature on the subject, found that:

> . . . social relationships, or the relative lack thereof, constitute a major risk factor for health-rivaling the effects of well-established health risk factors such as cigarette smoking, blood pressure, blood lipids, obesity, and physical activity.[xvi]

AoA's survey found that 96% of respondents like to visit with friends at the site; 73% like to participate in activities at the meal site; and 60% reported that their social opportunities have increased since they started receiving congregate nutrition services.

Over the life of the ENP program, all formal and less formal evaluations have found the same results; the program does exactly what it was designed to do.

Other Nutrition Interventions

As America's consciousness of the needs of older people grew, old programs were redesigned, others scaled back, and new programs implemented to meet the nutritional needs of the elderly. The government appropriates about $1 billion annually for all food and nutrition intervention programs for older adults.[xvii] The largest of these is AoA's Older Americans Nutrition Program. Although AoA's program may be the most visible nutrition intervention in the public's mind, it is not the only federal program designed to improve the nutritional well-being of older persons. Other federal interventions include Food Stamps, Commodity Supplemental Food Program, Child and Adult Care Food Program, Farmers' Market Nutrition Program, waivers under the Medicaid program, and Medical Nutrition Therapy (MNT) for Medicare beneficiaries. Nutrition education activities carried out in the various states, under the Cooperative Extension Service, can also be added to this list. (Medicare and the other government programs are also discussed in subsequent chapters.)

Food Stamp Program

By far the largest of these programs in both numbers of participants and cost is the Food Stamp Program administered by the U.S. Department of Agriculture. The program provides older people with food coupons or electronic benefit transfer cards that can be used to purchase food items at retail stores. The purpose of the program is to assist low-income families, including the elderly, to buy food that is nutritionally adequate. The USDA Food and Nutrition Service estimated that 1.5 million elderly households received about $1 billion in benefits ($59 monthly, per household) in 1998.[xviii]

The Commodity Supplemental Food Program

The Commodity Supplemental Food Program provides packaged food (such as juice, powdered milk, canned vegetables, and meat) to low-income participants, including older persons. Older persons must have a household income at or below 130% of the poverty level. In fiscal year 2000, $88.3 million was appropriated for this program. In 1999, about 71% (270,000 of the total enrollment of almost 382,000 people) of those enrolled in this program were older.[xix] Only 33 states and 2 reservations participate in the program.[xx]

The Child and Adult Care Food Program

The Child and Adult Care Food Program serves any person 60 years of age or older, and any person 18 years of age or older who also has a functional impairment and attends a nonresidential daycare facility. The program provides meal reimbursements to the daycare facility, if licensed or approved by the state. The Food and Nutrition Service, which administers this program, does not maintain statistics on those aged 60 or older. But, in fiscal year 1999, 1,855 facilities served an average of 62,500 adults aged 18 or over. This program received $1.6 billion in federal funds in fiscal year 1999.[xxi]

Seniors Farmers' Market Nutrition Program

In 2000, the USDA created the Seniors Farmers' Market Nutrition Program to improve nutrition and food security among low-income senior citizens by helping them to purchase more fresh fruits and vegetables at farmers' markets.[xxii] This program is modeled after the Market Coupon Program developed by the Massachusetts Department of Food and Agriculture in 1986, which had as its focus participants in the WIC program. Seniors at nutritional risk were added in 1987.[xxiii]

This program provides coupons to low-income seniors, which can be exchanged for eligible foods at farmers' markets, roadside stands, and community-supported agriculture programs. Besides providing fresh and nutritious foods for the elderly, the program is also designed to increase the domestic consumption of agricultural commodities and to help expand the network of farmers' markets. Fifteen million dollars in direct funding is available to the states each year. About 700,000 older people were served in fiscal year 2003.[xxiv]

The Future

It is impossible to predict how the federally funded nutrition program for the elderly will evolve in the future, but it will change. Those familiar with the program anticipate that issues centered around wellness, lifestyle, health promotion, nutrition education, and exercise will become more important among an aging population as they try to stay healthy and fit as long as possible.

Some nutrition practitioners, disappointed with the poor results of traditional nutrition education strategies whereby older people sit through information-filled lectures, are experimenting with promising new strategies. One model is the Healthy Eating for Successful Living in Older Adults program, an evidence-based healthy eating program developed by an expert advisory panel under the supervision of the Lahey Clinic in Massachusetts. This project is part of the Model Programs Project sponsored by the National Council on the Aging (NCOA) with funding from the John A. Hartford Foundation.[xxv] It is both an educational and support program designed to help older Americans take control of their nutritional health. The program stresses self-management strategies using behavior modification approaches.

Another opportunity that holds promise for improving the health of seniors is the Internet. Although less than a third (31%) of older Americans have ever gone online, their numbers can be expected to increase dramatically over the next few years. A recent survey of seniors who use the Internet, released in 2005 by the Kaiser Family Foundation, found that topics related to prescription drugs were the most popular issue, followed by searches for information on nutrition, exercise or weight control, cancer, heart disease, and arthritis. This survey found that seniors say that they consider e-mail and the Internet an important part of their lives that "they wouldn't want to do without."[xxvi]

The future of the Older Americans Nutrition Program, and other federally supported nutrition programs, can be expected to be a valuable part of this nation's "safety net" for ensuring the independence, health, and longevity of America's aging population. To ensure that these programs are efficient and effective, program managers at all levels—federal, state, and community—must continually assess the nutrition needs of the elderly, modify the programs to meet those needs, and periodically evaluate the program to ensure that it is doing what it was designed to do. If these tried and true methods are followed, there is no reason why all Americans can't grow old, knowing that there will be a program to meet their nutrition needs if they ever need it.

Issues for Discussion

1. Compare a nutrition program that is available in another country (if known) to the present nutrition program for elders in the United States. What are the similarities and differences?
2. Discuss the ethical implications of a government-funded nutrition program for the elderly.
3. Discuss possible improvements for future nutrition programs for the great number of elders the United States will experience by 2010.

References

i. National Center for Health Statistics. (2004). *Health, U.S., 2004 with chartbook on trends in the health of Americans.* Hyattsville, MD: U.S. Department of Health and Human Services, Centers for Disease Control and Prevention, 21. (DHHS Pub. No. 2004-1232)
ii. National Center for Health Statistics. (2004). *Health, U.S., 2004 with chartbook on trends in the health of Americans.* Hyattsville, MD: U.S. Department of Health and Human Services, Centers for Disease Control and Prevention, 44. (DHHS Pub. No. 2004-1232)

iii. Frongillo, Edward & Horan, Claire M. (Fall 2004). Hunger and aging. *Generations: Journal of the American Society on Aging*, XXVIII(3), 28–33.

iv. Nord, Mark, Andrews, Margaret, & Carlson, Steven. (2004). *Household food security in the U.S., 2003*. Washington, DC: USDA Economic Research Service, i.

v. Nord, Mark, Andrews, Margaret, & Carlson, Steven. (2004). *Household food security in the US, 2003*. Washington, DC: USDA Economic Research Service, 9.

vi. Kotz, Nick. (1979). *Hunger in America: The federal response*. New York: The Field Foundation, 10–11.

vii. Carlin, Joseph M. (2004). Meals on Wheels. In (ed.), *Oxford Encyclopedia of Food and Drink in America*. New York: Oxford University Press.

viii. Bechill, William D. & Wolgamot, Irene. (1973). *Nutrition for the elderly. The program highlights of research and development nutrition projects funded under Title IV of the Older Americans Act of 1965*. Washington, DC: U.S. Department of Health, Education, and Welfare, Administration on Aging.

ix. Administration on Aging. Budget request for fiscal year 2003 by the Administration on Aging. *Federal Register*. (August 19, 1972). 37(162), 16848.

x. *Budget request for fiscal year 2003 by the Administration on Aging*. 2003. Washington, DC: U.S. Department of Health and Human Services.

xi. U.S. House of Representatives. *Older Americans Act of 1965 and the Native American Programs Act of 1974 as amended through December 31, 1992*. (June 15, 1993). Washington, DC: Committee on Education and Labor of the U.S. House of Representatives, Serial No. 103-E, 22–24.

xii. Millen, Barbara E., Ohls, James C., Ponza, Michael, & McCool, Audrey C. ( ). The Elderly Nutrition Program: An effective national framework for preventive nutrition interventions. *Journal of the American Dietetic Association*, 102(2), 234–240.

xiii. Ponza, Michael, Ohls, James C., & Millen, Barbara E. (1996). *Serving elders at risk*. Washington, DC: Mathematica Policy Research, Inc. for the U.S. Department of Health and Human Services, Administration on Aging, 12.

xiv. Administration on Aging. (2004). *2003 annual report—What we do makes a difference*. Washington, DC: U.S. Department of Health and Human Services.

xv. The Nutrition Screening Initiative. (1991). *Nutrition screening manual for professionals caring for older Americans*. Washington, DC: The American Academy of Family Physicians, 4–5.

xvi. House, James S., Landis, Karl R., & Umberson, Debra. (July 29, 1988). Social relationships and health. *Science*, 241, 541.

xvii. Wellman, Nancy S. & Kamp, Barbara. (Fall 2004). Federal food and nutrition assistance programs for older people. *Generations: Journal of the American Society on Aging*, 27(3), 78.

xviii. U.S. General Accounting Office. *Food assistance: Options for improving nutrition for older Americans*. (August 2000). Washington, DC: U.S. General Accounting Office, 6. (GAO/RCED-00-238)

xix. U.S. General Accounting Office. *Food assistance: Options for improving nutrition for older Americans.* (August 2000). Washington, DC: U.S. General Accounting Office. Washington, DC, 7-8. (GAO/RCED-00-238)

xx. Wellman, Nancy S. & Kamp, Barbara. (Fall 2004). Federal food and nutrition assistance programs for older people. *Generations: Journal of the American Society on Aging,* 27(3), 85.

xxi. U.S. General Accounting Office. *Food assistance: Options for improving nutrition for older Americans.* (August 2000). Washington, DC: U.S. General Accounting Office. Washington, DC, 8-9. (GAO/RCED-00-238)

xxii. Older Americans Report. Clinton's food security initiative will help seniors get fresh produce. (December 1, 2000). *Older Americans Report,* 403.

xxiii. Balsam, Alan, Webber, David, & Oehlke, Bonita. (1994). The farmers' market coupon program for low-income elders. *Journal of Nutrition for the Elderly,* 13(4), 35–42.

xxiv. Wellman, Nancy S. & Kamp, Barbara. (Fall 2004). Federal food and nutrition assistance programs for older people. *Generations: Journal of the American Society on Aging,* 27(3), 85.

xxv. *Healthy Eating for Successful Living in Older Adults.* (2004). Model Programs Project sponsored by the National Council on the Aging (NCOA) with funding from the John A. Hartford Foundation.

xxvi. *e-health and the elderly: How seniors use the Internet for health.* Press Release. (January 12, 2005). Menlo Park, CA: Kaiser Family Foundation in consultation with Princeton Survey Research Associates (PSRA).

CHAPTER 13

PROVIDING NUTRITION SERVICES IN PUBLIC HEALTH PRIMARY CARE

Arlene Spark, EdD, RD, FADA, FACN

Reader Objectives

After studying this chapter and reflecting on the contents, you should be able to:

1. Describe what primary healthcare is.
2. Understand where primary care is practiced.
3. Discuss who the providers and recipients of primary care are.
4. Explain how primary care services are financed.
5. Describe the scope and breadth of nutrition services available in primary care settings, why barriers exist to providing nutrition services in primary healthcare, and how those barriers may be overcome.

Primary Care: Setting, Practice, Providers

There tends to be a lack of clarity and consensus about the term *primary care*. The confusion may be attributed to the numerous meanings of the word *primary*. Among its many meanings are main, chief, most important, key, prime, principal, crucial, fundamental, core, central, essential, basic, and important, as well as first, initial, leading, top, and foremost. If *primary* is understood to connote *first, initial,* or *leading* in time or order, this leads to a relatively narrow concept of primary care as "first contact" or the entry point of healthcare delivery. This narrow definition of primary care connotes only a triage function in which patients are then passed on to a higher level of care. If, on the other hand, *primary* is understood in its sense of *chief, principal,* or *main,* then *primary care* is understood as central and fundamental to health care. This latter idea supports the multidimensional view of primary care envisioned in the Institute of Medicine's (IOM) report, *Primary Care: America's Health in a New Era* (1996).[1] That primary care is fundamental to healthcare is also the view envisioned in this chapter.

The IOM defines primary care as:

> . . . the provision of integrated, accessible healthcare services by clinicians who are accountable for addressing a large majority of personal health needs, developing a sustained partnership with patients, and practicing in the context of family and community.[2]

According to this definition, primary care is a function predicated on relationships and collaboration (rather than boundaries between specialties and disciplines). It emphasizes the clinician's role as the patient's partner and advocate, as the patient navigates his or her way through the healthcare system. The IOM recommends that primary care should be viewed as a central mission of the healthcare system (not as a feeder to tertiary care), and that it should be provided by teams that bring:

> . . . different kinds of expertise . . . to bear on the patient's needs through collaborative activity, and . . . permit the delegation of some tasks by broadening the range of professionals involved in primary care.[3]

Primary care is *continuing, comprehensive*, and *preventive* personal medical care. The primary care setting includes all public and/or private outpatient clinics and private practices that offer office-based general medical care. (Although not considered here, primary care settings also include emergency rooms, acute care facilities, chronic care facilities, and addiction treatment facilities.) Typically, primary care practice is defined within the categories of pediatrics, adolescent medicine, general internal medicine, family practice, geriatrics, and obstetrics and gynecology. Providers of primary care include allopathic physicians or medical doctors (MDs) and osteopathic physicians or doctors of osteopathy (DOs). Primary care physicians often work with other healthcare providers, such as physician assistants (PAs), nurse practitioners (NPs), registered nurses (RNs), social workers, nutritionists/registered dietitians (RDs), and behavioral health practitioners. MDs and DOs are described in the accompanying sidebar.

Medical Doctors and Doctors of Osteopathy[a]

MDs practice allopathic medicine. Allopathy is defined as the system of medical practice that treats disease by using remedies that produce effects different from those produced by the disease itself. The Association of American Medical Colleges (AAMC) (http://www.aamc.org/medicalschools.htm) reports that there are 125 allopathic medical schools in the United States and an additional 17 in Canada. In 2000, the American Medical Association (AMA) estimated there were almost three-quarters of a million (737,504) active MDs in the United States, including physicians-in-training (residents and fellows), 238,734 of whom were in primary care. One-half of the physicians were located in just 10 states.[b]

In contrast, there are approximately 52,000 osteopathic physicians (DOs) in the United States,

(Continues)

The concept of primary care is so fundamental to public health that objectives to address primary care appear in the very first chapter of Healthy People 2010.[4,7] You will recall that HP 2010 is the prevention agenda for the nation. It consists of national health objectives for the most significant preventable threats to health. The primary care objectives called for in Chapter 1 of HP 2010 include:[3]

- *Objective 1.4:* Increasing the proportion of people who have a specific source of ongoing care, from 87% of the U.S. population in 1998 to 96% in 2010. (By 2001, no significant progress had been made toward this target; only 88% had ongoing care. The rate for Hispanic Americans with a regular source of ongoing care was 10% lower than for the population overall.)[5]

- *Objective 1.5:* Increasing the proportion of persons with a usual primary care provider, from 77% of the U.S. population in 1996 to 85% in 2010.

- *Objective 1.6:* Reducing the proportion of families that experience difficulties or delays in obtaining healthcare, or do not receive needed care for one or more family members, from 12% of the population in 1996 to 7% in 2010.

(Continued)

according to the American Osteopathic Association (AOA). Because osteopathic medical education places such a strong emphasis on primary medical care, two-thirds of all DOs practice in family practice, internal medicine, pediatrics, or obstetrics/gynecology. Many DOs fill the critical need for doctors by practicing in rural and medically underserved areas. In terms of education, the training of a DO is similar to that of an MD. Following graduation from one of the 20 osteopathic medical colleges in the United States, DOs complete a one-year internship, rotating through hospital departments including internal medicine, family practice, and surgery. Many then choose to complete a residency program in a specialty area, requiring 2 to 6 years of additional training. DOs are licensed for the full practice of medicine and surgery in all 50 states; in some states, the same tests are given to DOs and MDs, whereas others administer separate licensing exams.[c]

---

[a]Compiled by the author from http://www.aoa-net.org. Accessed June 28, 2003.

[b]American Medical Association. Physician Characteristics and Distribution in the United States 2002-2003 Edition, Chicago, 2002. Table "Number of Active Physicians (MDs) and Physician-to-Population Ratios by Specialty, Selected Years: 1970-2000." Available online at: http://www.healthworkforce.health.nsw.gov.au/amwac/amwac/pdf/US_health_system_overview_Anna_Kuta.pdf.

[c]Gutzler A, Kuta L. An Overview of the United States Healthcare System and Its Workforce. Presented at the International Medical Workforce Conference. Oxford, UK, 2003. Available at: http://www.healthworkforce.health.nsw.gov.au/amwac/amwac/pdf/US_health_system_overview_Anna_Kuta.pdf. Accessed April 12, 2004.

- *Objective 1.7:* Increasing the proportion of schools training doctors, nurses, and other health professionals, whose basic curriculum for healthcare providers includes the core competencies in health promotion and disease prevention.
- *Objective 1.8:* Increasing the proportion of all health professions, allied and associated health professions, and nursing degrees awarded to members of underrepresented ethnic minorities. (To achieve this objective, in 2002 the Surgeon General recommended expanding efforts to recruit minorities and people from disadvantaged backgrounds into health and allied health professions training, with an emphasis on reaching young people before they have made firm career decisions.)[6]
- Objective 1.9: Reducing hospitalization rates for ambulatory-care-sensitive conditions, such as uncontrolled diabetes, from 7.2 admissions per 10,000 persons in 1996 to 5.4 in 2010. (This objective can be accomplished by maintaining tighter glycemic control, an aim of diabetes self-management programs.)

Nutrition in Primary Care

During 2000, an estimated 823.5 million visits were made to physicians' offices in the United States. (DOs received 66.7 million office visits, or 8.1% of the total.) About 60% of the visits were to physicians in the primary care specialties. The most common nutrition-related diagnoses were essential hypertension, routine infant or child health check, type 2 diabetes mellitus, normal pregnancy, and general medical exam/prevention. Tests for blood pressure were the leading diagnostic screening tests (45.3% of office visits). Patient visits to doctors for preventive care in 2000 numbered only 6.8% of all office visits. Approximately one-third of office visits were for treatment of chronic conditions and another one-third of visits were for acute problems, such as sudden illness and accidents.

> View the complete statistics for office visits to primary care physicians and the most common diagnoses at http://www.cdc.gov/nchs/data/ad/ad328.pdf.

In today's healthcare climate, aging Americans are taking a more active role in their health, which translates into increasing numbers of visits to doctors. More than one-half of the patients who visited their physicians in 2000 were middle-aged or senior citizens. Although the number of people in the United States over 45 years of age rose 11% in the last decade, doctor visits by that age group increased 26% in the same time period. This increase in doctor visits is due primarily to the treatment of chronic diseases, which requires follow-up care.

Nutrition counseling is an appropriate component of treatment for such chronic conditions as diabetes and heart disease, and is also on the rise. Drugs for nutrition-related conditions of the heart and kidney (Lipitor, Zocor, Lasix) were among the top therapeutic classifications of drugs prescribed during physician office visits in 2000. Diagnostic and screening tests increased 28% from 1992 to 2001. Visits that included education or counseling increased by 34%. E-mail consultations were not common between doctors and their patients in 2000. Only 6% of physicians made any e-mail consultations, a percentage that is expected to increase over the next few decades. The proportion of visits to an office where a physician or physician group was the owner of the practice increased from 74.3% in 1997 to 88.1% in 2000.

Agency for Healthcare Research and Quality (AHRQ)

AHRQ is the lead U.S. federal agency for research on healthcare quality, costs, outcomes, and patient safety. It complements the biomedical research mission of its sister agency, the National Institutes of Health (NIH). AHRQ serves as a major source of funding and technical assistance for health services research and research training at leading U.S. universities and other institutions. It is home to research centers that specialize in such major areas of healthcare research as primary care (including preventive services), healthcare organization and delivery systems, and healthcare costs and sources of payment. Goals of AHRQ include supporting improvements in health outcomes by:

- Supporting research that addresses concerns of very high public priority, such as primary care practice and integrated healthcare delivery systems
- Supporting projects that test and evaluate successful methods that translate research into practice to improve patient care in diverse healthcare settings
- Translating the recommendations of the U.S. Preventive Services Task Force (USPSTF) into resources for providers, patients, and healthcare systems

The USPSTF is an independent panel of experts in primary care and prevention that systematically reviews the evidence of effectiveness and develops recommendations for clinical preventive services. Their health risk profiles and flow sheets include an Adult Health Risk Profile, a Child and Adolescent Health Risk Profile, an Adult Preventive Care Flow Sheet, and a Child and Adolescent Preven-

Health Risk Profiles and Flow Sheets are available at http://www.ahrq.gov/ppip/manual/appc.pdf.

Prevention Prescriptions are available at http://www.ahrq.gov/ppip/manual/appd.pdf.

tive Care Flow Sheet, all of which contain questions about diet. Also available from the USPSTF are Prevention Prescriptions for Adults, which consist of one-page sheets with generic strategies for prevention of a particular condition. By 2004, 15 different Prevention Prescriptions had been developed. Dietary recommendations are included in the prescriptions for weight, healthy weight, blood pressure, diabetes, colon and rectal cancer, cholesterol, and heart health.

The task force produced its first *Guide to Clinical Preventive Services* in 1989. The second edition,[8] released in 1996, provides recommendations on preventive interventions (screening tests, counseling, immunizations, and chemo prophylactic regimens) for more than 80 conditions. It includes assessments of more than 200 services offered in primary care settings for adults, pregnant women, and children. As the guide's introduction says:

> The patients for whom these services are recommended include asymptomatic individuals of all age groups and risk categories. Thus, the subject matter is relevant to all of the major primary care specialties: family practice, internal medicine, obstetrics-gynecology, and pediatrics. The recommendations in each chapter reflect a standardized review of current scientific evidence and include a summary of published clinical research regarding the clinical effectiveness of each preventive service.[8]

The third edition is available in hard copy and electronically.[9] Beginning in 2001, individual reports have been released in print and on the AHRQ website as they have been completed. The guide is used widely in medical, nursing, and nutrition education as a key reference for teaching preventive care.

A variety of clinical preventive services for normal-risk children[10] and adults[11] are recommended by the USPSTF. The recommended nutrition-related screening and counseling services include:

PKU (phenylketonuria)—A hereditary disease caused by the lack of an enzyme needed to convert an essential amino acid (phenylalanine) into a form usable by the body; can cause mental retardation unless detected early.

Sickle cell—An abnormal red blood cell that has a crescent shape and an abnormal form of hemoglobin.

Hemoglobinopathies—A group of disorders that cause changes in the type or amount of hemoglobin that is produced.

- Screening for PKU, sickle cell, hemoglobinopathies, and hypothyroidism at birth
- Measuring head circumference periodically from birth to 2 months
- Measuring height and weight periodically from birth to 18 years
- Screening for anemia and lead blood levels at 1 year
- Measuring blood pressure and determining dental health periodically, from 3 to 18 years
- Screening for alcohol use periodically, from 11 to 18 years

- Counseling parents and/or the child regarding development, nutrition, and physical activity, from birth to 18 years
- Screening blood pressure, height, weight, and obesity periodically, starting at age 18 years
- Screening cholesterol every 5 years in men starting at age 35 years and women starting at age 45 years (starting at age 20 in men and women at risk, according to a joint statement issued in 2004 by the American Cancer Society, the American Diabetes Association, and the American Heart Association)[12]
- Counseling women for calcium intake periodically, starting at 18 years of age
- Counseling women of childbearing age on folic acid
- Counseling women of childbearing age on breast-feeding after childbirth

> **Hypothyroidism**—Deficient production of thyroxin by the thyroid gland, as well as the resultant bodily condition characterized by a lowered metabolic rate, weight gain, and general loss of vigor, can cause growth and development problems in children.

To implement these recommendations, in 1994 the DHHS's Office of Disease Prevention and Health Promotion (ODPHP) launched Put Prevention Into Practice (PPIP).[13] PPIP is a national program to improve delivery of appropriate clinical preventive services, such as the screening tests and counseling recommendations listed above. The purpose of the PPIP initiative is to enable doctors and other healthcare providers to determine which services their patients should receive, facilitate the implementation of the delivery of clinical preventive services, and make it easier for patients to understand and keep track of their own preventive care. The PPIP program also works to increase the appropriate use of clinical preventive services through a variety of resources and tools for clinicians, healthcare systems, patients, and the public. For example, growth charts developed by the Centers for Disease Control and Prevention (CDC) are recommended to measure head circumference periodically from birth to 2 months and measure height and weight periodically from birth to 18 years.

> Growth Charts. Available at http://www.cdc.gov/growthcharts/.

Barriers to Providing Nutrition Services in Primary Care and Strategies for Increasing Services

Despite the myriad opportunities to offer the nutrition services described in the previous section of this chapter, multiple factors[14] hamper the fulfillment of this potential. The mitigating factors include characteristics of the physician, the healthcare establishment, financial considerations, and the patient's readiness for change. The physician may be hampered by a lack of confidence and competence in nutrition counseling, and have limited time available to spend with each patient. In addition, the organization of the medical office may not be conducive to supporting nutrition services. There may be inadequate third-party reimbursement for nutrition consultation services. Finally, the patient may have a low level of motivation or interest in changing.

Physician Confidence and Skills

Practicing physicians report a lack of confidence and related proficiency in nutrition counseling skills because of inadequate training.[15,16] Despite concerted scientific, educational, and congressional calls to increase nutrition coverage in medicine for more than half a century, most graduating medical students report an inadequate quality and quantity of nutrition training.[17,18]

Strategies to Improve Confidence and Skills

In 1997 the National Heart, Lung, and Blood Institute (NHLBI) developed the Nutrition Academic Award (NAA) Program, an initiative to improve nutrition training across a network of U.S. medical schools. The purpose of this funding was to support the development and enhancement of nutrition curricula so that medical students, residents, and practicing physicians could learn principles and practice skills in nutrition. The first 10 NAA awards were funded by NHLBI for the period 1998–2003. In 2000, nine more grants were funded by NHLBI, plus the National Institute of Diabetes and Digestive and Kidney Diseases (NIDDK) funded an additional two more. Although NHLBI has supported a number of other academic award programs addressing various topics in medical school curricula since 1970, this is the first academic award to focus primarily on nutrition.

NAA Awards—The medical schools that have received NAA awards are located at Albert Einstein College of Medicine, Brown University, Northwestern University, Tufts University, University of Alabama, University of Iowa, University of Pennsylvania, University of Rochester, University of Texas Southwestern Medical Center, the University of Washington (1998–2003), Columbia University, Harvard University, Mercer University, Stanford University, University of Arkansas, University of Colorado, University of Maryland, University of Nevada, University of Texas/Houston, University of Vermont, and the University of Wisconsin (2000–2005).

NAA recipients at the Albert Einstein College of Medicine identified the need for brief, user-friendly tools to make it possible for physicians to quickly determine a patient's diet and exercise habits, as well as provide information to aid in the delivery of effective nutrition counseling. The Einstein team developed WAVE and REAP, acronyms for tools to help physicians and other healthcare providers conduct nutrition assessments and counseling with their patients in as little as one minute. Weight, Activity, Variety and Excess (WAVE) was designed to encourage provider-patient dialogue about the pros and cons of the patient's status regarding weight, diet, and activity. The Rapid Eating and Activity Assessment for Patients (REAP) is a questionnaire designed to aid providers in performing a quick assessment of diet and physical activity. An accompanying key aids the provider in discussing the patient's answers and provides guidelines for counseling.[19] REAP and WAVE are examples of tools that facilitate nutrition assessment and counseling in the provider's office.

> REAP and WAVE are available at http://www.nutrition.org/cgi/content/full/133/2/556S.

Physician's Time Constraints

The frequency, time spent, and factors associated with nutrition counseling in primary care are not well studied. The investigation reported in this chapter suggests that the amount of time spent on nutrition by the physician is a function of the reason for the visit and the patient's age. Presented here are summaries of four surveys that were conducted in order to answer which patients receive nutrition counseling and how much time primary care physicians spend discussing diet.

- *Study 1*: A cross-sectional study of 84 family physician practices in northeast Ohio in 1998 revealed that the average primary care office visit lasted 16 to 17 minutes (17 minutes for patients in non-prepaid insurance plans and 16 minutes for patients in prepaid insurance plans), with physicians spending 20 seconds longer, on average, with elderly patients.[20]
- *Study 2*: In 1995, a questionnaire was mailed to a random sample of 2,250 primary care physicians selected from the American Medical Association (AMA) master file of general practice, internal medicine, and pediatrics, representing self-employed, group, hospital, and health maintenance organization (HMO) practices. A 49% response rate ($n = 1,103$) was obtained, with 70%

> **Health Maintenance Organization (HMO)**—A plan that provides health care from specific doctors and hospitals that contract with the plan. Usually there are no deductibles to be met, no claim forms to be completed by the enrollee, and a geographically restricted service area.

of the respondents in private practice. Over two-thirds of the physicians reported providing dietary counseling to 40% or less of their patients and spending 5 or fewer minutes discussing dietary changes during those sessions.[21]

- *Study 3*: In 2002, nutrition counseling was measured by direct observation on 2 days for visits to family physicians. Nutrition counseling occurred in 24% of all office visits, 17% of visits for acute illnesses, 30% of chronic illness visits, and 41% of well-care visits. The average time spent on nutrition counseling was 55 seconds (with a range of less than 20 seconds to more than 6 minutes). Nutrition counseling occurred in 45% of visits for diabetes, 33% of visits by obese patients, 31% of visits for hypertension, 26% of prenatal visits, and 25% of visits for cardiovascular disease (CVD). Nutrition counseling was more likely to occur during visits by patients who were older or had diabetes mellitus, during visits for well care or chronic illness, and during longer visits.[22]

- *Study 4*: According to a report published in 2004, when trained medical students observed physician, office, and patient characteristics in 4,344 patient visits in 38 non-metropolitan primary care physician offices, they found that counseling rates ranged from 0% in some offices to 55% in others. Physicians counseled patients on dietary habits in 25% of visits and exercise in 20% of visits. New patients were counseled 30% more often than established ones. When counseling occurred, physicians (rather than patients) initiated both dietary and exercise counseling 61% of the time. Counseling for dietary habits was associated with counseling for exercise.[23]

Strategies to Reduce Time Constraints

Given the time constraints of primary care practice, nutrition counseling needs to be brief and part of an organized office system that is conducive to supporting nutrition services. When necessary, the physician must be able to refer appropriate patients to qualified nutrition professionals. Strategies targeting both physicians and the healthcare system may improve the consistency of physician preventive counseling practices.[24]

AHRQ recommends that primary care physicians utilize the 5 A's to deliver nutrition counseling.[25] The 5 A's—assess, advise, agree, assist, and arrange—is a mnemonic algorithm that outlines minimal contact interventions that may be provided by a variety of clinical staff in primary care settings.

Strategies for using the 5 A's are available at http://www.ahrq.gov/clinic/3rduspstf/behavior/behsum1.htm.

Nutrition Curriculum Guide for Training Physicians—Available at http://www.nhlbi.nih.gov/funding/training/naa/curr_gde/index.htm.

NAA recipients developed the Nutrition Curriculum Guide for Training Physicians. Dissemination of this and other NAA materials is facilitated by a website with presentations, publications, consultants, and advisors from the NAA nutrition education programs. The NAA program constitutes a major government-sponsored effort to enhance nutrition knowledge and skills among healthcare providers and to effectively apply the science of human nutrition to clinical medicine.[26]

Cost

In the past, nutrition counseling was covered by insurance only for adult patients with a diagnosis of hypercholesterolemia, hypertension, or diabetes.[27] Until the mid-1970s, most people in the United States had traditional indemnity coverage, which is also referred to as fee-for-service. Indemnity plans were similar to automobile insurance in that one pays a certain amount of one's medical expenses up front, in the form of a deductible, and afterwards the insurance company pays the majority of the bill.

As advances in modern medicine increased the cost of providing healthcare and made it possible for people to live longer, many insurance companies developed plans to reduce their cost of doing business. This led to the birth of managed care systems. Current health insurance market options include traditional fee-for-service health insurance and managed care plans. Some forms of coverage are highly specialized and others are more comprehensive. The more comprehensive and inclusive the health insurance becomes, the higher the premiums. It is generally in the individual's best interest to purchase group coverage (mostly through an employer or association), when available. Group coverage is generally more comprehensive and group rates are generally lower because there is strength in numbers. Group plans are almost always managed care programs, which contain many restrictions. If group coverage is not available, then the individual will need to purchase an individual plan. Individual plans are medically underwritten, and there are no guarantees that an insurer will approve the application. Premiums for individual policy holders may be more in line with their expected healthcare costs than in group coverage. These premiums may also be higher for those who are older or less healthy.

Systemwide Change Strategies for Reducing the Cost of Medical Care

Population-based medicine and chronic disease management are of particular importance to public health nutritionists. Population-based medicine addresses the healthcare of whole populations rather than of individual patients. It represents a community-based strategy for disease management and health promotion, and places each patient within the context of the larger community, made up of both sick and healthy people. The community may be as small as an individual physician's private medical practice or as comprehensive as a multi-site HMO. In population-based medicine, disease groups within a given patient population are identified, and new levels of disease monitoring and patient education are used to ensure that best practice is systematically applied across the group. This is accomplished within the traditional relationship of doctor and patient, but with integral support from nurses, nutritionists, pharmacists, health educators, and other members of the healthcare team who are employed by the medical practice.

Chronic Disease Management and Self-Management

Disease management is a system of coordinated healthcare interventions and communications for populations with conditions in which patient self-care efforts are significant. Disease management supports the physician or practitioner-patient relationship and plan of care; emphasizes prevention of exacerbations and complications utilizing evidence-based practice guidelines and patient empowerment strategies; and evaluates clinical, humanistic, and economic outcomes on an ongoing basis with the goal of improving overall health. To improve health outcomes for the chronically ill, system change interventions that involve primary care and cut across chronic conditions are needed. Chronic disease improvement efforts must create care systems that are designed to meet the needs of patients and their families. The AHRQ and the Robert Wood Johnson (RJW) Foundation have funded research directed at improving the care of patients with major chronic illnesses. Additionally, valuable experience has been accrued in implementing evidence-based system change ideas in large-scale chronic disease quality improvement programs, sponsored by the Bureau of Primary Healthcare (BPHC), the CDC, and Improving Chronic Illness Care (ICIC), which is a 5-year national demonstration project sponsored by the RWJ Foundation and other organizations.

> View information on grants for improving healthcare, available at http://www.gold.ahrq.gov/PrintView.cfm?GrantNumber=R13%20HS12091.

> A recommended website for disease management is available at http://www.dmaa.org/definition.html.

> A component of population medicine is chronic disease management (CDM). CDM is a systematic approach to improving health care for people with chronic disease. Healthcare can be delivered more effectively, efficiently, and at lower cost if patients with chronic diseases take an active role in their own care and if experienced providers are supported with the necessary resources to assist their patients in managing their illness.

CDM is now a major component of primary healthcare. The population is aging, and older adults have many chronic conditions. In addition, medicine has helped transform conditions such as HIV/AIDS, once treated as acute self-limited disease states, into chronic diseases that can be lived with for decades. As indicated in

Chapter 11, the leading causes of death in the United States include the chronic diseases, CVD, and type 2 diabetes. Nutrition is fundamental in the self-management of these conditions. A cost-effective way of delivering nutrition services is through group (or cluster) visits.

Group visits are a cost-effective means of providing self-care guidance and support to chronically ill patients who need more dietary advice than physicians have the resources (skill and time) to deliver. Group (or cluster) visits are designed to help patients manage their health, adhere to their physicians' plans of care, and assure that they seek or obtain medical care they need to reduce their health risks. The term is applied to groups of patients with similar characteristics, rather than individual patient-provider appointments. In this model, the healthcare team facilitates an interactive process of care delivery in a periodic group visit program. The group can be conceptualized as an extended doctor's office visit. Invitations are extended by the healthcare team to specific patients on the basis of chronic disease history and utilization patterns. Variations of this group format have been used for disease-specific populations, such as diabetes, hypertension, and weight control. Group visits offer the staff a means to interact with patients that makes efficient use of resources, improves access, and uses group process to help motivate behavior change and improve outcomes. Guidelines for planning and implementing group visits have been developed by Improving Chronic Illness Care (ICIC), a national program of the RWJ Foundation.

> Improving Chronic Illness Care (ICIC) guidelines are available at http://www.improvingchroniccare.org/tools/criticaltools.html.

Martha M. Funnell, MS, RN, CDE, and Robert M. Anderson, EdD, describe an urban, community-based diabetes self-management education program for African Americans that uses a culturally appropriate problem-based curriculum. The diabetes self-management program is led by a nurse and a dietitian, who are Certified Diabetes Educators (CDEs). The program consists of a series of six 2-hour sessions held in a community location. Participants are recruited through flyers, postings, and newspaper advertisements near the location where the education is to be provided. Group sessions are held with 6 to 18 participants.[28]

> Diabetes education materials are available at no cost from the National Diabetes Information Clearinghouse. A list of publications for consumers, professionals, school personnel, and organizations can be found at http://www.ndep.nih.gov/diabetes/pubs/catalog.htm.

Chronic diseases have a long course of illness. They rarely resolve spontaneously and are generally not cured by medication. Today, chronic diseases such as CVD (primarily heart disease and stroke), cancer, and diabetes are among the most prevalent, costly, and preventable of all health problems. The prolonged course of illness and disability from such chronic diseases as diabetes and arthritis has resulted in extended pain and suffering and decreased quality of life for millions of Americans. These and other chronic, disabling conditions are discussed in Chapter 11.

Representative Public Health Nutrition Programs in Primary Care Settings

The Indian Health Service

The Indian Health Service (IHS), an agency within the DHHS, is responsible for providing federal health services to Native American Indians and Alaska Natives (AI/AN). As the principal federal healthcare provider and health advocate for indigenous populations, the goal of the IHS is to assure that comprehensive, culturally acceptable public health services are available and accessible. The IHS provides health services to 1.5 to 2 million individuals who belong to more than 557 federally recognized tribes in 35 states, mostly in the western United States and Alaska. In 2003, Congress appropriated $2.9 billion to help provide healthcare services to AI/AN.[29]

IHS services are provided directly through tribally contracted and operated health programs. Health services include healthcare purchased from more than 9,000 private providers annually. The federal system consists of hospitals, health centers, health stations, and residential treatment centers. In addition, Native American tribes and Alaska Native corporations administer hospitals, health centers, residential treatment centers, health stations, and Alaska village clinics. Most of the care supported by the IHS is administered through community-oriented primary care (COPC), an approach to healthcare delivery that undertakes responsibility for the health of a defined population. COPC is practiced by combining epidemiologic study and social interventions with clinical care of individual patients, so that the primary care practice itself becomes a community medicine program. Both the individual patient and the community in which the patient lives are the focus of diagnosis, treatment, and ongoing surveillance.

The IHS employs approximately 15,000 people, including members of virtually every discipline involved in providing health care and social and environmental health services. Approximately 88% of IHS staff are of AI/AN descent. Nutritionists and others who have health-related degrees can join the IHS as civil servants or as commissioned officers in the Public Health Service (PHS). To become familiar with the IHS agency and its programs, the following section contains information found on the IHS website (http://www.ihs.gov).

Most IHS funds are appropriated for Native Americans who live on or near reservations, but Congress also supports programs that provide care for Native Americans who live in urban areas, rather than on reservations or in Alaska Native villages. The National Council of Urban Indian Health was founded in 1998 to meet the unique healthcare needs of the urban Native American population through education, training, and advocacy. Title V of Public Law 94-437, the Indian Healthcare Improvement Act, authorizes the appropriation of funds for urban Indian health organizations. Title V funds are but one source of funding for urban Native American health organizations. There are 36 urban Native American health organizations operating at 41 sites located in cities throughout the United States. Urban Native American primary care clinics and outreach programs provide culturally acceptable, accessible, affordable, and accountable health services to an underserved off-reservation urban Native American population. These urban health organizations engage in a variety of activities, ranging from the provision of outreach and referral services to the delivery of comprehensive ambulatory healthcare.

The IHS's Patient Education Protocols and Codes (PEPC) were developed to standardize the provision of health services and documentation of patient education encounters from one health professional to another. Among the nutrition-related topics included in the 2003 edition of the manual are gestational diabetes, type 2 diabetes, obesity, wellness, exercise, and medical nutrition therapy.

> Patient Education Protocols and Codes (PEPC) are available at http://www.ihs.gov/NonMedicalProg rams/HealthEd/index.cfm?module=in itiative&option=protocols&newquer y=dsp_NatlPatientEd_Protocols.cfm.

Type 2 Diabetes

Almost 15% of Native Americans and Alaska Natives, age 20 or older who are receiving care from IHS, have diabetes. At the regional level, diabetes is least common among Alaska Natives (8.2%) and most common among Native Americans in the southeastern United States (27.8%) and southern Arizona (27.8%). On average, Native Americans and Alaska Natives are 2.3 times as likely to have diabetes as non-Hispanic American Caucasians of similar age.[30]

Current evidence suggests that modifiable risks for type 2 diabetes mellitus include obesity and lack of breast-feeding.[31] Primary prevention efforts can focus on the prevention of obesity in children and the promotion of breast-feeding. Preventing obesity in women of childbearing age is another primary prevention goal, because exposure to the environment of a diabetic pregnancy places the fetus at increased risk of future onset of diabetes. Early diagnosis and optimal medical care are the keys to effective secondary prevention. When type 2 diabetes mellitus is the established diagnosis, secondary prevention efforts by primary healthcare professionals are important for the prevention of complications (e.g., vascular, neural, renal, and retinal).

The American Academy of Pediatrics (AAP) Committee on Native American Child Health, in collaboration with the IHS Diabetes Program, the CDC, and the AAP Section on Endocrinology, developed guidelines to improve medical care for AI/AN children with type 2 diabetes mellitus and those at risk of type 2 diabetes mellitus. The guidelines are consistent with the 2000 American Diabetes Association (ADA) consensus statement on type 2 diabetes mellitus in children and adolescents.[32] The guidelines support the role of the general pediatrician or other primary healthcare professional as being at the front line for care. The treatment of most AI/AN children with type 2 diabetes mellitus should be managed by primary healthcare professionals with specialty consultation. The guidelines are intended to serve as a framework for the development of diabetes care programs and strategies aimed at decreasing the impact of type 2 diabetes mellitus in AI/AN children and their families and communities.

Prevention should focus on decreasing the risk, incidence, and consequences of type 2 diabetes mellitus among AI/AN children. Primary prevention efforts by primary healthcare professionals are recommended in two arenas: 1) general community health promotion and health education, and 2) activities in the primary care clinic. Clinically based health promotion activities should not duplicate community-wide health promotion, but instead should offer additive benefits. For example, if significant health education is offered at the community level, then motivational interviewing and collaborative problem solving can be offered in the clinical setting.

The *IHS Standards of Care for Patients with Type 2 Diabetes* was developed and updated by the IHS National Diabetes Program and Area Diabetes Consultants in 2003 to help provide consistent, quality care to AI/AN patients with diabetes. The IHS Diabetes Program supports the American Diabetes Association position that everyone with diabetes should receive regular nutrition counseling and should be seen by an RD every 6 to 12 months. Some people may require more frequent evaluation and counseling.

> Information about the IHS National Diabetes Program is available at http://www.ihs.gov/medicalprograms/diabetes/.

Health Resources and Services Administration, Bureau of Primary Healthcare Community Health Centers[33]

Technically known as federally qualified health centers (FQHCs), community health centers are nonprofit healthcare providers that serve the communities in which they are located. Health centers serve as the medical home and family physician to 15 million people nationally. Health center patients are among the nation's most vulnerable populations who, even if insured, would nonetheless remain isolated from traditional forms of medical care because of where they live, who they are, the language they speak, and their higher levels of complex healthcare needs. About half of health center patients reside in rural areas, while the other half tend to live in economically depressed inner-city communities. In addition, health centers serve one in five low-income children.

Two-thirds of health center patients have family incomes at or below the U.S. poverty level. Moreover, nearly 40% of health center patients are uninsured and another 36% depend on Medicaid, which is much higher than the national rates of 12% and 15%, respectively. These centers provide care to more than 1 million medically underserved Medicare beneficiaries. In many cases, health centers may be the only source of primary and preventive services to which these beneficiaries have access. Two-thirds of health center patients are members of ethnic minorities. The 2002 appropriation for this program was $1.3 billion.

Migrant Health Program[34]

Since 1962, the Migrant Health Program (MHP) has provided grants to community nonprofit organizations for a broad array of medical and support services to migrant and seasonal farm workers and their families. The program was originally authorized by the Migrant Health Act, Public Law 87-692, enacted in September 1962, and is currently authorized under section 330(g) of the Public Health Service Act. The vision of the MHP is the universal accessibility to quality and appropriate health care for our nation's migrant and seasonal farm workers (MSFW) and their families. The MHP provides MSFWs and their families access to comprehensive, culturally competent primary care services. The MHP supports the delivery of migrant health services, including primary and preventive healthcare, transportation, outreach, dental, pharmaceutical, occupational health and safety, and environmental health. These programs use health personnel; bilingual, bicultural, lay outreach workers; and culturally sensitive appropriate protocols. They also provide prevention-oriented and pediatric services such as immunizations, well baby care, and developmental screenings. Currently the MHP provides grants to 125 public and nonprofit organizations that support the development and operation of 400 migrant clinic sites throughout the United States and Puerto Rico. In 2001, migrant health centers served over 650,000 migrant and seasonal farm workers. MHP funding in 2002 was $107 million.

Public Housing Primary Care Program[35]

Access to health care is a concern for many residents of publicly assisted housing. The Public Housing Primary Care (PHPC) Program is a federal grant program created under the Disadvantaged Minority Health Improvement Act of 1990. In 1996, the PHPC Program was reauthorized under the Health Centers Consolidation Act as Section 330(i) of the Public Health Service Act. The PHPC is administered by the Bureau of Primary Healthcare (BPHC), a branch of the Health Resources and Services Administration (HRSA). The mission of PHPC is to provide accessible, comprehensive primary health care and supportive services in order to improve the overall health and well-being of the public housing community, and to eliminate health disparities.[36]

In 1997, 2.9 million people lived in public housing. On average, there were 2.16 individuals per household; the average income per household was $8,900. Sixty-eight percent of the families were minority, and 45% of the families had children under 18 years of age.[37] The PHPC Program supports health centers and other health delivery systems in providing services in partnership with other community-based providers in public housing developments or at other locations immediately accessible to residents of public housing. PHPC grantees provide primary healthcare services, including direct medical care, health screening and education, dental, prenatal and perinatal, preventive health, and case management; conduct outreach services to inform residents about health services availability; aid residents in establishing eligibility for assistance under entitlement programs and in obtaining government support for health care, mental and oral health, or social services; and train and employ residents of public housing to provide health screenings and health education services.

The PHPC budget in 2003 was $18.5 million. In 2002, 33 PHPC grantees in 18 states were awarded program funds to provide primary healthcare services. Over 70,000 clients with hypertension (20%), asthma (11%), diabetes (13%), ear infections (13%), and severe mental disorders (21%) were served. At least one-third of the primary diagnoses were nutrition-related (high blood pressure and diabetes), suggesting the need for nutrition services in this federally sponsored initiative.

Recommendations/Conclusions

Medical caregivers should be able to increase their patients' motivation to improve their diet (just as counseling by medical caregivers has been found to profoundly increase smokers' motivation to stop using tobacco[38]). Unfortunately, physicians may not have the time or the expertise to perform detailed nutrition counseling. The single most important barrier to providing adequate nutrition services in primary care is money. Although there is general consensus regarding the importance of prevention and early detection of the nutrition-related chronic diseases, inadequacies in the structure and organization of healthcare delivery detract from the adequate delivery of primary and preventive care and recommendations and support of requisite lifestyle changes.

Strategies to improve the delivery of nutrition services in the primary healthcare setting include, at a minimum: increased third-party reimbursement for preventive nutrition counseling; training physicians so they feel confident about delivering nutrition advice and are aware of the full armamentarium of nutrition materials that have been developed and will help with the delivery of dietary advice; and reorganizing the primary care office so that self-management is incorporated into disease management.

Issues for Discussion

1. Discuss methods for convincing primary care physicians that nutrition counseling is a necessary part of disease prevention.
2. Discuss methods for convincing medical schools that nutrition should be a part of the curriculum.
3. How should the public health nutrition department approach primary care physicians for assistance with nutrition counseling?
4. Should the federal government enact policies that primary care physicians must comply with concerning the public's right to receive nutritional counseling where warranted? When should nutrition counseling be warranted?

References

1. Donaldson MS, Yordy KD, Lohr KN, Vanselow NA, eds. *Committee on the Future of Primary Care, Division of Healthcare Services.* Washington, DC: Institute of Medicine National Academy Press; 1996.
2. Donaldson MS, Yordy KD, Lohr KN, Vanselow NA, eds. *Committee on the Future of Primary Care, Division of Healthcare Services.* Washington, DC: Institute of Medicine National Academy Press; 1996, p. 31.
3. U.S. Department of Health & Human Services—Public Health Service. Progress Review. Diabetes. June 4, 2002. Available at: http://www.healthypeople.gov/data/2010prog/focus05/. Accessed June 8, 2004.
4. U.S. Department of Health and Human Services. *Healthy People 2010: Understanding and Improving Health.* 2nd ed. Washington, DC: U.S. Government Printing Office; November 2000.
5. U.S. Department of Health & Human Services—Public Health Service. Progress Review. Diabetes. June 4, 2002. Available at: http://www.healthypeople.gov/data/2010prog/focus05/. Accessed June 8, 2004.

6. U.S. Department of Health & Human Services—Public Health Service. Progress Review. Diabetes. June 4, 2002. Available at: http://www.healthypeople.gov/data/2010prog/focus05/. Accessed June 8, 2004.

7. Cherry DK, Woodwell DA. *National Ambulatory Medical Care Survey: 2000 Summary. Advance Data from Vital and Health Statistics; No. 328.* Hyattsville, Md: National Center for Health Statistics; 2002.

8. U.S. Preventive Services Task Force. Guide to Clinical Preventive Services, 2nd ed. 1996. Electronic archive available at: http://www.ahrq.gov/clinic/cpsix.htm. Accessed April 11, 2004.

9. U.S. Preventive Services Task Force. Guide to Clinical Preventive Services. 3rd ed. Periodic Updates. Available at: http://www.ahrq.gov/clinic/gcpspu.htm. Accessed April 3, 2005.

10. Agency for Healthcare Policy and Research. Child Health Guide: Put Prevention into Practice. Consumer Information. Available at: http://www.mdadvice.com/topics/prevention/info/ppchild.htm. Accessed April 3, 2005.

11. Agency for Healthcare Research and Quality. Clinical Preventive Services for Normal-Risk Adults Recommended by the U.S. Preventive Services Task Force. Put Prevention into Practice, January 2004. Available at: http://www.ahrq.gov/ppip/adulttm.htm. Accessed April 11, 2004.

12. Eyre H, Kahn R, Robertson RM, et al. Preventing cancer, cardiovascular disease, and diabetes: a common agenda for the American Cancer Society, the American Diabetes Association, and the American Heart Association. Circulation. 2004 Jun 29;109(25):3244–3255. Epub 2004 Jun 15. Available at: http://circ.ahajournals.org/cgi/reprint/109/25/3244. Accessed June 30, 2004.

13. Agency for Healthcare Research and Quality. About PPIP. Put Prevention Into Practice, May 2000. Available at: http://www.ahrq.gov/ppip/ppipabou.htm. Accessed April 11, 2004.

14. Kushner RF. Barriers to providing nutrition counseling by physicians: a survey of primary care practitioners. *Prev Med.* 1995;24:546–552.

15. Eaton CB, McBride PE, Gans KA, Underbakke GL. Teaching nutrition skills to primary care practitioners. *J Nutr.* 2003;133:563S–566S.

16. Mihalynuk TV, Scott CS, Coombs JB. Self-reported nutrition proficiency is positively correlated with the perceived quality of nutrition training of family physicians in Washington State. *Am J Clin Nutr.* 2003;77(5):1330–1336.

17. Mihalynuk TV, Scott CS, Coombs JB. Self-reported nutrition proficiency is positively correlated with the perceived quality of nutrition training of family physicians in Washington State. *Am J Clin Nutr.* 2003;77(5):1330–1336.

18. Schulman JA. Nutrition education in medical schools: trends and implications for health educators. *Med Educ Online* [serial online] 1999;4:4. Available at: http://www.Med-Ed-Online.org. Accessed June 23, 2004.

19. Gans KM, Ross E, Barner CW, Wylie-Rosett J, McMurray J, Eaton C. REAP and WAVE: new tools to rapidly assess/discuss nutrition with patients. *J Nutr.* 2003;133:556S–562S.

20. Mechanic D, McAlpine DD, Rosenthal M. Are patients' office visits with physicians getting shorter? *N Eng J Med.* 2001;344:198–204.

21. Kushner RF. Barriers to providing nutrition counseling by physicians: a survey of primary care practitioners. *Prev Med.* 1995;24:546–552.

22. Eaton CB, Goodwin MA, Stange KC. Direct observation of nutrition counseling in community family practice. *Am J Prev Med.* 2002;23: 174–179.

23. Anis NA, Lee RE, Ellerbeck EF, Nazir N, Greiner KA, Ahluwalia JS. Direct observation of physician counseling on dietary habits and exercise: patient, physician, and office correlates. *Prev Med.* 2004;38: 198–202.

24. Eaton CB, McBride PE, Gans KA, Underbakke GL. Teaching nutrition skills to primary care practitioners. *J Nutr.* 2003;133:563S–566S.

25. Whitlock EP, Orleans T, Pender N, Allan J. Evaluating primary care behavioral counseling interventions: an evidence-based approach. Originally in *Am J Prev Med.* 2002;22(4):267–284. Available at: http://www.ahrq.gov/clinic/3rduspstf/behavior/behsum1.htm. Accessed July 1, 2004.

26. Pearson TA, Stone EJ, Grundy SM, McBride PE, Van Horn L, Tobin BW, NAA Collaborative Group. Translation of nutritional sciences into medical education: the Nutrition Academic Award Program. *Am J Clin Nutr.* 2001;74:164–170.

27. Kushner RF. Barriers to providing nutrition counseling by physicians: a survey of primary care practitioners. *Prev Med.* 1995;24:546–552.

28. Funnell MM, Anderson RM. *HSTAT: Guide to Clinical Preventive Services,* 3rd ed.: Recommendations and Systematic Evidence Reviews, Guide to Community Preventive Services. Available at: http://www.ncbi.nlm.nih.gov/books/bv.fcgi?call=bv.View..ShowSection&rid=hstat3. Accessed June 28, 2004.

29. Indian Health Service. Fact Sheet. March 29, 2004. Available at: http://www.ihs.gov/PublicInfo/PublicAffairs/Welcome_Info/ThisFacts.asp. Accessed June 22, 2004.

30. National Institute of Diabetes and Digestive and Kidney Diseases. *National diabetes statistics fact sheet: general information and national estimates on diabetes in the United States, 2003.* Bethesda, Md: U.S. Department of Health and Human Services, National Institutes of Health; 2003. Rev. ed. Bethesda, MD: U.S. Department of Health and Human Services, National Institutes of Health; 2004.

31. Pettitt DJ, Knowler WC. Long-term effects of the intrauterine environment, birth weight, and breast-feeding in Pima Indians. *Diabetes Care.* 1998;21(Suppl 2):B138–B141.

32. American Diabetes Association. Type 2 diabetes in children and adolescents. *Pediatrics.* 2000;105:671–680.

33. Bureau of Primary Healthcare. Program Information. (Community Health Centers). Available at: http://bphc.hrsa.gov/programs/chcprograminfo.asp#accomplishments. Accessed July 1, 2004.

34. Bureau of Primary Healthcare. Migrant Health Program. Available at: http://bphc.hrsa.gov/programs/MHCProgramInfo.htm. Accessed July 1, 2004.

35. Bureau of Primary Healthcare. Public Housing Primary Care Program. Available at: http://bphc.hrsa.gov/phpc/. Accessed March 30, 2005.

36. Department of Health and Human Services. Health Resources and Services Administration. Bureau of Primary Healthcare. Public Housing Primary Care Program fact sheet. Available at: http://bphc.hrsa.gov/phpc/phpc_program/fact_sheet.htm. Accessed June 30, 2004.

37. NAHRO (National Association of Housing and Redevelopment Officials). Building Communities Together. 1997 Picture of Subsidized Households. Available at: http://www.nahro.org/reference/stats_picture97.html. Accessed April 4, 2005.

38. Fiore MC, Bailey WC, Cohen SJ, et al. *Clinical Practice Guideline: Treating Tobacco Use and Dependence.* Rockville, MD: U.S. Department of Health and Human Services, Public Health Service; 2000. Available at: http://www.surgeongeneral.gov/tobacco/treating_tobacco_use.pdf. Accessed July 1, 2004.

CHAPTER 14

THE BABY BOOMERS: IDENTIFICATION OF WELLNESS NEEDS

Stacey Chappa, RD

Shirley Chao, MS, RD, LDN

Sari Edelstein, PhD, RD

Reader Objectives

After studying this chapter and reflecting on the contents, you should be able to:

1. Describe the demographic characteristics of the baby boomer population.
2. Discuss the wellness concerns of baby boomers.
3. Identify how public health can best address these wellness concerns.

Baby Boomer Demographics and Characteristics

One-third of the United States' population is composed of baby boomers. A literature review suggests that boomers have different characteristics, needs, and demands than the elderly population currently served by the public health community. Taking into account the research on education level, family complexity, diversity, income, and health conditions, the major needs for baby boomers have begun to surface. To sum up current research simply, the baby boomers' needs center on quality of life.

> Baby boomers are those persons born between the years 1946 and 1964. There are currently 78 million baby boomers in the United States.

Aging is a multidimensional process influenced by health, desires, family roles, and productivity. Sensitivity to family dynamics and diversity are important considerations when serving baby boomers. The well-being of the boomer generation encompasses screening, assessment, diet, supplement usage, exercise, sexual vitality, pain management, and health condition. Boomers need health information through education by academia, public health programs, comprehensive health packages offered by the private sector, and personal inquiries. Health packages must integrate alternative and traditional medicine. To ensure quality of life and overall wellness of boomers, their needs must be addressed and met. This responsibly falls on the community at large composed of the private, public, government/regulatory, and academic/research sectors. These factors and more are the discussion topics of this chapter.

Growing up after World War II, baby boomers were better educated and better paid than previous American generations. And boomers are soon to become our nation's elders; the youngest baby boomer will turn 46 years old in 2010, while the oldest will turn 64. Between 2011 and 2029, the over-65 population will grow by 77 million people.[1] By 2010, there will be between 5 and 6 million people in their 90s.[3]

Boomers have different characteristics, needs, and demands than the elderly population currently served by the community sectors. Boomers' heritage and family structure, formal education, income, employment, and health conditions are different from that of today's elders. Assessing the characteristics of boomers' needs and demands provides a portrait of who they are; these needs are shown in Table 14-1.

TABLE 14-1   Characteristics of the Boomer Generation (1945–1965)

Characteristic	Definition
Heritage and family structure	More racially and ethnically diverse than generations before them. Have fewer children than their parents' generation. Have higher rates of divorce and remarriage than their parents' generation. Grandparents are often raising grandchildren.
Formal education	More formal education than today's senior citizens.
Income (median or household)	Higher median family and household incomes than today's senior citizens (although the cost of living is much higher today than it was 20 to 40 years ago).
Employment	Longer working hours than their parents' generation and more women working.
Health condition	Much more likely to smoke, be overweight, and have a sedentary lifestyle than their parents' generation. Sedentary lifestyle is a risk factor of heart disease, cancer, and diabetes.

As stated previously, the general needs of boomers center on maintaining the quality of their lives. Health-related quality of life is a scientific concept that describes a person's perception of their health, well-being, and ability to function. Aging is a multidimensional process characterized by biological changes, evolving wants and needs, family roles, and productivity. Another goal of this chapter is to identify boomers' needs so that public health professionals can help to promote a smooth transition into their golden years.[2]

Family Structure

Boomers have complex family structures and greater diversity than previous generations. Family dynamics are an important consideration when working with boomers. Many are still caring for their elderly parents. Due to the high divorce rate and number of single parents, boomers may also be caring for their grandchildren.[16] Census data from 2000 stated that 5.6 million grandparents nationwide had grandchildren living with them, and 42% of these people reported being the primary caregiver of their grandchildren. Therefore, public health programs must appeal to dynamic families. Public health professionals also need to customize and adjust existing programs, materials, and means of communication to fit the demographic diversity of age, language, and ethnic culture of the boomer population.[16] It is important to have culturally sensitive and knowledgeable workers on staff to best serve this population.

Boomers have more formal education than their elders. According to the 2000 U.S. census summary, about 84% of people between the ages of 35 and 64 graduated high school, compared to only 65% of people over 64 years of age. About 26% of people aged 35 to 64 have a bachelor's degree or higher, whereas only 15% of people over age 64 have a bachelor's degree or higher. The average household income for boomers is $80,000 annually. Boomers are expected to retire later in life and slowly shift from full-time employment to retirement. For them, jobs provide a source of income, add meaning to life, and may prevent social isolation. By creating new identities and roles, boomer women are becoming a strong force in the workplace. Women, as a whole, contribute about 40% of all household income.[17] The health conditions of boomers will directly affect their quality of life, their wellness needs, and their ability to seek these new roles.

State of Health

The leading causes of death in the United States in the year 2000 were heart disease, cancer, stroke, respiratory disease, accidents, diabetes mellitus, influenza and pneumonia, Alzheimer's disease, and kidney failure.[18-27] Heart disease and cancer accounted for over one-half of all deaths, when combined.[4] Tobacco use, lack of physical activity, and poor nutrition are major contributors to heart disease and cancer.[5] Obesity and lack of physical activity are risk factors for developing type 2 diabetes. According to NHANES III (Third National Health and Nutrition Examination Survey), an estimated 29 million persons (14.4%) aged ≥ 20 years had either been diagnosed with diabetes, had undiagnosed diabetes, or had an impaired fasting glucose blood level. Diabetes is also the leading cause of kidney failure. More than 193,000 deaths and 60% of all lower-limb amputations occur annually due to diabetes.[5] Behavior modification through diet and exercise, as well as smoking cessation, can decrease the prevalence of heart disease, cancer, and diabetes. One in every five deaths is caused by tobacco.[5] Smokers who die of tobacco-related usage lose about 12 years of expected life.[5] About 25% of American adults, or about 47 million, smoke.[5] Elderly smokers who quit can obtain significant health benefits and risk reduction of death, which justify the need for smoking cessation programs. Arthritis and back pain are other health conditions that affect quality of life and functionality. Some arthritis and back pain may be attributed to carrying excess body weight.

Several factors have contributed to the surge in weight among U.S. adults. Boomers value generous portion sizes and value, as they grew up at the same time the fast food industry was created. Convenience foods were introduced, as well as meal replacement drinks and bars, to accommodate the busy lifestyles of boomers. Fast food and snacks replaced home-cooked meals. And, boomers adopted a sedentary lifestyle. According to data from NHANES III, approximately one-third of Americans aged 20 to 74 (58 million) are overweight. (These numbers are derived from NHANES III, 1988–1991. NHANES III defines overweight as a BMI value of 27.3% or more for women and 27.8% or more for men.) A study from 2003 showed that more than half the adults in the state of Massachusetts were overweight, which is a 30% increase since 1990.[9] The study defined obesity as having a BMI score of 30 or more. In Massachusetts, 16.1% of adults were obese in 2002.[5] In 2000, the prevalence of obesity among U.S. adults was 19.8%, which accounted for 38.8 million people. Between 2000 and 2001, obesity prevalence climbed from 19.8% to 20.9% in U.S. adults. Currently, more than 44 million Americans are considered obese.[5] This reflects an increase of 74% since 1991.

A report done by the Centers for Disease Control in 2000 assessed the level of physical activity among adults in the United States. The results indicated that about one-fifth of adults engaged in a high level of physical activity and one-quarter engaged in a medium level of physical activity. Most adults, 75%, did not achieve the recommended amount of physical activity during leisure time.[5]

Arthritis is one of the most prevalent diseases in the United States and affects 43 billion people. Arthritis limits the boomer's ability to be mobile and perform daily activities without assistance. The ability to function is a component of quality of life. One out of six people have arthritis in the United States, which means that more than 7 million Americans' daily activities are limited by arthritis. Arthritis and other rheumatoid conditions are the leading cause of disability in the United States and will affect an estimated 60 million people by 2020.[5] Low back pain is also prevalent among Americans. According to the American Academy of Orthopedic Surgeons, 80% of Americans will experience back pain at some time in their life.

In the United States, elderly people of all ethnicities are experiencing a proportionately greater rate of new AIDS cases than any other age group. Between 1991 and 1996, there was a 22% rise in new AIDS cases in Americans over 50 years of age.[8] A report published in the April issue of *AIDS Patient Care* and STDs indicated that more than 10% of AIDS patients in the United States are over 50 years old and that the HIV rate is rising among people 60 to 70 years old. Mortality is high among older persons who contract the virus. About 37% of patients over the age of 80 years are dying within 1 month of diagnosis.[7] Public health educational materials and risk reduction are needed to halt HIV/AIDS infection among the boomers.

> STD stands for sexually transmitted disease and can refer to other diseases besides HIV and AIDS, such as syphilis and gonorrhea.

Educational Demands

Boomers have a need for health education through many sources, as stated previously. The academic sector must continue to conduct research and publish results of trials and studies. Boomers also need more Internet navigation sites to help them sift through the health information online.

More public health programs that promote the health and well-being of boomers through education are needed. Preventative health measures need to be taken to reduce the prevalence of chronic, preventable diseases in the boomer population. Community and public health classes on diet and exercise should be given that discuss the relationship between lifestyle behaviors and the development of heart disease, cancer, obesity, and diabetes. Smoking cessation programs can be initiated for boomers. Also, sexual health and vitality affect quality of life, and boomers need programs that promote healthy sexual practices. This area, relatively ignored in recent years, has been brought to the forefront with the creation of sexual stimulants marketed to boomers. Americans have already spent over $2 billion on sexual stimulants, and the sales continue to climb.[6] Safe sex education needs to be provided for boomers as they age. With pregnancy no longer a risk, boomers may not practice safe sexual behavior and could be in danger of contracting a sexually transmitted disease, which can include HIV/AIDS.

Public health programs also need to address the accuracy of health information provided by the media. Trained, knowledgeable employees who are familiar with various supplements and their claims are needed to assist boomers in making informed, smart decisions. Boomers must be careful when purchasing and taking supplements. They need to be aware of possible drug/nutrient interactions and supplement reactions with prescription drugs. Independent companies need to be available to provide test results of health claims for products marketed to the public and help consumers and healthcare professionals evaluate health, wellness, and nutrition practices of those products currently found in the marketplace.

The Food and Drug Administration (FDA) has launched an initiative to help consumers obtain accurate, up-to-date information about the health consequences of dietary supplements with a grading system. The FDA will assign health claims letters ranging from A to D. This will have a significant impact on products because health claims will now be supported with various degrees of scientific agreement. For example, grade A indicates the health claim meets the significant scientific agreement standard, whereas a grade D means that very limited and preliminary scientific research has been done, suggesting that the FDA concludes that there is little evidence supporting this claim.[10]

Because many boomers seek health information through magazines, newspapers, and the Internet, they need to be educated on which sources are accurate and credible. More than 70% of people who are online access health information.[17] It would be helpful if boomers were knowledgeable about peer-reviewed journal articles and able to identify quality research designs and studies.

Health Insurance and Screening

The baby boomers need a comprehensive health package that meets their nutritional and physical needs by integrating medically sound alternative and traditional medicine. Vitamins, supplements, pharmaceuticals, hormone therapies, and other anti-aging substances are abundant and widely used by boomers. For example, supplements and homeopathic remedies are used to manage nutritional status and pain. It is estimated that consumers spend about $14 billion on complementary or integrative medicine in the course of one year.[1]

In 1998, homeopathic remedy expenditures exceeded all past dollar spending totals in the public sector. Thus, employers and health maintenance organizations (HMOs) should offer comprehensive health programs to boomers, which include medically recog-

nized homeopathic and complementary services. These
services can be included in a
health package that should
contain screening, education
and private consulting, and
intervention.

> Homeopathic remedies may include chiropractic, massage, vitamins, yoga, herbals, hypnosis, acupuncture, and many other complementary therapies.

Screening efforts for breast cancer, colorectal cancer, cervical
cancer, high blood pressure, arthritis, cholesterol levels, and diabetes mellitus are crucial for the boomer population and need to be
continued as a part of traditional medicine as boomers age. Screening by health professionals must also include nutritional intakes,
eating patterns, supplement usage, physical activity patterns, and
preferred modes of exercise. During this process health professionals should also inquire about the boomer's interests or participation
in alternative medicine therapies.

Once screening is completed, education through private consultation may be needed. Boomers may want to have several meetings
with dietitians or personal trainers to improve their general condition and adopt a healthier lifestyle. Interventions can be developed
through these private consultations.

Interventions for Baby Boomers

Intervention efforts for boomers include cultivating healthy nutrition behaviors and identifying appealing modes of exercise.

Nutrition

A challenge for the nutritionist is to teach boomers proper, balanced
nutrition and motivate them to make changes in their lifestyles.
A top trend of Americans is consuming functional foods, that is,
nutrient-enhanced, fortified foods, as well as nutriceuticals and
phytochemicals. Many boomers seek out these types of foods. People want to manage their health through the foods they eat and
make selections based on health benefits. Instead of focusing on
components of food, nutritionists may need to focus on the benefits of eating certain foods.

Supplements, as discussed briefly, are another intervention. Supplement use is prevalent among baby boomers. In 2001, those 55 and
older spent $1.4 billion on vitamins and supplements.[10] Consumers
spent $6.2 billion on vitamins and another $1.5 billion on minerals
in 2002. The top five vitamins were multivitamins, B vitamins, and
vitamins E, C, and A.[11] The top five minerals were calcium, magnesium, iron, chromium, and a zinc/potassium/selenium combination.[11]

Prebiotics and probiotics are also gaining popularity. *Prebiotics* are substances that promote the growth or activity of a limited number of bacterial species in the gut. Prebiotics produce short-chain fatty acids that are critical to gut integrity, immune system functioning, calcium absorption, and cholesterol maintenance.[13] *Probiotics* are live organisms that confer a health effect on the host.[12] Probiotics can be used to fight common female health problems such as urinary tract and vaginal infections. Some studies showed the lactobacillus GG strain helped manage Crohn's disease and irritable bowel syndrome.[12] Lactobacillus is found in about 80% of the U.S.'s yogurt.[12] Dairy products are often supplemented with probiotics because they buffer stomach acid and increase the chance the bacteria will survive.

Exercise

Programs, classes, and facilities are needed that will attract boomers to engage in physical fitness. Needs assessment and surveys can articulate where the boomers' interests lie and can help frame programs. In adults, regular physical activity has been associated with decreased risk of coronary heart disease, obesity, non-insulin dependent diabetes, osteoporosis, and post-endometrial cancer. Physical activity has also been associated with increased longevity and lower rate of disability.[14]

Exercise, both cardiovascular and resistance, can help maintain the muscle masses of aging adults. Encouraging strength training for both men and women is important. Circuit training that combines cardiovascular fitness and resistance training is popular among boomers. Boomers need to know about how to train prior to exercise, as the most common injuries affecting aging athletes are ankle and knee sprains; strains in the hamstring, calf, and back muscles; rotator-cuff tendonitis; tennis elbow; stress fractures; and heel spurs.[15] Health professionals also need to encourage regular activity and discourage "weekend warriors." Poor conditioning and stiff bones and muscles in older adults may increase their risk for injuries.

America is a market-driven country, and boomers want to choose which services and products they spend money on. Wellness programs need to be affordable and managed by credible, educated professionals. Such programs need to be located near the boomers' homes in order to be accessible, and they must have flexible hours to accommodate boomers' work schedules and family commitments. Finally, programs need to be diverse in order to adapt to each individual's demands. Boomers need a variety of gym options, the choice of meeting with a dietitian or personal trainer, and the option of utilizing medically recognized homeopathic remedies. Dietitians need to package their materials differently to appeal to the boomers and be successful in establishing healthy eating habits.

Time is a crucial factor for many boomers, who need an effective workout in a short amount of time. Boomers are seeking not only physical benefits from exercise, but also mind/spirit benefits. This reflects the shift from traditional, Western healthcare to a more integrative, holistic model.

Recommendations for the Future

America's baby boomers have different health needs and demands than the elderly population being served today. These differences, due to increased longevity, will produce health needs related to a higher incidence of arthritis, obesity, and diabetes. Baby boomers will demand more medical education and intervention than past generations.

A public health needs assessment (as discussed in Chapter 3) should be designed and distributed to boomers across the United States in order to collect information on their wellness needs and wants. California and New York have done preliminary research, and other states need to follow so that appropriate resources may be allocated, desired programs developed, and adequate facilities and staff provided to serve the boomers when they are elderly. In addition to surveying the boomers, existing programs and facilities must be mapped out and inspected so they do not duplicate what is already in place. Once gaps are identified, program planning and development can begin.

Issues for Discussion

1. Given that there are more and more demands made on the public health system, do you think that the baby boomer demands are feasible?
2. Make suggestions as to how the public health system can meet baby boomer demands.

References

1. Bartlett D. The new healthcare consumer. *J Healthcare Finance.* 1999; 25:46–51.
2. Age power, how the new-old will transform medicine in the 21st century. *Geriatrics.* 1999;54(12):22–27.
3. Mycek S. We're not in Kansas anymore. *Trustee.* 1999;52(8):22–24.
4. Centers for Disease Control and Prevention. *National Vital Statistics Report.* 2002;50(15).
5. Centers for Disease Control and Prevention. The CDC home page. Available at: http://www.cdc.gov. Accessed October 14, 2003.

6. Greenwald J. Drug quest: magic bullets for boomers. *Time.* 1998;151 (17):54–55.

7. Reuters Health Information Services. *HIV/AIDS in the Elderly on the Rise.* 1998. Available at: www.ruetershealth.com. Accessed on October 14, 2003.

8. Waysdorf S. The aging of the AIDS epidemic: emerging legal and public health issues for elderly persons living with HIV/AIDS. *Elder Law Journal.* 2002;10:28–30; 33-34; 36–38.

9. Gotbaum R. Good fat, bad fat, and fighting a looming fat epidemic. Available at: http://wbur.org. Accessed September 29, 2003.

10. Perry J. Staving off the many aches of age. *U.S. News & World Report.* 2002;132(19):84.

11. Madley-Wright R. Vitamins and minerals. *Nutraceuticals World.* September 1, 2003.

12. Skovsende A. Probiotics: good for what's bugging you. *Nutraceuticals World.* September 1, 2003.

13. Douglas L. Prebiotics overview. *Nutraceuticals World.* November 1, 2003.

14. Barnes PM. Physical activity among adults: U.S., 2000. *Advance Data,* CDC. May 14, 2003: 333.

15. Clark J. A pain in the back for boomers. *Kiplinger's Personal Finance Magazine.* 1997;51:98.

16. Project 2015, White Paper for Discussion. The New York State Office for the Aging page. Available at: http://www.aging.state.ny.us/ explore/project2015/report02. Accessed October 15, 2003.

17. Institute for the Future. Fault lines in the shifting landscape: the future of growing older in California 2010. Available at: http://www.archstone.org/publications2292/ publications_show.htm?doc_id=33534. Accessed March 31, 2005.

18. Dougherty K, Senelick R. *Baby Boomers' Guide to Women's Health: Living Great the Next 50 Years.* Health South Press; 2003.

19. Naditz A. Coming of age. As the baby boomer ages, long-term care must gear up for its own "boom." *Contemporary, Long-Term Care.* 2003;26(10):18-19.

20. Hartman-Stein PE, Potkanowicz FS. Behavioral determinants of healthy aging: good news for the baby boomer generation. *Online J Issues Nurs.* 2003;8(2):6.

21. Rosenbloom AA Jr. New aged and old aged: impact of the baby boomer. *Optometry.* 2003;74(4):211–213.

22. Bertholf L, Loveless S. Baby boomers and Generation X: strategies to bridge the gap. *Semin Nurse Manag.* 2001;9(3):169-172.

23. Mangino M. The aging employee. Impact on occupational health. *AAOHN J.* 2000;48(7):349–357.

24. Wagner L. Meeting the baby boomer challenge. How will a generation of 70 million elders reshape and redirect long-term care? *Provider.* 2000;26(1):28–30, 33-34, 36–38.

25. Dunn-Cane KM, Gonzalez JL, Stewart HP. Managing the new generation. *AORN J.* 1999 May;69(5):930, 933-936, 939–940.

26. Mangino M. Mid-life is upon us. Preventative care for the baby boomer. *Mich Health Hosp.* 1996;32(4):22–24.

27. Wilson M. The future of telemedicine. *Stud Health Technol Inform.* 2002;80:129-136.

CHAPTER 15

MAINTAINING NUTRITION AND FOOD SERVICE STANDARDS IN GROUP CARE

Thelma B. Baker, PhD, RD, LD

Reader Objectives

After studying this chapter and reflecting on the contents, you will be able to:

1. Recognize the role of public health nutrition in setting food service standards in acute, long-term, group, and home care facilities.
2. Address the role of the nutrition professional in providing services for individuals in group care settings.
3. Be aware of governmental licensing and monitoring agencies that govern nutrition and food service in group care settings.
4. Discuss how nutrition professionals can position themselves as specialists who are responsible for disseminating nutrition and food service information in healthcare facilities.
5. Discuss the information needed by administrators in order to enable the nutrition professional to provide quality nutrition care and food service management.

Within the last 30 years there has been a marked increase in the need for community group care. This is due to the de-institutionalization of residents in homes for mentally and physically disabled individuals, group homes for persons undergoing alcohol and drug rehabilitation, shelters for battered and abused women, and emergency shelters that provide residential and food services to homeless families with children, among other institutions. As a result, the need for a number of different healthcare service professionals, such as occupational and physical therapists, social services caseworkers, and nutritionists, has increased. Some of the community institutions that require these services may be denominational, not-for-profit, or for-profit organizations. Although the provision of nutrition and food service production are guided by public health nutrition federal and state laws and are carefully monitored at some newer institutions, the food service operation is not designed and monitored as closely as established healthcare institutions. The purpose of this chapter is to help the reader to learn how to apply public health nutrition regulations from traditional healthcare settings to these newer types of facilities.

With the expansion of group care to community-based practice, new employment opportunities for nutrition professionals have come into focus. Nutrition professionals can now be found in non-traditional agencies and organizations that provide primary care, promote health, and prevent chronic diseases in the community or in community groups. Thus, they are making an additional contribution to securing the nutrition health of the public.

The Role of the Nutritionist

In some group care organizations, dietitians or nutritionists may be involved only in services such as menu writing, whereas other organizations may need full-time personnel for more complex nutritional services. Listed below are some group care organizations that serve three or more meals each day, and thus require the skills of a nutrition specialist.

Healthcare organizations:

- Hospitals for acute, long-term, or mental health care
- Nursing homes
- Rehabilitation centers
- Assisted living facilities

Community care organizations:

- Group homes for mentally and physically disabled individuals
- Halfway houses for individuals undergoing alcohol and/or drug rehabilitation
- Retirement homes
- Halfway houses for previously incarcerated individuals
- Male and female shelters

Child-care organizations:

- Head Start and preschool programs
- Family daycare homes
- Family foster homes
- Schools

Later in this chapter, we will discuss the evolving role of the nutritionist in group care situations.

Licensure, Regulation, and Accreditation

In order to protect the health and safety of consumers, community and healthcare organizations must be licensed by at least one government public health agency. Organizations that provide healthcare services, including nutrition, and that receive funding from Medicaid and/or Medicare must adhere to specific regulations. These regulations are established by the Healthcare Financing Administration (HCFA) of the U.S. Department of Health and Human Services (DHHS). In addition, these institutions are licensed by states and counties as warranted. Licensure ensures that the institutions maintain clean and sanitary conditions and staffing patterns that are sufficient to meet the needs, including nutritional needs, of the clients being served. Although hospitals and nursing facilities must be state licensed, in some instances they require additional accreditation by the Joint Commission on Accreditation of Healthcare Organizations (JCAHO). Even though some of the requirements of the various agencies overlap, the goal is to ensure that clients receive appropriate care.

The state health agency, in addition to county government in some instances, is responsible for licensing group care agencies. Licensure laws cover sanitation, safety of facilities, staffing, quality of care, and clients' rights. Regulations cover the safety and sanitation of the food services and the nutritional adequacy of the menu in addition to other requirements. Some of the nutrition requirements specific to hospitals are that clients should be seen by a dietitian/nutritionist and a nutrition assessment must be completed within a specified period of time following admission. The diet recommendation should address the disease state and ultimately should be prescribed by the admitting physician. Follow-up assessments by the dietitian/nutritionist must also be completed within a specific period of time.

> **JCAHO**—An independent, not-for-profit organization that is a standards-setting and accrediting body in healthcare. Learn more about JCAHO at http://www.jcaho.org.

Evolving Nutrition Standards in Healthcare Organizations

The role of nutrition professionals in healthcare institutions continues to evolve. Once upon a time, nutrition professionals in healthcare settings were responsible for assessing clients' nutritional status based on laboratory parameters and clinical observations, educating clients and family regarding dietary modifications, and making recommendations to physicians for dietary changes. However, in addition to these duties, nutrition professionals, particularly registered dietitians, now serve as active members of the healthcare team and make substantial contributions regarding nutrition and patient care in the area of specialized feedings such as enteral and parenteral nutrition. Registered dietitians teach resident physicians and medical students about nutrition and are responsible for developing and implementing nutrition programs pertaining to lifestyle changes.

Following admission to a healthcare institution, a client's nutrition status must be addressed within a specified period of time and monitored continuously. In situations requiring specialized dietary modifications, daily assessment may be warranted. In addition, nutrition professionals are required to conduct internal audits and patient satisfaction surveys periodically to assure that dietary standards are being maintained.

As rules for the funding for healthcare become more stringent, and length of in-hospital stays decrease, dietitians need to develop and implement more outpatient programs to ensure that dietary needs are being met following discharge. Some of the outpatient programs the dietitians are responsible for are classes in diabetic care and bariatric and cardiovascular management. In some states and cities, hospital dietitians are required to make house calls to clients in order to provide continuous nutrition care. In these situations, the nutrition professional must take into consideration the client's ability and desire to prepare meals, the living situation, and other conditions that may impact nutrition status.

> **Bariatric**—Refers to the management of morbid obesity by surgery; dietitians assist in educating patients about how to eat properly. Learn more about bariatrics at http://www.asbs.org.

Evolving Nutrition Standards in Community Organizations

Group Homes for People Who Are Mentally and Physically Disabled

People who are mentally and physically disabled, as a group, are at high nutritional risk for many reasons. This population may have problems with eating and swallowing, limited eating skills, mechanical feeding difficulties or neuromotor dysfunctions, inborn errors of metabolism, problems with underweight and overweight, and malabsorption problems. Additionally, there may be a mixture of older and younger clients with developmental disabilities and clients with additional nutritional needs associated with aging. The basic goal of nutrition management for all clients is to provide adequate calories and other nutrients for proper growth and development in addition to resolving any nutritional problems related to aging. In this capacity, the role of the nutrition specialist is very challenging due in part to age range of clients, limited or a lack of communication skills on the part of the client, unusual food habits or eating behaviors, multiple medical problems, and physical disabilities that complicate the implementation of nutritional intervention.

Determining the client's nutritional status is essential because people with disabilities may be malnourished. A comprehensive assessment must include diet information, physical assessment data, laboratory data, and medications affecting nutritional status. Information should be obtained from the direct care staff, as well as a parent or guardian. A nutrition care plan with clearly defined goals for managing each client should be identified in medical charts and adjustments made as necessary. In addition, the nutrition professional should serve as a member of the interdisciplinary healthcare team to address nutrition-related problems, other problems that affect nutrition status, and the client's progress. Appendix B provides some good examples of nutritional assistance for those people with challenging disabilities.

Adult Outplacement Homes: Drug and Alcohol Rehabilitation

Adults living in outplacement homes may include otherwise healthy individuals who are undergoing drug or alcohol rehabilitation. These individuals may include adults living with a chronic condition, such as diabetes or hypertension. Homes providing treatment for these recovering individuals are required to be licensed by the state and/or county, and all regulations must be met in order to provide service. In order to ensure that clients receive nutritious meals, a dietitian or nutritionist must be engaged either part-time or as a consultant. Here, the dietitian's role is to ensure that the client's diet satisfies the Dietary Reference Intakes (DRIs). The DRIs provide quantitative estimates of nutrient intake that can be used when planning and assessing diets for healthy individuals. Modified diets must be devised for clients requiring them. For example, diets for diabetes, hypertension, obesity, or another condition should be provided by the home. The diet must be adequate in energy and other macronutrients, and additional vitamins and minerals may need to be provided in order to correct deficiencies created as a result of drug and alcohol problems. Clients should also be monitored for weight gain due to prescribed medications. Workers should be educated on drug-nutrient interactions, and meals should be timed in order to prevent problems associated with drug-nutrient interactions.

Evolving Nutrition Standards in Retirement Homes

As the older population increases in number, accommodations for individuals not wishing to or unable to care for themselves are increasing. Among these accommodations are assisted living facilities, retirement homes with skilled care services, and nursing homes. Assisted living offers some independence and is a combination of safe housing and supportive social and healthcare services. It is designed to meet the needs of individuals requiring assistance with activities of daily living. Individuals who are unable to care for themselves and require skilled care, or those who have lost the capacity to function independently due to illness, may reside in skilled nursing facilities or skilled care units in retirement communities. These facilities must undergo certification by the Centers for Medicare and Medicaid Services (CMS) and follow established guidelines. In order to receive funding under the federal and state Medicaid program, nursing facilities must have in place a quality care team that assesses patients and establishes measurable clinical goals, outcomes assessments, and approaches to management. This team must include a nutrition professional who assesses clients upon admission and at least 30 days following admission. Clients are reassessed for weight changes, changes in dietary consumption, laboratory parameters affected by nutrition intake, and other clinical incidences. In addition, they must conduct an annual assessment on each resident in order to determine if goals are being met.

Older individuals may suffer from multiple chronic diseases, and data from the third National Health and Nutrition Examination Survey (NHANES) suggest that the older adult is also at risk for malnutrition because of the presence of disease, physical disabilities, poor dental and oral health, many medications (prescribed and over the counter), social isolation, financial limitations, or impaired mental health. Physiological changes that accompany aging also place this population at additional risk. Some older adults enter residential homes in order to remove themselves from social isolation and to relieve themselves of the responsibilities associated with their daily care.

In caring for this population, the nutrition professional must take into consideration their unique needs. For example, energy requirements generally decrease with age because of changes in body composition, a reduction in physical activity, and a decrease in the basal energy expenditure. Although the energy requirement is decreased in older adults, the requirements for protein, vitamins, and minerals remain the same or increase in some cases. Adequate sources of carbohydrate-rich foods should be consumed and should be provided in the form of complex carbohydrates, such as whole grains and legumes, in addition to fruits, in order to provide fiber. An adequate supply of water also must be provided.

As people age and experience a loss of skeletal mass, dietary intake of protein becomes more important. Although the Dietary Reference Intakes (DRI) for protein remains the same, in some instances, protein needs may have to be decreased due to some physiological illness; therefore, it is incumbent on the nutrition professional to carefully evaluate the client's nutrition status and any conditions that affect dietary planning. A common marker for nutrition status is the serum albumin level; in acute cases, pre-albumin measures may be required. If depleted albumin stores are exhibited, clients should be evaluated carefully to determine if there are contributing factors, other than diet, that affect albumin levels.

In older adults, intakes of vitamins and minerals should be monitored. It is especially important to provide some sources of calcium other than milk for clients who may have a lactase deficiency, and to offer foods that are low in sodium content.

Individuals requiring skilled care should be serviced meals based on their disease states. Where possible, nutrient-dense foods should be served in situations where a poor appetite exists. Adequate fiber and fluid should be incorporated into the menu in order to prevent dehydration and constipation. Serving attractive and palatable meals in an atmosphere that encourages independent eating helps clients to maintain a sense of self-confidence. Assistance should be provided when necessary to promote the nutritional well-being of the individuals.

Evolving Nutrition Standards for Children in Group Care

School and Head Start Programs

Food service in group settings such as Head Start programs, daycare centers, and preschool programs in elementary schools is regulated by standards established by federal and/or state agencies. These standards, which are administered by regulatory programs, are science-based and are necessary to ensure that childcare food service is of uniformly high quality. Many facilities and some daycare homes participate in the U.S. Department of Agriculture (USDA) Child and Adult Care Food Programs. These programs provide reimbursement on a sliding scale for meals served to children, and each program has nutrient requirements. The programs are designed to assist childcare programs in providing nutritious and healthful meals.

> See meal patterns for the Child and Adult Care Food Programs at http://www.nutrition.gov.

Consuming nourishing, wholesome, and attractive food is a foundation for developmentally appropriate learning experiences and contributes to health, well-being, and physical growth. Therefore, in order to provide children with optimal nutrients, a program should offer food that is appealing, wholesome, safely prepared, and age-appropriate.

These programs should plan cycle menus, which offer seasonal and cultural foods, and should include foods that are colorful and texture-appropriate. When possible, family-style meals should be encouraged in order to promote independence and self-confidence.

Through focus groups, families could be consulted about the inclusion of some food items on menus. Young children do not enjoy mixed dishes and foods that are unidentifiable. Although children usually eat well in group settings, peer influence could have a negative effect on food intake. Refusal of foods by one or more children can affect the entire group. To discourage problem eaters and to strengthen family-style eating, teachers and parents should sit at the table and share the same meal with children. The presence of an adult at the table with children while they are eating also encourages social interactions and conversations about the food.

The nutrition professional can develop nutrition education projects that teachers can incorporate into the lesson plans; mealtime can be an ideal environment for this. Some helpful learning activities include experiencing new foods through identifying and tasting, describing size and shapes, and participating in simple food preparation. Federal guidelines require families who participate in the Head Start program to receive nutrition education, so periodic nutrition classes should be planned for families and teachers.

The latest information on child health has resulted in a shift in emphasis for the child nutrition program from the prevention of dietary deficiencies to the promotion of healthful food practices for prevention of chronic diseases, which are appearing in young children today. (See Chapter 5 on childhood obesity.) In an effort to promote growth and development and good dietary habits that may reduce the incidence of chronic diseases later in life, MyPyramid (formerly called the Food Guide Pyramid) was developed by the USDA. When planning meals, this guide should be utilized in conjunction with the Dietary Guidelines for Americans. Also incorporated into the pyramid is a physical activity regimen, which should be encouraged. (Both are available at www.MyPyramid.gov.)

The Mission of Food Service

In group care organizations, whether healthcare or community care, the mission of the institution guides the food-service delivery system. In healthcare organizations, the mission is to provide food and nutrition that will help to alleviate illnesses and restore health. In community organizations, the mission is to provide meals that meet the nutrient needs of clients; although modified diets may be provided, the emphasis is on maintaining health. In group care for children, the emphasis is on providing food and nutrition that promote growth and development as well as maintain cognitive and emotional health.

If food is not prepared and held in sanitary conditions or if infection control factors are not enforced, the food service delivery system can have a deleterious effect on an individual's nutrition status. If incorrect diets are presented to clients, this can also affect nutrition and health status.

In large conventional healthcare organizations such as hospitals and nursing facilities, a multi-layer system for providing meals exists. The first layer is the food service systems staff, who are responsible for ensuring that foods served to clients are safe and wholesome. In this layer, an administrative dietitian or food service director administers the food service department and may report to an administrative officer of the institution or an officer of a food service company. The next layer of food service is the food production area. The production area is usually well designed with adequate resources to promote meal preparation and to ensure that acceptable sanitation procedures are adhered to. The recommendations of the Hazard Analysis and Critical Control Point (HACCP) are followed to ensure safety in food handling, cooking, and storage.

> Read more about HACCP at http://vm.cfsan.fda.gov/~lrd/haccp.html.

The next layer of food service is the menu, which is overseen by a registered dietitian. The cycle menu, designed for a specific period of time, serves as the basis for procurement and food production. All menus must meet the DRIs except for nutrient-modified menus, which the dietitian modifies by altering nutrients where necessary. Diet manuals, authored by nutrition professionals, are available for use by staff.

In privately owned group care facilities for mentally and physically disabled persons, it is mandated that a nutrition specialist be employed for food service oversight. In some states, the professional must be a registered dietitian. Depending on the size of the facility, a full-time, part-time, or consulting dietitian may be employed to ensure that the dietary needs of the clients are met.

The nutrition professional may find problems associated with overseeing a food service operation. There may be limited storage in the production area, resulting in improperly stored foods. Also, the staff may have limited knowledge of meal preparation using a standardized menu. This may result in inconsistencies in taste, appearance, and nutritive value of the meals. Proper measures must be in place to ensure that food is received, stored, and prepared according to acceptable sanitation procedures in order to preserve the nutritive value. Workers should be trained to understand the importance of following menus and recipes as prescribed, the relationship of food storage and sanitation to health, and the reason for safe food handling and preparation. In addition, a reduction in the use of sodium, total fat, saturated fats, and trans-fatty acids should be incorporated into staff training sessions. Alternative methods for the use of seasoning should also be taught. In order to control food costs and decrease waste, recipes for combination dishes should be provided, and detailed shopping lists with quantities for each menu item should be attached.

A daily routine for meal service should be planned into the schedule. Meals should be served at approximately the same time each day. Regulations require that dining space should be adequate to accommodate wheelchairs, and furnishings should be comfortable to serve the number and types of clients for which they are intended. Clients' self-feeding skill can affect their nutritional status;

therefore, if necessary, adaptive feeding devices should be provided with comfortable positioning to maximize ingestion. It is also important to ensure that clients are given the correct portions and that all meals including desserts are consumed. Clients who are self-feeders may spill portions of their food, and it is important to replace foods in order to provide adequate nutrition. Although every effort should be made to promote independence, adequate help should be available at mealtime to assist clients who may need to be assisted with feeding when necessary.

Counseling Clients and Families

Clients and family members should be encouraged to participate in nutrition education programs so that they understand the reasons for meals being served to children or relatives in group care facilities. Lessons should be simple, interactive, and fun so that participants do not feel threatened. The provision of basic nutrition information should assist in planning healthy and attractive meals. Good food preparation techniques such as storing, handling, and proper temperature control should also be included in the nutrition education. One of the requirements of the Head Start Program is that parents receive basic nutrition education so that there can be some continuity in meal planning and preparation. Parents should be made aware of the link between nutrition and health so that they may become more amenable to practicing healthful nutrition habits for themselves and their families. Where modified diets are served, families should be educated regarding the diets so that they can understand the purpose and, therefore, promote compliance.

What Administrators and Staff Need to Know

Although community-based residences are beneficial for many individuals, they result in staff training and management issues that are not encountered in institutional settings. One staff training issue unique to community residences is dietary management. In a traditional institution, trained personnel are responsible for menu development, food storage, and meal preparation. In community residences, these responsibilities fall to the direct-care staff, who may have little or no training or experience in institutional food production. Unlike traditional settings (e.g., hospitals), where supervisory personnel are usually present, employees in community-based group homes usually lack continuous on-site supervision for long periods and must make decisions that may affect nutrition status. Evolving nutrition standards promote that administrators should:

- Be knowledgeable about state and local laws governing nutrition and food service management to ensure appropriate staffing.
- Participate in policy development and implementation that promote and support community nutrition services.
- Take advantage of available resources, such as a local chapter of the American Dietetic Association, registered dietitians at hospitals, and local and state nutritionists in health departments.

Staff in community-based homes:

- Should be provided ongoing education, especially in the area of food production, to include receiving, sanitation, storage, food handling, and preparation.
- Who are preparing meals should not be caring for clients simultaneously, to prevent contamination.
- Should be knowledgeable of the effect of food preparation on nutrient content.
- Should consult with nutrition specialists prior to making menu changes that may affect nutrient intake.

To ensure that safe nutrition and food services standards are maintained in group care, the dietitian/nutritionist should:

- Keep abreast of local and state regulations that affect the clients who are being served. This should include being knowledgeable about public health regulations for group care situations, inclusive of menu patterns.
- Serve as members of the public health advisory boards that formulate regulations and guidelines for food service in group care, where possible.
- Where possible, serve as a team member of an organization that conducts inspections and regulates licensure in group care.
- Monitor food guidance systems and public health nutrition education resources to ensure that they are useful and accessible to caregivers at group care facilities.
- Encourage administrators and staff to participate in public health nutrition education training to ensure safe nutrition practices.
- Work in partnership with public health licensing agencies in order to keep abreast of changes in regulations affecting nutrition standards.
- Provide simple references for staff in community sites, such as posters of the appropriate MyPyramid and Dietary Guidelines for Americans.

Issues for Discussion

1. In order to ensure that nutrition services are being met, should community group organizations be held to the same food and nutrition standards as other healthcare organizations that provide nutrition services?

2. Discuss how dietitians/nutritionists should be proactive by ensuring that adequate nutrition services are being provided to clients by means of increasing the ratio of dietitians/nutritionists to clients and increasing the role of the dietitian/nutritionist in these facilities.

3. Discuss how dietitians/nutritionists should position themselves politically to better impact the lives of those living in group care situations.

References

American Dietetic Association. (1999). Position of The American Dietetic Association: Nutrition standards for child-care programs. *Journal of the American Dietetic Association*, 99, 981–988.

Briley, M. E., Roberts-Gray, C., & Simpson, D. (1994). Identification of factors that influence the menu at childcare centers. A grounded theory approach. *Journal of the American Dietetic Association*, 94, 276–281.

Drake, M. A. (1992). Menu evaluation, nutrient intake of young children, nutrition knowledge of menu planners in childcare centers in Missouri. *Journal of Nutrition Education*, 24, 145–148.

Dyer, K., Kneringer, M. J., & Luce, S. C. (1996). An efficient method of ensuring program quality for adults with developmental disabilities in community-based settings. *Journal of Clinical and Consulting Psychology*, 48, 171–179.

Kneringer, M. J. & Pace, M. J. (1999). Improving staff nutritional practices in community-based group homes: Evaluation, training, and management. *Journal of Applied Behavior Analysis*, 32, 221–224.

Mahan, K. & Escott-Stump, S. (Eds.). (2004). *Krause's food, nutrition, and diet therapy*. Philadelphia: Saunders.

U.S. Department of Agriculture. (1999). *Food guide pyramid for young children: A daily guide for 2 to 6 year olds*. Washington, DC: Department of Agriculture, Center for Policy and Promotion.

PART V

PROTECTING THE PUBLIC'S NUTRITIONAL HEALTH

Part V includes *Nutrition in Public Health's* newest additions. Although Chapter 16 appeared in the first edition, it has now been greatly enriched. However, Chapters 17 and 18 bring us to a whole new frontier of public health nutrition. Chapter 17 discusses securing adequate food for those who still live in poverty. Despite the present outreach of public health nutrition, a hefty percentage of Americans still live without adequate food and/or live in a constant state of fear of being without food, showing that we have far to go in reaching those at highest risk. Chapter 18 discusses the fact that we must protect ourselves from potential bioterrorism plots directed at our food supply. Our food must be kept secure because it can be a potent avenue for terrorism. Public health nutrition will now have to meet the challenge of keeping food safe from many forms of invasion.

CHAPTER 16

SAFEGUARDING THE FOOD SUPPLY

Paul N. Taylor, PhD

Reader Objectives

After studying this chapter and reflecting on the contents, you should be able to:

1. List and describe the roles of federal, state, and local agencies responsible for the safety of the U.S. food supply.
2. List and describe the hazards to food safety.
3. Identify current national food safety issues.
4. Explain why food safety education should be integrated into public health nutrition programs and describe possible approaches.
5. Understand the importance of keeping informed about food safety.

America's food supply is among the safest in the world. The federal food safety system was recently strengthened in many areas, with new surveillance systems, better prevention programs, faster outbreak responses, enhanced education programs, more focused and coordinated research initiatives, and better risk assessment activities. According to officials, federal food safety agencies are improving their working relationships with each other.[1]

Despite these efforts, every year approximately 76 million Americans contract a foodborne illness, and 5,000 die from it.[2] Causative factors include transportation and refrigeration issues, an increasing volume of imported foods, and more people eating more meals away from home. Among those at greatest risk for foodborne illness are children, the elderly, pregnant women, and immunocompromised persons. Children and the elderly comprised approximately 38% of the population in 1999, and are expected to comprise 41% of the population by 2020.[3,4]

Americans demand nutritious, wholesome, and safe food that is plentiful, varied, and at reasonable cost. In a rapidly changing world, food producers, processors, vendors, and regulators must constantly adapt to the changing expectations and demands of consumers.

The basic framework of today's federal food safety system was developed early in the twentieth century. President Theodore Roosevelt's investigation of Chicago's meat packing industry and Upton

Sinclair's exposé of conditions there[5] prompted passage of the Meat Inspection Act of 1906 (concomitant with the Pure Food and Drug Act). Early in this century, terrorist attacks in the United States prompted increased scrutiny of the various food safety regulatory systems and procedures, and passage of antibioterrorism legislation.[6] The new Department of Homeland Security absorbed some food safety functions.[7] Against this backdrop, the full range of food safety issues continues to demand vigilance by industry, government, and consumers.

Public health professionals, nutritionists, and consumers must not become (or remain) complacent about the safety of the nation's food supply. Significant challenges have not been overcome and new challenges emerge frequently (e.g., globalization of food production, manufacturing, and marketing; geographic centralization and consolidation of food processing; some foodborne pathogens' ability to overcome traditional hurdles such as acidity, temperature, or oxygen, employed against them; new foodborne pathogens evolving or being discovered; and bioterrorism directed at food and water supplies). Old paradigms are increasingly irrelevant; yet, as is human nature, powerful forces resist the changes necessary to keep pace with a dynamic system of food production and supply and to ensure safety at all points in the system. The new paradigm for the 21st century should make this chapter's opening line, "America's food supply is among the safest in the world," obsolete by ensuring global food safety.

Food Safety Defined

Stier defines "food safety" in terms of hazards and risks:

> A safe food may be defined as a product which contains no physical, chemical or microbial organisms or by-products of those organisms which if consumed by man will result in illness, injury, or death (an unacceptable consumer health risk). The definition purposely does not use the term contaminants because many of the potential hazards in food . . . are typically found in or on the food. It is their concentration, numbers or size that creates potential safety problems.[8]

"Hazard" expresses a food's capacity to cause harm (i.e., "Any biological, chemical, or physical property that may cause an unacceptable consumer health risk"[8]). The food does not always cause harm; rather, hazard indicates that the food might cause a specified harm. The probability that the specified harm will occur is the hazard's associated "risk."[9]

To evaluate food safety, scientists must first attempt risk assessment (i.e., to "identify hazards related to foods or food components and then estimate the size of the risk that the hazard will occur"[9]).

"When conducting hazard analysis, the [food processor] looks at potential hazards that could realistically cause illness or injury."[8] Risk management involves deciding whether an identified risk is acceptable. ". . . Note that the process outlined . . . considers all foods to have some degree of risk," that is, "no food is absolutely safe."[9]

Public health nutritionists must understand food safety issues, using critical thinking to evaluate scientific literature and the press, in order to keep consumers informed in today's environment of "junk science" and pseudo-science. Always a dynamic field, food technologies and food safety regulations are changing at an increasingly rapid rate. Food scientists, environmental health specialists, health educators, and other public health colleagues may be consulted to help educate consumers about food safety issues. These professionals can help consumers sort through the many government and scientific Websites that are available. Lists of websites are maintained by organizations which include The Food Safety Consortium[10] (http://www.uark.edu/depts/fsc/fslinks.htm) and the Simmons College Center for Hygiene and Health in Home and Community (http://www.simmons.edu/hygieneandhealth/links.shtml),[11] and more than 100 websites are listed as references to this chapter.

Protecting the Food Supply

Federal Agencies

Several federal agencies, with sometimes overlapping jurisdictions, share responsibility for the safety of the U.S. food supply (Table 16-1). The following sections describe the principal federal agencies and their roles.

The Food and Drug Administration

The Department of Health and Human Services' (DHHS) Food and Drug Administration (FDA) oversees all domestic and imported food (except meat and poultry) sold in interstate commerce, including seafood, shell eggs, bottled water, and wine beverages containing < 7% alcohol.[12] The FDA enforces food safety laws governing these foods through inspections; food analysis; safety reviews of food and color additives and animal drugs; monitoring of the safety of food-animal feeds; developing model codes, ordinances, guidelines, and interpretations; working with states to implement such models; establishing good food manufacturing practices (GMP); establishing sanitation and packaging requirements; establishing Hazard Analysis and Critical Control Points (HACCP) programs; collaborating with foreign governments to ensure imported foods safety; requesting and monitoring voluntary recalls of unsafe foods; enforcement; research; and industry and consumer food safety education.[12]

TABLE 16-1   Federal Agencies with Food Safety Responsibilities

Agency	Unit	Mission	Internet
Department of Agriculture (USDA)	Animal and Plant Health Inspection Service (APHIS)[1]	Protects and promotes U.S. agricultural health	USDA: http://www.usda.gov APHIS: http://www.aphis.usda.gov
	Food Safety and Inspection Service (FSIS)	Ensures that the nation's commercial supply of meat, poultry, and egg products is safe, wholesome, and correctly labeled and packaged	http://www.fsis.usda.gov
	Agricultural Research Service (ARS), National Animal Disease Center (NADC)	Conducts research on animal health and food safety problems	http://www.nadc.ars.usda.gov
Department of Commerce (USDC)	National Oceanic and Atmospheric Administration (NOAA)	Administers National Seafood Inspection Program (NSIP) offering seafood inspection, grading, certification, and other services to the seafood industry (voluntary, fee-for-service)	USDC: http://www.commerce.gov NOAA: http://www.noaa.gov NSIP: http://seafood.nmfs.noaa.gov
Department of Health and Human Services (DHHS)	Centers for Disease Control and Prevention (CDC)	Tracks foodborne illness incidents and outbreaks; provides data and information to the other food safety agencies	DHHS: http://www.os.dhhs.gov CDC: http://www.cdc.gov
	Food & Drug Administration (FDA)	Approves food and drugs for widespread use; its Center for Food Safety and Applied Nutrition (CFSAN) ensures that food is safe, nutritious, and wholesome	FDA: http://www.fda.gov CFSAN: http://vm.cfsan.fda.gov/list.html
Department of Homeland Security (DHS)	Customs & Border Protection (CBP)	Inspects agricultural goods arriving in the U.S. at ports and borders	DHS: http://www.dhs.gov/dhspublic/ CBP: http://www.customs.ustreas.gov Introducing the new CBP Agriculture Specialist: http://www.cbp.gov/xp/CustomsToday/2004/May/agSpec.xml

Agency	Unit	Mission	Internet
Department of the Treasury	Bureau of Alcohol, Tobacco, Firearms and Explosives	Regulates qualification and operations of distilleries, wineries, breweries, importers, and wholesalers	Treasury: http://www.ustreas.gov ATF: http://www.atf.gov
Federal Trade Commission	Bureau of Consumer Protection (BCP); Division of Advertising Practices (DAP); Division of Consumer Protection (DCP); Division of Enforcement (DE)	Protects consumers against unfair, deceptive, or fraudulent practices; protects consumers from deceptive and unsubstantiated advertising (advertising claims for food, particularly those relating to nutritional or health benefits of foods); conducts law enforcement activities to protect consumers	FTC: http://www.ftc.gov BCP: http://www.ftc.gov/bcp/bcp.htm DAP: http://www.ftc.gov/bcp/bcpap.htm DE: http://www.ftc.gov/bcp/bcpenf.htm

[1]Some APHIS functions and personnel transferred to the Department of Homeland Security, Customs and Border Protection, on March 1, 2003.

Source: Compiled by the author.

The Food Safety and Inspection Service

The U.S. Department of Agriculture's (USDA) Food Safety and Inspection Service (FSIS) oversees domestic and imported meat, poultry and related products (e.g., meat- or poultry-containing stews, pizzas and frozen foods), and processed egg products (generally liquid, frozen, and dried pasteurized egg products). FSIS enforces food safety laws governing these foods through antemortem and postmortem inspections of food animals, meat and poultry slaughter and processing plant inspections, monitoring and inspecting processed egg products (together with the USDA Agricultural Marketing Service), food analysis, establishing additive and ingredient standards, inspections of foreign meat and poultry processing plants exporting to the United States, requesting and monitoring unsafe meat/poultry products recalls, meat/poultry safety research, and industry and consumer food safety education.[12]

The U.S. Environmental Protection Agency

The Environmental Protection Agency (EPA) regulates pesticides and oversees drinking water quality. Its food safety role for foods made from plants, seafood, meat, and poultry includes regulating toxic substances and wastes to prevent entry into the environment or foods, determining new pesticide safety, setting tolerance levels for pesticide residues in foods, and promoting safe use of pesticides (enforcement of these standards is an FDA function).[12] The EPA also establishes safe drinking water standards and assists states in protecting and monitoring drinking water quality.

Customs and Border Protection

In 2003, the Department of Homeland Security (DHS), Customs and Border Protection (CBP) assumed responsibility for inspecting agricultural goods arriving in the United States. Previously, this was a function of the USDA's Animal and Plant Health Inspection Service (APHIS).[13,14] The transfer "linked and integrated the . . . scientific mission of agriculture border inspection to the expertise and operational capabilities of the primary CBP mission: to prevent terrorists and terrorist weapons from entering the United States."[13] CBP expects to "play an important role in the Department of Homeland Security's multi-layered approach to protect the food supply from the threats of agroterrorism and bioterrorism,"[13] while also detecting and denying entry to animal and plant pests and diseases that could harm U.S. agriculture.

The Centers for Disease Control and Prevention

DHHS's Centers for Disease Control and Prevention (CDC) oversees and directs prevention efforts against foodborne and waterborne infections. Collaborating with other domestic and international agencies, the CDC recently expanded its mission to work toward effective global surveillance and control of foodborne and waterborne pathogens. In the United States, the CDC participates in the National Food Safety Initiative (NFSI) with the FDA, USDA, and other agencies to address food safety problems, and collaborates with the EPA and the drinking water industry to improve drinking water safety.[12,15] The CDC also initiated and participates in addressing emerging infectious diseases and preventing future emergent infectious diseases worldwide.[16]

The National Oceanic and Atmospheric Administration

The Department of Commerce, National Oceanic and Atmospheric Administration (NOAA) administers a Seafood Inspection Program offering seafood inspection, grading, and certification; vessel and plant sanitation; label review; laboratory analysis; training; and consultative and information services to the seafood industry on a voluntary fee-for-service basis.[17,18] Processors may use official marks on complying products, indicating that they are federally inspected. (Note: All seafood processors must participate in the FDA's seafood HACCP program,[19,20] under which FDA inspects the processors annually. In 2001 the FDA refocused on seafood products presenting the highest risk to consumers by intensifying inspection, laboratory testing, enforcement, and education efforts on processors not controlling for pathogens, processors not controlling for histamines, and processors without HACCP plans.[21])

The Bureau of Consumer Protection

The Federal Trade Commission's (FTC) Division of Advertising Practices, Bureau of Consumer Protection protects consumers from deceptive and unsubstantiated advertising. It enforces laws pertaining to advertising claims for food (particularly those claims relating to nutritional or health benefits of foods), television infomercials (to ensure that format and content are non-deceptive), and general advertising.[22]

The Bureau of Alcohol, Tobacco, Firearms and Explosives

The U.S. Department of Justice's Bureau of Alcohol, Tobacco, Firearms and Explosives (ATF) regulates distilleries, wineries, breweries, and importers and wholesalers in the industry. ATF tests new alcohol products, determines whether products currently marketed pose a health risk to consumers, and ensures that alcohol beverage labels are not misleading.[23]

State and Local Collaboration

State and local governmental agencies oversee all food products within their jurisdictions, in cooperation with federal agencies. Usually, public health departments and state agriculture departments are the delegated authorities, with responsibilities at the state, county, and city level varying by state. Registered sanitarians, environmental health specialists, and sometimes other classes of employees in-

spect restaurants, food stores, supermarkets, other retail food establishments, dairy farms, milk processing plants, grain mills, and food
manufacturing plants within local jurisdictions. They may also collaborate with federal agencies to develop and implement food safety
standards for foods produced within state borders, and seize unsafe
food products made or distributed within their jurisdictions.[12] State
food sanitation codes usually meet or exceed model federal standards, and for those states maintaining their own commodity inspection programs (e.g., at least 29 states have state meat inspection
programs[24]), the state program must be equivalent to the corresponding federal program and operates under federal oversight.

Public health nutritionists should know their jurisdiction's regulatory authorities for sanitation and food safety and develop working relationships with them to identify and serve the needs of their
communities. Inviting these officials to attend or speak at regional,
state, and local dietetic or other association meetings is one way to
build networking relationships. Nutritionists will find opportunities
to assist these officials during natural disasters, in investigating outbreaks of food- and waterborne disease, and during other civil disturbances.[25-27] During the severe acute respiratory syndrome (SARS)
crisis in China, for example, "Qualified nutritionists supervised
preparations of meals" that were then delivered to quarantined residents in Nanking.[28] Civil emergency preparedness and response organizations should include public health nutritionists and/or
registered dietitians on their teams. (Find out who is on your local
team—see the American Civil Defense Association's website at
http://www.tacda.org/defensenow/.[29]) Nutritionists are also needed
to participate in emergency nutrition and food aid research.[30,31]

Food Safety Laws

Major food safety legislation in the United States began in 1906
with the Pure Food and Drug Act (which created the FDA) and the
Meat Inspection Act. Table 16-2 lists several federal laws with ap-
plicability to food safety. Some of these laws are discussed in the
following sections.

The Federal Meat Inspection Act of 1906

The Federal Meat Inspection Act (amended by the Wholesome Meat
Act in 1967) requires continuous inspection (antemortem, during
slaughter, and postmortem) by USDA or USDA-sanctioned state
meat inspection programs of all cattle, sheep, swine, goats, and
horses at slaughter. Additionally, a federal (or state equivalent) in-
spector must be present for at least part of every shift while meat
products are processed for human or animal consumption. Meat and
meat products meeting federal standards are stamped "United States

TABLE 16-2   Selected Federal Regulations Important to Food Safety

1906	Pure Food and Drug Act[1]
1906	Federal Meat Inspection Act[2]
1967	Wholesome Meat Act
1968	Wholesome Poultry Products Act
1938	Federal Food, Drug, and Cosmetic Act[3]
1958	Food Additives Amendment
1960	Color Additives Amendment
1938	Federal Trade Commission Act (amended for food)[4]
1957	Federal Poultry Products Inspection Act[5]
1966	Fair Packaging and Labeling Act[6]
1980	Infant Formula Act[7]
1990	Nutrition Education and Labeling Act[8]
1990	Organic Foods Production Act[9-13]
1994	Dietary Supplement Health and Education Act[14]
1996	Food Quality Protection Act[15]
1996	Safe Drinking Water Act[16]
2002	Homeland Security Act[17]
2002	Public Health Security and Bioterrorism Preparedness and Response Act[18]
2004	Food Allergen Labeling and Consumer Protection Act[19]

Source: Compiled by the author. For more information, see:

[1] http://vm.cfsan.fda.gov/~lrd/history1.html#toc

[2] http://www.fda.gov/opacom/laws/meat.htm

[3] http://vm.cfsan.fda.gov/~lrd/histor1a.html

[4] http://www.fda.gov/opacom/laws/ftca.htm

[5] http://www.fda.gov/opacom/laws/pltryact.htm

[6] http://www.fda.gov/opacom/laws/fplact.htm

[7] http://vm.cfsan.fda.gov/~dms/inf-guid.html

[8] http://www.fda.gov/ora/inspect_ref/igs/nleatxt.html

[9] http://www.ams.usda.gov/nop/archive/OFPA.html

[10] http://www.ams.usda.gov/nop/indexNet.htm

[11] http://www.nal.usda.gov/afsic/ofp/

[12] Olsson, F. & Weeda, P. C. (2001). A primer on the U.S. Department of Agriculture national organic program. Elmwood Park, NJ: Food Institute.

[13] Fishman, S. (1990). The guide to the U.S. Organic Foods Production Act of 1990. Greenfield, MA: Organic Foods Production Association of North America.

[14] http://www.fda.gov/opacom/laws/dshea.html

[15] http://www.fda.gov/opacom/laws/foodqual/fqpatoc.htm

[16] http://www4.law.cornell.edu/uscode/42/300f.html

[17] http://www.dhs.gov/dhspublic/interweb/assetlibrary/hr_5005_enr.pdf

[18] http://www.fda.gov/oc/bioterrorism/bioact.html

[19] Bush signs food allergen labeling bill. (August 4, 2004). IFT Newsletter. Available at: http://www.ift.org/cms/?pid=1001085. Accessed August 5, 2004.

Inspected and Passed by Department of Agriculture" (or state equivalent program). Products bearing the federal mark may be shipped and sold in interstate commerce; whereas, products bearing state marks may only be shipped and sold in intrastate commerce. State (and city) meat inspection programs must meet federal standards.[32,33]

The Federal Food, Drug, and Cosmetic Act of 1938

The Federal Food, Drug, and Cosmetic Act (FDCA) prohibits entry into interstate commerce of any food that is adulterated containing poisonous or deleterious substances that may make the food unhealthful; containing filth; decomposed; prepared or handled under unsanitary conditions; from a diseased animal; subjected to radiation except as permitted; having a valuable constituent omitted; having an unauthorized ingredient substitution; having a concealed defect; increased in bulk weight or decreased in strength to deceptively improve appearance; or containing an unapproved or uncertified coloring agent or misbranded (not honestly labeled). The FDA establishes guidance and regulatory requirements under the law, codified in Title 21, Code of Federal Regulations. Although the FDA uses inspections to monitor whether food manufacturers adhere to their legal responsibility of producing safe, wholesome foods, the agency's budget and personnel are insufficient and inspections are infrequent. (The USDA, also lacking funding, and the FDA jointly adopted an industry-operated food safety and inspection system, Hazard Analysis and Critical Control Points.)[32,33]

Food Additives Amendment, 1958

The FDA regulates food additives under the 1958 Food Additives Amendment to the FDCA. The FDA must approve an additive before it can be included in food and requires the additive's manufacturer to prove its safety for the ways it will be used in food. Food additives include substances intentionally added for specific purposes, such as carrageenan (a red seaweed gum used to emulsify, stabilize, or thicken foods)[34] or ozone (as an antimicrobial agent in contact with food),[35] and substances unintentionally added to foods, such as acetone (a component of adhesives) or mineral oil (a lubricant, not to exceed 10 ppm in food).[36]

The Food Additives Amendment provided two exemptions:

1. Those additives in use before 1958, which had been determined by the FDA or USDA to be safe for use in specific foods, were given "prior sanctioned" status.[37] For example, sodium nitrite as a preservative in red meats is prior sanctioned and regulated by the USDA, whereas sodium nitrite when added to fish products is an additive regulated by the FDA.[33]

2. Those additives (such as salt and sugar) whose use in foods is Generally Recognized As Safe (GRAS) by experts,[38-40] based on

either an extensive history of common use in food before 1958 or published scientific evidence.[41] Chemicals may be added to or removed from either list as necessary whenever scientific knowledge of the chemical so warrants. The FDA and USDA continuously monitor substances on both lists.[42,43]

The Color Additives Amendment, 1960

The Color Additives Amendment to the FDCA brought all colors, natural and synthetic, under federal regulation. The FDA must approve all colors used in foods, drugs, and cosmetics before they can be marketed. Some colors (primarily coal-tar dyes) must be batch-certified (the manufacturer submits samples from each batch produced to the FDA for testing and pays a fee for service); whereas, others (mostly from plant, animal, or mineral sources) are exempt from batch certification.[44,45] Manufacturers and food processors may not use color additives to deceive consumers or to conceal blemishes or inferiorities in food products, and must declare color additives by their common or usual names on labels (e.g., FD&C Yellow 5 or carotene) rather than collectively as "colorings."[46]

The Nutrition Labeling and Education Act of 1990

The Nutrition Labeling and Education Act (NLEA) requires most foods to carry a nutrition label expressing nutrients as a percentage of Daily Values (DVs) for a 2,000-calorie diet rather than the now outdated Recommended Dietary Allowances (RDAs). The act also: 1) mandates more specific definitions for words such as "free," "light," or "reduced"; 2) restricts the use of the terms "sodium free" and "cholesterol free" to products normally containing sodium and/or cholesterol; 3) defines and regulates health claims, such as calcium helping to prevent osteoporosis; and 4) mandates that the total percentage of juice in juice drinks be declared.[47]

The Dietary Supplement Health and Education Act of 1994

The Dietary Supplement Health and Education Act (DSHEA) mandates premarket manufacturer responsibility for dietary supplement safety and requires truthful supplement label information. After supplements reach the market, the FDA monitors supplement safety, including voluntary dietary supplement adverse event reporting; monitors product information (e.g., labeling and claims); and takes action against unsafe supplements. The law does not provide for manufacturer registration, nor does it require manufacturers to seek FDA approval before producing or marketing supplements.[48] The law is controversial because, unlike foods or food additives, which must be proven safe by manufacturers before they are marketed, neither the safety nor the efficacy of supplements needs to be proven by producers.[49] Rather, the FDA must prove that a supplement is unsafe, after marketing, before any action may be taken to remove the product from the market. (For example, it took more than 10 years for the FDA to accumulate enough evidence to ban ephedra.[50]) Legislation is pending to address problems with DSHEA and supplement safety.

The Food Quality Protection Act of 1996

The Food Quality Protection Act of 1996 (FQPA)[50] amended the FDCA and the Insecticide, Fungicide, and Rodenticide Act (IFRA),[51] changing the way the EPA regulates pesticides (also see the 2003 Pesticide Registration Improvement Act[51]). The zero-tolerance provision of the FDCA's food additives anticancer clause ("Delaney Clause"[33]) was replaced with a new safety standard, "reasonable certainty of no harm resulting from aggregate exposure," to be applied to all pesticides used on foods. With no provision for phasing in the new requirements, the EPA faced enforcing the new regulations while simultaneously learning to evaluate pesticides under the new rules and developing or approving new, scientifically tested methodologies for evaluating aggregate and cumulative risks.[52-55] Not surprisingly, this led to controversy among the EPA, environmental advocates, and public health organizations.[56,57] In 1993, the EPA was sued by four states and several environmental and public health groups "for allegedly failing to adequately protect children from pesticides used on food . . . contend[ing] that the EPA set inadequate limits on several organophosphate insecticides."[58]

Public Health Security and Bioterrorism Preparedness and Response Act of 2002

The Bioterrorism Act's Title III specifically addresses food safety, directing:

> . . . federal agencies, the food industry, consumer and producer groups, scientific organizations, and the States, [to] develop a crisis communications and education strategy with respect to bioterrorist threats to the food supply. Such strategy shall address threat assessments; technologies and procedures for securing food processing and manufacturing facilities and modes of transportation; response and notification procedures; and risk communications to the public.[59]

Title II covers security strategy, food adulteration, detention, registration, records maintenance, prior notice, and marking.[60] Bioterrorism and food is covered in length in Chapter 18.

The Food Allergen Labeling and Consumer Protection Act, 2004

The Food Allergen Labeling and Consumer Protection Act (FALCP, effective 2006) will provide improved food labeling information to consumers who suffer from food allergies. FALCP will require food labels to identify the presence of any of eight major food allergens: milk, eggs, fish, crustaceans, peanuts, tree nuts, wheat, and soybeans. Concomitant with expanding the number of allergens to be identified, the new requirements represent improvements over present labeling standards:

> ... if a product contains the milk-derived protein casein, the product's label would have to use the term "milk" in addition to the term "casein" so that those with milk allergies would clearly understand the presence of an allergen they need to avoid.[61]

Hazard Analysis and Critical Control Points (HACCP)

The HACCP protocol was developed by the Pillsbury Corporation in 1971 to ensure food safety for astronauts in outer space. Its principles focus on preventing hazards that could cause foodborne illness by identifying and correcting hazards before they develop, following foods from raw materials to finished products.[62,63] HACCP consists of seven principles:

1. Identify hazard(s).
2. Identify critical control point(s) (CCPs) for controlling each hazard identified.
3. Define limits for each CCP.
4. Establish specific procedures for monitoring each CCP.
5. Establish a procedure for taking corrective action whenever a CCP's limits have been exceeded.
6. Implement procedures to verify that the HACCP program is working as intended.
7. Thoroughly document the HACCP program and maintain records of CCP monitoring data. Examples of HACCP plans and flowcharts are easily obtained.[9,64,65]

HACCP programs are used in the seafood industry (since 1995, FDA oversight), meat and poultry processing plants (since 1998, USDA oversight), and the juice industry (since 2001, FDA oversight). Other segments of the food industry, such as food service, also use HACCP programs,[66,67] and the FDA is developing HACCP protocols for use in other segments of the food industry.[62]

Good Manufacturing Practices

Some regulations published by the FDA are collectively called good manufacturing practices (GMPs), or the Code of GMPs.[68] These specify sanitation, safety, and quality assurance procedures to be followed by food processors.[69] For example, the FDA specifies safe procedures for manufacturing, thermally processing, and packing low-acid canned foods to avoid growth of *Clostridium botulinum* and subsequent toxin formation by the pathogen.[70] The FDA also recognizes that it is impossible to manufacture, process, and package foods that are 100% free of poisonous, deleterious, or aesthetically unpleasant substances, and it has established specific tolerances and rules relating to these substances (e.g., fresh, frozen, and canned clams, mussels, and oysters must not contain > 80 μg paralytic shellfish poisoning toxin/100 g meat;[71] ground nutmeg poses no inherent hazard to health if it contains 100 insect fragments and/or ≤ 1 rodent hair/10 g.[72]

Hazards to Food Safety

Biological Hazards

Biological hazards include bacteria, viruses, parasites, and fungi (Table 16-3). Although several previously unknown or lesser-known pathogens have emerged in recent years,[73] bacterial pathogens remain the primary cause of foodborne illnesses.[74] These microbes cause either infections or intoxications. In infections, pathogens are ingested and multiply in the body, causing illness; in intoxications, toxins made by pathogens cause illness. Intoxications result from ingesting live pathogens that go on to multiply and produce toxin in the body, or they can occur without ingesting the live pathogens, if the pathogens are allowed to grow on food and produce heat-stable toxins. Food processing then kills the organisms, but does not damage the toxin.

In 1996–97, the CDC's Emerging Infections Program's Foodborne Diseases Active Surveillance Network (FoodNet) began collecting data from 10 states for laboratory-diagnosed cases of foodborne illness caused by bacterial pathogens *Campylobacter*, Shiga toxin-producing *Escherichia coli* (STEC) O157, *Listeria*, *Salmonella*, *Shigella*, *Vibrio*, and *Yersinia*, and protozoan parasites *Cryptosporidium* and *Cyclospora cayetanensis*. Although the incidence of infections caused by *Campylobacter*, *Cryptosporidium parvum*, *E. coli* O157, *Salmonella*, and *Y. enterocolitica* declined substantially since 1996, infants and young children continue to suffer a high incidence of infections from several of these nine organisms, and this is a major public health concern.[75] Despite this, 7-year data trends indicate that meeting the 2010 national health objectives of reducing the incidence of foodborne infections is possible.[75,76]

Bacteria

Campylobacter jejuni subsp. jejuni, one of about 14 species of *Campylobacter*,[77] is responsible for most cases of foodborne bacterial infection in the United States.[78] It is found in the intestinal tracts of farm livestock (especially poultry),[77,79] wild birds,[80–82] and rodents,[83,84] and in drinking water[85,86] and unchlorinated water[87,88]—it can also be car-

TABLE 16-3   Some Biological Hazards Associated with Food[1,2]

Hazard Type	Organism	Examples of Food Vehicles
Bacteria	*Bacillus cereus*	Chicken fried rice[3]
	Campylobacter jejuni	Unpasteurized milk[4]
	Clostridium botulinum	Muktuk (whale meat)[5]
	Clostridium perfringens	Corned beef[6]
	Escherichia coli	Ground beef[7]
	Listeria monocytogenes	Sliceable turkey deli meat[8]
	Salmonella Typhi	Prob. asymptomatic carrier/cook[9]
	Salmonella Enteriditis	Turkey & stuffing w/raw eggs[10]
	Shigella dysenteriae	Raw vegetables from salad bar[11]
	Staphylococcus aureus	Precooked packaged ham[12]
	Streptococcus pyogenes	Macaroni and cheese/cook[13]
	Vibrio cholerae	Seafood[14]
	Yersinia enterocolitica	Pork chitterlings[15]
Viruses	Hepatitis A	Green onions/foodhandlers[16]
	Rotavirus	Deli sandwiches[17]
	Noroviruses	Oysters, raspberries, et al.[18]
Fungi	*Alternaria* spp	Grain[19]
	Aspergillus spp.	Prob. Kombucha tea[20]
	Byssochlamys spp.	Fruits, vegetables[21]
	Fusarium spp.	Corn; sorghum[22]
	Penicillium spp.	Chestnuts[23]
Parasites: Flatworms	*Clonorchis sinensis*	Fish (frozen, raw, or salted)[24, 25]
	Diphyllobothrium latum	Fish[26]
	Fasciola hepatica	Watercress[27]
	Fasciolopsis buski	Raw aquatic plants; untreated water[28]
	Paragonimus spp.	Raw crayfish;[29] undercooked crayfish[30]
	Taenia spp.	Fecal/oral[31]
Parasites: Protozoans	Cryptosporidium parvum	Chicken salad[32]
	Cyclospora cayetanensis	Guatemalan raspberries[33]
	Entamoeba histolytica	Prob. ice and ice cream[34]
	Giardia lamblia	Prob. taco ingredients[35]
	Sarcocystis spp.	Raw beef and pork[36]
	Toxoplasma gondii	Raw and undercooked venison[37]

(Continues)

TABLE 16-3   Some Biological Hazards Associated with Food (Continued)

Hazard Type	Organism	Examples of Food Vehicles
Parasites: Roundworms	*Anisakis simplex*	Raw fish[38]
	Ascaris lumbricoides	Fecal/oral[39]
	Pseudoterranova decipiens	Raw fish[40]
	Trichinella spiralis	Bear, cougar, wild boar meats; pork[41]
Prions	Abnormal prion proteins	Wild game[42]

[1]This is not a complete listing.

[2]For excellent reviews of most of these organisms, see: Hui, Y. H., Pierson, M. D., & Gorham, M. D. (Eds.). (2000). *Foodborne disease handbook* (2nd ed., Vol. 1: Bacterial Pathogens, Vol. 2: Viruses, Parasites, Pathogens, and HACCP, Vol. 3: Plant Toxicants, & Vol. 4: Seafood and Environmental Toxins). New York: Marcel Dekker; Jay, J. M. (2000). *Modern food microbiology* (6th ed.). Gaithersburg, MD: Aspen.

[3]Epidemiologic notes and reports Bacillus cereus food poisoning associated with fried rice at two child day care centers—Virginia, 1993. (1994). *MMWR*, 43(10), 177.

[4]Outbreak of *Campylobacter jejuni* infections associated with drinking unpasteurized milk procured through a cow-leasing program—Wisconsin, 2001. (2002). *MMWR*, 51(25), 548.

[5]Outbreak of botulism type E associated with eating a beached whale—Western Alaska, July 2002. (2003). *MMWR*, 52(2), 24.

[6]*Clostridium perfringens* gastroenteritis associated with corned beef served at St. Patrick's Day meals—Ohio and Virginia, 1993. (1994). *MMWR*, 43(08), 137, 143.

[7]Multistate outbreak of *Escherichia coli* O157:H7 infections associated with eating ground beef—U.S., June–July 2002. (2002). *MMWR*, 51(29), 637.

[8]Public health dispatch: Outbreak of listeriosis—Northeastern U.S., 2002. (2002). *MMWR*, 51(42), 950.

[9]Epidemiologic notes and reports typhoid fever—Skagit County, Washington. (1990). *MMWR*, 39(42), 749.

[10]Salmonellosis associated with a Thanksgiving dinner—Nevada, 1995. (1996). *MMWR*, 45(46), 1016.

[11]Hospital-associated outbreak of *Shigella dysenteriae* type 2—Maryland. (1983). *MMWR*, 32(19), 250.

[12]Outbreak of staphylococcal food poisoning associated with precooked ham—Florida, 1997. (1997). *MMWR*, 46(50), 1189.

[13]Farley, T. A., Wilson, S. A., Mahoney, F., Kelso, K. Y., Johnson, D. R., & Kaplan, E. L. (1993). Direct inoculation of food as the cause of an outbreak of group a streptococcal pharyngitis. *Journal of Infectious Diseases*, 167(5), 1232.

[14]Crump, J. A., Bopp, C. A., Greene, K. D., Kubota, K. A., Middendorf, R. L., Wells, J. G., et al. (2003). Toxigenic *Vibrio cholerae* serogroup O141-associated cholera-like diarrhea and bloodstream infection in the U.S. *Journal of Infectious Diseases*, 187(5), 866.

[15]*Yersinia enterocolitica* gastroenteritis among infants exposed to chitterlings—Chicago, Illinois, 2002. (2003). *MMWR*, 52(40), 956.

[16]Hepatitis A outbreak associated with green onions at a restaurant—Monaca, Pennsylvania, 2003. (2003). *MMWR*, 52(47), 1155.

[17]Foodborne outbreak of group a rotavirus gastroenteritis among college students—District of Columbia, March–April 2000. (2000). *MMWR*, 49(50), 1131.

[18]Bresee, J. S., Widdowson, M.-A., Monroe, S. S., & Glass, R. I. (2002). Foodborne viral gastroenteritis: Challenges and opportunities. *Clinical Infectious Diseases*, 35(6), 748.

[19]Liu, G. T., Qian, Y. Z., Zhang, P., Dong, W. H., Qi, Y. M., & Guo, H. T. (1992). Etiological role of *Alternaria alternata* in human esophageal cancer. *Chinese Medical Journal*, 105(5), 394.

[20]Unexplained severe illness possibly associated with consumption of Kombucha tea—Iowa, 1995. (1995). *MMWR*, 44(48), 892, 899.

[21]Frank, H. K. (1977). Occurrence of patulin in fruit and vegetables. *Annales de la Nutrition et de l'Alimentation*, 31(4–6), 459.

[22]Bhat, R. V., Shetty, P. H., Amruth, R. P., & Sudershan, R. V. (1997). A foodborne disease outbreak due to the consumption of moldy sorghum and maize containing fumonisin mycotoxins. *Journal of Toxicology. Clinical Toxicology*, 35(3), 249.

[23]Overy, D. P., Seifert, K. A., Savard, M. E., & Frisvad, J. C. (2003). Spoilage fungi and their mycotoxins in commercially marketed chestnuts. *International Journal of Food Microbiology*, 88(1), 69.

[24]Fan, P. C. (1998). Viability of metacercariae of *Clonorchis sinensis* in frozen or salted freshwater fish. *International Journal for Parasitology*, 28(4), 603.

[25]Choi, D. W. (1984). *Clonorchis sinensis*: Life cycle, intermediate hosts, transmission to man and geographical distribution in Korea. *Arzneimittel-Forschung*, 34(9B), 1145.

[26]Curtis, M. A. & Bylund, G. (1991). Diphyllobothriasis: Fish tapeworm disease in the circumpolar north. *Arctic Medical Research*, 50(1), 18.

[27]LaPook, J. D., Magun, A. M., Nickerson, K. G., & Meltzer, J. I. (2000). Sheep, watercress, and the internet. *Lancet*, 356(9225), 218.

[28]Graczyk, T. K., Gilman, R. H., & Fried, B. (2001). Fasciolopsiasis: Is it a controllable food-borne disease? *Parasitology Research*, 87(1), 80.

[29]DeFrain, M. & Hooker, R. (2002). North American paragonimiasis: Case report of a severe clinical infection. *Chest*, 121(4), 1368.

[30]Procop, G. W., Marty, A. M., Scheck, D. N., Mease, D. R., & Maw, G. M. (2000). North American paragonimiasis. A case report. *Acta Cytologica*, 44(1), 75.

[31]Locally acquired neurocysticercosis—North Carolina, Massachusetts, and South Carolina, 1989–1991. (1992). *MMWR*, 41(1), 1.

[32]Foodborne outbreak of diarrheal illness associated with *Cryptosporidium parvum*—Minnesota, 1995. (1996). *MMWR*, 45(36), 783.

[33]Update: Outbreaks of *Cyclospora cayetanensis* infection—U.S. and Canada, 1996. (1996). *MMWR*, 45(28), 611.

[34]de Lalla, F., Rinaldi, E., Santoro, D., Nicolin, R., & Tramarin, A. (1992). Outbreak of *Entamoeba histolytica* and *Giardia lamblia* infections in travellers returning from the tropics. *Infection*, 20(2), 78.

[35]Epidemiologic notes and reports common-source outbreak of giardiasis—New Mexico. (1989). *MMWR*, 38(23), 405.

[36]Wilairatana, P., Radomyos, P., Radomyos, B., Phraevanich, R., Plooksawasdi, W., Chanthavanich, P., et al. (1996). Intestinal sarcocystosis in Thai laborers. *Southeast Asian Journal of Tropical Medicine and Public Health*, 27(1), 43.

[37]Ross, R. D., Stec, L. A., Werner, J. C., Blumenkranz, M. S., Glazer, L., & Williams, G. A. (2001). Presumed acquired ocular toxoplasmosis in deer hunters. *Retina*, 21(3), 226.

[38]Bouree, P., Paugam, A., & Petithory, J. C. (1995). Anisakidosis: Report of 25 cases and review of the literature. *Comparative Immunology, Microbiology and Infectious Diseases*, 18(2), 75.

[39]Hughes, R. G., Sharp, D. S., Hughes, M. C., Akau'ola, S., Heinsbroek, P., Velayudhan, R., et al. (2004). Environmental influences on helminthiasis and nutritional status among Pacific schoolchildren. *International Journal of Environmental Health Research*, 14(3), 163.

[40]Adams, A. M., Murrell, K. D., & Cross, J. H. (1997). Parasites of fish and risks to public health. *Revue Scientifique et Technique*, 16(2), 652.

[41]Trichinellosis surveillance—U.S., 1997–2001. (2002). *MMWR*, 52(SS06), 1.

[42]Fatal degenerative neurologic illnesses in men who participated in wild game feasts—Wisconsin, 2002. *MMWR*, 52(7), 125.

Source: Compiled by the author.

ried by insects.[89,90] Most cases of *campylobacteriosis* can be traced to eating undercooked poultry or to other foods contaminated by raw poultry.[91] The next most common route of infection is via unpasteurized milk,[77,91-93] but the largest outbreak, where about 2,000 people were infected, was traced to contaminated water.[77,94] Symptoms include abdominal pain, diarrhea, headache, and fever, and infection rates are higher in immunocompromised individuals (e.g., HIV/AIDS patients, infants, the elderly)[91,95-97] In severe cases of campylobacteriosis there may be bloody diarrhea.[77,97] Among the sequelae to infection are Guillain-Barré syndrome[98,99] and Reiter syndrome.[100]

> **Guillain-Barré syndrome**—An inflammatory disorder of the peripheral nerves that is characterized by the rapid onset of weakness and, often, paralysis of the legs, arms, breathing muscles, and face.
>
> **Reiter syndrome**—A peripheral arthritis lasting longer than 1 month.

E. coli

Escherichia coli, a known human pathogen since the 18th century,[101] gained widespread recognition in 1971 after an enteritis outbreak was traced to contaminated imported cheeses.[102] *E. coli* is one of four genera of coliform bacteria used as indicators of food safety (microbiological coliform test), and *E. coli* is often specifically assayed because it is more indicative of fecal contamination than are the other three genera.[103] Within the genus *Escherichia* there are some 200 O and 30 H serotypes.[102] *E. coli* O157 inhabit the intestinal tracts of cattle; other *E. coli* are normal inhabitants of human intestinal tracts. When people become ill from *E. coli*, the usual transmission vehicles are raw or undercooked ground beef and other red meats, and occasionally prepared foods such as mashed potatoes and cream pies. Untreated water, raw milk, cheeses, and fish have also been implicated. Shiga toxin-producing *E. coli* (STEC) O157:H7 (a toxin similar to that of *Shigella dysenteriae*) was first recognized in 1982.[104-108] Causing either infection or intoxication, symptoms of illness resemble those of shigellosis, including, for infection, bloody diarrhea and colitis, and for intoxication, severe abdominal pain, nausea, vomiting, diarrhea, and sometimes fever.[109,110] Hemolytic uremic syndrome (HUS) and hemorrhagic colitis are especially severe and are particularly serious for children; several fatalities have occurred in the last 20 years. Although STEC is the organism monitored by the CDC, other strains of *E. coli* cause diarrhea (e.g., enteroaggregative *E. coli*[111]). E. coli is among the leading causes of travelers' diarrhea (others include Noroviruses, *Campylobacter jejuni/coli*, and *Giardia lamblia*[103]). To prevent foodborne illness caused by *E. coli* (and other pathogens), nutritionists should advise that foods be cooked thoroughly and that a thermometer be used to ensure that proper temperatures are reached. Avoiding cross-contamination, proper handling/reheating of leftovers, and handwashing/personal hygiene are also appropriate control measures against *E. coli*.

> See Cook It! (http://vm.cfsan.fda.gov/~fsg/fs-cook.html) and "FightBAC" (http://www.fightbac.org/cook_facts.cfm), for current temperature guidance.[112,113]

Listeria

The genus Listeria has six recognized species. *Listeria monocytogenes*, the primary pathogen, has 13 serovars.[114] For many years listeriosis was recognized as an animal disease, but *Listeria's* association with foodborne illness in humans is a recent phenomenon. The organisms are widespread in nature, in wild and domestic animals and birds, in water and soil, and in vegetation. Found in raw milk, soft cheeses, raw meats, and poultry, it can also contaminate raw soil-grown vegetables such as lettuce. Symptoms of listeriosis include nausea, vomiting, and headache, but the health of the host determines the course and severity of the disease—many healthy people never develop clinical manifestations.[114] However, infants may be congenitally infected, and infected pregnant women (often with no or mild symptoms) may spontaneously abort, deliver prematurely, or deliver a stillborn infant.[114] Immunocompromised

individuals, such as those with HIV/AIDS, are particularly susceptible, and neoplasms, alcoholism, diabetes (especially type 1), cardiovascular disease, renal transplant, and corticosteroid therapy
predispose individuals to clinical listeriosis, characterized by
meningitis, meningoencephalitis, or encephalitis.[114] *Listeria* can
grow at cold temperatures, so refrigeration is inadequate as a control. Thorough cooking, using pasteurized milk and dairy products,
avoiding cross-contamination, handwashing/personal hygiene, and
maintaining clean, dry food storage and preparation areas are all
effective against *Listeria*.

Salmonella

The salmonellae are a large group of bacteria, but there are only two
species, *Salmonella enterica* and *S. Bongori*. These species are further classified into four subspecies and one subspecies, respectively,
and further into 2,324 serovars—these are commonly treated as separate species.[115] *Salmonella* spp. (spp. is defined as all individual
species within a genus) are found in animal intestinal tracts, including birds, livestock, humans, reptiles, and some insects. Shed in
feces, they may then be spread by insects and other vermin.[115] Animal feeds may serve as routes of infection for livestock,[116] and animal carcasses may be contaminated with gastrointestinal
salmonellae during slaughter and processing. People who eat undercooked *Salmonella*-contaminated meats, poultry, or eggs, or
drink *Salmonella*-contaminated water develop nausea, vomiting,
abdominal pain, diarrhea, headache, and fever. The strains most
commonly responsible for human illness are *S. Typhimurium* and
S. Enteritidis. (The incidence of cases of non-typhoid *Salmonella*
infections has increased substantially since about 1950.[73]) *S. Enteritidis* infections have been increasing since the 1970s and are often
associated with eggs, egg products, or egg-containing foods.[115,117-119]
Because *S. Enteritidis* may be present in fresh, uncracked shell
eggs,[120-122] eating undercooked or raw eggs is ill-advised unless the
eggs have been pasteurized in the shell.[123,124]

Shigella

The genus Shigella has four species, *S. dysenteriae*, *S. flexneri*, *S.
boydii*, and *S. sonnei*. Although *S. dysenteriae* causes bacillary
dysentery and can be carried in food or water, it is not considered
a food-poisoning organism.[115] The other three species cause shigellosis infection, characterized by diarrhea, abdominal pain, fever,
and chills. *Shigella* is unique among the bacteria discussed thus far,
because there are no known non-human reservoirs.[115] Thus, poor
personal hygiene is usually behind outbreaks, with shellfish, raw
produce, chicken, and salads the usual vehicles.[115] People may carry
Shigella for several weeks, excreting the bacteria in their stool. Flies
and other vermin may also transmit the bacteria to foods. Control

measures include fastidious handwashing/personal hygiene, rapid cooling of foods, vermin control, and use of potable water.

Vibrio

The genus *Vibrio* includes about 28 species, 5 being of public health significance: *V. parahaemolyticus*, *V. vulnificus*, *V. hollisae*, *V. alginolyticus*, and *V. cholerae*.[77] These are marine organisms, so the usual vehicle for foodborne illness is seafood, especially shellfish and dried fish, or other foods cross-contaminated by seafood.[77] *V. parahaemolyticus* is the leading cause of foodborne illness in Japan, and in the United States it has been responsible for many outbreaks, usually associated with eating raw oysters or clams. *V. vulnificus* causes soft-tissue infections and primary septicemia, particularly affecting immunocompromised individuals and those with liver cirrhosis. The organism consumed via raw oysters is responsible for about 95% of seafood-associated mortality in the United States.[77] *V. hollisae* causes gastroenteritis via shellfish consumption, and *V. alginolyticus* can cause gastroenteritis, but is more often implicated in soft-tissue and ear infections among swimmers.[77] *V. cholerae* is well known as the causative agent of cholera. Several foodborne gastroenteritis infections have been recorded in the United States, all in patients who had eaten raw oysters. Other foods implicated in small outbreaks (one to six individuals) were raw seaweed, palm fruit, and coconut milk.[77] Control measures against vibriosis include avoiding raw shellfish and seafood, purchasing shellfish/seafood from approved sources, avoiding cross-contamination, and good handwashing/personal hygiene habits.

Yersinia

The genus *Yersinia* includes 11 species, among them the plague-causing *Y. pestis*. *Y. enterocolitica* is the primary organism of importance to food safety.[77] Swine are the usual reservoirs, but *Yersinia* is also associated with milk, seafood, and vegetables.[77] Foodborne yersiniosis manifestations include gastroenteritis, pseudoappendicitis, lymphadenitis, and many others.[77] The gastroenteritis is characterized by abdominal pain and diarrhea, and the illness may progress to a variety of systemic syndromes.[77] Children are more susceptible than adults.

Viruses

Viruses differ from bacteria in that they require a vector (i.e., virus-contaminated food or hands) in order to enter the body and cause disease. Pathogenic viruses have always been associated with foods, but some such as the Norwalk viruses,[125] newly renamed "Noroviruses,"[126] have been known as food-associated pathogens only since the 1970s.[127-129] Before then, causative agents for most gastroenteritis cases could not be identified. Noroviruses are responsible for most of the cases of acute gastroenteritis in the United States.[130] Norwalk virus is "the prototype strain of genetically and antigenically diverse single stranded RNA (ribonucleic acid) viruses,"[125] formerly known as small, round structural viruses. It was first identified as the causative agent for a school outbreak of gastroenteritis in 1968, in Norwalk, Ohio.[130] Norovirus outbreaks have been associated with contaminated water, fruits, raw oysters, and scallops,[130-132] and are notorious for their association with acute gastroenteritis outbreaks on cruise ships.[133]

In the United States, food- and waterborne hepatitis A outbreaks are relatively uncommon. However, transmission via the fecal-oral route is possible; food handler carriers of hepatitis A are often identified, and raw or undercooked shellfish may carry the virus, so prevention and control measures (see *Vibrio* previously) are necessary.[134,135]

Parasites

Parasites include flatworms, roundworms, tapeworms, protozoans, and other organisms that use the body as a host in order to live and multiply. Some familiar parasites are listed in Table 16-3. These are usually ingested in raw or undercooked foods or water in which the parasites live; for example, *Trichinella spiralis* (roundworm of pork, also found in game, like bear or walrus) causes trichinellosis,[116] and *Giardia lamblia*, a waterborne protozoan, causes giardiasis ("beaver fever").[136] Parasites emerging recently as significant to food safety include *Cryptosporidium* and *Cyclospora*, and liver flukes (e.g., *Fasciola hepatica* and *F. gigantica*).[137]

Cryptosporidium parvum, a protozoan found in mammals, reptiles, and birds, causes diarrhea in humans (it is particularly severe in immunocompromised individuals). Abdominal pain, nausea, vomiting, and fever are often reported.[138] Cryptosporidiosis is "acquired by at least one of five known transmission routes: zoonotic, person to person, water, nosocomial, or food."[138] People are infected by ingesting oocysts of the parasite, which are shed in the feces of the host.[138] Major outbreaks of cryptosporidiosis have occurred in Maine (1993, unpasteurized apple cider),[139] Minnesota (1995, chicken salad),[140] New York (1996, unpasteurized apple cider),[141] and Washington (1997, raw green onions).[142]

Cyclospora cayetanensis, a protozoan similar to *Cryptosporidium*, causes symptoms similar to cryptosporidiosis in infected humans. Like cryptosporidiosis, cyclosporiasis is much more serious in immunocompromised individuals.[143] The most notorious foodborne cyclosporiasis outbreak "occurred in 1996 in 20 U.S. states and two Canadian provinces, infecting 1,465 people who had eaten imported Guatemalan raspberries."[138]

Prions

Problems in the British beef industry in the 1980s brought prion diseases under increased scientific scrutiny and public curiosity.[130,144-146] Prions, the etiologic agents of, among others, Creutzfeldt-

Jacob disease (CJD) and kuru in humans[147,148] and chronic wasting disease and sheep scrapie in animals, are physiological cellular glycoproteins. The bovine spongiform encephalopathy (BSE; "mad cow disease") prion (PrPSc) is an infectious variant of a normal copper-binding prion (PrPC) on cell surfaces.[149] BSE is one of several transmissible spongiform encephalopathies (the human form of BSE is variant Creutzfeldt-Jakob disease, vCJD[150]) that are emerging, serious public health concerns.[151,152] Critics of U.S. regulatory policies regarding BSE cite half-hearted efforts to monitor for the disease, lack of research funding, and undue meat industry pressure.[153] After two BSE-infected cows were detected in the United States, one each in 2003 and 2004, public, professional, and Congressional lobbying for changes in regulatory oversight ensued. The FDA and USDA have strengthened safeguards protecting consumers from PrPSc, prohibiting "the use of certain cattle-derived materials in human food (including dietary supplements) and cosmetics."[154-156]

Chemical Hazards

Nutritionists understand that foods consist of chemicals, but the public grossly misunderstands the word "chemicals." Several chemical hazards are associated with foods, some naturally occurring (e.g., aflatoxin, alkaloids, histamine), some indirectly added (e.g., pesticides, compounds that migrate from packaging materials, lubricants from food processing machinery), and others directly added (e.g., colors, preservatives).[9]

Naturally Occurring Toxicants

Many foods contain natural toxins that may be harmful when consumed at certain levels, such as aflatoxin and mushroom toxins, whereas others contain toxins that are harmful over time, such as mercury. Mycotoxins, potato glycoalkaloids, shellfish toxins, and methylmercury are illustrative of this group, but there are many others, including oxalic acid, goitrogens, hemagglutinens, and protease inhibitors.

Mycotoxins are mold-produced toxins, many of which are of public health importance. The aflatoxins (*Aspergillus flavus* toxin), highly substituted coumarins, are the most studied.[157] Usually associated with corn, cottonseed, peanuts, and products made from them, aflatoxins are also found in milk, cheese,[158] meats, and other foods. Aflatoxins produce liver cancer in animals.[159] Developing countries in Africa and Asia have the greatest incidence of aflatoxin-related cancers.[160] The FDA specifies limits for aflatoxins in animal feeds and foods for human consumption, currently 20 ppb for food, feeds, Brazil nuts, peanuts, peanut products, and pistachios, and 0.5 ppb for milk.[160,161] At the international level, the Codex Alimentarius Commission[162] recommends maximums of 15 μg/kg of aflatoxin in peanuts for further processing and 0.05 μg/kg of aflatoxin in milk.[163]

Other molds, such as *Aspergillus, Alternaria, Fusarium,* and *Penicillium,* produce toxins in foods. *Aspergillus* spp. produce ochratoxins, found in corn, nuts, grains, meats, and other foods.[157] These heat-stable toxins are hepatotoxic and nephrotoxic in rats.[157] Alternariol and other *Alternaria*-produced toxins have been found in grains and fruits.[164,165] Fumonisins are *Fusarium*-produced toxins found in corn and other grains. These are associated with high rates of esophageal cancer in Africa and Asia.[166,167] Citrinin and patulin are toxins produced by *Penicillium* spp. Citrinin is found in many foods, including bread, rice, other cereal grains, and country-cured hams, and patulin has been found in bread, sausage, fruits, and juices.[157] The Codex Alimentarius Commission recommends maximums of 50 μg/kg of patulin in apple juice and apple juice as an ingredient in other beverages, and 5 μg/kg ochratoxin A in cereals and cereal products.[163]

Mycotoxins survive food-processing methods,[168] but continuous monitoring for them ensures safety of the foods affected. Although mycotoxins are not formed (or are formed in very small quantities) at refrigerator temperatures (generally, 36-41° F),[169] consumers should be advised to throw out foods that develop molds. Preformed toxins are not affected by refrigeration, freezing, or cooking. Consumers should also be advised to store foods to minimize mold growth, by storing foods in small quantities, under refrigeration, and dry.

Alkaloids are found in many food products. Various glycoalkaloids are present in potatoes and potato products[170-176] and can increase with exposure to light,[177-179] heat,[180,181] and insect damage during the growing season.[182] Toxic effects of glycoalkaloids include abdominal pain, diarrhea, and vomiting at low doses; fever, hypotension, neurological disorders, tachycardia, tachypnea,[183] and death[184] at higher doses. Glycoalkaloid poisoning is uncommon, however, and individual responses to glycoalkaloids vary. For many years nutritionists and other health professionals merely cautioned people to avoid eating the green parts of potatoes. The generally accepted safe limit for potato glycoalkaloids is 200 mg/kg.[185] Recently, as scientists have broadened their understanding of the biochemistry of glycoalkaloids, warnings about chronic versus acute effects of ingested glycoalkaloids have become more strident.[186] Glycoalkaloids increase risk for some cancers;[187] are teratogenic, embryotoxic, and genotoxic;[188,189] and may interfere with or interact with commonly prescribed pharmaceuticals.[190] With the food industry's interest in developing value-added products from potato peels[191,192] (and in reducing the glycoalkaloid content[193]) and the increasing likelihood that nutritionists will encounter clients (such as Bangladeshis[172]) for whom potato leaves and potato peels are acceptable food choices, regular monitoring of the scientific literature pertaining to potato glycoalkaloids is warranted.

Toxins causing amnesic shellfish poisoning (ASP), ciguatera poisoning, and paralytic shellfish poisoning (PSP) are not produced by shellfish or fish. Rather, they are produced by microscopic phytoplankton (diatoms and dinoflagellates) consumed by the shellfish and fish. The diatom *Pseudonitzschia pungens* produces domoic acid, which acts as a glutamic acid antagonist in the human central nervous system,[130] producing sometimes fatal ASP.[194] Several outbreaks have occurred since 1988.[195-198]

Ciguatoxin is produced by the dinoflagellate *Gambierdiscus toxicus.* Humans ingest the toxin in predatory fish, such as barracuda, groupers, and sea bass, which in turn have ingested herbivorous fish in which the toxin is concentrated in organs and muscles. Symptoms of ciguatoxin poisoning are similar to those of PSP (nausea, oral paresthesia, and respiratory paralysis), but the onset of symptoms is somewhat longer (3–6 hours vs. 2 hours for PSP). Long considered an illness of the tropics,[199,200] modern food transportation systems can deliver ciguatoxic fish to locations far removed from their home waters.[201-204]

PSP is caused by ingesting toxins (decarbamoyl saxitoxin, neosaxitoxin, gonyautoxins, and others[205, 206]) in bivalve mollusks that have eaten dinoflagellates such as *Gonyaulax catenella* and *G. acatenella* (Pacific Coast) and *G. tamarensis* (Atlantic Coast), among others. The toxins are heat-stable and can cause cardiovascular collapse and respiratory failure.[130] PSP mortality can reach 22%.[207]

The National Shellfish Sanitation Program (NSSP),

> . . . a voluntary, tripartite program composed of state officials, the shellfish industry, and Federal agencies . . . is designed to prevent human illness associated with the consumption of fresh and frozen shellfish (oysters, clams, and mussels) through the establishment of sanitary controls over all phases of the growing, harvesting, shucking, packing and distribution of fresh and frozen shellfish.[208]

The FDA oversees the NSSP and, together with state agencies, manages the sanitation programs at the state level. Foreign countries (e.g., Canada, Chile, Korea, Mexico, New Zealand) may import shellfish into the United States by agreeing to abide by the provisions of the NSSP as set forth in a Memorandum of Understanding between countries. Public health nutritionists should consult the Interstate Certified Shellfish Shippers List (ICSSL),[209] published monthly by the FDA, because under the NSSP all states require that shellfish be from a certified source, proof of which is dealer listing in the ICSSL.

Metals such as mercury are persistent environmental pollutants and can cause foodborne illness. Foods usually implicated are fish, shellfish, and marine mammals. These animals ingest and accumulate methylmercury from their foods. Mercury enters the environment and food chains from both human activities (coal-fired power plant emissions, medical and electronics wastes, etc.) and natural processes.[210] Methylmercury is neurotoxic[210] and possibly immunomodulating[211] in humans, usually over time with chronic exposure. The human fetus is particularly susceptible to methylmercury poisoning. The FDA's seafood website (http://vm.cfsan.fda.gov/seafood1.html) has links to population-specific seafood advisories[212,213] and data on mercury levels in commonly consumed fish and shellfish.[214,215] Recently methylmercury and its association with fish, shellfish, and fish-eating human populations; and the possible role of nutrition in modulating the effects of methylmercury ingestion have received more attention.[216-218] Until more is known, some authorities question current recommendations to eat more fish to improve cardiovascular health.[219]

Directly Added Chemicals

Food Additives

Humans have added chemicals to food since before recorded history. Primitive food preservation methods included salting, smoking, and fermentation, all still in use today, and herbs and spices were used to retard spoilage and to mask off flavors caused by spoilage. Today, with fewer people cooking meals "from scratch" and with fewer meals eaten in the home, consumers are increasingly leaving decisions about which chemicals are added to foods to the food industry and its government regulators. Nutritionists are likely to encounter ignorance of the purposes of food additives in foods consumed by their clients, as well as fear of the chemical names listed on ingredient labels (at least from those who read the labels; some believe that many do not read food labels,[220,221] and among those who do read labels, comprehension is not what it should be[222,223]). Many people are influenced by the popular press and news media, where innuendo, half-truths, and patently false statements compete with sound science on issues surrounding chemical use in foods. The food and chemical industries and government regulatory agencies often exacerbate the confusion by offering platitudes in response to accusations. Recently, however, steps have been taken to restore public confidence in food safety and in the industries themselves.[224-229] This constant interchange between science and pseudo-science is one of the most daunting obstacles a nutritionist is likely to face. We must regularly evaluate the scientific literature and government policy to better inform clients and to provide guidance in critically evaluating claims made about food additives.

Chemicals are added to foods for many reasons: to increase nutritional quality; to aid in food processing; to increase, decrease, or neutralize certain sensory characteristics of foods; to prolong storage stability; and to inhibit microbial growth. Within broad categories of additives (Table 16-4) there are usually several alternatives available to gain the same desired effect. For some applications, combinations of additives are applied to meet specific requirements (e.g., a manufacturer may use a blend of acesulfame-K and aspar-

TABLE 16-4   Examples of Chemical Food Additives[1]

Class	Representative Chemicals	Purposes
Antioxidants	Ascorbic acid (vitamin C) butylated hydroxyanisole, butylated hydroxytoluene, sulfur dioxide, tocopherols (vitamin E)	Retard deterioration, rancidity, discoloration from oxidation; free radical scavengers
Flour bleaching agents, flour maturing agents, starch bleaching agents, starch modifiers	Acetone peroxides, calcium bromate, sodium hypochlorite, adipic anhydride (esterifier), propylene oxide (etherifier)	Enhance whiteness of flour or starch; enhance baking qualities of flour; modify starch functional characteristics to applications desired
Buffers, acids, alkalis	Acetic acid, ammonium hydroxide, citric acid, fumaric acid, malic acid, oxalic acid, sodium carbonate, succinic acid, tartaric acid	Lower or raise pH; buffer pH against change
Colors (exempt from batch certification)[2]	Annatto extract, caramel, carmine, grape skin extract, turmeric	Impart, enhance, or preserve food color or shading
Colors (must be batch certified)[3]	FD&C Blue No. 1, FD&C Green No. 3, Orange B, Citrus Red No. 2, FD&C Yellow No. 5	Impart, enhance, or preserve food color or shading
Flavors, chemical	2-acetyl thiazole, 3-heptanone, benzaldehyde, cresyl acetate, decanal, eugenol, quinine sulfate	Impart or enhance a flavor or flavor "note" in food
Nutritional additives	Amino acids (e.g., DL-leucine), beta-carotene, kelp, minerals (e.g., ferrous sulfate), vitamins (e.g., biotin)	Necessary for the body's nutritional and metabolic processes
Preservatives	Benzoic acid, butyl P-hydroxybenzoate, calcium benzoate, calcium disodium EDTA, calcium sorbate, cupric sulfate, heptylparaben	Retard microbial spoilage; block ripening and enzymatic processes; antioxidation
Sequestrants	Calcium acetate, calcium disodium EDTA, citric acid, disodium EDTA, glucono delta-lactone	Combine with polyvalent metal ions to form a soluble metal complex; improve product quality and stability
Stabilizers and thickeners	Carrageenan, carob bean gum, dammar gum, dextrin, edible gelatin, modified starches, tara gum	Increase viscosity of solutions; produce/improve dispersions; impart body, improve consistency, or stabilize emulsions

Class	Representative Chemicals	Purposes
Surface-active agents:		Modify surface properties of liquid food components
detergents;	TERG-A-ZYME™[4]	
dispersants;	microcrystalline cellulose	
defoaming agents;	decanoic acid	
foaming agents;	acacia	
solubilizing agents;	1,3-butylene glycol	
wetting agents;	dioctyl sodium sulfosuccinate	
whipping agents	calcium polyphosphates	
Miscellaneous additives:		For specific applications
alternative sweeteners;	aspartame, sucralose, tagatose	
anti-caking agents;	aluminum silicate	
anti-sticking agents;	castor oil	
clarifying agents;	polyvinylpolypyrrolidone	
fat replacers[5]	dextrins, whey protein, olestra	
firming agents;	aluminum sulfate	
growth promoters;	calcium lactate (yeast food)	
lubricants;	mineral oil	
solvents	ethylene dichloride	

[1]Not a complete list. For extensive lists, see the NutritionData Food Additive Identifier, http://www.nutritiondata.com/food-additives.html; "Food Additives Permitted for Direct Addition to Food for Human Consumption," *Code of Federal Regulations*, Title 21, Vol. 3, (U.S. Government Printing Office, April 1, 2003), Ch. 1, Part 172; "Secondary Direct Food Additives Permitted in Food for Human Consumption," *Code of Federal Regulations*, Title 21, Vol. 3, (U.S. Government Printing Office, April 1, 2003), Ch. 1, Part 173; "Indirect Food Additives," *Code of Federal Regulations*, Title 21, Vol. 3, (U.S. Government Printing Office, April 1, 2003), Ch. 1, Parts 174–178.

[2]See "Color Additives Approved for Use in Human Food. Part 73, Subpart A: Color Additives Exempt from Batch Certification," http://www.cfsan.fda.gov/~dms/opa-col2.html#table1A.

[3]See "Color Additives Approved for Use in Human Food. Part 74, Subpart A: Color Additives Subject to Batch Certification," http://www.cfsan.fda.gov/~dms/opa-col2.html#table1A.

[4]TERG-A-ZYME consists of sodium linear alkylaryl sulfonate, phosphates, carbonates, and protease enzyme (*Bacillus licheniformis subtilisin Carlsberg*). See Document #123, "TERG-A-ZYME Technical Bulletin" (White Plains NY: Alconox, http://www.alconox.com/static/section_customer/ind_fooddairy.asp).

[5]For a current list of fat replacers, see the Calorie Control Council's website, http://www.caloriecontrol.org/frgloss.html.

Source: Compiled by the author.

tame to obtain an optimum low-calorie sweetener for hot coffee
and tea beverages[230]). Development, testing, and approval of new
chemical food additives continue at a rapid pace.

Antioxidants

Foods containing fats are subject to oxidative rancidity during storage. To enable foods such as crackers, nuts, and potato chips to be
packaged and stored while retaining freshness, antioxidant chemicals
such as ascorbic acid (vitamin C), butylated hydroxyanisole (BHA),
butylated hydroxytoluene (BHT), sulfur dioxide, and tocopherols (vitamin E), among others, are used, singly or in combinations.[9]

Alternative Sweeteners

Sweeteners may be classified as nutritive (or caloric, e.g., sucrose,
honey, corn syrups) or non-nutritive (or noncaloric, e.g., acesulfame-K, saccharin). Some nutritive alternative sweeteners are so
much sweeter than sucrose that they are essentially reduced-calorie sweeteners (e.g., aspartame, 4 kcal/g but approximately 200
times sweeter than sucrose,[231] thus calorically negligible in foods to
which it has been added). Reduced-calorie or noncaloric alternatively sweetened foods are popularly used in weight-reducing diets
and weight-maintenance plans to reduce incidence of dental caries,
or to manage diabetes. Food scientists and food technologists continue to research and develop alternative sweeteners (the most recently approved sweetener is tagatose, a natural sugar[232]).

Nutritionists can help consumers recognize the various sugars
(e.g., corn syrup, dextrose, fructose, high fructose corn syrup [HFCS],
honey, lactose, sucrose) and alternative sweeteners[233] listed on food
labels, and to choose foods sweetened with additives that are suited
to their individual health profiles, diets, and lifestyles. Nutritionists
may also be asked about alternative sweeteners that, although
legally used abroad, are not approved for additive use in the United
States, such as stevia (powdered extract of the plant *Stevia rebaudi-
ana Bertoni*),[234] currently regulated and sold as a food supplement.
(Stevia is purported to have antihyperglycemic[235] and antihypertensive properties.[236-238]) Finally, nutritionists must thoroughly understand the controversial aspects of some additive sweeteners (e.g., the
alleged association of HFCS with the increasing worldwide prevalence of obesity;[239] the purported carcinogenicity of sodium saccharin;[240,241] and the alleged adverse health effects of dietary
aspartame[242-247] and sucralose[248-251]) and critically evaluate the evidence available to make the best possible recommendations to consumers. The Dietary Guidelines for Americans,[252] the Dietary
Reference Intakes,[253] and the position statement on sweeteners of the
American Dietetic Association[254] are useful guidelines.

Bleaching Agents, Maturing Agents, and Starch Modifiers

Oxidizing agents such as benzoyl peroxide and chlorine dioxide are
used to bleach flour color and to mature flour to improve baking

properties. Modified food starches are used to improve the appearance, stability, texture, and quality of food products.[9] Starches may be cross-linked with phosphates or adipates, stabilized by etherification or esterification (acetate- or hydroxypropyl-modified), or thinned by dextrinization or acid hydrolysis.[255]

Buffers, Acids, and Alkalis

Buffers (e.g., acetic acid/sodium acetate), acids (e.g., acetic, malic, tartaric acids), and alkalis (e.g., ammonium hydroxide, carbonates) are used in foods to control or adjust pH. They may be from natural sources, fermentation-derived, or chemically synthesized.[9,256]

Colors

Natural and synthetic colors are added to foods to enhance visual appeal. Natural colors may be obtained from plant (e.g., beets, grapes, saffron), mineral (e.g., iron oxide, titanium dioxide), and animal (e.g., cochineal extract or carmine from female scale insects, Coccus cacti) sources.[9]

Flavors

Flavoring agents constitute the largest group of food additives. Natural flavor substances include spices (e.g., anise, paprika, vanilla), herbs (e.g., basil, parsley, thyme), essential oils (e.g., clove, lime, rose), and plant extracts (e.g., almond, garlic, rosemary). Some natural flavor substances may appear in multiple categories; for example, chervil may be added to foods as a spice, an oil, or an extract, among other designations.[257] Synthetic flavoring agents are also used (e.g., allyl disulfide, isopropyl alcohol, thymol). Flavoring agents may be listed on food labels as "flavorings," "natural flavors," "artificial flavors," and "spices." Monosodium glutamate (MSG), a flavor enhancer, is associated with adverse reaction symptoms (chest pain, edema, facial or oral numbness, headache, perspiration, and cranial or facial pressure such as "Chinese Restaurant Syndrome"[258–264] and MSG-induced asthma[265,266]) in some people, but is listed GRAS by the FDA and is reported safe by the Joint Food and Agriculture Organization/World Health Organization (FAO/WHO) Expert Committee on Food Additives,[267] in the absence of conclusive proof that it is harmful. Many health professionals do, however, recognize a subpopulation of MSG-sensitive individuals. Nutritionists should be prepared to help these consumers identify MSG-containing foods (MSG may be hidden in general ingredient label statements, such as "hydrolyzed vegetable protein," "natural flavorings," "seasonings") and to suggest alternatives.

Nutritional Additives

Vitamins and minerals are added as enrichments and fortifiers to several foods. Although there is no legal distinction between enrichment and fortification in the United States (the FDA uses the terms interchangeably[268]), enrichment usually signifies replacement of nutrients lost in flour and cereal processing. Enriched flour has had B vitamins and iron added, most breakfast cereals are vitamin and mineral enriched, and polished rice is usually enriched. Fortification also signifies the replacement of lost nutrients, usually in foods other than flour and cereals, as well as the addition of nutrients to commonly used foods to redress deficiency of the nutrient(s) in most diets. Thus, milk may be fortified with vitamin D because the diet of children and older adults is often deficient in vitamin D;[269] no-fat and low-fat milks have vitamins A (by law) and D (optional) added because these vitamins are lost when fat is removed; salt may be fortified with iodine to prevent goiter; and cereal and grain products are fortified with folic acid to prevent neural tube defects.[270]

Food fortification is one of the leading research areas in food technology today.[271-273] For example, consumers can buy calcium-fortified and vitamin D–fortified orange juice[274] and vitamin-and-herb-fortified spring water (e.g., Kraft Foods' Fruit$_2$O Plus™). Unfortunately, most people purchase fortified foods with little or no knowledge of bioavailability or potential toxicities of the substances used to fortify the foods.[275,276]

Preservatives

Preservatives (e.g., butylated hydroxyanisole [BHA], butylated hydroxytoluene [BHT], sodium propionate, sulfur dioxide) are used as antimicrobial agents to retard microbial spoilage of foods, as metal chelators to block ripening and enzymatic processes that continue in foods after harvest, and as antioxidants to retard rancidity and browning, allowing consumers to enjoy a variety of foods, from global sources, year-round.[277, 278] Nutritionists may receive questions from consumers concerning the safety of BHA,[279-282] BHT,[279,280,282] sulfites,[283,284] nitrites,[285-287] and food irradiation ("cold pasteurization," considered a food additive by the FDA).[288-297] Currently, several classes of foods may be irradiated in the United States, including some fresh fruits and vegetables, spices and seasonings, meats, poultry, and prepackaged foods, at doses between 4.5 and 7.0 kGy.[298]

Sequestrants

Chelating agents (e.g., ethylenediamine tetraacetic acid [EDTA], citric acid) are used to sequester metal ions in foods. Left alone, metals such as iron and copper contribute to off colors and catalyze oxidation reactions in foods.[9]

Stabilizers and Thickeners

Processed foods, such as gravies, puddings, and salad dressings, are stabilized and thickened by substances such as carboxymethyl cellulose, gums, and pectin.[9] Foods containing little or no fat, such as low-fat salad dressings, are formulated using stabilizers and thickeners to resemble their full-fat counterparts.

Surface-Active Agents

Emulsifiers, defoaming agents, and detergents are all active at molecular surfaces. Emulsifiers (e.g., lecithin, mono- and diglycerides, and fatty acids) are used to keep food mixtures, such as oil in water and water in oil, stable.[9]

Miscellaneous Additives

Many other additives (e.g., anti-caking and anti-sticking agents, clarifying agents, firming agents, growth promoters, lubricants, solvents) are used for very specific applications.[9] Macrocomponents, such as fat replacers, are added to foods to replace some or all of a food component. Thus, bean pastes, fruit pastes, or microparticulated whey protein concentrates (e.g., Simplesse®) and emulsifiers may be used to replace some or all of the fat in baked goods.[299,300]

Agricultural Chemicals

Agricultural chemicals include antibiotics, growth hormones, herbicides, fertilizers, fungicides, insecticides, and rodenticides, all of which may enter the food supply. Antibiotics at subtherapeutic doses are used to promote animal growth (in the United States) and to prevent disease. Evidence that antibiotic-resistant strains of bacteria develop in food animals and might be passed on to humans, and that consuming antibiotic residues in food might inhibit the efficacy of therapeutic antibiotic use in humans, is controversial.[301,302] Growth hormones, such as recombinant bovine growth hormone (rbGH or BGH) or recombinant bovine somatotropin (rbST or BST), are considered safe when used as directed.[303,304] However, product labeling is controversial, particularly the use of label statements such as "BST-free."[305-308] Herbicides, fertilizers, fungicides, insecticides, and other pesticides are regulated by the EPA. Residues of these chemicals in food[309-312] are under FDA jurisdiction.

Physical Hazards

Physical hazards include extraneous objects or foreign materials in food that may cause illness or injury if consumed. The most common physical hazards found in foods are:

- Metal (from fields, equipment, premises), bullets and BB shot (from animals shot in the field), and hypodermic needles (broken off when treating animals)
- Jewelry (buttons, earrings, rings, etc.)
- Stones and rocks (from fields, ceilings, walls), wood (from fields, ceilings, walls, boxes, pallets), and insulation (from buildings)
- Glass (from bottles, jars, light fixtures, utensils, equipment)
- Insects, insect parts, and other filth (from fields, premises, entry after processing)
- Bone (from improper processing; also from fields and premises)

- Plastic (from fields, packaging and packing, employees)
- Personal effects (bandages, pens, pencils, thermometers, etc.)[8]

Less common physical hazards include capsules, crystals (e.g., struvite), paper, pits, scum, shells, and slime.[313] Food processors must identify potential physical hazards and determine procedures to control each hazard; if warranted, control points should be implemented as part of the facility HACCP plan.[314]

Agroterrorism and Bioterrorism

For centuries, humans have targeted agricultural crops and employed biological agents in adversarial confrontations with each other,[315] but for most of the 20th century, these methods were thought unlikely to be employed. In the 1990s, government and public health professionals began to assess vulnerabilities and to prepare countermeasures against acts of warfare or terrorism directed against the agricultural, food, and water systems of the national infrastructure.[316-318] The CDC identified many biological and chemical agents that could be used for these purposes.[319,320] The effects of several of these, such as mercury, could be insidious, whereas others, such as *Salmonella*, would make it difficult to distinguish disease outbreaks due to bioterrorism from those due to mundane incidents. (In *1984*, a bioterrorist act was perpetrated by a religious cult attempting to gain political control of Wasco County, Oregon. More than 700 people were sickened after *Salmonella* was sprinkled over salad bars in 10 restaurants. What was most frightening about this incident was that it went unrecognized as bioterrorism until disgruntled members of the cult told their stories.)[321,322]

Public health nutritionists will most likely be involved with bioterrorism directed at food and water systems. A consensus is forming that preventing and detecting these incidents will require more than the usual precautions taken by government and the food and water industries, and that improvements made or contemplated by these entities will be inadequate. Rather, the focus should be on improving surveillance systems with the aim of detecting outbreaks early enough to intervene.[323-325] Consumers are an integral part of this plan, but currently do not seek medical care for gastrointestinal illnesses.[325] This is one area where nutritionists can help. Public health nutritionists are routinely involved in educating consumers and should actively seek ways to expand their roles to encompass antibioterrorism. (As noted earlier, nutritionists should be involved in investigating and monitoring outbreaks of foodborne disease and in emergency preparedness planning and response.)[326,327] Bioterrorism and the food supply are discussed at length in the Chapter 18.

Food Safety in the 21st Century

Among the food safety issues that will occupy the nation in the 21st century, expect these to be prominent in the early years:

1. *Federal regulation/oversight by a single agency:* Government and some industry groups contend that the current array of federal (as discussed previously in Table 16-1), state, and local agencies results in overlapping jurisdictions and in duplicated efforts that often impede the progress of new food safety initiatives and slow responses to emerging food safety issues.[328-332] Limited resources end up being divided among the several federal agencies, reducing the effectiveness of each tax dollar. Others in government and industry contend that creating a single food safety agency is unnecessary, pointing out that the United States sets the international standard for food safety.[333-335] Proponents favor increasing cooperation and collaboration among agencies, increasing funding for the agencies, and adopting a single national food safety policy.

2. *Safety of bioengineered foods:* Genetically engineered food crops and animals are controversial.[336-338] Whereas most scientists agree that bioengineered foods are safe,[339, 340] some make persuasive opposing arguments,[340-342] and consumers hold strong views at either extreme.[342-346] There are also those who question labeling of foods with respect to consumers' right to know what they are buying.[347]

3. *Chronic health effects of natural and synthetic chemicals ingested in foods:* As synthesis of new food additives, pesticides, and antibiotics continues, and as new uses for these chemicals and combinations of them continue to be found, the need for research on chronic effects of low-level exposure to these chemicals will be needed. Studies of interactions among additives, naturally occurring chemicals and toxicants, environmental chemicals and toxicants, and their acute and chronic effects on humans are also needed. Research addressing these issues in specific subpopulations, such as children, pregnant and lactating women, the elderly, and the immunocompromised, must be accomplished.[348-353]

4. *Prions as infective agents of foodborne disease:* The experience with BSE and vCJD in the United Kingdom initiated intense research efforts into prions as infective agents.[145] When a "mad cow" was thought to have entered the food supply in the United States, a series of reforms in regulating the meat industry were undertaken.[150,354] As research on prions and prion diseases[146,355] (as well as other issues concerning emerging microbial pathogens) continues, public health nutritionists should be prepared to assist consumers in understanding this issue within the context of hazards and risks.

5. *Home food safety:* Today, more meals than ever before are eaten outside the home. Ready-prepared meals for home consumption have never been more popular. Despite these trends, a significant number of foodborne illnesses result from hygiene errors committed at home.[356–362] In the area of home hygiene alone, the public health nutritionist can make a difference in consumer habits affecting individual and community health. For example, workshops and individual training could be offered to reinforce the food safety messages that should have been received in elementary and high school health classes. Occasional focused articles can be submitted to newspapers to reach a broader audience. Through partnerships with other professionals, such as sanitarians and school health teachers, consumers can be apprised of the many resources available to them in their communities. For all of the various federal, state, and local food safety initiatives, present and future, to succeed, food safety must begin at home.

Issues for Discussion

1. How can nutritionists help consumers understand food safety hazards and risks?
2. How should nutritionists approach other health agency staff to offer expertise on food safety issues? How is the nutritionist's perspective likely to differ from other health professionals' perspectives?
3. What possible roles exist for nutritionists to identify and combat bioterrorism directed against the food supply system?
4. Considering risks versus benefits, what specific recommendations should be made to clients concerned about bovine growth hormones in milk?
5. How can nutritionists help to instill a sense of individual responsibility for food safety?

References

1. Schwetz, B. A. (October 10, 2001). Statement before the Committee on Governmental Affairs, Subcommittee on Oversight of Government Management, Restructuring and the District of Columbia. Available at: http://www.fda.gov/ola/2001/foodsafety1010.html. Accessed June 19, 2004.
2. Mead, P. S., Slutsker, L., Dietz, V., McCaig, L. F., Bresee, J. S., Shapiro, C., et al. (1999). Food-related illness and death in the United States. *Emerging Infectious Diseases*, 5, 607.

3. Interagency Forum on Child and Family Statistics. America's Children: Key National Indicators of Well-Being, 2000. Available at http://www.childstats.gov/ac2000/Intro.asp#atr. Accessed June 22, 2004.

4. Anderson, G. F. & Hussey, P. S. (October 1999). *Health and population aging: A multinational comparison.* Baltimore MD: Johns Hopkins University, 6.

5. Sinclair, U. (1906). *The Jungle.* Available at: http://sunsite.berkeley.edu/Literature/Sinclair/TheJungle/. Accessed June 19, 2004.

6. Dingell, J. D. (April 23, 2002). Food safety and the bioterrorism legislation. Remarks before the Consumer Federation of America's 26th Annual National Food Policy Conference 2002. Available at: http://www.house.gov/commerce_democrats/press/107rm4.shtml. Accessed April 26, 2005.

7. Veneman, A. M. (February 27, 2003). Testimony before the Subcommittee on Agriculture, Rural Development, Food and Drug Administration, and Related Agencies Committee on Appropriations, U.S. House of Representatives. Available at: http://www.usda.gov/news/special/ctc33.htm. Accessed June 22, 2004.

8. Stier, R. F. (April/May 2003). The dirty dozen: Ways to reduce the 12 biggest foreign materials problems. *FoodSafety.* Available at: http://www.foodsafetymagazine.com/issues/0304/feat0304-2.htm. Accessed July 30, 2004.

9. Potter, N. N. & Hotchkiss, J. H. (1998). *Food science* (5th ed.). Gaithersburg, MD: Aspen Publishers, 533.

10. University of Arkansas. The Food Safety Consortium. Available at: http://www.uark.edu/depts/fsc/fslinks.htm. Accessed June 24, 2004.

11. Simmons College. Simmons Center for Hygiene and Health. Available at: http://www.simmons.edu/hygieneandhealth. Accessed August 1, 2004.

12. U.S. Food and Drug Administration. (September 24, 1998). Food safety: A team approach. *FDA Backgrounder.* Available at: http://vm.cfsan.fda.gov/~lrd/foodteam.html. Accessed June 21, 2004.

13. Department of Homeland Security, Customs and Border Protection. (July 13, 2004). U.S. Customs and Border Protection Graduates First Class of CBP Agriculture Specialists. Available at: http://www.cbp.gov/xp/cgov/newsroom/press_releases/archives/2004_press_releases/07302004/07132004.xml. Accessed April 4, 2005.

14. Kushner, G. J., Silverman, R. S., Steinborn, S. B., & Ungvarsky, A. M. (December 2002). *Update. Food industry and U.S. homeland security.* Washington DC: Hogan & Hartson LLP.

15. DHHS, CDC, National Center for Infectious Diseases. (1998). Addressing the Problem of Foodborne and Waterborne Diseases. Available at: http://www.cdc.gov/ncidod/emergplan/Foodborne/index.htm. Accessed July 29, 2004.

16. DHHS, CDC. (October 1998). Preventing Emerging Infectious Diseases. A Strategy for the 21st Century. Available at: http://www.cdc.gov/ncidod/emergplan/plan98.pdf. Accessed July 29, 2004.

17. Office for Seafood Inspection. (2002). Organization Handbook. NOAA Circular 02-15. Available at: http://www.rdc.noaa.gov/~ohb/F/FKA500.html. Accessed July 29, 2004.

18. NOAA Fisheries. Seafood Inspection Program. Available at: http://seafood.nmfs.noaa.gov. Accessed July 29, 2004.

19. 21 CFR Parts 123 and 1240. Procedures for the Safe and Sanitary Processing and Importing of Fish and Fishery Products; Final Rule. (December 18, 1995). *Federal Register,* 60(242), 65095.

20. Foulke, J. (December 5, 1995). Seafood safety regulations announced. *HHS News, P95-9.* Available at: http://www.cfsan.fda.gov/~lrd/hh-seareg.html. Accessed June 27, 2004.

21. FDA, CFSAN, Office of Seafood. (February 13, 2001). FDA's Seafood HACCP Program: Mid-Course Correction. Available at: http://www.cfsan.fda.gov/~comm/shaccp1.html. Accessed July 15, 2004.

22. Federal Trade Commission. For Consumers: Division of Advertising Practices. Available at: http://www.ftc.gov/bcp/bcpap.htm. Accessed July 29, 2004.

23. ATF. Alcohol/Tobacco Programs. Available at: http://www.atf.gov/about/programs/proal.htm. Accessed July 29, 2004.

24. USDA, FSIS. (2001). State Officials. Cooperative Meat and Poultry Inspection Programs. Available at: http://www.fsis.usda.gov/Regulations_&_Policies/State_Inspection_Programs/index.asp.htm. Accessed April 27, 2005.

25. Landman, J. (1999). Food aid in emergencies: A case for wheat? *Proceedings of the Nutrition Society, 58,* 355.

26. Stevens, S. (1990). Just a matter of time. *Food Management,* 25(11), 116.

27. Gemperlein, J. (1990). When the earth moved. . . . *Food Management,* 25(1), 130.

28. *The China Post.* (March 23, 2003). Over 200 Taipei citizens quarantined over SARS. Available at: http://www.chinapost.com.tw/taiwan/detail.asp?ID=36279&GRP=B. Accessed June 27, 2004.

29. The American Civil Defense Association. (2004). Civil/Homeland Defense and Emergency Management Resource Library. Available at: http://www.tacda.org/resources/index.php. Accessed April 27, 2005.

30. Marchione, T. J. (2002). Foods provided through U.S. government emergency food aid programs: Policies and customs governing their formulation, selection and distribution. *Journal of Nutrition, 132*(7), 2104S.

31. Reed, B. A., Habicht, J.-P., & Garza, C. (2002). Translating nutrition research into action in humanitarian emergencies. *Journal of Nutrition, 132*(7), 2112S.

32. Vogt, D. U. (2001). Food safety issues in the 107th Congress. *Congressional Research Service Issue Brief for Congress,* IB98009, 4.

33. Potter, N. N. & Hotchkiss, J. H. (1998). *Food Science* (5th ed.). Gaithersburg, MD: Aspen, 562.

34. Food additives permitted for direct addition to food for human consumption. *Code of Federal Regulations* (Title 21, Vol. 3, April 1, 2003), Ch. 1, Part 172.

35. Secondary direct food additives permitted in food for human consumption. *Code of Federal Regulations* (Title 21, Vol. 3, April 1, 2003), Ch. 1, Part 173.

36. Indirect food additives. *Code of Federal Regulations* (Title 21, Vol. 3, April 1, 2003), Ch. 1, Parts 174–178.

37. Prior-sanctioned food ingredients. *Code of Federal Regulations* (Title 21, Vol. 3, April 1, 2003), Ch. 1, Part 181.

38. Substances generally recognized as safe. *Code of Federal Regulations* (Title 21, Vol. 3, April 1, 2003), Ch. 1, Part 182.

39. Direct food substances affirmed as generally recognized as safe. *Code of Federal Regulations* (Title 21, Vol. 3, April 1, 2003), Ch. 1, Part 184.

40. Indirect food substances affirmed as generally recognized as safe. *Code of Federal Regulations* (Title 21, Vol. 3, April 1, 2003), Ch. 1, Part 186.

41. Burdock, G. A. & Carabin, I. G. (2004). Generally recognized as safe (GRAS): History and description. *Toxicology Letters, 150*, 3.

42. Rados, C. (2004). GRAS: Time-tested, and trusted, food ingredients. *FDA Consumer, 38*, 20.

43. A primer on food additives. (November 1988). *FDA Consumer*, 44.

44. Henkel, J. (December 1993). From shampoo to cereal. Seeing to the safety of color additives. *FDA Consumer*, 1.

45. FDA, CFSAN, Office of Cosmetics and Colors. (2001). Color Additives Fact Sheet. Available at: http://www.cfsan.fda.gov/~dms/cos-221.html. Accessed June 22, 2004.

46. USDA, FSIS. (2001). Additives in Meat and Poultry Products. Available at: http://www.fsis.usda.gov/OA/pubs/additive.htm. Accessed June 22, 2004.

47. The Food Label. (May 1999). *FDA Backgrounder BG 99-5*. Available at: http://www.fda.gov/opacom/backgrounders/foodlabel/newlabel.html. Accessed July 29, 2004.

48. FDA. (2004). Dietary Supplements. Overview. Available at: http://www.cfsan.fda.gov/~dms/supplmnt.html. Accessed July 29, 2004.

49. Hileman, B. (2004). Reining in dietary supplements. Food additives critics demand changes in the law governing supplement. *Chemical and Engineering News, 82*(25), 21.

50. FDA. Food Quality Protection Act. Available at: http://www.fda.gov/opacom/laws/foodqual/fqpatoc.htm. Accessed July 29, 2004.

51. EPA. (2004). Laws. Available at: http://www.epa.gov/pesticides/regulating/laws.htm. Accessed July 29, 2004.

52. EPA. Food Quality Protection Act (FQPA) of 1996. Available at: http://www.epa.gov/opppsps1/fqpa/. Accessed July 29, 2004.

53. Tomerlin, J. R. (2000). The U.S. Food Quality Protection Act-Policy implications of variability and consumer risk. *Food Additives and Contaminants, 17*(7), 641.

54. Sumner, D. (2000). The Food Quality Protection Act: A public health perspective. *Neurotoxicology, 21*(1–2), 183.

55. DiFonzo, C. (1997). Food Quality Protection Act. In: *Pesticide Policy and Michigan Specialty Crops Food Quality Protection Act*. East Lansing, MI: Michigan State University. Available at: http://ipmworld.umn.edu/chapters/fqpa96.htm. Accessed July 29, 2004.

56. Measure continues ban on human tests. (2003). *Chemical & Engineering News, 81*(31), 21.

57. Wagner, J. M. (1997). Food Quality Protection Act: Its impact on the pesticide industry. *Quality Assurance, 5*(4), 279.

58. EPA sued over pesticide standards. (2003). *Chemical & Engineering News, 81*(38), 25.

59. FDA. (2002). Public Health Security and Bioterrorism Preparedness and Response Act of 2002. Available at: http://www.fda.gov/oc/bioterrorism/PL107-188.html#title3. Accessed July 29, 2004.

60. FDA. (2002). The Bioterrorism Act of 2002. Available at: http://www.fda.gov/oc/bioterrorism/bioact.html. Accessed July 29, 2004.

61. FDA. (July 20, 2004). FDA commends passage by the House of Representatives of S. 741, a bill providing improved consumer protection and incentives for animal drug development. *FDA News P04-72.* Available at: http://www.fda.gov/bbs/topics/news/2004/ NEW01094.html. Accessed July 29, 2004.

62. FDA. (October 2001). HACCP: A state-of-the-art approach to food safety. *FDA Backgrounder.* Available at: http://www.cfsan.fda.gov/ ~lrd/bghaccp.html. Accessed July 28, 2004.

63. National Restaurant Association. (1995). *Applied foodservice sanitation: A certification coursebook.* (4th ed.). Chicago, IL: The Educational Foundation of the National Restaurant Association, 80.

64. Spears, M. C. (2000). *Foodservice organizations: A managerial and systems approach* (4th ed.). Englewood Cliffs, NJ: Prentice-Hall, 156.

65. FDA and USDA, National Advisory Committee on Microbiological Criteria for Foods. (August 14, 1997). Hazard Analysis and Critical Control Point Principles and Application Guidelines. Available at: http:// www.cfsan.fda.gov/~comm/nacmcfp.html. Accessed July 29, 2004.

66. Dulen, J. (1998). HACCP becomes reality. *Restaurants and Institutions, 108*(3), 90.

67. King, P. (1992). Implementing a HACCP program. *Food Management, 27*(12), 54.

68. Current good manufacturing practice in manufacturing, packing, or holding human food. *Code of Federal Regulations* (Title 21, Vol. 2, Part 110, April 1, 2003 [Revised]), 215.

69. Gould, W. A. (1994). *Current Good Manufacturing Practices/Food Plant Sanitation* (2nd ed.). Cockeysville, MD: CTI Publications, Ch. 2.

70. Potter, N. N. & Hotchkiss, J. S. (1998). *Food science* (5th ed.). Gaithersburg, MD: Aspen, 161.

71. FDA. (2000). Action levels for poisonous or deleterious substances in human food and animal feed. *Industry Activities Staff Booklet.* Available at: http://www.cfsan.fda.gov/~lrd/fdaact.html. Accessed June 25, 2004.

72. FDA, CFSAN. (1995, revised 1997 and 1998). The food defect action levels. Levels of natural or unavoidable defects in foods that present no health hazards for humans. Available at: http://www.cfsan.fda.gov/ ~dms/dalbook.html. Accessed June 25, 2004.

73. Tauxe, R. V. (1997). Emerging foodborne diseases: An evolving public health challenge. *Emerging Infectious Diseases, 3,* 425.

74. Altekruse, S. F. & Swerdlow, D. L. (1996). The changing epidemiology of foodborne diseases. *American Journal of the Medical Sciences. 311,* 23.

75. Preliminary FoodNet data on the incidence of infection with pathogens transmitted commonly through food—selected sites, United States, 2003. (2004) *Morbidity and Mortality Weekly Report, 53*(16), 338.

76. U.S. Department of Health and Human Services. (November 2000). *Healthy people 2010: Understanding and improving health* (2nd ed.). Washington, DC: Government Printing Office, Objective 10.

77. Jay, J. M. (2000). *Modern food microbiology* (6th ed.). Gaithersburg, MD: Aspen, 560.

78. Tauxe, R. V. (1992). Epidemiology of Campylobacter jejuni infections in the United States and other industrialized nations. In: I. Nachamkin, M. J. Blaser, & L. S. Tompkins (eds.), *Campylobacter jejuni: Current status and future trends.* Washington, DC: American Society of Microbiology, 9–19.

79. Blaser, M. J. (1982). *Campylobacter jejuni* and food. *Food Technology, 36*, 89.

80. Moore, J. E., Gilpin, D., Crothers, E., Canney, A., Kaneko, A., & Matsuda, M. (2002). Occurrence of *Campylobacter* spp. and *Cryptosporidium* spp. in seagulls (Larus spp.). *Vector Borne and Zoonotic Diseases, 2*, 111.

81. Yogasundram, K., Shane, S. M., & Harrington, K. S. (1989). Prevalence of *Campylobacter jejuni* in selected domestic and wild birds in Louisiana. *Avian Diseases, 33*, 664.

82. Stelzer, W., Mochmann, H., Richter, U., & Dobberkau, H. J. (1989). A study of *Campylobacter jejuni* and *Campylobacter coli* in a river system. *Zentralblatt fur Hygiene und Umweltmedizin, 189*, 20.

83. Pacha, R. E., Clark, G. W., Williams, E. A., Carter, A. M., Scheffelmaier, J. J., & Debusschere, P. (1987). Small rodents and other mammals associated with mountain meadows as reservoirs of *Giardia* spp. and *Campylobacter* spp. *Applied and Environmental Microbiology, 53*, 1574.

84. Rosef, O., Gondrosen, B., Kapperud, G., & Underdal, B. (1983). Isolation and characterization of *Campylobacter jejuni* and *Campylobacter coli* from domestic and wild mammals in Norway. *Applied and Environmental Microbiology, 46*, 855.

85. Cools, I., Uyttendaele, M., Caro, C., D'Haese, E., Nelis, H. J., & Debevere, J. (2003). Survival of *Campylobacter jejuni* strains of different origin in drinking water. *Journal of Applied Microbiology, 94*, 886.

86. Moore, J., Caldwell, P., & Millar, B. (2001). Molecular detection of Campylobacter spp. in drinking, recreational and environmental water supplies. *International Journal of Hygiene and Environmental Health, 204*, 185.

87. Skirrow, M. B. (1991). Epidemiology of *Campylobacter* enteritis. *International Journal of Food Microbiology, 12*, 9.

88. Palmer, S. R., Gully, P. R., White, J. M., Pearson, A. D., Suckling, W. G., Jones, D. M., et al. (1983). Water-borne outbreak of *Campylobacter* gastroenteritis. *Lancet, 1*, 287.

89. Bates, C. Hiett, K. L., & Stern, N. J. (2004). Relationship of *Campylobacter* isolated from poultry and from darkling beetles in New Zealand. *Avian Diseases, 48*, 138.

90. Gregory, E., Barnhart, H., Dreesen, D. W., Stern, N. J., & Corn, J. L. (1997). Epidemiological study of *Campylobacter* spp. in broilers: Source, time of colonization, and prevalence. *Avian Diseases, 41*, 890.

91. Altekruse, S. F., Stern, N. J., Fields, P. I., & Swerdlow, D. L. (1999). *Campylobacter jejuni*—An emerging foodborne pathogen. *Emerging Infectious Diseases, 5*, 28.

92. Birkhead, G., Vogt, R. L., Heun, E., Evelti, C. M., & Patton, C. M. (1988). A multiple-strain outbreak of *Campylobacter* enteritis due to consumption of inadequately pasteurized milk. *Journal of Infectious Diseases, 157*, 1095.

93. Hudson, P. J., Vogt, R. L, Brondum, J., & Patton, C. M. (1984). Isolation of *Campylobacter jejuni* from milk during an outbreak of *campylobacteriosis*. *Journal of Infectious Diseases, 150*, 789.

94. Vogt, R. L., Sours, H. E., Barret, T., Feldman, T. A., Dickinson, R. J., & Witherell, L. (1982). *Campylobacter* enteritis associated with contaminated water. *Annals of Internal Medicine, 96*, 292.

95. Manfredi, R., Nanetti, A., Ferri, M., & Chiodo, F. (1999). Fatal *Campylobacter jejuni* bacteraemia in patients with AIDS. *Journal of Medical Microbiology, 48*, 601.

96. Meier, P. A., Dooley, D. P., Jorgensen, J. H., Sanders, C. C., Huang, W. M., & Patterson, J. E. (1998). Development of quinolone-resistant *Campylobacter* fetus bacteremia in human immunodeficiency virus-infected patients. *Journal of Infectious Diseases, 177*, 951.

97. Tauxe, R. V., Pegues, D. A., & Hargrett-Bean, N. (1987). *Campylobacter* infections: The emerging national pattern. *American Journal of Public Health, 77*, 1219.

98. Bereswill, S. & Kist, M. (2003). Recent developments in *Campylobacter* pathogenesis. *Current Opinion in Infectious Diseases, 16*, 487.

99. Tsang, R. S. (2002). The relationship of *Campylobacter jejuni* infection and the development of Guillain-Barré syndrome. *Current Opinion in Infectious Diseases, 15*, 221.

100. Locht, H. & Krogfelt, K. A. (2002). Comparison of rheumatological and gastrointestinal symptoms after infection with *campylobacter jejuni/coli* and enterotoxigenic Escherichia coli. *Annals of the Rheumatic Diseases, 61*, 448.

101. Neill, M. A., Tarr, P. I., Taylor, D. N., & Wolf, M. (2000). *Escherichia coli*. In: Y. H. Hui, M. D. Pierson, & J. R. Gorham (eds.), *Foodborne disease handbook* (2nd ed., Vol. 1: *Bacterial pathogens*). New York: Marcel Dekker, 196.

102. Jay, J. M. (2000). *Modern food microbiology* (6th ed.). Gaithersburg, MD: Aspen, 531.

103. Jay, J. M. (2000). *Modern food microbiology* (6th ed.). Gaithersburg, MD: Aspen, 387–406.

104. Besser, R. E., Griffin, P. M., & Slutsker, L. (1999). *Escherichia coli* 0157:H7 gastroenteritis and the hemolytic uremic syndrome: An emerging infectious disease. *Annual Review of Medicine, 50*, 355.

105. Nauschuetz, W. (1998). Emerging foodborne pathogens: Enterohemorrhagic *Escherichia coli*. *Clinical Laboratory Science, 11*(5), 298.

106. Qadri, S. M. & Kayali, S. (1998). Enterohemorrhagic Escherichia coli. A dangerous food-borne pathogen. *Postgraduate Medicine, 103*(2), 179.

107. Isolation of E. coli 0157:H7 from sporadic cases of hemorrhagic colitis— U.S. 1982. (1997). *Morbidity and Mortality Weekly Report, 46*(30), 700.

108. Doyle, M. P. (1991). *Escherichia coli* 0157:H7 and its significance in foods. *International Journal of Food Microbiology, 12*(4), 289.

109. Griffin, P. M., Ostroff, S. M., Tauxe, R. V., Greene, K. D., Wells, J. G., Lewis, J. H., et al. (1988). Illnesses associated with *Escherichia coli* 0157:H7 infections. A broad clinical spectrum. *Annals of Internal Medicine, 109*(9), 705.

110. Riley, L. W., Remis, R. S., Helgerson, S. D., McGee, H. B., Wells, J. G., Davis, B. R., et al. (1983). Hemorrhagic colitis associated with a rare Escherichia coli serotype. *New England Journal of Medicine, 308*(12), 681.

111. Nataro, J. P., Steiner, T., & Guerrant, R. L. (1998). Enteroaggregative *Escherichia coli*. *Emerging Infectious Diseases, 4*(2), 251.

112. USDA, FSIS. (August 1999). COOK IT! Cooking Temperature. Available at: http://vm.cfsan.fda.gov/~fsg/fs-cook.html. Accessed July 29, 2004.

113. Partnership for Food Safety Education. Safe Cooking Fact Sheet. Available at: http://www.fightbac.org/cook_facts.cfm. Accessed July 29, 2004.

114. Jay, J. M. (2000). *Modern food microbiology* (6th ed.). Gaithersburg, MD: Aspen, 488.

115. Jay, J. M. (2000). *Modern food microbiology* (6th ed.). Gaithersburg, MD: Aspen, 511–513.

116. Orriss, G. D. (October–December 1997). Animal diseases of public health importance. *Emerging Infectious Diseases, 3,* 497.

117. Hogue, A., White, P., Guard-Petter, J., Schlosser, W., Gast, R., Ebel, E., et al. (1997). Epidemiology and control of egg-associated salmonella enteritidis in the United States of America. *Revue Scientifique et Technique, 16,* 542.

118. Barnhart, H. M., Dreesen, D. W., Bastien, R., & Pancorbo, O. C. (1991). Prevalence of *Salmonella enteritidis* and other serovars in ovaries of layer hens at time of slaughter. *Journal of Food Protection, 54,* 488.

119. St. Louis, M. E., Morse, D. L., Potter, M. E., DeMelfi, T. M., Guzewich, J. J., Tauxe, R. V., et al. (1988). The emergence of grade A eggs as major source of *Salmonella enteritis* infections: New implications for the control of salmonellosis. *Journal of the American Medical Association, 259,* 2103.

120. Guard-Petter, J. (2001). The chicken, the egg and *Salmonella enteritidis*: Minireview. *Environmental Microbiology, 3,* 421.

121. Humphrey, T. J. (1994). Contamination of egg shell and contents with *Salmonella enteritidis*: A review. *International Journal of Food Microbiology, 21,* 31.

122. Perales, I. & Audicana, A. (1988). *Salmonella enteritidis* and eggs. *Lancet, 2,* 1133.

123. USDA, FSIS. (February 2003). Focus on shell eggs. *Food Safety Focus.* Available at: http://www.fsis.usda.gov/OA/pubs/shelleggs.htm. Accessed July 29, 2004.

124. Mermelstein, N. H. (2001). Pasteurization of shell eggs. *Food Technology, 55*(12), 72.

125. Parashar, U., Quiroz, E. S., Mounts, A. W., Monroe, S. S., Fankhauser, R. L., Ando, T., et al. (2001). "Norwalk-like viruses": Public health consequences and outbreak management. *Morbidity and Mortality Weekly Report. Recommendations and Reports, 50*(RR-9), 1.

126. CDC, National Center for Infectious Diseases, Division of Viral and Rickettsial Diseases, Respiratory and Enteric Viruses Branch. (January 21, 2003). Norovirus: Q&A. Available at: http://www.cdc.gov/ncidod/dvrd/revb/gastro/norovirus-qa.htm. Accessed July 29, 2004.

127. Goldrick, B. A. (2003). Foodborne diseases: More efforts needed to meet the Healthy People 2010 objectives. *American Journal of Nursing, 103,* 105–106.

128. Mao, Y., Zhu, C., & Boedeker, E. C. (2003). Foodborne enteric infections. *Current Opinion in Gastroenterology, 19,* 11–22.

129. Lasky, T. (2002). Foodborne illness—Old problem, new relevance. *Epidemiology, 13,* 59–598.

130. Jay, J. M. (2000). *Modern food microbiology* (6th ed.). Gaithersburg, MD: Aspen, 614–615.

131. Norovirus activity—U.S., 2002. (2003). *Morbidity & Mortality Weekly Report, 52*(3), 41.

132. Bresee, J. S., Widdowson, M. A., Monroe, S. S., & Glass, R. I. (2002). Foodborne viral gastroenteritis. *Clinical Infectious Diseases, 35*(6), 748.

133. Outbreaks of gastroenteritis associated with noroviruses on cruise ships—U.S. (2002). *Morbidity & Mortality Weekly Report, 51,* (49), 1112.

134. DHHS, CDC, National Center for Infectious Diseases, Division of Viral Hepatitis. (July 1, 2004). Viral hepatitis A. Available at: http://www.cdc.gov/ncidod/diseases/hepatitis/a. Accessed July 29, 2004.

135. Fiore, A. E. (2004). Hepatitis A transmitted by food. *Clinical Infectious Diseases, 38*, 705.

136. Furness, B. W., Beach, M. J., & Roberts, J. M. (2000). Giardiasis surveillance—U.S., 1992–1997. (2000). *Morbidity and Mortality Weekly Report, 49*, 1.

137. Slifko, T. R., Smith, H. V., & Rose, J. B. (2000). Emerging parasite zoonoses associated with water and food. *International Journal for Parasitology, 30*, 1379.

138. Jay, J. M. (2000). *Modern food microbiology* (6th ed.). Gaithersburg, MD: Aspen, 576–578.

139. Millard, P. S., Gensheimer, K. F., Addiss, D. G., Sosin, D. M., Beckett, G. A., Houck-Jankoski, A., & Hudson, A. (1994). An outbreak of cryptosporidiosis from fresh-pressed apple cider. *Journal of the American Medical Association, 272*(20), 1592.

140. Foodborne outbreak of diarrheal illness associated with *Cryptosporidium parvum*—Minnesota, 1995. (1996). *Morbidity and Mortality Weekly Report, 45*(36), 783.

141. Outbreaks of Escherichia coli O157:H7 infection and cryptosporidiosis associated with drinking unpasteurized apple cider—Connecticut and New York, October 1996. (1997). *Morbidity and Mortality Weekly Report, 46*(1), 4.

142. Foodborne outbreak of cryptosporidiosis-Spokane, Washington, 1997. (1998). *Morbidity and Mortality Weekly Report, 47*(27), 565.

143. Soave, R. (1996). Cyclospora: An overview. *Clinical Infectious Diseases, 23*(3), 429.

144. Harris, D. A. (Ed.). (2004). *Mad cow disease and related spongiform encephalopathies.* (Vol. 284 in *Current Topics in Microbiology and Immunology Series*). New York: Springer-Verlag, 1–219.

145. Yam, P. (2003). *The pathological protein: Mad cow, chronic wasting, and other deadly prion diseases.* New York: Copernicus Books, 1–284.

146. Brown, P., Will, R. G., Bradley, R., Asher, D. M., & Detwiler, L. (2001). Bovine spongiform encephalopathy and variant Creutzfeldt-Jakob disease: Background, evolution, and current concerns. *Emerging Infectious Diseases, 7*(1), 6.

147. Pedersen, N. S. & Smith, E. (2002). Prion diseases: Epidemiology in man. *Acta Pathologica, Microbiologica, et Immunologica Scandinavica, 110*(1), 14.

148. Ironside, J. W. (1998). Prion diseases in man. *Journal of Pathology, 186*(3), 227.

149. Kretzschmar, H. A. (1999). Molecular pathogenesis of prion diseases. *European Archives of Psychiatry and Clinical Neuroscience, 249*(Suppl. 3), 56.

150. Scott, M. R., Will, R., Ironside, J., Nguyen, H. O., Tremblay, P., DeArmond, S. J., & Prusiner, S. B. (1999). Compelling transgenetic evidence for transmission of bovine spongiform encephalopathy prions to humans. *Proceedings of the National Academies of Sciences USA, 96*(26), 15137–15142.

151. FDA. Bovine Spongiform Encephalopathy (BSE). Also Known as "Mad Cow Disease. Available at: http://www.fda.gov/oc/opacom/hottopics/bse.html. Accessed July 29, 2004.

152. Brown, P. The risk of bovine spongiform encephalopathy ("mad cow disease") to human health. *Journal of the American Medical Association, 278*(12), 1008.

153. Hileman, B. (2004). Mad cow disease. Regulatory changes stemming from discovery of one diseased cow create new conflicts spawned in part by gaps in scientific understanding. *Chemical & Engineering News, 82*(22), 21.

154. USDA, FSIS and APHIS, and DHHS, FDA. (July 9, 2004). USDA and HHS Strengthen Safeguards Against Bovine Spongiform Encephalopathy. Available at: http://www.fda.gov/bbs/topics/news/2004/ NEW01084.html. Accessed July 29, 2004.

155. FDA, CFSAN. (July 9, 2004). Fact Sheet: I. FDA's New Interim Final Rule Prohibiting Use of Certain Cattle Materials That May Carry the Risk of Bovine Spongiform Encephalopathy in Human Foods and Cosmetics and II. FDA's Proposed Rule on Recordkeeping Requirements for Human Food and Cosmetics Manufactured from, Processed with, or Otherwise Containing Material from Cattle. Available at: http:// www.cfsan.fda.gov/~comm/bsefact2.html. Accessed July 29, 2004.

156. FDA, USDA propose mad cow regulations. (July 19, 2004). *Chemical & Engineering News, 82*(29), 15.

157. Jay, J. M. (2000). *Modern food microbiology* (6th ed.). Gaithersburg, MD: Aspen, 595–600.

158. Lie, J. L. & Marth, E. H. (1967). Formation of aflatoxin in cheddar cheese by Aspergillus flavus and Aspergillus parasiticus. *Journal of Dairy Science, 50*, 1708.

159. Van Rensburg, S. J. (1974). Primary liver cancer rate and aflatoxin intake in a high cancer area. *South African Medical Journal, 48*, 2508a.

160. Park, D. L. (1993). Controlling aflatoxin in food and feed. *Food Technology, 47*, 92.

161. Labuza, T. P. (1983). Regulation of mycotoxins in food. *Journal of Food Protection, 46*, 260.

162. FAO/WHO. FAO/WHO Food Standards. Codex Alimentarius. Available at: http://www.codexalimentarius.net/web/index_en.jsp. Accessed July 25, 2004.

163. Newsome, R. (1999). Issues in international trade: Looking to the Codex Alimentarius Commission. *Food Technology, 53*, 26.

164. Stinson, E. E., Osman, S. F., Heisler, E. G., Siciliano, J., & Bills, D. D. (1981). Mycotoxin production in whole tomatoes, apples, oranges, and lemons. *Journal of Agricultural and Food Chemistry, 29*, 790.

165. Stinson, E. E., Bills, D. D., Osman, S. F., Siciliano, J., Ceponis, M. J., & Heisler, E. G. (1980). Mycotoxin production by Alternaria species grown on apples, tomatoes, and blueberries. *Journal of Agricultural and Food Chemistry, 28*, 960.

166. Marasas, W. F. O., Jaskiewicz, K., Venter, F. S., & Van Schalkwyk, D. J. (1988). Fusarium moniliforme contamination of maize in oesophageal cancer areas in Transkei. *South African Medical Journal, 74*, 110.

167. Yoshizawa, T., Yamashita, A., & Luo, Y. (1994). Fumonisin occurrence in corn from high- and low-risk areas for human esophageal cancer in China. *Applied and Environmental Microbiology, 60*, 1626.

168. Bennett, G. A. & Richard, J. L. (1996). Influence of processing on Fusarium mycotoxins in contaminated grains. *Food Technology, 50*, 235.

169. Mycotoxins and food safety. (1986). *Food Technology, 40*, 59.

170. Friedman, M., Roitman, J. N., & Kozukue, N. (2003). Glycoalkaloid and calystegine contents of eight potato cultivars. *Journal of Agricultural and Food Chemistry, 51*(10), 2964.

171. Friedman, M. & McDonald, G. M. (1996). Glycoalkaloids in fresh and processed potatoes. In: Lee, T.-C., Kim, H.-J., (eds.), *Chemical Markers for Processed and Stored Foods* (p. 189). Washington, DC: American Chemical Society.

172. Phillips, B. J., Hughes, J. A., Phillips, J. C., Walters, D. G., Anderson, D., & Tahourdin, C. S. M. (1996). A study of the toxic hazard that might be associated with the consumption of green potato tops. *Food and Chemical Toxicology, 34*(5), 439.

173. Hellenas, K. E., Branzell, C., Johnsson, H., & Slanina, P. (1995). Glycoalkaloid content of early potato varieties. *Journal of the Science of Food and Agriculture, 67*(1), 125.

174. Zhao, J., Camire, M. E., Bushway, R. J., & Bushway, A. A. (1994). Glycoalkaloid content and in vitro glycoalkaloid solubility of extruded potato peels. *Journal of Agricultural and Food Chemistry, 42*(11), 2570.

175. Friedman, M. (1992). Composition and safety evaluation of potato berries, potato and tomato seeds, potatoes, and potato alkaloids. *ACS Symposium Series, 484*, 429.

176. Friedman, M. & Dao, L. (1992). Distribution of glycoalkaloids in potato plants and commercial potato products. *Journal of Agricultural and Food Chemistry, 40*(3), 419.

177. Edwards, E. J. & Cobb, A. H. (1999). The effect of prior storage on the potential of potato tubers (*Solanum tuberosum* L) to accumulate glycoalkaloids and chlorophylls during light exposure, including artificial neural network modelling. *Journal of the Science of Food and Agriculture, 79*(10), 1289.

178. Griffiths, D. W., Bain, H., & Dale, M. F. B. (1998). Effect of storage temperature on potato (*Solanum tuberosum* L.) tuber glycoalkaloid content and the subsequent accumulation of glycoalkaloids and chlorophyll in response to light exposure. *Journal of Agricultural and Food Chemistry, 46*(12), 5262.

179. Percival, G., Dixon, G. R., & Sword, A. (1996). Glycoalkaloid concentration of potato tubers following exposure to daylight. *Journal of the Science of Food and Agriculture, 71*(1), 59.

180. Coria, N. A., Sarquis, J. I., Penalosa, I., & Urzua, M. (1998). Heat-induced damage in potato (*Solanum tuberosum*) tubers: Membrane stability, tissue viability, and accumulation of glycoalkaloids. *Journal of Agricultural and Food Chemistry, 46*(11), 4524.

181. Griffiths, D. W., Bain, H., & Dale, M. F. B. (1997). The effect of low-temperature storage on the glycoalkaloid content of potato (*Solanum tuberosum*) tubers. *Journal of the Science of Food and Agriculture, 74*(3), 301.

182. Hlywka, J. J., Stephenson, G. R., Sears, M. K., & Yada, R. Y. (1994). Effects of insect damage on glycoalkaloid content in potatoes (*Solanum tuberosum*). *Journal of Agricultural and Food Chemistry, 42*(11), 2545.

183. Rayburn, J. R., Bantle, J. A., & Friedman, M. (1994). Role of carbohydrate side chains of potato glycoalkaloids in developmental toxicity. *Journal of Agricultural and Food Chemistry, 42*(7), 1511.

184. Friedman, M. & McDonald, G. M. (1997). Potato glycoalkaloids chemistry analysis, safety and plant physiology. *Critical Reviews in Plant Science, 16*(1), 55.

185. New safeguards against glycoalkaloids. (1997). *Agricultural Research Magazine 45*(12), 14.

186. Korpan, Y. I., Nazarenko, E. A., Skryshevskaya, L. V., Martelet, C., Jaffrezic-Renault, N., & El'skaya, A. V. (2004). Potato glycoalkaloids: True safety or false sense of security. *Trends in Biotechnology, 22*(3), 147.

187. Friedman, M., Henika, P. R., & Mackey, B. E. (2003). Effect of feeding solanidine, solasodine, and tomatidine to non-pregnant and pregnant mice. *Food and Chemical Toxicology, 41*(1), 61.

188. Smith, D. B., Roddick, J. G., & Jones, J. L. (1996). Potato glycoalkaloids: Some unanswered questions. *Trends in Food Science and Technology, 7*(4), 126.

189. Nigg, H. H. & Beier, R. C. (1995). Evaluation of food for potential toxicants. In *Phytochemicals and Health: Proceedings, Tenth Annual Penn State Symposium in Plant Physiology*, May 18-20, 1995, 192-201.

190. Tanne, J. H. (1998). Foods and drugs alter response to anaesthesia. *British Medical Journal, 317*(7166), 1102.

191. Arora, A. & Camire, M. E. (1994). Performance of potato peels in muffins and cookies. *Food Research International, 27*(1), 15.

192. Camire, M. E. & Flint, S. I. (1991). Thermal processing effects on dietary fiber composition and hydration capacity in corn meal, oat meal, and potato peels. *Cereal Chemistry, 68*(6), 645.

193. Surjawan, I., Dougherty, M. P., Bushway, R. J., Bushway, A. A., Briggs, J. L., & Camire, M. E. (2001). Sulfur compounds reduce potato toxins during extrusion cooking. *Journal of Agricultural and Food Chemistry, 49*(6), 2835.

194. Teitelbaum, J. S., Zatorre, R. J., Carpenter, S., Gendron, D., Evans, A. C., Gjedde, A., et al. (1990). Neurologic sequelae of domoic acid intoxication due to the ingestion of contaminated mussels. *New England Journal of Medicine, 322*, 1781.

195. Perl, T. M., Bédard, L., Kotsatsky, T., Hockin, J. C., Todd, E. C., & Remis, R. S. (1990). An outbreak of toxic encephalopathy caused by eating mussels contaminated with domoic acid. *New England Journal of Medicine, 322*, 1775.

196. Stewart, G. R., Zorumski, C. F., Price, M. T., & Olney, J. W. (1990). Domoic acid: A dementia-inducing excitotoxic food poison with kainic acid receptor specificity. *Experimental Neurology, 110*, 127.

197. Zatorre, R. J. (1990). Memory loss following domoic acid intoxication from ingestion of toxic mussels. *Canada Diseases Weekly Report, 16*(Suppl 1E), 101.

198. Iverson, F., Truelove, J., Nera, E., Tryphonas, L., Campbell, J., & Lok, E. (1989). Domoic acid poisoning and mussel-associated intoxication: Preliminary investigations into the response of mice and rats to toxic mussel extract. *Food and Chemical Toxicology, 27*, 377.

199. Pottier, I., Vernoux, J. P., & Lewis, R. J. (2001). Ciguatera fish poisoning in the Caribbean islands and Western Atlantic. *Reviews of Environmental Contamination and Toxicology, 168*, 99.

200. Ting, J. Y., Brown, A. F., & Pearn, J. H. (1998). Ciguatera poisoning: An example of a public health challenge. *Australian and New Zealand Journal of Public Health, 22*, 140.

201. Pearn, J. (2001). Neurology of ciguatera. *Journal of Neurology, Neurosurgery, and Psychiatry, 70*, 4.

202. Bruneau, A., Mahanty, S., al-Azraqui, T., MacLean, J., Bourque, M., & Desroches, F. (1997). Ciguatera fish poisoning linked to the ingestion of barracuda in a Montreal restaurant—Quebec. *Canada Communicable Disease Report, 23*, 153.

203. Klemme, T. M. & Lösch, R. R. (1997). Ciguatera-Eine Tückische Fischvergiftung. Durch Fischimporte ist das Risiko Potentiell auch Hierzulande Gegeben. *Fortschritte der Medizin, 115*, 39.

204. Sanders, Jr., W. E., (1987). Intoxications from the seas: Ciguatera, scombroid, and paralytic shellfish poisoning. *Infectious Disease Clinics of North America, 1*, 665.

205. Lawrence, J. F., Niedzwiadek, B., & Menard, C. (2004). Quantitative determination of paralytic shellfish poisoning toxins in shellfish using prechromatographic oxidation and liquid chromatography with fluorescence detection: Interlaboratory study. *Journal of AOAC International, 87*, 83.

206. Biré, R., Krys, S., Frémy, J. M., & Dragacci, S. (2003). Improved solid-phase extraction procedure in the analysis of paralytic shellfish poisoning toxins by liquid chromatography with fluorescence detection. *Journal of Agricultural and Food Chemistry, 51*, 6386.

207. Lehane, L. (2001). Paralytic shellfish poisoning: A potential public health problem. *Medical Journal of Australia, 175*, 29.

208. FDA, CFSAN. (February 6, 2001). The National Shellfish Sanitation Program. A Protocol for International Participation. Available at: http://vm.cfsan.fda.gov/~ear/nsspprot.html. Accessed June 22, 2004.

209. FDA, CFSAN. Interstate Certified Shellfish Shippers List. Available at: http://www.cfsan.fda.gov/~ear/shellfis.html. Accessed June 22, 2004.

210. Castoldi, A. F., Coccini, T., & Manzo, L. (2003). Neurotoxic and molecular effects of methylmercury in humans. *Reviews on Environmental Health, 18*(1), 19.

211. Sweet, L. I. & Zelikoff, J. T. (2001). Toxicology and immunotoxicology of mercury: A comparative review in fish and humans. *Journal of Toxicology and Environmental Health. Part B, Critical Reviews 4*(2), 161.

212. DHHS and EPA. (March 2004). What You Need to Know About Mercury in Fish and Shellfish. 2004 EPA and FDA Advice For: Women Who Might Become Pregnant, Women Who Are Pregnant, Nursing Mothers, Young Children. EPA-823-R-04-005. Available at: http://www.cfsan.fda.gov/~dms/admehg3.html. Accessed July 15, 2004.

213. Crawford, L. M. (March 2004). Fish Is an Important Part of a Balanced Diet. Available at: http://www.fda.gov/oc/opacom/hottopics/mercury/mercuryop-ed.html. Accessed July 15, 2004.

214. DHHS and EPA. (March 19, 2004). Mercury Levels in Commercial Fish and Shellfish. Available at: http://www.cfsan.fda.gov/~frf/sea-mehg.html. Accessed July 15, 2004.

215. FDA, CFSAN. (March 19, 2004). Mercury in Fish: FDA Monitoring Program (1990-2003). Available at: http://www.cfsan.fda.gov/~frf/seamehg2.html. Accessed July 15, 2004.

216. Clarkson, T. W. & Strain, J. J. (2003). Nutritional factors may modify the toxic action of methyl mercury in fish-eating populations. *Journal of Nutrition, 133*(5 Suppl 1), 1539S.

217. Shipp, A. M., Gentry, P. R., Lawrence, G., Van Landingham, C., Covington, T., Clewell, H. J., et al. (2000). Determination of a site-specific

reference dose for methylmercury for fish-eating populations. *Toxicology and Industrial Health, 16*(9–10), 335.

218. Chapman, L. & Chan, H. M. (2000). The influence of nutrition on methyl mercury intoxication. *Environmental Health Perspectives, 108*(Suppl 1), 29.

219. Chan, H. M. & Egeland, G. M. (2004). Fish consumption, mercury exposure, and heart diseases. *Nutrition Reviews, 62*(2), 68.

220. Smith, S. C., Taylor, J. G., & Stephen, A. M. (2000). Use of food labels and beliefs about diet-disease relationships among university students. *Public Health Nutrition, 3*(2), 175.

221. Elbon, S. M., Johnson, M. A., Fischer, J. G., & Searcy, C. A. (2000). Demographic factors, nutrition knowledge, and health-seeking behaviors influence nutrition label reading behaviors among older American adults. *Journal of Nutrition for the Elderly, 19*(3), 31.

222. Joshi, P., Mofidi, S., & Sicherer, S. H. (2002). Interpretation of commercial food ingredient labels by parents of food-allergic children. *Journal of Allergy and Clinical Immunology, 109*(6), 1019–1021.

223. Levy, L., Patterson, R. E., Kristal, A. R., & Li, S. S. (2000). How well do consumers understand percentage daily value on food labels? *American Journal of Health Promotion, 14*(3), 157.

224. Institute of Food Technologists. (2004). Office of Science, Communications, and Government Relations. Available at: http://www.ift.org/cms/?pid=1000316. Accessed June 22, 2004.

225. Institute of Food Technologists. (2003). IFT's New Strategic Plan: Changing Direction. Available at: http://www.ift.org/cms/?pid=1000258. Accessed June 22, 2004.

226. Institute of Food Technologists. (March 2002). The Long-Range Strategic Plan. Available at: http://www.ift.org/cms/?pid=1000257. Accessed June 22, 2004.

227. Reisch, M. S. (2004). Track us, trust us. American Chemistry Council says will supply the facts to earn the public's trust. *Chemical & Engineering News, 82*, 24.

228. Thayer, A. (2003). ACC convenes amid upheaval. Industry group wrestles with issues of money, resignations, and image. *Chemical & Engineering News, 81*, 10.

229. Storck, W. (2001). ACC tests new ad image program. By stressing "chemistry" not "chemicals," group hopes to change public's view of industry. *Chemical & Engineering News, 79*, 13.

230. Pszczola, D. E. (2003). Sweetener + sweetener enhances the equation. *Food Technology, 57*, 48.

231. Homler, B. E. (1984). Properties and stability of aspartame. *Food Technology, 38*, 50.

232. Levin, G. V. (2002). Tagatose, the new GRAS sweetener and health product. *Journal of Medicinal Food, 5*, 23.

233. Gilman, V. (2004). Artificial sweeteners. No-calorie sugar substitutes provide options for enjoying the sweet life. *Chemical & Engineering News, 82*, 43.

234. Geuns, J. M. (2003). Stevioside. *Phytochemistry, 64*, 913.

235. Gregersen, S., Jeppesen, P. B., Holst, J. J., & Hermansen, K. (2004). Antihyperglycemic effects of stevioside in type 2 diabetic subjects. *Metabolism: Clinical and Experimental, 53*, 73.

236. Hsieh, M. H., Chan, P., Sue, Y. M., Liu, J. C., Liang, T. H., Huang, T. Y., et al. (2003). Efficacy and tolerability of oral stevioside in patients with mild essential hypertension: A two-year, randomized, placebo-controlled study. *Clinical Therapeutics, 25,* 2797.

237. Jeppesen, P. B., Gregersen, S., Rolfsen, S. E., Jepsen, M., Colombo, M., Agger, A., et al. (2003). Antihyperglycemic and blood pressure-reducing effects of stevioside in the diabetic Goto-Kakizaki rat. *Metabolism: Clinical and Experimental, 52*(3), 372.

238. Chan, P., Tomlinson, B., Chen, Y. J., Liu, J. C., Hsieh, M. H., & Cheng, J. T. (2000). A double-blind placebo-controlled study of the effectiveness and tolerability of oral stevioside in human hypertension. *British Journal of Clinical Pharmacology, 50*(3), 215.

239. Bray, G. A., Nielsen, S. J., & Popkin, B. M. (2004). Consumption of high-fructose corn syrup in beverages may play a role in the epidemic of obesity. *American Journal of Clinical Nutrition, 79,* 537.

240. Chappel, C. I. (1992). A review and biological risk assessment of sodium saccharin. *Regulatory Toxicology and Pharmacology, 15,* 253.

241. Ellwein, L. B. & Cohen, S. M. (1990). The health risks of saccharin revisited. *Critical Reviews in Toxicology, 20,* 311.

242. Butchko, H. H., Stargel, W. W., Comer, C. P., Mayhew, D. A., Benninger, C., Blackburn, G. L., et al. (2002). Aspartame: Review of safety. *Regulatory Toxicology and Pharmacology, 35,* S1.

243. Potenza, D. P. & el-Mallakh, R. S. (1989). Aspartame: Clinical update. *Connecticut Medicine, 53,* 395.

244. Yost, D. A. (1989). Clinical safety of aspartame. *American Family Physician, 39,* 201.

245. Garriga, M. M. & Metcalfe, D. D. (1988). Aspartame intolerance. *Annals of Allergy, 61,* 63.

246. Janssen, P. J. & van der Heijden, C. A. (1988). Aspartame: Review of recent experimental and observational data. *Toxicology, 50,* 1.

247. Stegink, L. D. (1987). The aspartame story: A model for the clinical testing of a food additive. *American Journal of Clinical Nutrition, 46*(Suppl 1), 204.

248. Finn, J. P. & Lord, G. H. (2000). Neurotoxicity studies on sucralose and its hydrolysis products with special reference to histopathologic and ultrastructural changes. *Food and Chemical Toxicology, 38*(Suppl 2), S7.

249. Goldsmith, L. A. (2000). Acute and subchronic toxicity of sucralose. *Food and Chemical Toxicology, 38*(Suppl 2), S53.

250. Grice, H. C. & Goldsmith, L. A. (2000). Sucralose-An overview of the toxicity data. *Food and Chemical Toxicology, 38*(Suppl 2), S1.

251. Knight, I. (1994). The development and applications of sucralose, a new high-intensity sweetener. *Canadian Journal of Physiology and Pharmacology, 72,* 435.

252. DHHS and USDA. (May 2000). Dietary Guidelines for Americans (5th ed.). Available at: http://www.health.gov/dietaryguidelines/. Accessed June 25, 2004.

253. USDA, National Agricultural Library, Food and Nutrition Information Center. (July 12, 2004). Dietary Reference Intakes (DRI) and Recommended Dietary Allowances (RDA). Available at: http://www.nal.usda.gov/fnic/etext/000105.html. Accessed July 29, 2004.

254. American Dietetic Association. (2004). Position of the American Dietetic Association: Use of nutritive and nonnutritive sweeteners. *Journal of the American Dietetic Association, 104*, 255.

255. Tate & Lyle PLC. (2004). About Food Starches. Available at: http://www.amylum.com/TateAndLyle/products_applications/_products/food_starches/default.htm. Accessed April 27, 2005.

256. Wittrig, B. (2003). Preservative analysis by liquid and gas chromatography. State College, PA: Restek Corp. Available at: http://www.restek.com/fantasia/pdfCache/pres-2003-preserv.pdf. Accessed July 27, 2004.

257. Duke, J. Module 19. Botanicals Generally Recognized As Safe. Available at: http://www.ars-grin.gov/duke/syllabus/gras.htm. Accessed July 28, 2004.

258. Geha, R. S., Beiser, A., Ren, C., Patterson, R., Greenberger, P. A., Grammer, L. C., et al. (2000). Review of alleged reaction to monosodium glutamate and outcome of a multicenter double-blind placebo-controlled study. *Journal of Nutrition, 130*(Suppl 4S), 1058S.

259. Yang, W. H., Drouin, M. A., Herbert, M., Mao, Y., & Karsh, J. (1997). The monosodium glutamate symptom complex: Assessment in a double-blind, placebo-controlled, randomized study. *Journal of Allergy and Clinical Immunology, 99*, 757.

260. Tarasoff, L. & Kelly, M. F. (1993). Monosodium l-glutamate: A double-blind study and review. *Food and Chemical Toxicology, 31*, 1019.

261. Scher, W. & Scher, B. M. (1992). A possible role for nitric oxide in glutamate (MSG)-induced Chinese restaurant syndrome, glutamate-induced asthma, "hot-dog headache," pugilistic Alzheimer's disease, and other disorders. *Medical Hypotheses, 38*, 185.

262. Pulce, C., Vial, T., Verdier, F., Testud, F., Nicolas, B., & Descotes, J. (1992). The Chinese restaurant syndrome: A reappraisal of monosodium glutamate's causative role. *Adverse Drug Reactions and Toxicological Reviews, 11*, 19.

263. Sands, G. H., Newman, L., & Lipton, R. (1991). Cough, exertional, and other miscellaneous headaches. *Medical Clinics of North America, 75*, 733.

264. Scopp, A. L. (1991). MSG and hydrolyzed vegetable protein induced headache: Review and case studies. *Headache, 31*, 107.

265. Stevenson, D. D. (2000). Monosodium glutamate and asthma. *Journal of Nutrition, 130*(Suppl 4S), 1067S.

266. Woods, R. K., Weiner, J. M., Thien, F., Abramson, M., & Walters, E. H. (1998). The effects of monosodium glutamate in adults with asthma who perceive themselves to be monosodium glutamate-intolerant. *Journal of Allergy and Clinical Immunology, 101*, 762.

267. Walker, R. & Lupien, J. R. (2000). The safety evaluation of monosodium glutamate. *Journal of Nutrition, 130*(Suppl 4S), 1049S.

268. FDA, Office of Public Affairs. (February 29, 1996). Folic Acid Fortification Fact Sheet. Available at: http://www.cfsan.fda.gov/~dms/wh-folic.html. Accessed July 28, 2004.

269. FDA, CFSAN. (May 15, 2002). Appendix O. Vitamin Fortification of Fluid Milk Products, in Grade "A" Pasteurized Milk Ordinance, 2001 Revision. Available at: http://www.cfsan.fda.gov/~ear/pmo01o.html. Accessed July 28, 2004.

270. Kurtzweil, P. (February 1999). How Folate Can Help Prevent Birth Defects. *FDA Consumer*. Available at: http://vm.cfsan.fda.gov/~dms/fdafolic.html. Accessed July 28, 2004.

271. Global trends. (Market trends): Fortified beverages. (2002). *Prepared Foods, 171*, 9.

272. Health sells!!! Refrigerators, etc. (May 27, 2002). *Business World*, 38.

273. Fortifying sales: Lifestyle choices support demand for fortified foods. (2002). *Gourmet Retailer, 23*, 42.

274. Food additives permitted for direct addition to food for human consumption; vitamin D3. (February 27, 2003). *Federal Register, 68*, 9000.

275. Penniston, K. L. & Tanumihardjo, S. A. (2003). Vitamin A in dietary supplements and fortified foods: Too much of a good thing? *Journal of the American Dietetic Association, 103*, 1185.

276. Greger, J. L. (1987). Food, supplements, and fortified foods: Scientific evaluations in regard to toxicology and nutrient bioavailability. *Journal of the American Dietetic Association, 87*, 1369.

277. Dalton, L. (2002). What's that stuff? Food preservatives. *Chemical & Engineering News, 80*, 40.

278. Foulke, J. E. (1993). A Fresh Look at Food Preservatives. *FDA Consumer*. Available at: http://vm.cfsan.fda.gov/~dms/fdpreser.html. Accessed July 28, 2004.

279. Williams, G. M., Iatropoulos, M. J., & Whysner, J. (1999). Safety assessment of butylated hydroxyanisole and butylated hydroxytoluene as antioxidant food additives. *Food and Chemical Toxicology, 37*(9-10), 1027.

280. Whysner, J. & Williams, G. M. (1996). Butylated hydroxyanisole mechanistic data and risk assessment: Conditional species-specific cytotoxicity, enhanced cell proliferation, and tumor promotion. *Pharmacology & Therapeutics 71*(1-2), 137.

281. Iverson, F. (1995). Phenolic antioxidants: Health protection branch studies on butylated hydroxyanisole. *Cancer Letters, 93*(1), 49.

282. Huang, M. T. & Ferraro, T. (1992). Phenolic compounds in food and cancer prevention. *ACS Symposium Series, 507*, 8.

283. Lester, M. R. (1995). Sulfite sensitivity: Significance in human health. *Journal of the American College of Nutrition, 14*(3), 229.

284. Lecos, C. (1985). Reacting to sulfites. *FDA Consumer, 19*(10), 17.

285. Skovgaard, N. (1992). Microbiological aspects and technological need: Technological needs for nitrates and nitrites. *Food Additives and Contaminants, 9*(5), 391.

286. Mirvish, S. S. (1991). The significance for human health of nitrate, nitrite and n-nitroso compounds. NATO ASI Series: Series G: *Ecological Sciences, 30*, 253.

287. Nitrate, nitrite, and nitroso compounds in foods. *Food Technology, 41*(4), 127.

288. FDA, CFSAN. (February 16, 2001). FDA broadens use of packaging materials for irradiation of prepackaged foods. Available at: http://www.cfsan.fda.gov/~dms/fsiupd24.html. Accessed August 1, 2004.

289. FDA. (January 2000). Food Irradiation: A Safe Measure (Publication No. 00-2329). Available at: http://www.fda.gov/opacom/catalog/irradbro.html. Accessed August 1, 2004.

290. American Dietetic Association. (2000). Position of the American Dietetic Association: Food irradiation. *Journal of the American Dietetic Association, 100*(2), 246.

291. Tritsch, G. L. (2000). Food irradiation. *Nutrition, 16*(7-8), 698.

292. Pauli, G. H. (May 1999). U.S. Regulatory Requirements for Irradiating Foods. FDA, CFSAN, Office of Premarket Approval. Available at: http://www.cfsan.fda.gov/~dms/opa-rdtk.html. Accessed August 1, 2004.

293. Farkas, J. (1998). Irradiation as a method for decontaminating food. A review. *International Journal of Food Microbiology, 44*(3), 189.

294. Morehouse, K. M. (1998). Food irradiation: The treatment of foods with ionizing radiation. *Food Testing & Analysis, 4*(3), 9.

295. Loaharanu, P. (1996). Irradiation as a cold pasteurization process of food. *Veterinary Parasitology, 64*(1-2), 71.

296. Dodd, N. J. (1995). Free radicals and food irradiation. *Biochemical Society Symposium, 61*, 247.

297. Lagunas-Solar, M. C. (1995). Radiation processing of foods: An overview of scientific principles and current status. *Journal of Food Protection, 58*(2), 186.

298. Irradiation in the production, processing and handling of food. (December 3, 1997). *Federal Register, 62*(232), 64107.

299. Swanson, R. B. & Munsayac, L. J. (1999). Acceptability of fruit purees in peanut butter, oatmeal, and chocolate chip reduced-fat cookies. *Journal of the American Dietetic Association, 99*(3), 343.

300. Blends reduce fat in bakery products. *Food Technology, 48*(6), 168.

301. Phillips, I., Casewell, M., Cox, T., De Groot, B., Friis, C., Jones, R., et al. (2004). Does the use of antibiotics in food animals pose a risk to human health? A critical review of published data. *Journal of Antimicrobial Chemotherapy, 53*(1), 28.

302. Wegener, H. C. (2003). Antibiotics in animal feed and their role in resistance development. *Current Opinion in Microbiology, 6*(5), 439.

303. Bauman, D. E. (1992). Bovine somatotropin: Review of an emerging animal technology. *Journal of Dairy Science, 75*(12), 3432.

304. Juskevich, J. C. & Guyer, C. G. (1990). Bovine growth hormone: Human food safety evaluation. *Science, 249*(4971), 875.

305. Bradley, T. (December 30, 2003). Monsanto's victory in Maine rBGH lawsuit a setback for consumers. Portland Press Herald, 10A.

306. Mohl, B. (September 28, 2003). Got growth hormone? Dairies play on fear in marketing milk without the additive. The Boston Globe, J1.

307. Centner, T. J. & Lathrop, K. W. (1997). Legislative and legal restrictions on labeling information regarding the use of recombinant bovine somatotropin. *Journal of Dairy Science, 80*(1), 215.

308. Food Marketing Institute. (1994). Backgrounder: Bovine Growth Hormone or Bovine Somatotropin. Available at: http://www.fmi.org/media/bg/bst.htm. Accessed April 27, 2005.

309. Hamilton, D., Ambrus, A., Dieterle, R., Felsot, A., Harris, C., Petersen, B., et al. (2004). Pesticide residues in food-Acute dietary exposure. *Pest Management Science, 60*(4), 311.

310. Potter, T. L., Marti, L., Belflower, S., & Truman, C. C. (2000). Multiresidue analysis of cotton defoliant, herbicide, and insecticide residues in water by solid-phase extraction and GC-NPD, GC-MS, and HPLC-diode array detection. *Journal of Agricultural and Food Chemistry, 48*(9), 4103.

311. Cabras, P. & Angioni, A. (2000). Pesticide residues in grapes, wine, and their processing products. *Journal of Agricultural and Food Chemistry, 48*(4), 967.

312. Mukherjee, I. & Gopal, M. (1996). Insecticide residues in baby food, animal feed, and vegetables by gas liquid chromatography. *Bulletin of Environmental Contamination and Toxicology, 56*(3), 381.

313. Hyman, F. N., Klontz, K. C., & Tollefson, L. (1993). Food and Drug Administration surveillance of the role of foreign objects in foodborne injuries. *Public Health Reports, 108*, 54.

314. Folks, H. & Burson, D. (2001). Physical hazards. Lincoln, NE: University of Nebraska-Lincoln, Institute of Agriculture and Natural Resources. Available at: http://www.foodsafety.unl.edu/html/physicalhazards.html. Accessed July 30, 2004.

315. Jacobs, M. K. (2004). The history of biologic warfare and bioterrorism. *Dermatologic Clinics, 22*(3), 231.

316. Martin, W. (2004). Legal and public policy responses of states to bioterrorism. *American Journal of Public Health, 94*(7), 1093.

317. Hassler, K. E. (2003). *Agricultural bioterrorism: Why it is a concern and what we must do.* Carlisle Barracks, PA: U.S. Army War College, 1-44.

318. Pellerin, C. (2000). The next target of bioterrorism: Your food. *Environmental Health Perspectives, 108*(3), A126.

319. CDC, Emergency Preparedness and Response. (November 19, 2003). Bioterrorism Agents/Diseases. Available at: http://www.bt.cdc.gov/agent/agentlist.asp. Accessed July 31, 2004.

320. CDC, Emergency Preparedness and Response. (May 26, 2004). Chemical Emergencies. Available at: http://www.bt.cdc.gov/agent/agentlistchem.asp. Accessed April 29, 2005.

321. Grossman, L. K. (2001). The story of a truly contaminated election. *Columbia Journalism Review, 39*(5), 65.

322. Török, T. J., Tauxe, R. V., Wise, R. P., Livengood, J. R., Sokolow, R., Mauvais, S., et al. (1997). A large community outbreak of salmonellosis caused by intentional contamination of restaurant salad bars. *Journal of the American Medical Association, 278*(5), 389.

323. American Dietetic Association. (2003). Position of the American Dietetic Association: Food and water safety. *Journal of the American Dietetic Association, 103*(9), 1203.

324. Sobel, J., Khan, A. S., & Swerdlow, D. L. (2002). Threat of a biological terrorist attack on the U.S. food supply: The CDC perspective. *Lancet, 359*(9309), 874.

325. Khan, A. S., Swerdlow, D. L., & Juranek, D. D. (2001). Precautions against biological and chemical terrorism directed at food and water supplies. *Public Health Reports, 116*, 3.

326. Bruemmer, B. (2003). Food biosecurity. *Journal of the American Dietetic Association, 103*(6), 687.

327. Peregrin, T. (2002). Bioterrorism and food safety: What nutrition professionals need to know to educate the American public. *Journal of the American Dietetic Association, 102*(1), 14.

328. Food Marketing Institute. Position Paper: It's Time to Designate a Single Food Safety Agency. Available at: http://www.fmi.org/media/bg/singlefoodagency.htm. Accessed August 1, 2004.

329. Committee to Ensure Safe Food from Production to Consumption (Institute of Medicine and National Research Council). (2003). *Ensuring safe food: From production to consumption.* Washington, DC: National Academies Press, 1-206.

330. Government Accountability Office. (October 10, 2001). Food Safety and Security: Fundamental Changes Needed to Ensure Safe Food. GAO-02-47T. Available at: http://www.gao.gov/new.items/d0247t.pdf. Accessed July 18, 2004.

331. Government Accountability Office. (May 14, 1998). Food Safety: Federal Efforts to Ensure Imported Food Safety Are Inconsistent and Unreliable. T-RCED-98-191. Available at: http://www.gao.gov/archive/1998/rc98191t.pdf. Accessed July 18, 2004.

332. Government Accountability Office. (October 8, 1997). Food Safety: Fundamental Changes Needed to Improve the Nation's Food Safety System. T-RCED-98-24. Available at: http://www.gao.gov/archive/1998/rc98024t.pdf. Accessed July 18, 2004.

333. Brackett, R. E. (March 30, 2004). Statement before the Committee on Government Reform, Subcommittee on Civil Service and Agency Organization, U.S. House of Representatives. Available at: http://www.fda.gov/ola/2004/foodsafety0330.html. Accessed August 1, 2004.

334. Zawel, S. A. (1999). GMA Testimony, Senate Committee on Governmental Affairs, Subcommittee on Oversight of Government Management, Restructuring, and the District of Columbia, "Overlap and Duplication in the Federal Food Safety System." Available at: http://www.gmabrands.com/news/docs/Testimony.cfm?DocID=626. Accessed April 29, 2005.

335. GMA: Food Safety Report Shows Need for Better Coordination, Planning But No Reason Shown to Create Single Food Safety Bureaucracy. (1999). Available at: http://www.gmabrands.com/news/docs/NewsRelease.cfm?DocID=231. Accessed April 29, 2005.

336. Polkinghorne, J. C. (2000). Ethical issues in biotechnology. *Trends in Biotechnology, 18*(1), 8.

337. Serageldin, I. (1999). Biotechnology and food security in the 21st century. *Science, 285*, 387.

338. Burke, D. (1998). Why all the fuss about genetically modified food? Much depends on who benefits. *British Medical Journal, 316*(7148), 1845.

339. Kuiper, H. A., König, A., Kleter, G. A., Hammes, W. P., & Knudsen, I. (2004). Safety assessment, detection and traceability, and societal aspects of genetically modified foods. European Network on Safety Assessment of Genetically Modified Food Crops (ENTRANSFOOD). Concluding remarks. *Food and Chemical Toxicology, 42*(7), 1195.

340. Perr, H. A. (2002). Children and genetically engineered food: Potentials and problems. *Journal of Pediatric Gastroenterology and Nutrition, 35*(4), 475.

341. Leeder, S. R. (2000). Genetically modified foods—Food for thought. *Medical Journal of Australia, 172*(4), 173.

342. Macilwain, C. (1999). U.S. food-safety body hears protests over genetically modified food. *Nature, 402*(6762), 571.

343. Finucane, M. L. (2002). Mad cows, mad corn and mad communities: The role of socio-cultural factors in the perceived risk of genetically modified food. *Proceedings of the Nutrition Society, 61*(1), 31.

344. Hino, A. (2002). Safety assessment and public concerns for genetically modified food products: The Japanese experience. *Toxicologic Pathology, 30*(1), 126.

345. Moseley, B. E. (2002). Safety assessment and public concern for genetically modified food products: The European view. *Toxicologic Pathology, 30*(1), 129.

346. Harlander, S. K. (2002). Safety assessments and public concern for genetically modified food products: The American view. *Toxicologic Pathology, 30*(1), 132.

347. Consumer protection from an EU regulation on the mandatory labelling of genetically modified food. (2004). *Clinical Laboratory, 50*(5-6), 380.

348. Breakey, J. (2004). Is food intolerance due to an inborn error of metabolism? *Asia Pacific Journal of Clinical Nutrition, 13*(Suppl.), S175.

349. Schafer, K. S. & Kegley, S. E. (2002). Persistent toxic chemicals in the U.S. food supply. *Journal of Epidemiology and Community Health, 56*(11), 813.

350. Goldman, L. R. & Koduru, S. (2000). Chemicals in the environment and developmental toxicity to children: A public health and policy perspective. *Environmental Health Perspectives, 108*(3), 443.

351. Käferstein, F. & Abdussalam, M. (1999). Food safety in the 21st century. *Bulletin of the World Health Organization, 77*(4), 347.

352. Bro-Rasmussen, F. (1996). Contamination by persistent chemicals in food chain and human health. *Science of the Total Environment, 188*(Suppl. 1), S45.

353. Abbott, P. J. (1992). Carcinogenic chemicals in food: Evaluating the health risk. *Food and Chemical Toxicology, 30*(4), 327.

354. USDA, FSIS and APHIS, and DHHS, FDA. (July 9, 2004). USDA and HHS Strengthen Safeguards Against Bovine Spongiform Encephalopathy. Press Release. Available at: http://www.fda.gov/bbs/topics/news/2004/NEW01084.html. Accessed July 29, 2004.

355. Legname, G., Baskakov, I. V., Nguyen, H. O., Riesner, D., Cohen, F. E., DeArmond, S. J., et al. (2004). Synthetic mammalian prions. *Science, 305*(5684), 673.

356. Anderson, J. B., Shuster, T. A., Hansen, K. E., Levy, A. S., & Volk, A. (2004). A camera's view of consumer food-handling behaviors. *Journal of the American Dietetic Association, 104*(2), 186.

357. Sharp, K. & Walker, H. (2003). A microbiological survey of communal kitchens used by undergraduate students. *International Journal of Consumer Studies, 27*(1), 11.

358. Scott, E. (2000). Relationship between cross-contamination and the transmission of foodborne pathogens in the home. *Pediatric Infectious Disease Journal, 19*(10 Suppl.), S111.

359. Sattar, S. A., Tetro, J., & Springthorpe, V. S. (1999). Impact of changing societal trends on the spread of infections in American and Canadian homes. *American Journal of Infection Control, 27*(6), S4.

360. Scott, E. (1999). Hygiene issues in the home. *American Journal of Infection Control, 27*(6), S 22.

361. Bloomfield, S. F. & Scott, E. (1997). Mini review: Cross-contamination and infection in the domestic environment and the role of chemical disinfectants. *Journal of Applied Microbiology, 83*(1), 1.

362. Scott, E. (1996). A review of foodborne disease and other hygiene issues in the home. *Journal of Applied Bacteriology, 80*, 5.

CHAPTER 17

SECURING ADEQUATE FOOD FOR THE PUBLIC

David Holben, PhD, RD, LD

Reader Objectives

After studying this chapter and reflecting on the contents, you should be able to:

1. Define food security and hunger.
2. Discuss and carry out food security measurement.
3. Interpret food security data from nutrition monitoring and research studies.
4. Understand the consequences of food security and its relationship to selected health issues.
5. Apply food security knowledge to program and client assessment strategies.
6. Discuss programs that assist the public in securing adequate food.

Healthy People 2010 goals relate to increasing the quality and years of healthy life and eliminating health disparities among Americans.[1] Securing adequate food for the public is paramount to achieving and maintaining health; therefore, Healthy People 2010 objectives include increasing food security among U.S. households to 94%.[1] Food insecurity persists at an unacceptable rate in the United States, with the most recent estimates indicating that only about 89% of households were food secure throughout the entire year in 2002.[2]

Food security exists when all people, at all times, have access to sufficient food for an active and healthy life without resorting to emergency food supplies or socially unacceptable ways of obtaining food, including begging, stealing, or scavenging.[3] On the other hand, food insecure families or individuals have limited resources and ability to acquire food, which often leads them to resort to socially unacceptable means of food acquisition.[3,4] A possible consequence of food insecurity is hunger, the uneasy or painful sensation caused by a lack of food or the recurrent and involuntary lack of access to food.[3] Common definitions of food security and related terms are summarized in Table 17-1.

TABLE 17-1   Definitions of Food Security and Related Terms

Term	Definition
Community food security	"The state in which all persons obtain a nutritionally-adequate, culturally acceptable diet at all times through local non-emergency sources."[a]
Food security	"Access by all people, at all times to sufficient food for an active and healthy life . . . [and] includes at a minimum: the ready availability of nutritionally adequate and safe foods, and an assured ability to acquire acceptable foods in socially acceptable ways."[b]
Food insecurity	"Limited or uncertain availability of nutritionally adequate and safe foods or limited or uncertain ability to acquire acceptable foods in socially acceptable ways."[b]
Food insufficiency	"An inadequate amount of food intake due to a lack of resources."[c]
Hunger	"The uneasy or painful sensation caused by a lack of food. The recurrent and involuntary lack of access to food . . . [which] may produce malnutrition over time."[b]
Nutrition security	"The provision of an environment that encourages and motivates society to make food choices consistent with short- and long-term good health."[d]

[a]Gottlieb R, Fisher A. Community food security and environmental justice: Searching for a common discourse. *Agriculture Hum Values*. 1996;3(3):23–32.

[b]Life Science Research Office. Federation of American Societies for Experimental Biology. Core indicator of nutritional state for difficult to sample populations. *J Nutr*. 1990;102:1599–1600.

[c]Briefel R, Woteki C. Development of the food sufficiency questions for the Third National Health and Nutrition Examination Survey. *J Nutr Educ*. 1992;24:24S–28S.

[d]*Nutrition Action Themes for the United States: A Report in Response to the International Conference on Nutrition*. Washington, DC: U.S. Department of Agriculture Center for Nutrition Policy and Promotion; 1996. CNPP-2 Occasional Paper.

Source: Compiled by the author.

Securing adequate food for the public is paramount. Public health nutrition professionals must not only be aware of programs that can assist the public in securing adequate food, but also know how to assess:

- The proportion of the public that is food secure
- The consequences of food insecurity
- If a particular program designed to improve food security is actually doing so

Therefore this chapter was designed to:

- Review the definitions of food security and hunger
- Outline food security measurement strategies
- Summarize the food security status of the United States
- Highlight the consequences of food security and its relationship to selected health issues
- Review how food security measurement can be used for program and client assessment strategies
- Discuss public health programs designed to improve food access by the public

Measuring the Food Security Status of the Public

Although food insecurity is broad in scope, its primary dimension is food insufficiency, which can be measured along a continuum of successive stages. These stages, as noted by Bickel and others,[4] each have specific characteristics, that is, conditions and experiences related to being unable to fully meet the basic needs of household members followed by the behavioral responses to those conditions and experiences. Public health nutrition professionals must be able to understand the federal, state, and local reports related to food security and their implications on public health issues. In addition, they need to be able to develop strategies in order to measure the effectiveness of interventions intended to improve food security.

Household food security status is one outcome measure that provides insight into the public's ability to secure adequate food. Bickel and colleagues have summarized food security measurement for U.S. households in *Guide to Measuring Household Food Security, Revised 2000*.[4]

> *Guide to Measuring Household Food Security, Revised 2000* can be conveniently accessed through the Food Security Briefing Room of the Economic Research Service at http://www.ers.usda.gov/briefing/foodsecurity/.[5]

The National Nutrition Monitoring and Related Research Act of 1990 (Table 17-2) prompted the development of the Food Security Measurement Project.[5] This project is an ongoing collaboration among federal agencies, academic researchers, and private commercial and nonprofit organizations. Standardized questionnaires for measuring household food security status and methods for editing and scoring those instruments have been one outcome of the project.[5]

The foundation for measuring the public's food security was laid through work conducted by Radimer and colleagues[6,7] and Wehler and others[8]; their work led to the development of an instrument capable of measuring the food security status of U.S. house-

TABLE 17-2   The National Nutrition Monitoring and Related Research Act of 1990

Facts About This Legislation

- Public Law 101-445.
- Enacted October 22, 1990.
- Leadership/Responsibility: U.S. Department of Health and Human Services and U.S. Department of Agriculture.
- Reports are filed at least every 5 years on the dietary, nutritional, and health-related status of people in the United States.
- Purposes of the Act
  1. "Make more effective use of Federal and State expenditures for nutrition monitoring, and enhance the performance and benefits of current Federal nutrition monitoring and related research activities."
  2. "Establish and facilitate the timely implementation of a coordinated National Nutrition Monitoring and Related Program, and thereby provide a scientific basis for the maintenance and improvement of the nutritional status of the people of the United States and the nutritional quality . . . of food consumed in the United States."
  3. "Establish and implement a comprehensive plan for the National Nutrition Monitoring and Related Research Program to assess, on a continuing basis, the dietary and nutritional status of the people of the United States and the trends with respect to such status, the state of the art with respect to nutrition monitoring and related research, future monitoring and related research priorities, and the relevant policy implications."
  4. "Establish and improve the quality of national nutritional health status data related data bases and networks, and stimulate research necessary to develop uniform indicators, standards, methodologies, technologies, and procedures for nutrition monitoring."
  5. "Establish a central Federal focus for the coordination, management, and direction of Federal nutrition monitoring activities."
  6. "Establish mechanisms for addressing the nutrition monitoring needs of Federal, State, and local governments, the private sector, scientific and engineering communities, healthcare professionals, and the public in support of the foregoing purposes."
  7. "Provide for the conduct of such scientific research and development as may be necessary or appropriate in support of such purposes."

Source: Adapted with permission from the National Nutrition Monitoring and Related Research Act of 1990. Available at: http://www.reeusda.gov/1700/legis/nutmontr.htm. Accessed on April 5, 2004.

holds. This instrument[4] is called the Food Security Survey Module (Table 17-3). The federal estimates of household food security status are measured using this instrument as part of the Census Bureau's Current Population Survey.[9] Other national surveys that contain the Food Security Survey Module include:

> See the Census Bureau's Current Population Survey at http://www.bls.gov/cps/home.htm.

- Early Childhood Longitudinal Study (http://nces.ed.gov/ecls/index.asp)[10]
- National Health and Nutrition Examination Survey (http://www.cdc.gov/nchs/nhanes.htm)[11]
- Panel Study of Income Dynamics (http://psidonline.isr.umich.edu)[12]
- Survey of Program Dynamics (http://www.sipp.census.gov/spd/)

Table 17-4 provides a brief summary of each of these national surveys. In addition to these, states, academic and private researchers, and public health nutrition professionals use the Food Security Survey Module to measure household food security status.

The Food Security Survey Module poses questions to respondents about:

- Anxiety related to food budget or supply and whether the budget is able to meet basic needs
- Experiences relating to running out of food without being able to obtain more due to financial constraints
- Perceptions of intake adequacy by themselves or other household members
- Food use[4]

This instrument measures only the "sufficiency" dimension of food security, and does not measure other aspects of food security, including the nutritional adequacy or safety of diets.[4] Therefore, other instruments must be used to capture this information in a research project or programmatic evaluation. As seen in Table 17-3, all of the questions in the Food Security Survey Module specify financial limitations as the reason for the reported behaviors or conditions and ask about circumstances that occurred within the past 12 months; however, shorter time periods can be utilized.[4] For example, if a public health nutrition intervention (e.g., community gardening project) was initiated in the spring and concluded in the early fall, the food security status of participating households could be measured in the spring and remeasured after 4 months when the program ends.

Responses to the Food Security Survey Module questions are tabulated, as summarized by Bickel,[4] resulting in a scale that meas-

TABLE 17-3   Food Security Survey Module

- "(I/We) worried whether (my/our) food would run out before (I/we) got money to buy more." Was that *often* true, *sometimes* true, or *never* true for (you/your household) in the last 12 months?

- "The food that (I/we) bought just didn't last, and (I/we) didn't have money to get more." Was that *often*, *sometimes*, or *never* true for (you/your household) in the last 12 months?

- "(I/We) couldn't afford to eat balanced meals." Was that *often*, *sometimes*, or *never* true for (you/your household) in the last 12 months?

- "(I/We) relied on only a few kinds of low-cost food to feed (my/our) (child/children) because (I was/we were) running out of money to buy food." Was that *often*, *sometimes*, or *never* true for (you/your household) in the last 12 months?

- "(I/We) couldn't feed (my/our) (child/children) a balanced meal, because (I/we) couldn't afford that." Was that *often*, *sometimes*, or *never* true for (you/your household) in the last 12 months?

- "(My/our) (child was/children were) not eating enough because (I/we) just couldn't afford enough food." Was that *often*, *sometimes*, or *never* true for (you/your household) in the last 12 months?

- In the last 12 months, since last (name of current month), did (you/you or other adults in your household) ever cut the size of your meals or skip meals because there wasn't enough money for food? Yes No
  – If yes, how often did this happen—almost every month, some months but not every month, or in only 1 or 2 months?

- In the last 12 months, did you ever eat less than you felt you should because there wasn't enough money to buy food? Yes No

- In the last 12 months, were you ever hungry but didn't eat because you couldn't afford enough food? Yes No

- In the last 12 months, did you lose weight because you didn't have enough money for food? Yes No

- In the last 12 months, did (you/you or other adults in your household) ever not eat for a whole day because there wasn't enough money for food? Yes No
  – If yes, how often did this happen—almost every month, some months but not every month, or in only 1 or 2 months?

- In the last 12 months, since (current month) of last year, did you ever cut the size of (your child's/any of the children's) meals because there wasn't enough money for food? Yes No

- In the last 12 months, did (CHILD'S NAME/any of the children) ever skip meals because there wasn't enough money for food? Yes No
  – If yes, how often did this happen—almost every month, some months but not every month, or in only 1 or 2 months?

- In the last 12 months, (was your child/were the children) ever hungry but you just couldn't afford more food? Yes No

- In the last 12 months, did (your child/any of the children) ever not eat for a whole day because there wasn't enough money for food? Yes No

Note: Questions relating to children are only asked if there are children under 18 in the household. Specific guidelines for using the Core Module, including screening techniques, can be found in the source below.

Source: Adapted with permission from Bickel G, Nord M, Price C, Hamilton W, Cook J. *Guide to Measuring Household Food Security, Revised 2000.* Alexandria, Va.: U.S. Department of Agriculture, Food and Nutrition Service; 2000.

TABLE 17-4   National Surveys That Include Food Security Measurement

Survey	Website	Brief Summary
Current Population Survey	http://www.bls.gov/cps/home.htm	A nationally representative study of employment and unemployment experiences. Used to provide U.S. food security estimates.
Early Childhood Longitudinal Study	http://nces.edu.gov/ecls/	National data with two overlapping cohorts, birth (birth through first grade) and kindergarten (kindergarten through fifth grade), on children's status at birth and thereafter. Includes family, school, community, and individual variables on development, early learning, and early performance in school.
National Health and Nutrition Examination Survey	http://www.cdc.gov/nchs/nhanes.htm	A nationally representative health and dietary study of the non-institutionalized civilian population.
Panel Study of Income Dynamics	http://psidonline.isr.umich.edu	A nationally representative longitudinal study of U.S. families on economic, health, and social behavior.
Survey of Program Dynamics	http://www.sipp.census.gov/spd/	A nationally representative longitudinal, demographic survey on the economic, household, and social characteristics of the United States.

Source: Compiled by the author.

ures the degree of the severity of food insecurity and hunger experienced by a household. In addition to being assigned a score ranging from 0–10, with larger numbers corresponding to a greater level of food insecurity, households can be categorized into three groupings of food security status, each representing a range of severity on the food security scale (Table 17-5).[1]

As summarized by Bickel and colleagues,[4] food-secure households show no or minimal evidence of food insecurity; that is, they are able to secure nutritionally adequate, safe foods in socially ac-

**TABLE 17-5   Food Security Survey Module Categories
of Food Security Status**

Food secure
• Households show no or minimal evidence of food insecurity.

Food insecure without hunger
• Food insecurity is evident in household members' concerns about adequacy
  of the household food supply and in adjustments to household food
  management, including reduced quality of food and increased unusual
  coping patterns. Little or no reduction in members' food intake is reported.

Food insecure with hunger
• *Moderate hunger:* Food intake for adults in the household has been reduced
  to an extent that implies that adults have repeatedly experienced the
  physical sensation of hunger. In most (but not all) food-insecure households
  with children, such reductions are not observed at this stage for children.
• *Severe hunger:* At this level, all households with children have reduced the
  children's food intake to an extent indicating that the children have
  experienced hunger. For some other households with children, this already
  has occurred at an earlier stage of severity. Adults in households with and
  without children have repeatedly experienced more extensive reductions in
  food intake.

Source: Adapted with permission from Bickel G, Nord M, Price C, Hamilton W, Cook J.
Guide to Measuring Household Food Security, Revised 2000. Alexandria, Va.: U.S.
Department of Agriculture, Food and Nutrition Service; 2000.

ceptable ways. On the other hand, households that are food insecure without hunger have members concerned about the adequacy
of the household food supply and management. This may include
reduced quality of food and increased use of unusual coping patterns. However, in this category, little or no reduction in members'
food intake is reported. When hunger is present at the most severe
level, household members may go one or more entire days with no
food due to lack of resources, or food intake may be reduced to an
extent that members have repeatedly experienced the physical sensation of hunger. In hungry households with children, typically at
the early stages, food reductions are not observed for children.
However, at the most severe level, even children have reduced food
intake to an extent that hunger has been experienced. For some
households with children, the children's food intake may have been
reduced at a less severe stage of food insecurity; however, children
are often protected from hunger by other family members.[14] Finally,
at the most severe stages of food insecurity, adults in households
with and without children have repeatedly experienced extensive
reductions in food intake.[4]

Generally, the Food Security Survey Module takes less than 4
minutes to administer, unless screening is performed, which would

decrease the time needed to administer the survey instrument to approximately 2 minutes.[4] Less time is needed because when screening is performed, all questions may not be asked if responses inconsistent with food insecurity are provided for the initial survey questions.

Some public health nutrition professionals may find it difficult to administer the 18-question module for a variety of reasons, but are still interested in food security status as an outcome or factor impacting public health program development and delivery. Therefore, if utilizing the entire Food Security Survey Module (all 18 questions) is not possible due to time constraints, an agency can use an abbreviated 6-item subset that is available at http://www.ers.usda.gov/briefing/foodsecurity/.[15] This tool also provides food security scale scores for classifying households by level of food security status.[4] However, use of this six-item subset does have limitations. Overall, researchers[15] were able to demonstrate that the abbreviated instrument correctly classified 98% of households correctly, but the abbreviated food security instrument was not able to differentiate the more severe range of food insecurity where child hunger had been experienced. This is because the abbreviated version does not include questions about these more extreme experiences and behaviors. Consequently, if a public health nutrition professional intends to utilize this tool, it is important for him or her to have a preliminary idea of what levels of food insecurity are likely to exist in the target population before choosing the abbreviated subset.

When the entire Food Security Survey Module is used, a subset of the questions can be employed to assess the extent to which children were hungry in the household.[16] Table 17-6 highlights these questions.

Food Security in the United States

The agricultural bounty of the United States has not completely overcome the problem of hunger. In 2002, almost 89% of U.S. households were food secure. However, 11.1%—that is, over 12 million households—were food insecure at some time during the year,[2] as shown in Figure 17-1. About two-thirds of the insecure avoided hunger; however, almost 4 million U.S. households (3.5% of all households) were food insecure, with one or more household members experiencing hunger at least sometime during the year.[2] Households with children had a higher level of food insecurity than the total population, with 16.5% being food insecure. Overall, the prevalence of hunger among children was 0.7% of all households with children.

The trends in food insecurity and prevalence in the United States are pictured in Figure 17-2. From 1995 to 2000, a consistent downward trend was noted; however, the following 2-year upward

TABLE 17-6   Child Hunger Food Security Survey Module

- "(I/We) relied on only a few kinds of low-cost food to feed (my/our) (child/children) because (I was/we were) running out of money to buy food." Was that *often*, *sometimes*, or *never* true for (you/your household) in the last 12 months?

- "(I/We) couldn't feed (my/our) (child/children) a balanced meal, because (I/we) couldn't afford that." Was that *often*, *sometimes*, or *never* true for (you/your household) in the last 12 months?

- "(My/our) (child was/children were) not eating enough because (I/we) just couldn't afford enough food." Was that *often*, *sometimes*, or *never* true for (you/your household) in the last 12 months?

- In the last 12 months, since (current month) of last year, did you ever cut the size of (your child's/any of the children's) meals because there wasn't enough money for food? Yes No

- In the last 12 months, did (CHILD'S NAME/any of the children) ever skip meals because there wasn't enough money for food? Yes No

    If yes, how often did this happen—almost every month, some months but not every month, or in only 1 or 2 months?

- In the last 12 months, (was your child/were the children) ever hungry but you just couldn't afford more food? Yes No

- In the last 12 months, did (your child/any of the children) ever not eat for a whole day because there wasn't enough money for food? Yes No

Source: Adapted with permission from Nord M, Bickel G. *Measuring Children's Food Security in the United States, 1995–1999* (FANRR-25). Alexandria, Va.: Food and Rural Economics Division, Economic Research Service, U.S. Department of Agriculture; 2002.

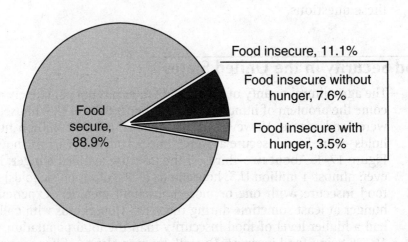

FIGURE 17-1   U.S. Households by Food Security Status, 2002
Source: Reprinted with permission from Nord M, Andrews M, Carlson S. *Household Food Security in the United States, 2002* (FANRR35). Alexandria, Va.: Food and Rural Economics Division, Economic Research Service, U.S. Department of Agriculture; 2003.

trend appeared to be secondary to a seasonal influence, which is hoped to be avoided in subsequent years by maintaining a consistent data collection month for the national surveys.[17] Overall, food insecurity rose from 10.7% to 11.1% from 2001 to 2002 (a 4.7% increase). Similarly, prevalence of hunger rose from 3.3% to 3.5% of U.S. households (an 8.2% increase). The prevalence of hunger among children was essentially unchanged from 2001 to 2002.[2]

Table 17-7 summarizes the 1998–2002 food security data. Table 17-8 summarizes the prevalence of food insecurity and hunger in 2001 and 2002. Overall, food insecurity was greater than the national average among: 1) households with incomes below the official poverty line (38.1%); 2) households with children headed by a single woman (32.0%); 3) African American households (22.0%); 4) Hispanic American households (21.7%); 5) households located in central cities (14.4%) or non-metropolitan areas (11.6%) (Note: households in suburban and metropolitan areas outside central cities = 8.8%); and 6) households in the South (12.4%) and West (12.1%) (Note: households in the Northeast and Midwest = 9.2% and

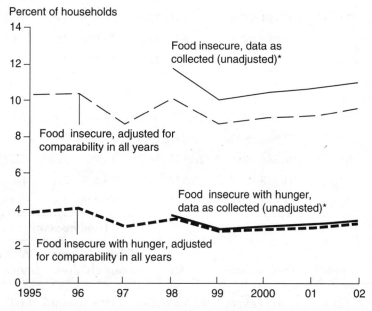

*Data as collected in 1995–97 are not directly comparable with data collected in 1998–2002.
Source: Calculated by ERS using data from Current Population Survey Food Security Supplements.

FIGURE 17-2 Trends in Prevalence of Food Insecurity and Hunger in U.S. Households, 1995–2002
Source: Reprinted with permission from Nord M, Andrews M, Carlson S. *Household Food Security in the United States, 2002* (FANRR35). Alexandria, Va.: Food and Rural Economics Division, Economic Research Service, U.S. Department of Agriculture; 2003.

TABLE 17-7   Prevalence of Food Security, Food Insecurity, and Hunger by Year

Unit	Total[1]	Food secure		All		Without hunger		With hunger	
					Food insecure				
	1,000	1,000	Percent	1,000	Percent	1,000	Percent	1,000	Percent
Households									
1998	103,309	91,121	88.2	12,188	11.8	8,353	8.1	3,835	3.7
1999	104,684	94,154	89.9	10,529	10.1	7,420	7.1	3,109	3.0
2000	106,043	94,942	89.5	11,101	10.5	7,786	7.3	3,315	3.1
2001	107,824	96,303	89.3	11,521	10.7	8,010	7.4	3,511	3.3
2002	108,601	96,543	88.9	12,058	11.1	8,259	7.6	3,799	3.5
All individuals (by food security status of household):[2]									
1998	268,366	232,219	86.5	36,147	13.5	26,290	9.8	9,857	3.7
1999	270,318	239,304	88.5	31,015	11.5	23,237	8.6	7,779	2.9
2000	273,685	240,454	87.9	33,231	12.1	24,708	9.0	8,523	3.1
2001	276,661	243,019	87.8	33,642	12.2	24,628	8.9	9,014	3.3
2002	279,035	244,133	87.5	34,902	12.5	25,517	9.1	9,385	3.4
Adults (by food security status of household):[2]									
1998	197,084	174,964	88.8	22,120	11.2	15,632	7.9	6,488	3.3
1999	198,900	179,960	90.5	18,941	9.5	13,869	7.0	5,072	2.5
2000	201,922	181,586	89.9	20,336	10.1	14,763	7.3	5,573	2.8
2001	204,340	183,398	89.8	20,942	10.2	14,879	7.3	6,063	3.0
2002	206,493	184,718	89.5	21,775	10.5	15,486	7.5	6,289	3.0

	Total[1]	Food secure		All		Without hunger among children		With hunger among children	
					Food insecure				
	1,000	1,000	Percent	1,000	Percent	1,000	Percent	1,000	Percent
Households with children:									
1998	38,036	31,335	82.4	6,701	17.6	6,370	16.7	331	.9
1999	37,884	32,290	85.2	5,594	14.8	5,375	14.2	219	.6
2000	38,113	31,942	83.8	6,171	16.2	5,916	15.5	255	.7
2001	38,330	32,141	83.9	6,189	16.1	5,978	15.6	211	.6
2002	38,647	32,267	83.5	6,380	16.5	6,115	15.8	265	.7

	Total[1]	Food secure		Food insecure		
			All		Without hunger among children	With hunger among children

	Total[1]	Food secure		All		Without hunger among children		With hunger among children	
Children (by food security status of household):[2]									
1998	71,282	57,255	80.3	14,027	19.7	13,311	18.7	716	1.0
1999	71,418	59,344	83.1	12,074	16.9	11,563	16.2	511	.7
2000	71,763	58,867	82.0	12,896	18.0	12,334	17.2	562	.8
2001	72,321	59,620	82.4	12,701	17.6	12,234	16.9	467	.6
2002	72,542	59,415	81.9	13,127	18.1	12,560	17.3	567	.8

[1]Totals exclude households whose food security status is unknown because they did not give a valid response to any of the questions in the food security scale. In 2002, these represented 336,000 households (0.3 percent of all households).

[2]The food security survey measures food security status at the household level. Not all individuals residing in food-insecure households are appropriately characterized as food insecure. Similarly, not all individuals in households classified as food insecure with hunger, nor all children in households classified as food insecure with hunger among children, were subject to reductions in food intake or experienced resource-constrained hunger.

Source: Reprinted with permission from: Nord M, Andrews M, Carlson S. *Household Food Security in the United States, 2002* (FANRR35). Alexandria, Va.: Food and Rural Economics Division, Economic Research Service, U.S. Department of Agriculture; 2003.

9.6%, respectively). Overall, households with children (16.5%) had more than double the rate of food insecurity as those without children (8.1%), and among households with children, those with married-couple families showed the lowest rate of food insecurity (10.4%).[2] Hunger patterns were similar.[2]

In most cases, when the U.S. public experiences food insecurity with hunger, it is occasional or episodic, rather than being chronic.[2] Overall, data support that about 3.5% of households experienced hunger anytime during the year and 2.7% of households experienced hunger during the 30 days prior to the survey, with an estimated daily average of household food insecurity with hunger being 0.5%–0.7%.[2] On average, among households experiencing food insecurity with hunger at some time during the year, this condition occurred in 8 or 9 months, while those reporting hunger during a month experienced it from 1 to 7 days.[2]

Although these national estimates paint a picture of the United States as a whole, regions within the United States and particular states may vary with regard to food security status. The prevalence of food security and hunger by state is summarized in Table 17-9. Again, although a particular state may experience food insecurity and hunger below the national average, a community within a state may exceed the state and national averages, necessitating the need for programmatic intervention.

In the United States, food insecurity is evident when families have limited resources, lack access to food (due to limited resources, lack of transportation, living in remote areas, or limited access to

Table 17-8   Prevalence of Food Security, Food Insecurity, and Hunger, by Selected Household Characteristics, 2002

Category	Total[1]		Food secure		Food insecure All		Without hunger		With hunger	
	1,000		1,000	Percent	1,000	Percent	1,000	Percent	1,000	Percent
All households	108,601		96,543	88.9	12,058	11.1	8,259	7.6	3,799	3.5
Household composition:										
With children <18	38,647		32,268	83.5	6,379	16.5	4,899	12.7	1,480	3.8
With children <6	17,073		14,039	82.2	3,034	17.8	2,450	14.4	584	3.4
Married-couple families	26,069		23,357	89.6	2,712	10.4	2,204	8.5	508	1.9
Female head, no spouse	9,496		6,456	68.0	3,040	32.0	2,212	23.3	828	8.7
Male head, no spouse	2,375		1,855	78.1	520	21.9	381	16.0	139	5.9
Other household with child[2]	707		599	84.7	108	15.3	102	14.4	6	.8
With no children <18	69,954		64,276	91.9	5,678	8.1	3,360	4.8	2,318	3.3
More than one adult	41,538		38,929	93.7	2,609	6.3	1,651	4.0	958	2.3
Women living alone	16,174		14,472	89.5	1,702	10.5	985	6.1	717	4.4
Men living alone	12,242		10,875	88.8	1,367	11.2	724	5.9	643	5.3
With elderly	24,791		23,229	93.7	1,562	6.3	1,099	4.4	463	1.9
Elderly living alone	10,072		9,327	92.6	745	7.4	490	4.9	255	2.5
Race/ethnicity of households:										
White non-Hispanic	80,266		73,859	92.0	6,407	8.0	4,294	5.3	2,113	2.6
Black non-Hispanic	13,515		10,546	78.0	2,969	22.0	1,999	14.8	970	7.2
Hispanic[3]	10,344		8,099	78.3	2,245	21.7	1,654	16.0	591	5.7
Other non-Hispanic	4,475		4,038	90.2	437	9.8	313	7.0	124	2.8

Category	Total[1]	Food secure		Food insecure					
				All		Without hunger		With hunger	
	1,000	1,000	Percent	1,000	Percent	1,000	Percent	1,000	Percent
Household income-to-poverty ratio:									
Under 1.00	11,515	7,128	61.9	4,387	38.1	2,736	23.8	1,651	14.3
Under 1.30	17,010	11,272	66.3	5,738	33.7	3,681	21.6	2,057	12.1
Under 1.85	25,134	17,802	70.8	7,332	29.2	4,894	19.5	2,438	9.7
1.85 and over	64,263	60,997	94.9	3,266	5.1	2,321	3.6	945	1.5
Income unknown	19,204	17,744	92.4	1,460	7.6	1,044	5.4	416	2.2
Area of residence:									
Inside metropolitan area	87,617	77,997	89.0	9,620	11.0	6,528	7.5	3,092	3.5
In central city[4]	26,922	23,047	85.6	3,875	14.4	2,517	9.3	1,358	5.0
Not in central city[4]	45,552	41,542	91.2	4,010	8.8	2,791	6.1	1,219	2.7
Outside metropolitan area	20,983	18,545	88.4	2,438	11.6	1,731	8.2	707	3.4
Census geographic region:									
Northeast	20,242	18,372	90.8	1,870	9.2	1,266	6.3	604	3.0
Midwest	25,180	22,755	90.4	2,425	9.6	1,602	6.4	823	3.3
South	39,195	34,325	87.6	4,870	12.4	3,442	8.8	1,428	3.6
West	23,984	21,090	87.9	2,894	12.1	1,950	8.1	944	3.9

[1]Totals exclude households whose food security status is unknown because they did not give a valid response to any of the questions in the food security scale. In 2002, these represented 336,000 households (0.3 percent of all households).

[2]Households with children in complex living arrangements—e.g., children of other relatives or unrelated roommate or boarder.

[3]Hispanics may be of any race.

[4]Metropolitan area subtotals do not add to metropolitan area total because central-city residence is not identified for about 17 percent of households in metropolitan statistical areas.

Source: Caluclated by ERS using data from the December 2002 Current Population Survey Food Security Supplement.

TABLE 17-9   Prevalence of Household Food Insecurity and Hunger, by State, Average 2000–2002[1]

Average State	Number of Households		Food insecure (with or without hunger)		Food insecure with hunger	
	2000-02[2]	Interviewed	Prevalence	Margin of Error[3]	Prevalence	Margin of Error[3]
	Numbers		Percent	Percentage points	Percent	Percentage points
U.S. Total	107,489,000	138,152	10.8	0.22	3.3	0.09
AK	224,000	1,771	11.8	1.43	4.3*	.62
AL	1,774,000	2,064	12.5*	1.24	3.7	.73
AR	1,038,000	1,707	14.6*	1.61	4.4	1.15
AZ	1,917,000	1,925	12.5*	1.50	3.7	.82
CA	12,434,000	9,360	11.7*	.68	3.5	.38
CO	1,652,000	2,550	9.2*	.83	2.8	.48
CT	1,274,000	2,125	7.6*	.85	2.8	.49
DC	260,000	1,701	9.3*	1.04	2.3*	.53
DE	300,000	1,614	6.8*	1.42	1.9*	.76
FL	6,383,000	6,257	11.8*	.99	3.7	.55
GA	3,084,000	1,898	12.9*	1.32	3.5	.76
HI	408,000	1,399	11.9	1.93	3.6	1.03
IA	1,144,000	2,293	9.1*	1.17	2.8	.74
ID	484,000	1,937	13.7*	1.35	4.3*	.74
IL	4,666,000	5,040	8.6*	.77	2.7	.41
IN	2,421,000	2,489	8.9*	.97	2.8	.59
KS	1,054,000	2,294	11.7	1.35	3.9	.72
KY	1,606,000	1,932	10.8	1.34	2.9	.70
LA	1,660,000	1,522	13.1*	1.66	2.9	.75
MA	2,441,000	2,809	6.4*	1.13	2.1*	.71
MD	2,049,000	2,118	8.2*	1.40	2.9	.72
ME	535,000	2,278	9.0*	1.08	2.8	.62
MI	3,907,000	4,076	9.2*	.74	3.0	.50
MN	1,877,000	2,526	7.1*	1.02	2.2*	.84
MO	2,236,000	2,094	9.9	1.37	3.3	.63
MS	1,080,000	1,503	14.8*	1.17	4.5*	.81
MT	365,000	1,764	12.8*	1.16	4.1	.81
NC	3,129,000	3,071	12.3*	1.08	3.7	.55
ND	259,000	2,279	8.1*	1.17	2.0*	.53
NE	649,000	2,188	10.7	1.63	3.1	.67
NH	485,000	2,139	6.7*	.99	2.1*	.56
NJ	3,104,000	3,435	8.5*	.90	2.7	.65
NM	687,000	1,639	14.3*	1.36	3.8	.76
NV	727,000	2,402	9.3*	.89	3.3	.75
NY	7,003,000	7,210	9.4*	.57	2.9	.36
OH	4,544,000	4,762	9.8*	.76	3.3	.43

Average State	Number of Households		Food insecure (with or without hunger)		Food insecure with hunger	
	2000-02[2]	Interviewed	Prevalence	Margin of Error[3]	Prevalence	Margin of Error[3]
	Numbers		Percent	Percentage points	Percent	Percentage points
OK	1,361,000	1,962	14.3*	1.28	5.1*	.68
OR	1,341,000	2,071	13.7*	1.12	5.0*	.87
PA	4,742,000	5,298	9.4*	.68	2.7*	.48
RI	395,000	2,183	10.1	1.49	3.4	.66
SC	1,576,000	1,677	12.3*	1.49	4.3	1.16
SD	291,000	2,240	8.0*	.92	2.2*	.53
TN	2,190,000	1,690	11.3	1.25	3.3	.66
TX	7,542,000	5,734	14.8*	1.05	4.1*	.46
UT	714,000	1,701	15.2*	1.70	4.6*	.99
VA	2,778,000	2,239	7.3*	1.13	1.8*	.49
VT	249,000	1,920	9.0*	1.16	2.4*	.56
WA	2,362,000	2,348	12.3*	1.36	4.4*	.86
WI	2,122,000	2,711	8.1*	.74	3.3	.49
WV	764,000	2,190	9.4*	1.11	2.7*	.45
WY	202,000	2,017	10.7	1.47	4.3*	1.00

*Difference from U.S. total was statistically significant with 90 percent confidence (t > 1.645).

[1] Prevalence rates for 1996–98 reported in *Prevalence of Food Insecurity and Hunger, by State, 1996–1998* (Nord et al., 1999) are not directly comparable with the rates reported here because of differences in screening procedures in the CPS Food Security Supplements from 1995 to 1998. Comparable statistics for the earlier period are presented in Appendix D.

[2] Totals exclude households whose food security status is unknown because they did not give a valid response to any of the questions in the food security scale. These represented about 0.3 percent of all households in each year.

[3] Margin of error with 90 percent confidence (1.645 times the standard error of the estimated prevalence rate).

Source: Prepared by ERS using data from the Sept. 2000, Dec. 2001, and Dec. 2002 Current Population Survey Food Security Supplements.

food stores), depend on food assistance programs, skip meals, substitute nutritious foods with less expensive alternatives, and seek assistance from soup kitchens and food pantries.[18,19] A low income, coupled with high housing and healthcare costs, can result in hunger and food insecurity,[20] possibly leading to malnutrition and various health problems.[21]

Coping Strategies Used by the Public to Avoid Food Insecurity and Hunger

People often use coping strategies to minimize household food security. Food management practices used by people with limited resources have been identified by Kempson and others,[22] including:

- Strategizing food preparation (e.g., making low-cost dishes; removing mold, insects, and slime from cheese, grain, and meats)

- Rationing the household food supply
- Conserving food
- Inadequately preserving food
- Restricting personal food intake
- Overeating when food is available
- Obtaining food opportunistically
- Cycling monthly eating patterns
- Eating low-cost foods

The authors also demonstrated that several of the strategies posed food safety and nutrition risks, including the modification and consumption of rotten foods (removing slime, mold, insects, and spoiled parts from foods), limiting the amount of food, taking leftovers home, eating expired food, inappropriate storage of perishables, consumption of road kill and "found" meat, deprivation of personal food intake, and overeating when food is available.[22]

Supporting some of these ideas, Greder and Brotherson[23] and other researchers[24] have identified coping strategies used in households with low incomes. These tactics included depending upon others (family, friends, community resources),[23,24] adjusting resources and making trade-offs (securing multiple jobs, not paying bills or only paying a portion of them in order to have enough money to buy food and other basic needs),[23] adjusting food consumption,[23] decreasing budgets to pay rent and utilities,[23] and obtaining nutrition and shopping knowledge and skills through nutrition education programs like the Expanded Food and Nutrition Education Program and the Special Supplemental Nutrition Program for Women, Infants and Children (WIC).[23]

As noted by Nord and others,[2] households with limited resources employ a variety of methods to help meet their food needs, including participating in one or more federal food assistance programs or obtaining food from community emergency food providers to supplement the household food purchased. Nord and others[2] noted,

> Households that turn to federal and community food assistance programs typically do so because they are having difficulty in meeting their food needs. The use of such programs by low-income households and the relationship between the food security status and use of food assistance programs by these households provide insight into the extent of their difficulties in obtaining enough food and the ways they cope with those difficulties.

Food assistance programs in the United States, that is, the nutrition safety net, have been key in helping the U.S. public secure adequate food. In fact, federally funded and community-based programs are vital in helping households make ends meet. Several program summaries follow.

The Child and Adult Care Food Program

This program provides nutritious meals and snacks to children and adults who receive day care or after-school care away from home. It also provides these provisions to children residing in home-less shelters. This program is usually administered by the state education agency.

> More information about The Child and Adult Care Food Program can be found at http://www.fns.usda.gov/cnd/CARE/CACFP/cacfphome.htm.[25]

The Expanded Food and Nutrition Education Program

This program helps families with limited incomes acquire knowl-edge, skills, attitudes, and behavior changes necessary to maintain nutritionally sound diets and enhance personal development, including basic nutrition, food preparation, and resource manage-ment skills. There are several food distribution programs, including:

- Child Nutrition Commodity Support
- Nutrition Services Incentive Program (formerly the Nutrition Program for the Elderly)
- Commodity Supplemental Food Program
- Food Assistance in Disaster Situations
- Food Distribution Program on Native-American Reservations
- Emergency Food Assistance Program
- State Processing Program
- Nutrition Assistance Program for Puerto Rican Americans, Samoan Americans, and the Northern Marianas population
- Homeless Children Nutrition Program

Overall, these programs support the nutrition safety net through commodity distri-bution and other nutrition assistance to families with low incomes, emergency feeding programs, Native American reservations, and older adults. Local food banks and pantries or other agencies or organiza-

> More information about the Expanded Food and Nutrition Education Program can be found at http://www.csrees.usda.gov/nea/food/efnep/about.html.[26]
>
> More information about America's Second Harvest can be found at http://www.secondharvest.org, http://www.fns.usda.gov/fdd/.[27–29]

tions, including faith-based groups, typically receive supplemental foods. Local food banks can be accessed through America's Second Harvest. (See more about this program later in this section.)

The Food Stamp Program

This program enables families with low incomes to buy nutri-tious food with coupons and elec-tronic benefits transfer cards. Food

> More information about Food Stamps can be found at http://www.fns.usda.gov/fsp/.[30]

stamp recipients spend their benefits to buy eligible food in au-thorized retail food stores.

The National Meals on Wheels Foundation

More information about the
National Meals on Wheels
Foundation can be found at
http://www.nationalmealsonwheels
.org.[31]

This program delivers meals to home-bound older adults and those at congregate meal sites. A variety of organizations, including local communities, churches, charitable organizations, and concerned citizens administer this program.

The National School Lunch and School Breakfast Programs

These programs provide nutritionally balanced, low-cost or free breakfasts and lunches to children enrolled in public and nonprofit

More information about the National
School Lunch and School Breakfast
Programs can be found at
http://www.fns.usda.gov/cnd/lunch/
default.htm and http://www.fns.usda.gov/
cnd/breakfast/default.htm.[32,33]

private schools and residential childcare institutions. They also provide snacks served in after-school educational and enrichment programs for children through 18 years of age.

The Senior Farmers' Market Nutrition Program

This program provides older adults, with low incomes, coupons that can be exchanged for fresh, nutritious, unprocessed fruits, vegetables,

More information about the Senior
Farmers' Market Nutrition Program can
be found at http://www.fns.usda.gov/
wic/seniorFMNP/SFMNPmenu.htm.[34]

and fresh-cut herbs at farmers' markets, roadside stands, and community-supported agriculture programs during the harvest season.

WIC and the WIC Farmers' Market Nutrition Program

Both of these programs provide supplemental foods, nutrition education and counseling, and access to health services to low-income pregnant, breast-feeding, and non-breast-feeding postpartum women, and to infants and children up to 5 years of age who are

More information about WIC and
the WIC Farmers' Market Nutrition
Program can be found at
http://www.fns.usda.gov/wic and
http://www.fns.usda.gov/wic/FMNP/
FMNPfaqs.htm.[35,36]

found to be at nutritional risk. As part of the WIC Farmers' Market Nutrition Program, as in the Senior Farmers' Market Nutrition Program, a variety of fresh, nutritious, unprepared, locally grown fruits, vegetables, and herbs may be purchased with coupons.

The Summer Food Service Program

This program provides nutritious breakfasts, lunches, and snacks to ensure that children in areas with lower incomes continue to receive nutritious meals during long school vacations, when they typically would not have access to the school breakfast and lunch programs.

Programs vary by area and may be accessed through local summer programs or through schools.

> More information about the Summer Food Service Program can be found at http://www.summerfood.usda.gov.[37]

America's Second Harvest

This is the largest domestic hunger-relief organization in the United States.[1] Emergency food providers include food pantries, soup kitchens, shelters, and other charitable agencies that feed hungry people. America's Second Harvest is a national network of over 200 food banks and food-rescue programs. In 2001, it distributed 1.7 billion pounds of food to hungry Americans through thousands of charitable agencies, including over 26,000 pantries, almost 6,000 kitchens, and over 4,000 shelters operated by private nonprofit organizations, government-affiliated agencies, or faith-based agencies affiliated with churches, mosques, synagogues, and other organizations. In fact, the majority of the emergency food providers—that is, 76% of pantries, 71% of kitchens, and 43% of shelters—are operated by the faith-based groups.[27]

The Impact of Food Insecurity on the Public

Food insecurity can have grave consequences on health, including physical impairments such as illness and fatigue; psychological suffering such as feelings of constraint to go against norms and values, and stress at home; and sociofamilial disturbances such as modifications of eating patterns and ritual, disruption of household dynamics, and distortion of the means of food acquisition and management.[38] Dietary quality can also be negatively impacted by food insecurity or insufficiency, including lower dietary intakes of fruits and vegetables[41] and other foods containing essential nutrients.[39-41] Over time these suboptimal intakes could increase the public's risk of developing diet-related, chronic diseases.[40] In fact, oveweight/obesity has been associated with food insecurity.[42-44] It has been asserted that the relationship between obesity and food insecurity may be mediated by the low cost of energy-dense foods and reinforced by the pleasing taste of sugar and fat.[45] Poorer functional health status has also been associated with food insecurity.[46] Regarding children, evidence links food insecurity with grave consequences, including poor health status,[47] psychosocial problems,[48,49] lower cognitive and academic performance,[50] and poor nutritional status.[51,52]

Strategies to Assist the Public in Securing Adequate Food

Public health nutrition professionals, registered dietitians, and physicians, along with other members of the healthcare team, can assist the public in improving food security. This is paramount, because noncompliance with dietary suggestions may simply be due to poor access to food rather than a lack of understanding of the regimen. Practical suggestions have been published for incorporating food security principles into practice.[53,54] During an interview, health professionals should inquire about issues similar to those assessed in the food security survey module: 1) anxiety related to food budget or supply and whether the budget is able to meet basic needs; 2) experiences relating to running out of food without being able to obtain more due to financial constraints; 3) perceptions of intake adequacy; and 4) food use.[4]

For example, in the context of having inadequate resources, questions could be posed about eating balanced meals, cutting meal size or skipping meals, and experiencing unintentional weight loss. In addition, questions to include should be related to:

- Available resources, including household income, that the individual has for food to implement dietary and nutrition interventions
- Storage facilities for food, including having a refrigerator and/or freezer in the household
- Availability of utilities, including gas, electric, and water, to the household
- Participation in federal and non-federal food assistance programs in their community, including food pantries, soup kitchens, and community gardens
- How the household acquires food, including gardening practices, hunting for game or fish, and related food safety issues related to dressing fish and game
- Meal planning and purchasing tips related to preserving food resources and reducing food waste[53,54]

Although the educational needs of clients vary, such as in meal planning and purchasing tips, in the face of scarce resources, training may be necessary. In addition, being prepared to discuss the rationale for federal and non-federal food assistance programs and their benefits, as well as being able to assist clients in accessing these programs or referring them to another professional, should be considered; in fact, an educational resource could be developed and updated periodically.[53] Other educational strategies may include an explanation of manufacturers' expiration codes and other information found on packages, such as "use-by" and "sell-by" dates, to help clients preserve scarce resources. Food safety education related to food preservation methods, including canning and freezing, and food storage processes should be included,[53] as should those related to some of the unsafe practices discussed previously.[22]

Conclusions

Securing adequate food for the public is paramount to achieving and maintaining health. Food security exists when all people, at all times, have access to sufficient food for an active and healthy life without resorting to emergency food supplies or socially unacceptable ways of obtaining food, including begging, stealing, or scavenging.[3] Understanding food security measurement strategies for programmatic evaluation and inclusion in community needs assessments, as well as the consequences of food insecurity and programs designed to assist the public in securing adequate food, is vital for public health professionals. Several resources will assist public nutrition professionals in staying abreast of food security-related issues, including the Food Security Briefing Room of the Economic Research Service (http://www.ers.usda.gov/briefing/foodsecurity),[5] the Center on Hunger and Poverty (http://www.centeronhunger.org),[55] and the Food Research and Action Center (http://www.frac.org).[56]

Issues for Discussion

1. You are developing a public health nutrition program that you think will impact the food security status of households in the community. The intervention is planned to be 12 months in length. Develop an assessment/evaluation strategy to assess the impact of the program on food security status.

2. As a public health nutrition team, your agency is working with individuals in the local community who have had trouble securing adequate food for the household. During a meeting you plan to discuss how some of the clients are coping to minimize household food insecurity. Develop a list of strategies that you believe would be generated from such a discussion and the risks associated with those strategies that appear to be "risky."

3. Select a life span group, for example, older adults, and discuss food assistance programs that may be accessed in the community, noting what resources each program provides.

4. Develop an interviewing strategy that will assist you in identifying clients at risk for food insecurity.

References

1. Office of Disease Prevention and Health Promotion, U.S. Department of Health and Human Services. Healthy People 2010. Available at: http://www.healthypeople.gov. Accessed April 15, 2004.

2. Nord M, Andrews M, Carlson S. *Household Food Security in the United States, 2002* (FANRR35). Alexandria, Va.: Food and Rural Economics Division, Economic Research Service, U.S. Department of Agriculture; 2003.

3. Life Science Research Office. Federation of American Societies for Experimental Biology. Core indicator of nutritional state for difficult to sample populations. *J Nutr.* 1990;102:1599–1600.

4. Bickel G, Nord M, Price C, Hamilton W, Cook J. *Guide to Measuring Household Food Security, Revised 2000.* Alexandria, Va.: U.S. Department of Agriculture, Food and Nutrition Service; 2000.

5. Economic Research Service, U.S. Department of Agriculture. Briefing Room—Food Security in the United States. Available at: http://www.ers.usda.gov/briefing/foodsecurity/. Accessed April 15, 2004.

6. Radimer KL, Olson CM, Campbell CC. Development of indicators to assess hunger. *J Nutr.* 1990;120:1544–1548.

7. Radimer KL, Olson CM, Greene JC, Campbell CC, Habicht J-P. Understanding hunger and developing indicators to assess it in women and children. *J Nutr.* 1992;24:36S–45S.

8. Wehler CA, Scott RI, Anderson JJ. The Community Childhood Hunger Identification Project: A model of domestic hunger—Demonstration project in Seattle, Washington. *J Nurs Educ.* 1992;24:29S–35S.

9. Bureau of Labor Statistics, U.S. Department of Labor. Labor Force Statistics from the Current Population Survey. Available at: http://www.bls.gov/cps/home.htm. Accessed April 15, 2004.

10. National Center for Education Statistics. Early Childhood Longitudinal Study. Available at: http://nces.ed.gov/ecls/index.asp. Accessed April 15, 2004.

11. National Center for Health Statistics, Centers for Disease Control and Prevention. National Health and Nutrition Examination Survey. Available at: http://www.cdc.gov/nchs/nhanes.htm. Accessed April 15, 2004.

12. Institute for Social Research, University of Michigan. Panel Study of Income Dynamics. Available at: http://psidonline.isr.umich.edu. Accessed April 15, 2004.

13. U.S. Census Bureau. Survey of Program Dynamics. Available at: http://www.sipp.census.gov/spd/. Accessed April 15, 2004.

14. McIntyre L, Glanvill NT, Raine KD, Dayle JB, Anerson B, Battaglia N. Do low-income lone mothers compromise their nutrition to feed their children? *Can Med Assoc J.* 2003;168:686–691.

15. Blumberg SJ, Bialososky K, Hamilton WL, Briefel RR. The effectiveness of a short form of the household food security scale. *Am J Public Health.* 1999;89:1231–1234.

16. Nord M, Bickel G. *Measuring Children's Food Security in the United States, 1995–1999* (FANRR-25). Alexandria, Va.: Food and Rural Economics Division, Economic Research Service, U.S. Department of Agriculture; 2002.

17. Andrews M, Carlson S. *Household Food Security in the United States, 2001* (FANRR-29). Alexandria, Va.: Food and Rural Economics Division, Economic Research Service, U.S. Department of Agriculture; 2002.

18. Andrews M, Nord M, Bickel G, Carlson S. *Household Food Security in the United States, 1999* (FANRR-8). Alexandria, Va.: Food and Rural Economics Division, Economic Research Service, U.S. Department of Agriculture; 2000.

19. Holben DH, McClincy MC, Holcomb JP, Dean KL, Walker CE. Food security status of households in Appalachian Ohio with children in Head Start. *J Am Diet Assoc.* 2004;104:238–241.

20. LeBlanc C, McMurry K. Discussion paper on food security. *Fam Econ Nutr Rev.* 1998;2:49–78.

21. Olivera V. *The Food Stamp Program and Food Insufficiency.* Washington, DC: Economic Research Service; 1998.

22. Kempson KM, Keenan DP, Sadani PS, Ridlen S, Rosato NS. Food management practices used by people with limited resources to maintain food sufficiency as reported by nutrition educators. *J Am Diet Assoc.* 2002;102:1795–1799.

23. Greder K, Brotherson MJ. Food security and low-income families: Research to inform policy and programs. *J Fam Cons Sci.* 2002;94(2):40–47.

24. Holben DH, Shih K-P, Manoogian MM. Relationship of food insecurity to physical and mental health of women from rural, low-income households in West Virginia. *FASEB J.* In press.

25. Food and Nutrition Service, U.S. Department of Agriculture. Child and Adult Care Food Program. Available at: http://www.fns.usda.gov/cnd/CARE/CACFP/cacfphome.htm. Accessed April 15, 2004.

26. Cooperative State Research, Education, and Extension Service. Expanded Food and Nutrition Education Program. Available at: http://www.csrees.usda.gov/nea/food/efnep/about.html. Accessed April 15, 2004.

27. America's Second Harvest. Available at: http://www.secondharvest.org. Accessed April 15, 2004.

28. Food and Nutrition Service, U.S. Department of Agriculture. Food Distribution Programs. Available at: http://www.fns.usda.gov/fdd/. Accessed April 15, 2004.

29. Food and Nutrition Service, U.S. Department of Agriculture. Nutrition Assistance Programs. Available at: http://www.fns.usda.gov/fns/menu/programs.htm. Accessed April 15, 2004.

30. Food and Nutrition Service, U.S. Department of Agriculture. Food Stamp Program. Available at: http://www.fns.usda.gov/fsp/. Accessed April 15, 2004.

31. National Meals on Wheels Foundation. Available at: http://www.nationalmealsonwheels.org. Accessed April 15, 2004.

32. Food and Nutrition Service, U.S. Department of Agriculture. National School Lunch Program. Available at: http://www.fns.usda.gov/cnd/lunch/. Accessed April 15, 2004.

33. Food and Nutrition Service, U.S. Department of Agriculture. School Breakfast Program. Available at: http://www.fns.usda.gov/cnd/breakfast/. Accessed April 15, 2004.

34. Food and Nutrition Service, U.S. Department of Agriculture. Senior Farmers' Market Nutrition Program. Available at: http://www.fns.usda.gov/wic/SeniorFMNP/SFMNPmenu.htm. Accessed April 15, 2004.

35. Food and Nutrition Service, U.S. Department of Agriculture. Special Supplemental Nutrition Program for Women, Infants and Children (WIC). Available at: http://www.fns.usda.gov/wic/. Accessed April 15, 2004.

36. Food and Nutrition Service, U.S. Department of Agriculture. WIC Farmers' Market Nutrition Program. Available at: http://www.fns.usda.gov/wic/FMNP/FMNPfaqs.htm. Accessed April 15, 2004.

37. Food and Nutrition Service, U.S. Department of Agriculture. Summer Food Service Program. Available at: http://www.fns.usda.gov/cnd/summer/. Accessed April 15, 2004.

38. Hamelin A-M, Habicht J-P, Beaudry M. Food insecurity: Consequences for the household and broader social implications. *J Nutr.* 1999;129:525S–528S.

39. Rose D, Oliveira V. Nutrient intakes of individuals from food insufficient households in the United States. *Am J Public Health.* 1997;87:1956–1961.

40. Dixon LB, Winkleby M, Radimer K. Dietary intakes and serum nutrients differ between adults from food-insufficient and food-sufficient families: Third National Health and Nutrition Examination Survey, 1988–1994. *J Nutr.* 2001;131:1232–1246.

41. Kendell A, Olson CM, Frongillo EA Jr. Relationship of hunger and food insecurity to food availability and consumption. *J Am Diet Assoc.* 1996;96:1019–1024.

42. Frongillo EA Jr, Olson CM, Raschenbach BS, Kendall A. *Nutritional Consequences of Food Insecurity in a Rural New York County.* Madison, Wisc.: Institute for Research on Poverty, University of Wisconsin-Madison; 1997. Discussion Paper no. 1120-97.

43. Olson CM. Nutrition and health outcomes associated with food insecurity and hunger. *J Nutr.* 1999;129:521S–524S.

44. Holben DH, Pheley AM. Obesity, diabetes, and BMI are greater in food insecure households in rural Appalachian Ohio. *J Am Diet Assoc.* 2001;101:A-78.

45. Drewnowski A, Specter SE. Poverty and obesity: The role of energy density and energy costs. *Am J Clin Nutr.* 2004;79:6–16.

46. Pheley AM, Holben DH, Graham AS, Simpson C. Food security and perceptions of health status: A preliminary study in rural Appalachia. *J Rural Health.* 2002;18:447–454.

47. Alaimo K, Olson CM, Frongillo EA, Jr. Food insufficiency, family income, and health in U.S. preschool and school-aged children. *Am J Public Health.* 2001;91:781–786.

48. Kleinman RE, Murphy JM, Little M, Pagano J, Wehler CA, Regal K, Jellinek MS. Hunger in children in the United States: Potential behavioral and emotional correlates. *Pediatrics.* 1998;101:1–6.

49. Murphy JM, Wehler CA, Pagano ME, Little M, Kleinman RE, Jellinek MS. Relationship between hunger and psychosocial functioning in low-income American children. *J Am Acad Child Adolesc Psychiatry.* 1998;37:163–170.

50. Alaimo K, Olson CM, Frongillo EA, Jr. Food insufficiency and American school-aged children's cognitive, academic and psychosocial development. *Pediatrics.* 2001;108:44–53.

51. Casey PH, Szeto K, Lensing S, Bogle M, Weber J. Children in food-insufficient, low-income families. Prevalence, health and nutrition status. *Arch Pediatr Adolesc Med.* 2001;155:508–514.

52. Kaiser LL, Melgar-Quinonez H, Lamp CL, Johns MC, Sutherlin JM, Harwood JO. Food insecurity and nutritional outcomes of preschool-age Mexican-American children. *J Am Diet Assoc.* 2002;102:924–929.

53. Boeing KL, Holben DH. Self-identified food security knowledge and practices of licensed dietitians in Ohio: Implications for dietetics and clinical nutrition practice. *Top Clin Nutr.* 2003;18:185–191.

54. Holben DH, Myles W. Food insecurity in the United States: How it affects our patients. *Am Fam Physician.* 2004;69:1058–1063.

55. Center on Hunger and Poverty. Available at: http://www.centeronhunger.org. Accessed April 15, 2004.

56. Food Research and Action Center. Available at: http://www.frac.org. Accessed April 15, 2004.

CHAPTER 18

SECURITY OF THE FOOD SUPPLY AND BIOTERRORISM PREPAREDNESS

Barbara Bruemmer, PhD, RD, CD

Reader Objectives

After studying this chapter and reflecting on the contents, you should be able to:

1. Describe the scope of the bioterrorist threat to the food supply.
2. Identify organisms that may be disseminated by ingestion.
3. Describe the foods most at risk of intentional contamination.
4. Compare and contrast the challenges in distinguishing an intentional food contamination from an unintentional food contamination.
5. Summarize the strengths and weaknesses of our current food biosecurity efforts.
6. Recommend actions public health nutritionists can take to promote preparedness for the community and the consumer.

The safety and security of our food supply is essential for physical survival as well as social stability and economic prosperity. In a developed country such as the United States, individuals may live a life quite removed from the acts that produce, process, and transport food for various levels of home, retail, and restaurant preparation and presentation. This chapter will examine the complex risks from bioterrorism that are inherent in a stratified food economy.

There are many historical precedents for biological warfare as far back as 184 BC, when Hannibal had pots filled with serpents placed on the decks of enemy ships.[1] In modern history, the Biological and Toxin Weapons Convention was signed by over 140 countries in the early 1970s. This agreement addressed research on offensive biological weapons and destruction of existing weapons. Although such international agreement on the development of biological weapons is necessary, certain rogue states and terrorist groups have declared their intent to fight an economic and political war with the United States. It has been revealed that during the Persian Gulf War in 1995, Iraq not only had stocks of botulinum toxin, the deadliest know substance to man, but also had loaded 11,200 liters into Scud missile warheads.[2]

Historically, food has been a vehicle for terrorist attacks both nationally and internationally. In 1984, a religious cult contaminated salad bars at 10 restaurants with *Salmonella typhimurium*, sickening 751 people in The Dalles, Oregon.[3] Chemical agents, as well as biologic agents, have also been added to food. In 2003, 200 pounds of ground beef were contaminated with nicotine by a supermarket employee. This attack resulted in illness in 111 people, 40 of whom were children.[4] Mark Wheelis has noted "Every major state biological weapons program we know of has included an anti-agricultural component."[5]

The potential for causing sickness in larger populations has been demonstrated with unintentional foodborne illness. The largest reported incident of unintentional foodborne illness occurred in China in 1991, where 300,000 reported victims suffered from an outbreak of hepatitis A that was linked to tainted clams.[6] Thus, when contamination occurs at a central food processing or distribution point, food may be a vehicle for wide dissemination of a biologic or chemical agent.

Assessment and quantification of this risk has been considered by numerous government agencies, including the Center for Food Safety and Applied Nutrition of the FDA. Its report of October 2003 noted:

> Though the likelihood of a biological or chemical attack on the U.S. food supply is uncertain, significant scientific evidence documents the risk to public health of food that has been inadvertently contaminated. Notwithstanding the uncertainties described in this risk assessment, and given the broad range of agents that may contaminate the food supply that FDA regulates, the agency concludes that there is a *high likelihood*, over the course of a year, that a significant number of people will be affected by an act of food terrorism or by an incident of unintentional food contamination that results in serious foodborne illness.[7]

Terrorism—The unlawful use of force or violence against persons or property to intimidate or coerce a government, the civilian population, or any segment thereof, in furtherance of political or social objectives.

In light of the terrorism threat to the United States, how can we defend and protect public health and these vital resources? In the event of an attack, how can we assure an adequate supply of safe food for victims and minimize short-term and long-term impacts?

Food as a Target

Food is vulnerable not only because of the physical need for survival, but also because of the complex layers of societal involvement. As illustrated in Figure 18-1, both individual and societal factors may be profoundly impacted by an attack on the food supply. The individual components are both physical and psychological; societal components can be economic and political.

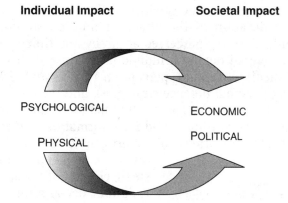

Individual Impact   **Societal Impact**

PSYCHOLOGICAL   ECONOMIC

PHYSICAL   POLITICAL

FIGURE 18-1   Potential Consequences of a Major Food Bioterrorism Event

Physical

The physical consequences start with our dependence on food for survival. Although this simple statement appears as a prima fascia tenet, so obvious that it should not need acknowledgment, it is our assumption that food is always available that contributes to our vulnerability. Our population does not regard food insufficiency as a risk that all may face; however, it is certainly recognized as a vulnerability of select groups, such as the homeless and poor. But the concept that a food shortage could occur is generally not considered a threat. The lack of food in the short term could cause physical discomfort, could be associated with mild malnutrition, or in an extreme situation could threaten life. Certain segments of the population could be more vulnerable to shortages, such as groups who may be isolated and unable to obtain emergency supplies, or those who by their physical limitations may have less reserves or increased needs, such as pregnant women, infants, small children, and older adults.

Another potential physical consequence includes the destruction or contamination of food that has been exposed to a biological weapon. This could potentially remove needed food supplies from circulation and cause disruption in the transportation and distribution of replacement food supplies to the public, retail outlets, restaurants, and institutional feeding sites.

Psychological

The events of 2001 demonstrated the widespread psychological impact of terrorist events, where millions of people experienced anxiety and distress. Individuals would understandably respond to attacks on the food supply in a similar fashion, but the degree of psychological harm may be very difficult to assess and control. Factors that may influence the magnitude of emotional response may include the weapon (the severity of the attack, the type of weapon used, the duration of the attack or multiple attacks), emergency communication (the perceived accuracy and timeliness of information, the level of detail on individual victims, the extent and duration of media coverage), perception of personal risk (uncertainty regarding personal defense strategies), and the coexistence of deprivation or discomfort. Factors that may contribute to public alarm and panic include rumors and misinformation that establish public mistrust, the appearance of favoritism for some individuals over others, a perception that there is a small chance of escape, requests for isolation, declarations of quarantine, social disruption, and civil discord and violence.[8] The psychological response to an attack on food would certainly be magnified for individuals who have inadequate food, suffer from hunger pains, or would be responsible for others, such as hungry children. Also, the majority of Americans are not accustomed to eating spoiled food, which might be a necessity in the situation of shortages.

> **Response**—Those activities and programs designed to address the immediate and short-term effects of the onset of an emergency or disaster.

The National Academy of Sciences (NAS) has published a report, *Preparing for the Psychological Consequences of Terrorism: A Public Health Strategy,*[9] that describes three spheres of psychological consequence: distress response, psychiatric illness, and behavioral change. The authors note the level of psychological response to terrorism may include "insomnia, fear, anxiety, vulnerability, anger, increased alcohol consumption or smoking; and, a minority will develop psychiatric illnesses, such as posttraumatic stress disorder or depression." Several elements related to food and psychological distress should be considered in public health preparedness. During an attack, availability of basic supplies including food is the responsibility of the public health infrastructure. The first of the 10 recommendations from the NAS report is the "Provision of basic resources including food, shelter, communication, transportation, information, guidance, and medical services." During a recovery phase we must recognize that attitudes toward a food or a food group may be altered as a psychological response, particularly if a food has been the vehicle to deliver a terrorist weapon.

> **Recovery**—Recovery, in this chapter, includes all types of emergency actions dedicated to the continued protection of the public or to promoting the resumption of normal activities in the affected area.

Such responses may result in short-term or long-term maladaptive behaviors, such as food aversions. Research on this area of behavioral change not only would help us to assure the return to psychological health, but also may help us avoid severe economic and/or nutritional consequences of long-term shifts in consumption patterns.

The final element to consider regarding psychological consequences is the amount of damage that potentially may result from small, sporadic terrorist attacks on food, where the main target is psychological health itself. Although few individuals were actually exposed to the anthrax bacterium in 2001, the uncertainty of the exposure and resulting perception created additional "victims" of this attack.

Economic

An attack on our food supply has the potential to cause tremendous economic damage both for domestic consumption and for our export markets and balance of trade. As described by Chalk, an agroterrorist attack would generate costs on three levels:

- *Direct losses:* From containment measures and the destruction of disease-ridden livestock
- *Indirect multiplier effects:* From compensation costs paid to farmers
- *International costs:* From protective trade embargoes imposed by major external trading partners[10]

In 2002, the total value of crop production in the United States was $94.7 billion, which included $71.3 billion in field and miscellaneous crops, $12.8 billion from fruits and nuts, and $10.6 billion in commercial vegetables. U.S. agricultural exports for 2001 included 1.9 billion bushels of corn, 961 million bushels of wheat, and 1.1 billion bushels of soybeans.[11] The gross domestic product for food was $1150 billion in 2004.[12] The food industry represents an estimated 20% of the gross national product.[13] The restaurant industry is also a major factor in our economy, with over $440 billion in sales forecast for 2004, with 878,000 locations serving more than 70 billion meals and snacks and employing 12 million individuals.[14] The Food Marketing Institute has estimated figures for grocery store sales in 2002 of $535.4 billion based on 166,135 grocery stores, which have 3.4 million employees. Americans are estimated to expend 6.1% of their disposable income on food prepared at home and 4.0% for food away from home.[15]

Following the events of September 2001, the food industry experienced:

> . . . a dramatic decline in some travel-dependent sectors of food service, a temporary slowdown in new grocery product introductions, impacts on transportation in small segments of the industry and increased security costs.[16]

Increased economic costs are continuing for agriculture and industry as preparedness plans are developed, implemented, evaluated, and revised. The consequences to our economy are difficult to estimate, but could potentially be profound with an agent delivered at a central distribution point with widespread contamination. Even random attacks on the food supply could have major economic impacts if consumers alter eating patterns, shopping habits, and food storage inventory. Also, a stigma with economic consequences may be associated with an industry or a food product. In 1993, after the outbreak of *E. coli* O157:H7 was traced to Jack in the Box restaurants in the Pacific Northwest, the parent company, Foodmakers, saw its stock value drop by 30%.[17]

Treatment costs following an outbreak may also be substantial. Trevejo et al. have reported that the median cost of hospitalization of patients with salmonellosis in 1990 to 1999 ranged from $160 to $3.2 million dollars (median 9.054).[18]

Political

How would these factors then impact the political situation? The outbreak of bovine spongiform encephalopathy (known as mad cow disease) led to a loss of confidence in the political system and political destabilization in Great Britain. Much of this fallout was due to communication missteps where the public was given assurances of safety that later proved to be unsubstantiated.[19] Certainly the election in Spain in the winter of 2004 was influenced by the bombings in Madrid. In the United States, the events of September 2001 and subsequent activities unmistakably influenced the political arena.

Public Health Preparedness for Food Biosecurity

In the face of these consequences of an attack on the food supply, federal agencies, state and local public health jurisdictions, emergency responders, academic institutions, researchers, and community groups have taken specific steps to safeguard the food supply and upgrade the public health infrastructure to lessen risk. The Centers for Disease Control and Prevention (CDC) uses a paradigm for preparedness that includes planning, surveillance, detection, and response. The Department of Health and Human Services also highlights the element of awareness in preparedness efforts.[20] Each of these components has unique challenges in regard to food biosecurity. The issue of awareness is particularly appropriate regarding food security. Although the events of September 2001 certainly maximized awareness of the potential for terrorist attacks, the risk to the food supply is still obscured by complacency that exists at various levels among institutions and individuals.

> Live agents cannot be detected by the human senses. Therefore, the first indication of a biologic attack is usually the first observed casualty, most often detected by local physicians who then report it to local public health officials.

The elements of effective planning include the identification of appropriate regulatory agencies, which are then responsible for the assessment of areas of risk; development of preparedness priorities, strategies, and plans to diminish risk; communication; training; and evaluation. Planning activities also depend on interagency cooperation. The FBI has prepared a *Concepts of Operations Plan (CONPLAN)*, which provides overall guidance on response to a potential or actual terrorist threat.[21]

To plan a strong defense system, it is important to assess those elements of our food environment that may be involved in a terrorist attack. There are two main approaches to our defense systems. First, we must recognize that food may be a vehicle to deliver a terrorist weapon; second, other types of terrorist activities may compromise the availability of safe food in adequate amounts. In both situations, we must provide defense, but also plan and empower local communities and individuals to be prepared with knowledge, skills, and reserves of necessary water and food.

Potential Agents

Food, as a vehicle for the delivery of a bioterrorist weapon, may be contaminated with either biological or chemical weapons that may be viable through the gastrointestinal tract. The CDC has created a list of agents that have been assigned to categories based on a number of criteria including:

> need for hospitalization, mortality rates for exposed untreated persons, potential for initial dissemination to a large population, potential for continued propagation by person-to-person transmission, potential for overall dissemination, capability for mass production, potential for rapid, large-scale dissemination including most effective route of infection and general environmental stability, source of the agent, i.e., soil, animal/insect, or plant source versus laboratory or clinical sources, and main routes of infection, i.e., respiratory versus gastrointestinal.[22]

This report notes several important aspects of this classification process. First, these agents are not ranked on their likelihood of use, but on their potential impact. Second, historically the presumed target for biological weapons was military person-

> **Virulence**—The relative severity of the disease produced by a pathogen.

nel and military capability. The virulence of these agents would be quite different in young, physically fit individuals in the military service compared to a cross-section of the population with varying levels of immune function and comorbidities.

The ingestion of biological agents may occur by:

- Contaminated food or drinking water (non-aerosols can contaminate food supplies or drinking water over long distances)

- Hand-to-mouth contact after touching contaminated surfaces
- Swallowing mucus that contains particles lodged in the nose and throat[23]

The potential targets include food crops, livestock (using aerosols, sprays, and crop dusters), food processing plants, imported foods and food additives, point of sale (i.e., grocery stores), restaurants, institutional feeding sites, and congregate meals.[23] Because the contaminants may be spread from hand to food, packaging may also be a target. Individual packages, such as milk cartons or other sealed containers, may be penetrated with a syringe.

Table 18-1 provides information on the category A and category B agents that may be viable through the gastrointestinal tract. Of these agents, botulism is certainly an agent that could potentially lead to substantial loss of life. It is considered the most toxic agent known. Arnon has stated that "one hundred grams of botulinum toxin evenly distributed in a food or beverage and ingested, could kill over one million people."[24] However, many of the traditional foodborne agents, such as salmonellosis, that do not have a high fatality rate may still cause significant morbidity, social disruption, and psychological damage, particularly in vulnerable populations.

Healthcare providers and public health professionals should be familiar with the latency periods and presenting symptoms of these agents to assist in communication for early detection and to provide informed responses to the public if one of these agents be suspected in an attack.

Foods at Risk

Two factors influence the magnitude of the impact of a foodborne bioweapon. First is the range of distribution of the vehicle (food), and second is the rate of introduction of the vehicle combined with the rate of clearance. Many of our current foods, including dietary staples, are centrally processed and widely distributed. Therefore, these foods would present a more attractive profile with which to deliver a bioweapon. A National Academy of Sciences (NAS) report has noted that food and water supply networks have a ready-made distribution system for the rapid and widespread introduction of biological and chemical weapons.[25] However, the rate of introduction of the vehicle into the food supply and the rate of clearance limits the effectiveness of many distribution systems. Foods that have a long shelf life would be less desirable, since the source of contamination may be identified and isolated before the food reaches many of the intended victims. Highly perishable foods with a large distri-

> **Perishable food**—Food that is not heat-treated, frozen, or otherwise preserved in a manner so as to prevent the quality of the food from being adversely affected if held longer than 7 days under normal shipping and storage conditions.

bution range would be most vulnerable to contamination. This category includes dairy products, fresh fruits and vegetables, and certain baked goods. These foods are staples for many of the most vulnerable in our population, such as children. The consequences of an attack on these foods would include a high level of publicity and the associated psychological impact, even though the actual human losses may be limited.

Food Biosecurity Triad: Food Systems Security, Public Health Vanguard, and Consumer Engagement

Our efforts to address the risks are focused on three areas, which are described as a triad: 1) the security of the food supply; 2) mobilizing public health and federal agencies as vanguards in preparedness; and 3) the engagement of individual consumers in this process. (See Figure 18-2.)

Food System Security

In this first area, actions have been taken to increase the security of the food supply with increased agency funding, expanded regulations, and revised guidelines for food producers and food importers. Title III of the Public Health Security and Bioterrorism Preparedness and Response Act of 2002 contained specific information related to protecting the food supply. The Food and Drug Administration (FDA), through the Center for Food Safety and Applied Nutrition (CFSAN), has implemented provisions for registration of food facilities and prior notice of imported food, as noted in Table 18-2. These actions will assist in communication regarding food that may have been contaminated, as well as serving as a deterrent.

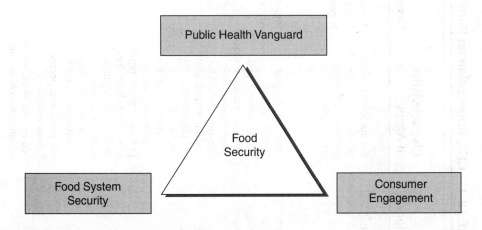

FIGURE 18-2   The Triad of Food Security

TABLE 18-1   CDC Information on Bioterrorism Agents and Diseases[54,55,56,57]

Category A	Characteristics of Agent	Dissemination	Incubation Period	Symptoms	Case Fatality Ratio (CFR) or Lethality
Anthrax[58,59] *Bacillus anthracis*	Encapsulated, aerobic, gram-positive, spore-forming, rod-shaped bacterium.	Aerosol Cutaneous **Ingestion**	1–7 days	GI: Nausea, anorexia, vomiting, and fever progressing to severe abdominal pain, hematemesis, and diarrhea that is almost always bloody.	Gastrointestinal has mortality rate of 50–100% despite treatment.
Botulism[60,61] Toxin of *Clostridium botulinum*	Most lethal agent known to man. Spore-forming, rod-shaped organisms that grow in anaerobic environments. The toxin interferes with the presynaptic release of acetylcholine at the neuromuscular junction. Seven types of toxin; A–F are toxic in humans. Victims with respiratory symptoms may require ventilatory support. No person-to-person transmission. No natural occurrence of inhalation botulism.	**Ingestion** Aerosol	18–36 hours (may range from 6 hours to 10 days, dose dependent)	Acute abdomen picture with rebound tenderness may develop. Initial: Blurred vision, double vision, drooping eyelids, slurred speech, difficulty swallowing, dry mouth, muscle weakness. Later: Descending neurologic impairment. GI: nausea, vomiting, abdominal cramps or abdominal pain, diarrhea.[62]	High mortality, 60% if untreated. Hospitalization rate 80%. Lethal dose 1 ng/kg.

(Continues)

Category A	Characteristics of Agent	Dissemination	Incubation Period	Symptoms	Case Fatality Ratio (CFR) or Lethality
Plague[63,64] *Yersinia pestis*	Pneumonic plague refers to respiratory infection. Person-to-person transmission from respiratory droplets.	Aerosols	2–6 days	Swollen and tender lymph gland accompanied by pain.	Untreated bubonic plague. CFR 50%.
Smallpox[64] *Variola major*	High transmissibility. Quarantine may be necessary for containment.	Aerosol	10–12 days	Fever, hypotension, rash.	Death occurs in 30% of cases.
Tularemia[65] *Francisella tularensis*	Bacterium found in animals. Highly infectious (10–50 organisms can cause disease). May remain alive for weeks in water.	Aerosol (most likely method for bioterrorism) **Ingestion**	3–5 days (may range 1–14 days)	Depends on site of exposure. Skin ulcers, swollen and painful lymph glands, sore throat, mouth sores, diarrhea, or pneumonia.	CFR for Jellison type A: 5–10%.
Viral hemorrhagic[66,67] fevers	Causes increased capillary permeability, leukopenia, and thrombocytopenia.	Contact Aerosol	4–16 days	Fever, easy bleeding, edema, malaise, headache, vomiting, diarrhea, jaundice, shock, sore throat, rash.	Lethality is moderate to high.

TABLE 18-1   CDC Information on Bioterrorism Agents and Diseases (Continued)

Category B (Those that may be ingested)	Characteristics of Agent	Dissemination	Incubation Period	Symptoms	Case Fatality Ratio (CFR) or Lethality
Brucellosis[68] *Brucella species*	Natural *Brucella* species affect sheep, goats, cattle, deer, elk, pigs, dogs, and several other animals.	**Ingestion** Aerosol Cutaneous through skin wounds	5–60 days	Acute form: Non-specific flu-like symptoms. Undulant form: Undulant fevers, arthritis, and epididymo-orchitis in males. Chronic form: Chronic-fatigue syndrome, depression, and arthritis	CFR: 5%. Hospitalization rate: 55%.
Epsilon toxin of *Clostridium perfringens*[69]	An anaerobic, gram-positive, spore-forming rod commonly found in the intestines of humans, domestic and feral animals [FDA]. The toxins bind to enterocytes and form protein complexes that alter cell permeability [Smedley].*	**Ingestion**	8–16 hours	Nausea, abdominal cramps, watery diarrhea.	CFR: 0.005%. Hospitalization rate: .3%.

Food Safety Threats	Characteristics of Agent	Dissemination	Incubation Period	Symptoms	Case Fatality Ratio (CFR) or Lethality
Salmonella species	Generally resolves in 5–7 days and does not usually require hospitalization. Victim may require rehydration. Estimated cases per year in U.S.: 400,000; mortality: 600. Person-to-person contact likely with fecal-oral transmission. Good hygiene and sanitation essential.	**Ingestion**	12–72 hours	Diarrhea, fever, abdominal cramps. 3–8 days with a median of 3–4 days.	Non-typhoidal. CFR: .8%. Hospitalization rate: 22%. Typhoid. CFR: .4%. Hospitalization rate: 75%. Severe bloody diarrhea and abdominal cramps.
Escherichia coli O:157:H7[71]	Gram-negative rod-shaped bacterium. Estimated cases per year in U.S.: 73,000; mortality: 61. Person-to-person contact likely with fecal-oral transmission. Good hygiene and sanitation essential. Children under 5 and the elderly are at risk of the complication of hemolytic uremia syndrome.	**Ingestion**	3–8 days	Severe bloody diarrhea and abdominal cramps.	CFR: 0.83%. Hospitalization rate: 29.5%.

TABLE 18-1   CDC Information on Bioterrorism Agents and Diseases (Continued)

Food Safety Threats	Characteristics of Agent	Dissemination	Incubation Period	Symptoms	Case Fatality Ratio (CFR) or Lethality
Dysentery *Shigella*[72]	Estimated cases per year in U.S.: 18,000. Person-to-person contact likely with fecal-oral transmission. Good hygiene and sanitation essential.	**Ingestion**	3 days.**	Diarrhea (often bloody), fever, stomach cramps.	CFR: 0.16%. Hospitalization rate: 0.14%.
Cholera[67–74] *Vibrio cholerae*	The disease is rare in industrialized nations. Person-to-person contact likely with fecal-oral transmission. Good hygiene and sanitation essential.	Aerosol **Ingestion**	12–72 hours	Sudden onset of profuse, watery diarrhea, cramps, vomiting, headache.	CFR: 0.6%. Hospitalization rate: 34%.
Cryptosporidium parvum[75,76]	Parasitic infection of the intestinal epithelium. Person-to-person contact likely with fecal-oral transmission. Good hygiene and sanitation essential.	**Ingestion**	7 days (range, 2–28 days)	Watery diarrhea, abdominal cramps, low-grade fever, malaise, fatigue, anorexia, occasionally nausea and vomiting.	CFR: 0.5%. Hospitalization rate: 0.05%.
Q Fever[77] *Coxiella burnetii*	Acute rickettsial disease.	Aerosol **Ingestion**	14–16 days	Fevers, chills, malaise, headache, myalgia, eye pain, hyperaesthesias, pulmonary syndrome, cough, chest pain.	Untreated CFR < 1%.

Food Safety Threats	Characteristics of Agent	Dissemination	Incubation Period	Symptoms	Case Fatality Ratio (CFR) or Lethality
Ricin toxin[77] From *Ricinus communis* (castor bean)	Causes damage to the liver and bone marrow.	Aerosol Ingestion	1–12 hours	Vomiting, nausea, diarrhea, cramps, bloody nose, fever, pulmonary edema 18–24 hours after inhalation, severe respiratory distress and death in 36–72 hours.	High lethality.
Staphylococcal enterotoxin B[77]	Causes damage to the gastrointestinal and respiratory systems.	Aerosol **Ingestion**	1 hour (range may be 3–12 hours)	Sudden onset of fever, chills, headache, nausea, muscle aches, pulmonary syndrome, vomiting, and diarrhea if ingested.	Fatality < 1%.

Agents that may be disseminated through ingestion are shown in bold type.

*Food and Drug Administration. *Bad Bug Book*. Available at: http://www.cfsan.fda.gov/~mow/chap11.html. Accessed April 25, 2005.

**Reference: Jojosky RA, Groseclose SL: Evaluation of reporting timeliness of public health surveillance systems for infectious diseases. BMC Public Health. 2004; 4: 29. Available at: http://www.biomedcentral.com/1471-2458/4/29. Accessed April 24, 2005.

Source: Compiled by author.

TABLE 18-2   Food Biosecurity Triad: Food Systems Security

Food and Drug Administration (FDA)

Center for Food Safety and Applied Nutrition	Activities related to Bioterrorism Act

Center for Food Safety and Applied Nutrition

Legislation: Public Health Security and Bioterrorism Preparedness and Response Act of 2002

Title III: Protecting Safety and Security of Food and Drug Supply

Implementation: December 12, 2003

Activities related to Bioterrorism Act

Title III, Section 305

- Registration of Food Facilities

  "Domestic and foreign facilities that manufacture, process, pack or hold food, as defined in the regulation, for human or animal consumption in the US must register with FDA."

  The purpose is to allow the FDA to: "determine the location and source of a potential bioterrorism incident or an outbreak of food-borne illness and to quickly notify facilities that may be affected."

  Examples provided by FDA:

  Included food:
  - Dietary supplements and dietary ingredients
  - Infant formulas
  - Beverages (including alcoholic beverages and bottled water)
  - Fruits and vegetables
  - Fish and seafood
  - Dairy products and shell eggs
  - Raw agricultural commodities for use as food or components of food
  - Bakery goods, snack food, and candy (including chewing gum)
  - Live food animals
  - Animal feeds and pet food

  Excluded food:
  - Food contact substances
  - Pesticides

  Facilities that do NOT need to register:
  - Private residences of individuals
  - Non-bottled water, such as municipal water systems
  - Transport vehicles that hold food only in the usual course of their business as carriers
  - Farms
  - Restaurants
  - Nonprofit food facilities [501(c)(3)]
  - Fishing vessels that harvest and transport fish
  - Facilities regulated exclusively and throughout the entire facility by the USDA—facilities that handle only meat, poultry, or egg products.

  For additional information and instructions on registration see http://www.cfsan.fda.gov/~dms/fsbtact.html.

Title III, Section 307

- Prior Notice of Imported Food

  "Act requires that FDA receive prior notice for food imported or offered for import into the U.S.

  The Act also provides that if an article of food arrives at the port of arrival with inadequate prior notice (i.e., no prior notice, inaccurate prior notice, or untimely prior notice), the food is subject to refusal of admission."

  http:www.cfsan.fda.gov/~pn/cpgpn.html

Issued Guidelines:

  CFSAN Guidance for Industry: Retail Food Stores and Food Service Establishments: Food Security Preventive Measures Guidance. http://www.cfsan.fda.gov/~dms/secgui11.html.

U.S. Department of Agriculture (USDA)

Food Safety and Inspection Service (FSIS)

Public Health Security and Bioterrorism Preparedness and Response Act of 2002. Responsible for the regulation of meat, poultry, and egg products.

Actions authorized under the legislation:

- "Enhance the ability of the Service to inspect and ensure the safety and wholesomeness of meat and poultry products.
- Improve the capacity of the Service to inspect international products at points of origin and ports of entry.
- Strengthen the ability of the Service to collaborate with relevant agencies within USDA and other entities within the Federal Government, States and Indian Tribes.
- Otherwise expand the capacity to protect against the threat of bioterrorism."[78]

Issued Guidelines:

FSIS Security Guidelines for Food Processors
Elements include:

1. Food security plan management: establish a team with a food security manager; develop and implement a plan; identify potential corrective action and recommendations for recall of adultered products; link to analytical labs; develop a procedure for notification of law enforcement; identify facility entry points; determine local emergency and public health contacts; provide for training, inspections, communication, and response to threats; and liaison with Homeland Security officials.
2. Checklists for: outside security, general inside security, slaughter and processing security, storage security, shipping and receiving security, water and ice security, mail handling security, and personnel security. See http://www.fsis.usda.gov.

FSIS Safety and Security Guidelines for the Transportation and Distribution of Meat, Poultry, and Egg Products:

Elements include:

1. Assess vulnerabilities
2. Emergency operations
3. Train and test
4. Screen and educate employees
5. Secure the facility

Industry Actions

National Food Processors Association

Alliance for Food Security

Includes government agencies, agricultural and food industry organizations.

Actions: Food Security Checklist, regarding food plant operations.

www.nfpa-food.org

Dietary Managers Association

Articles for Dietary Managers and Food Protection Publications.

www.dmaonline.org

Source: Compiled by the author.

The U.S. Department of Agriculture (USDA), through the Food Safety and Inspection Service (FSIS), has also taken action regarding meat, poultry, and egg products with guidelines for food processors and for the transportation and distribution of these foods. Many of these actions are also based on directives from the Public Health Security and Bioterrorism Preparedness and Response Act of 2002. Additional procedures have been added during times of heightened threat levels (orange or red) to enhance inspection activity, enhance surveillance of transportation, storage, retail sites, and import facilities, conduct random laboratory sampling for threat agents in high-risk commodities, and increase surveillance of human illness.[26] These actions should improve security at sites that could potentially serve as distribution points for an attack. The key to the success of these actions is consistent high standards for compliance and ongoing evaluations. Vigilance in this regard is essential.

Another tool that has been promoted in the food industry is the Hazard Analysis and Critical Control Point (HACCP) approach to food safety. The FSIS has reported a reduction in *Salmonella* prevalence on raw meat and poultry products with the enforcement of the Pathogen Reduction/HACCP rule.[27] The guidelines for HACCP procedures to diminish the risk of a bioterrorist attack include:

1. Evaluate significant food security hazards and evaluate the likelihood of these risks.
2. Develop and institute preventive or risk control measures to reduce hazards.
3. Determine the points in your operation that are critical for managing a specific risk. These could be locations, processes, functions, or times when your operation is at greatest risk.
4. Develop monitoring procedures for each critical point.
5. Develop a procedure to fix security problems or failures that occur if a critical control has been breached or compromised, similar to a corrective-action program in HACCP.
6. Verify or test your security program periodically.[28]

However, while these agencies are in a transition period to a higher state of preparedness, there are still many areas that have not been addressed and that result in serious weaknesses in protecting the food supply. In November 2003, the General Accounting Office (GAO) provided testimony to Congress on the bioterrorist threat to agriculture. The GAO found gaps in federal controls for protecting agriculture and the food supply, which it concludes renders the United States vulnerable to bioterrorism.[29] Four specific areas had been studied and found deficient: prevention of foot and mouth disease, improvements in the animal feed ban to prevent mad cow disease, food-processing security, and the Plum Island Animal Disease Center. Each of these areas represents opportunities for the introduction of a weapon into the food biosystem.

Another report from the GAO in March 2004 focused on the overlapping and inefficient partitioning of food service regulation among multiple agencies. As noted by Robin Strongin, 12 different federal agencies administer 35 different laws on food safety, with an additional 28 House and Senate subcommittees having food safety oversight.[30] The GAO review recommended fundamental changes with: 1) comprehensive, uniform, and risk-based food safety legislation; and 2) establishment of a single, independent food safety agency.[31] Its assessment of the hazards for attack is that terrorists would attack livestock and crops to cause severe economic harm, but would contaminate finished food products to cause harm to humans. As an example of the lapses in oversight, the report notes that neither the FDA nor the USDA considers itself to have the authority to require processors to adopt physical facility security measures. Taken together, these omissions and inefficiencies contribute to food system vulnerability.

Public Health Vanguard

In this second area, progress has been made to create bridge organizations that address interagency coordination, communication, and harmonization activities and to integrate technology into surveillance systems (Table 18-3).

TABLE 18-3   Food Biosecurity Triad: Public Health Vanguard

Department of Homeland Security	State Homeland Security and Emergency Services. http://www.dhs.gov/dhspublic/
FEMA	Antiterrorism hazard mitigation information. http://www.fema.gov/fima/antiterrorism/
	NEMB-CAP—National Emergency Management Baseline Capability Assessment Program. A program to assess, analyze, evaluate, and collectively review state capabilities against a national standard. http://www.fema.gov
Health and Human Services	
CDC	Epi-X, The Epidemic Information Exchange System A secure Web-based communication network for public health professionals. http://www.cdc.gov/mmwr/epix/epix.html
	PHLIS, Public Health Laboratory Information System An electronic reporting system.
	PHIN, Public Health Information Network. A framework to support communication and data exchange. http://www.cdc.gov/phin/
	CDC Surveillance Systems:
	BioNet Combines PulseNet and the Laboratory Response Network (LRN) to detect links between disease agents during terrorist attacks. http://www.bt.cdc.gov/surveillance/bionet.asp
	EARS, Early Aberration Reporting System A syndromic surveillance tool. http://www.bt.cdc.gov/surveillance/ears/

(Continues)

TABLE 18-3   Food Biosecurity Triad: Public Health Vanguard (Continued)

	FoodNet, Foodborne Diseases Active Surveillance Network A laboratory-based surveillance for foodborne illness. http://www.cdc.gov/foodnet/
	NEDSS, National Electronic Disease Surveillance System A component of PHIN. This system promotes standards for data and information systems. http://www.cdc.gov/nedss/index.htm
	NETSS, National Electronic Telecommunications System for Surveillance A computerized public health system that provides the CDC with weekly data on notifiable diseases. http://www.cdc.gov/epo/dphsi/netss.htm
	PulseNet National Molecular Subtyping Network for Foodborne Disease Surveillance is a network of public health laboratories that provides an early warning system for foodborne illness. http://www.cdc.gov/pulsenet/
	CDC Response Systems:
	HAN, Health Alert Network A system to link local health departments and other organizations for preparedness and response. Other partners for HAN include the National Association of County and City Health Officials (NACCHO) and the Association of State and Territorial Health Officials (ASTHO). http://www.bt.cdc.gov/documentsapp/HAN/han.asp
FDA	CBER, Center for Biologics Evaluation and Research "Responsible for the development of products to diagnose, treat or prevent outbreaks from exposure to the pathogens that have been identified as bioterrorist agents." http://www.fda.gov/cber/cntrbio/cntrbio.htm
	eLEXNET, Electronic Laboratory Exchange Network An Internet-based data exchange system for federal, state, and local government food safety laboratories.
U.S. Department of Agriculture	
Food Safety and Inspection Service (FSIS)	OFSEP, Office of Food Security and Emergency Preparedness Manages homeland security activities with FSIS. http://www.fsis.usda.gov/About_FSIS/OFSEP/index.asp
Multi-agency: FDA, CDC, USDA	FERN, Food Emergency Response Network Coordinates activities among federal, state, regional, and university laboratories to identify bioterrorist agents in food.
Industry	
Food Marketing Institute, Grocery Manufacturers of America	FoodElert Food Safety and Security Rapid Alert Database may be used in emergencies to obtain contains contact information and access a listserv to send e-mail messages. http://www.fmi.org/foodelert/

The Food Emergency Response Network (FERN) (the lead agency of the FDA) coordinates activities among federal, state, regional, and university laboratories to identify bioterrorist agents in food. The FERN Steering Committee has included representatives of the FDA, Office of Regulatory Affairs, CFSAN, CDC, USDA, FSIS, Animal and Plant Health Inspection Service, Agriculture Marketing Service, Grain Inspection Packers and Stockyards Administration, Customs, Department of Defense, FBI, Environmental Protection Agency, Association of Public Health Laboratories, the agriculture community, and public health.[32] Surveillance activities include federal and state sampling programs for domestic and imported food. The agency will also examine response and recovery capabilities. Surge capacity has previously been identified as a critical weakness in public health efforts. The potential large number of casualties, as well as the number of worried well, may indeed overwhelm current health facilities. Response issues specific to a foodborne attack include the rapid dissemination of information on the affected food; the tracking, isolation, and recall of tainted food; and the ability to maintain adequate food in circulation.

> **Lead agency**—The federal department or agency assigned lead responsibility under U.S. law to manage and coordinate the federal response in a specific functional area. For the purposes of the CONPLAN, there are two lead agencies: the FBI for crisis management and FEMA for consequence management.

The Department of Homeland Security and the USDA coordinate food security activities through the USDA Homeland Security Council. The Office of Food Security and Emergency Preparedness (OFSEP) (the lead agency of FSIS) functions with the FDA and CDC. It is the lead office for:

> emergency preparedness and response; federal/state/industry relations; continuity of operations; scientific expertise in biological, chemical, physical, and radiological terrorism; and security clearance and safeguarding classified information.[33]

It was created in 2002 and assumed the function of the Food Biosecurity Action Team (F-BAT).

While these agencies function to enhance planning, response, and recovery, the function of surveillance is divided among many groups. (See Table 18-3.) The challenge of surveillance of foodborne agents is unique because many of the potential agents (shown in Table 18-1) are common in unintentional foodborne illness. Thus, surveillance must distinguish between the background "noise" of seasonal incidents and sentinel events from a bioweapon. The CDC and other agencies have drawn on efforts to enhance food safety to link state and local laboratories with national databases. As noted by Sobel et al., "The adequacy of response will depend on the capacity of public-health officials to respond to all foodborne disease outbreaks."[33] Technology has greatly enhanced the ability to conduct passive, automated surveillance. *Syndromic surveillance* is an approach that is being tested to examine trends in various syndromic criteria that may be suggestive of a bioterrorist attack. In theory, this method would provide a more rapid alert system than conventional reporting systems.[34] Ashford et al. reviewed CDC outbreak investigations, including non-U.S., for agents with a high potential for bioterrorism. Of the 1,099 investigations, healthcare providers and infection control practitioners reported 36.3% and health departments reported 30.5%. The lag time for reporting had a range of up to 26 days.[35] The CONPLAN highlights specific differences between an attack with weapons of mass destruction and other incidents, noting that the situation may not initially be recognizable until there are multiple casualties, and there may be multiple events with the intent to influence another event's outcome.[36] Thus, time to detection is critical for tainted food to be identified and the threat neutralized.

> **Syndromic surveillance—**
> Surveillance activities that enable early detection of epidemics with data analysis for patterns of prodromal illnesses including the use of medications, illness syndromes, or events.[37]

To combat these challenges, our vanguard of public health agencies must have the resources and structure to respond. However, as noted by a report of the Trust for America's Health, there are many concerns regarding public health preparedness, including insufficient funds; unspent federal aid; agencies unprepared for stockpiling; the exclusion of local agencies, which are unprepared for natural as well as bioterrorist threats; and a workforce crisis.[38] A GAO report of 2003 notes that state and local jurisdictions have requested additional guidance from the federal government on preparedness standards, and specifically cited the example of a state that had ceased testing for foodborne or waterborne diseases until more guidance was provided.[39]

Consumer Engagement

The third element of the triad is the engagement of individuals/consumers. Table 18-4 outlines some of the recommendations to consumers to raise awareness and direct action for food reserves and disaster plans in the event of a bioterrorism attack. For example, the Federal Emergency Management Agency (FEMA) has prepared both educational brochures describing personal preparation for emergencies and recommendations for specific items that should be stored in the event of an emergency. This material needs to be reviewed and revised based on simulations and surveys. Recommendations should be founded on the best in evidence-based medicine and practice.

TABLE 18-4   Food Biosecurity Triad: Consumer Engagement

	Activity/Message for Consumers	Recommendations Regarding Food Preparedness
Department of Homeland Security		
Ready.gov	"Preparing makes sense" • "Make a Kit • Make a Plan • Be Informed" Web information: http://www.ready.gov[79]	Make a Kit: Supply Checklists: "Emergency supplies of water, food and clean air Recommendations include: • Water—One gallon of water per person per day, for drinking and sanitation • Food—At least a 3-day supply of non-perishable food • Can opener for food • Infant formula, if you have an infant"
FEMA Shelters	"Toolkit for managing the emergency consequences of terrorist incidents" Guidelines for stocking shelters following a terrorist incident.[77]	Water: Quantity required: • 1–2 gallons per person per day for drinking (infants may need more) • 1–2 gallons per person per day for sanitation needs Possible source: • Bottled water companies • Soft-drink companies • National Guard Food: Quantity required: • Three 800- to 1000-calorie meals per person per day (prepackaged or hot) • A 4- to 7-day supply should be readily accessible. Possible source: • Red Cross suppliers • Salvation Army suppliers • Local fast food vendors • Existing supplies in school and church kitchens • Local food growers, farmers, and co-ops
Individuals and families	"Food and Water in an Emergency"[80]	Short-term (2 weeks) food supply Comments: • "Eat at least one well-balanced meal each day. • Drink enough liquid to enable your body to function properly (2 quarts per day) • Take in enough calories to enable you to do any necessary work

(Continues)

TABLE 18-4   Food Biosecurity Triad: Consumer Engagement (Continued)

		• Include vitamin, mineral and protein supplements in your stockpile to assure adequate nutrition."
		Other comments and recommendations:
		• "If activity is reduced, healthy people can survive on half their usual food intake for an extended period and without any food for many days. Food, unlike water, may be rationed safely, except for children and pregnant women."
	"Your Family Disaster Supplies Kit"[81]	Recommendations:
		Food: "Include a selection of the following foods in your Disaster Supplies Kit:
		• Ready-to-eat canned meats, fruits and vegetables
		• Canned juices, milk, soup (if powdered, store extra water)
		• Staples—sugar, salt, pepper
		• High-energy foods—peanut butter, jelly, crackers, granola bars, trail mix
		• Vitamins
		• Foods for infants, elderly persons or persons on special diets
		• Comfort/stress foods—cookies, hard candy, sweetened cereals, lollipops, instant coffee, tea bags."
		Other recommendations:
		• Practice and maintain your plan.
		Long-term (greater than 2 weeks)
		Food: "Store large amounts of staples along with a variety of canned and dried foods
		Stock the following amounts per person per month:
		• Wheat—20 pounds
		• Powdered milk (for babies and infants)— 20 pounds*
		• Corn—20 pounds
		• Iodized salt—1 pound
		• Soybeans—10 pounds
		• Vitamin C—15 gms"
		Supplies: A hand-cranked grain mill to grind the corn and wheat
Department of Health and Human Services		
FDA Center for Food Safety and Applied Nutrition	"Food Tampering: An Extra Ounce of Caution"[82]	Recommendations:
		• Examine food packaging.
		• Check anti-tampering devices.
		• Do not eat food from a package that appears damaged.

| U.S. **Department of Agriculture** | "Food Safety and Food Security: What Consumers Need to Know"[83] | Recommendations:
• Examine all food product packaging.
• Be aware of the normal appearance of food containers.
• Contact local health department or law enforcement agency if tampering is suspected and preserve the evidence.
"Most of the food safety practices already in place apply equally to intentional contamination."
To report unusual characteristics of meat, poultry, and egg products: USDA Meat and Poultry Hotline: 1-888-674-6854. |

*Families with infants should stock infant formula as opposed to powered milk.

Source: Compiled by the author.

However, should we consider individuals as active or passive partners in preparedness? Government agencies and food industries engage in preparedness activities (e.g., awareness, planning, surveillance, response, and recovery), but do individuals? As Figure 18-1 illustrates earlier in the chapter, physical and psychological consequences to the individual are antecedents to economic and political outcomes. So how well prepared are our citizens?

Most families have some stockpile of food on hand, although the suitability for use during a crisis may be limited. An ironic resource is our high prevalence of overweight and obesity, certainly a reserve of energy stores. With over 50% of our population overweight, we may analytically recognize that these individuals may be able to tolerate short-term food deprivation with the provision of water and vitamin and mineral supplements. However, although discomfort may be acceptable during intentional dieting, we know that the perception of risk is altered when the situation is not voluntary. The estimates of the amount of calories that may be necessary to sustain individuals during food shortages varies from the estimates for refugees of 2,100 calories per day[40] to the levels that were available in Biosphere 2, which was 1,780 calories per day.[41] FEMA currently recommends that shelters plan on providing 2,400–3,000 calories per person/per day. (See Table 18-4.) Certainly, the estimated needs will vary with energy expenditure. Are we prepared to convey messages to individuals to assist them in distinguishing discomfort from true risk?

Our current food culture has substantially lessened the need for food preparation skills and familiarity with raw foods. Yet, the foods recommended by FEMA for long-term food supply (greater than 2 weeks) includes grinding corn and wheat. What data should be gathered to provide insight into the utility of these recommendations? Food preparation skills are rapidly diminishing in our population. Do we have a mechanism for disseminating information in a time of crisis? The actual endpoint may be more related to psychological well-being than actual food intake.

There is a lack of survey and observational data on consumer reaction to a bioterrorist attack. One study examined a simulated attack and found that 50% of residents said they would compete for vaccine for themselves and their families, and 75% said they would comply with a rumor of quarantine and not try to leave.[42] Overall, the sample indicated that before the bioterrorism agent was identified and implications were known, they would put more trust in local sources of information; after the bioterrorism was confirmed, no single source of information was preferred. The sample size for this exercise was small (n = 39), but the issues raised are very important, and additional scenarios involving contaminated food are necessary.

Should we challenge ourselves and our neighbors to engage in food preparedness by conducting drills? We recognize the need for first responders and public health officials to be familiar with response processes, yet consumers do not have specific events to increase food biosecurity awareness. It may be beneficial to have a "vanguard" exercise periodically, such as the last week of June leading up to the Fourth of July. This exercise might serve to raise awareness, build skills, and engage in the preparedness process. Such an exercise may have specific goals such as:

- Review food and water supplies, including dating and circulating food stocks.
- Stockpile the appropriate amount of water and food for short-term needs.
- Include the preparation of one raw food during the vanguard period.
- Do a food safety check of the home.

These activities could be integrated with other measures to improve preparedness. Families may then be better prepared, both physically and psychologically, for a disruption in food availability that may actually have the most benefit during natural disasters. It would also be an opportunity to raise awareness and support of food banks.

Currently, our citizens are not prepared to make reasonable decisions on food biosecurity. Can these limitations be overcome with central planning and resources? How much physical and psychological damage can be diminished with preparedness, and, therefore, how much can we safeguard against economic and political consequences?

From Awareness to Security

The events of September 2001 have reshaped our national awareness of food safety related to the potential of a bioterrorism attack. The accomplishments to date have focused on critically vulnerable areas, but given the scope of the challenge, significant risks remain. As previously noted, the FDA has summarized our current situation by concluding that there is a high likelihood of an attack on the food supply.[43] Of additional concern is the potential for engineered bioweapons, which may increase the ability of a virus to kill infected cells, overcome vaccine-induced immunity, increase the agent's ability to survive environmental stress, and increase the potential for dissemination.[44] The technology required to produce such weapons is not obscure, and Smith et al. note that "The distinction between good biology and its 'dark side' lies only in intent and application."

Public health nutritionists possess skills and competencies to support preparedness at all levels, including community interventions and consumer outreach. Consider their didactic and experiential training in food safety, nutritional requirements, nutrition education, and food service management. Professional associations may play a pivotal role in raising awareness among these individuals that they may serve as responders should a foodborne bioweapon or chemical weapon be suspected or confirmed. Such resources are vital to preserve and sustain food security.

Issues for Discussion

1. How well-prepared are our communities to provide food to individuals in the event of an intentional attack on the food supply? In the event of an attack that compromises access to food? In the event of a quarantine?

2. What research is necessary to identify community and consumer capacity to use food on hand in the event of food shortages?

3. What priority should food security receive in public health preparedness efforts?

4. What level of investment is appropriate for security of the food supply, and who should provide the funding?

5. Are public health nutritionists involved in preparedness activities?

6. What role should nutrition professionals assume for risk assessment, surveillance, planning, response, and recovery in the event of an attack?

Terms Relevant to Public Health Preparedness

Agroterrorism—The deliberate introduction of a disease agent, either against livestock or into the food chain, for purposes of undermining the socioeconomic stability and/or generating fear.[45]

Biologic toxin—The toxic material of plants, animals, microorganisms, viruses, fungi, or infectious substances of a recombinant molecule, whatever its origin or method of production, including 1) any poisonous substance or biological product engineered as a result of biotechnology produced by a living organism; or 2) any poisonous isomer of biologic products, homolog, or derivative of such a substance.[46]

Carriers—Infected humans who can transmit contagious diseases to other humans.[47]

CDC: Bioterrorism Agents/Diseases

Category A

- Can be easily disseminated or transmitted from person to person
- Result in high mortality rates and have the potential for major public health impact
- Might cause public panic and social disruption
- Require special action for public health preparedness

Category B

- Are moderately easy to disseminate
- Result in moderate morbidity rates and low mortality rates
- Require specific enhancements of the CDC's diagnostic capacity and enhanced disease surveillance

Category C: Emerging pathogens that could be engineered for mass dissemination in the future because of availability, ease of production and dissemination, and potential for high morbidity and mortality rates and major health impact.[48]

Consequence management—Includes measures to protect public health and safety; restore essential government services; and provide emergency relief to governments, businesses, and individuals affected by the consequences of terrorism. A consequence management response will be managed by FEMA using structures and resources of the Federal Response Plan (FRP).[49]

Crisis management—Crisis management is predominantly a law enforcement function and includes measures to identify, acquire, and plan the use of resources needed to anticipate, prevent, and/or resolve a threat or act of terrorism.

Debarment—Authorizes the FDA to debar (prohibit from importing food) persons who have been convicted of a felony relating to the importation of any food or who have engaged in a pattern of importing adulterated food that presents a threat of serious adverse health consequences or death to humans or animals.[50]

Disaster field office (DFO)–The office established in or near the designated area to support federal and state response and recovery operations. The disaster field office houses the federal coordinating officer (FCO), the emergency response team, and, where possible, the state coordinating officer and support staff.

Emergency operations center (EOC)–The site from which civil government officials (municipal, county, state, and federal) exercise direction and control in an emergency.

Emergency public information–Information that is disseminated primarily in anticipation of an emergency or at the actual time of an emergency; in addition to providing information, it frequently directs actions, instructs, and transmits direct orders.

Emergency response team–A team composed of federal program and support personnel, which FEMA activates and deploys into an area affected by a major disaster or emergency.

Emergency support function–A functional area of response activity established to facilitate coordinated federal delivery of assistance required during the response phase to save lives, protect property and health, and maintain public safety.

Evacuation–Organized, phased, and supervised dispersal of civilians from dangerous or potentially dangerous areas, and their reception and care in safe areas.

Federal coordinating officer (FCO)–The person appointed by the FEMA director, following a declaration of a major disaster or of an emergency by the president, to coordinate federal assistance.

Federal Response Plan (FRP)–The plan designed to address the consequences of any disaster or emergency situation in which there is a need for federal assistance.

First responder–Local police, fire, and emergency medical personnel who first arrive on the scene of an incident and take action to save lives, protect property, and meet basic human needs.

Incubation period–The time between exposure and appearance of symptoms.

Infectivity–The ease with which a microorganism establishes itself in a host species.

Joint information center (JIC)–A center established to coordinate the federal public information activity on-scene.

Lead federal agency (LFA)–The agency designated by the president to lead and coordinate the overall federal response. It is determined by the type of emergency.

Local government–Any county, city, village, town, district, or political subdivision of any state, Indian tribe or authorized tribal organization, or Alaska Native village or organization, including any rural community or unincorporated town or village or any other public entity.

Mitigate—To cause to become less harsh or hostile; to make less severe or painful.[51]

Public information officer—Official at headquarters or in the field responsible for preparing and coordinating the dissemination of public information in cooperation with other responding federal, state, and local agencies.

Recovery plan—A plan developed by each state, with assistance from the responding federal agencies, to restore the affected area.

Regional director—The director of one of FEMA's 10 regional offices and principal representative for working with other federal regions, state and local governments, and the private sector in that jurisdiction.

Regional operations center (ROC)—The temporary operations facility for the coordination of federal response and recovery activities, located at the FEMA regional office.

State coordinating officer—An official designated by the governor of the affected state, upon a declaration of a major disaster or emergency, to coordinate state and local disaster assistance efforts with those of the federal government, and to act in cooperation with the FCO to administer disaster recovery efforts.

Toxicity—The relative severity of the illness or incapacitation produced by a toxin.

Trace backward—Retailers, wholesalers, carriers, and others who have received products from federally inspected meat, poultry, or egg processing establishments should be able to identify the source of the products quickly and efficiently.[52]

Trace forward—Shippers (including operators of federally inspected meat, poultry, and egg processing establishments) and carriers should have systems in place for quickly and effectively locating products that have been distributed to wholesalers and retailers.[52]

Transmissibility—The ease with which disease is transmitted by victims. Methods may be direct (personal contact), indirect (through material contaminated by the infected person), or secondary (through particles spread by coughing or sneezing).

Vectors—Infected animals or insects that serve as hosts to the organism.

Weaponization for aerosol—As it pertains to the use of anthrax as a bioterrorist weapon, this generally involves use of a small particle size, a high concentration of spores, treatment to reduce clumping, neutralization of the electrical charge, and use of antimicrobial-resistant strains or genetic modification of the organism to increase virulence or escape vaccine protection.[53]

Weapon of mass destruction (WMD)—Any device, material, or substance used in a manner, in a quantity or type, or under circumstances evidencing an intent to cause death or serious injury to persons or significant damage to property.

References

1. Osterholm MT, Schwartz J. *Living Terrors: What America Needs to Know to Survive the Coming Bioterrorist Catastrophe*. New York, NY: Dalacort Press; 2000.

2. Sobel J, Khan AS, Swerdlow DL. Threat of a biological terrorist attack on the U.S. food supply: The CDC perspective. *Lancet*. 2002;359: 874–880.

3. Torok TJ, Tauxe RV, Wise RB, et al. A large community outbreak of salmonellosis caused by intentional contamination of restaurant salad bars. *JAMA*. 1997;278:389–395.

4. Center for Food Safety and Applied Nutrition, Food and Drug Administration. Risk Assessment for Food Terrorism and Other Food Safety Concerns. October 7, 2003. Available at: http://www.cfsan.fda.gov/~dms/rabtact.html. Accessed March 13, 2004.

5. Wheelis M. Agricultural Biowarfare & Bioterrorism: An Analytical Framework & Recommendations for the Fifth BTWC Review Conference. Available at: http://www.fas.org/bwc/agr/goals.htm. Accessed July 26, 2002.

6. Halliday ML, et al. An epidemic of hepatitis A attributable to the ingestion of raw clams in Shanghai China. *J Infect Dis*. 1991;164:852–859.

7. Center for Food Safety and Applied Nutrition, Food and Drug Administration. Risk Assessment for Food Terrorism and Other Food Safety Concerns. October 7, 2003. Available at: http://www.cfsan.fda.gov/~dms/rabtact.html. Accessed March 13, 2004.

8. Hall MJ, Norwood AE, Ursao RJ, Fullerton CS: The Psychological Impacts of Bioterrorism. *Biosecurity and Bioterrorism: Biodefense Strategy, Practice, and Science*. 2003;1:139–144.

9. Committee on Responding to the Psychological Consequences of Terrorism, National Research Council. *Preparing for the Psychological Consequences of Terrorism: A Public Health Strategy*. Washington, DC: National Academy Press; 2003.

10. Chalk P. *Hitting America's Soft Underbelly: The Potential Threat of Deliberate Biological Attacks Against the U.S. Agricultural and Food Industry*. Santa Monica, Calif.: RAND Publications; 2004.

11. U.S. Department of Agriculture, National Agricultural Statistics Service. Trends in U.S. Agriculture. Available at: http://www.usda.gov/nass/pubs/stathigh/2003/crops.pdf. Accessed March 27, 2004.

12. U.S. Department of Commerce, Bureau of Economic Analysis. Gross Domestic Product and Corporate Profits. Available at: http://www.bea.gov/bea/newsrel/gdpnewsrelease.htm. Accessed April 23, 2005.

13. Strongin RJ. *How Vulnerable Is the Nation's Food Supply? Linking Food Safety and Food Security*. The George Washington University, National Health Policy Forum Issue Brief No. 773; May 17, 2002.

14. National Restaurant Association. Restaurant Industry Facts. Available at: http://www.restaurant.org/research/ind_glance.cfm. Accessed April 10, 2004.

15. Food Marketing Institute. Supermarket Facts: Industry Overview 2003. Available at: http://www.fmi.org/facts_figs/superfact.htm. Accessed April 23, 2005.

16. Neff J. Food industry deals with crisis: from disruptions to previously unimaginable threats, the food industry braces for a new reality post-Sept. 11. *Food Processing* 2001; Nov 2.

17. Nestle M. *Safe Food: Bacteria, Biotechnology, and Bioterrorism.* Berkeley, Calif.: University of California Press; 2003.

18. Trevejo RT, Courtney JG, Starr M, Vugia DJ. Epidemiology of salmonellosis in California, 1990–1999: Morbidity, mortality, and hospitalization costs. *Am J Epidemiol.* 2003;157:48–57.

19. Center for Food Safety and Applied Nutrition. Food and Drug Administration. Risk Assessment for Food Terrorism and Other Food Safety Concerns. Available at: http://www.cfsan.fda.gov/(dms/rabtact.html. Accessed May 7, 2004.

20. Meadows M. The FDA and the fight against terrorism. *FDA Consumer Mag.* January-February 2004: Available at: http://www.fda.gov/fdac/features/2004/104_terror.html. Accessed April 23, 2005.

21. Federal Bureau of Investigation. U.S. Government Interagency Domestic Terrorism Concept of Operations Plan. January 2001. Available at: http://www.fbi.gov/publications/conplan/conplan.pdf. Accessed March 22, 2004.

22. Rotz LD, Khan AS, Lillibridge SR, Ostroff SM, Hughes JM. Public health assessment of potential biological terrorism agents. *CDC Emerging Infect Dis.* 2002;8(2). Available at: http://www.cdc.gov/ncidod/EID/vol8no2/01-0164.htm. Accessed April 12, 2005.

23. Federal Emergency Management Agency. Toolkit for Managing the Emergency Consequences of Terrorist Incidents. Available at: http://www.fema.gov/onp/toolkit.shtm. Accessed August 14, 2003.

24. Institute of Medicine. Biological Threats and Terrorism: Assessing the Science and Response Capabilities: Workshop Summary. 2002. Available at: http://www.nap.edu/openbook/0309082536/html/43.html. Accessed April 12, 2005.

25. Committee on Science and Technology for Countering Terrorism, National Research Council. *Making the Nation Safer, the Role of Science and Technology in Countering Terrorism.* Washington, DC: National Academy Press; 2002.

26. U.S. Department of Agriculture, Food Safety and Inspection Service. Protecting America's Meat, Poultry, and Egg Products: A Report to the Secretary on the Food Security Accomplishments of the Food Safety and Inspection Service, 2003. April 2004. Available at: http://www.fsis.usda.gov/PDF/Food_Security_Accomplishments_2003.pdf. Accessed April 23, 2005.

27. U.S. Department of Agriculture, Food Safety Inspection Service. Keynote Address, Taking Food Safety and HACCP to a New Level. May 17, 2002. Available at: http://www.fsis.usda.gov/OA/speeches/2002/mp_haccp.htm. Accessed April 23, 2005.

28. Bledsoe GE, Rasco BA. Addressing the risk of bioterrorism in food production. *Food Technol.* 2002;56:43–47.

29. Government Accounting Office. *Bioterrorism: A Threat to Agriculture and the Food Supply.* Testimony Before the Committee on Governmental Affairs, U.S. Senate. November 19, 2003. Washington, DC: GAO. GAO-04-259T.

30. Strongin RJ. How vulnerable is the nation's food supply? Linking food safety and food security. *Nat Health Policy Forum.* 2002;773:2–22.

31. Dyckman LJ. *Federal Food Safety and Security System: Fundamental Restructuring Is Needed to Address Fragmentation and Overlap.* Testimony Before the Subcommittee on Civil Service and Agency Organization, Committee on Government Reform, House of Representatives. Washington, DC: Government Accounting Office; March 30, 2004. GAO-04-588T.

32. Food and Drug Administration. FDA Science Board Advisory Committee. November 6, 2003. Available at: http://www.fda.gov/ohrms/dockets/ac/03/transcripts/4001t1.txt. Accessed May 7, 2004.

33. Sobel J, Khan AS, Swerdlow DL. Threat of a biological terrorist attack on the U.S. food supply: The CDC perspective. *Lancet.* 2002;359:874–880.

34. Buehler JW, Berkelman RL, Hartley DM, Peters CJ. Syndromic surveillance and bioterrorism-related epidemics. *Emerging Infect Dis.* 2003;9(10). Available at: http://www.cdc.gov/ncidod/EID/vol9no10/03-0231.htm. Accessed April 4, 2004.

35. Ashford DA, Kaiser RM, Bales ME, et al. Planning against biological terrorism: Lessons from outbreak investigations. *Emerging Infect Dis.* 2003;9:515–519.

36. Federal Bureau of Investigation. U.S. Government Interagency Domestic Terrorism Concept of Operations Plan. January 2001. Available at: http://www.fbi.gov/publications/conplan/conplan.pdf. Accessed March 22, 2004.

37. Buehler JW, Berkelman RL, Hartley DM, Peters CJ: Syndromic surveillance and bioterrorism-related epidemics. 9 *Emerg Infect Dis* (October 2003). Available at: http://www.cdc.gov/ncidod/EID/vol9no10/03-0231.htm. Accessed April 4, 2004.

38. Trust for America's Health. Ready or Not? Protecting the Public's Health in the Age of Bioterrorism. December 2003. Available at: http://www.healthyamericans.org. Accessed March 14, 2004.

39. General Accounting Office. *Bioterrorism: Preparedness Varied across State and Local Jurisdictions.* Report to Congressional Committees. Washington, DC: GAO; April 2003. GAO-03-373.

40. UN News Service, Relief Web. UN Appeals for $10 Million to Feed Refugees in Ethiopia This Year. February 24, 2004. Available at: http://www.reliefweb.int/w/rwb.nsf/s/42DD226AEE3B209285256E440069149D. Accessed March 28, 2004.

41. Walford RL, Harris SB, Gunion MW. The calorically restricted low-fat nutrient-dense diet in Biosphere 2 significantly lowers blood glucose, total leukocyte count, cholesterol, and blood pressure in humans. *Proc Natl Acad Sci.* 1992;89:11533–11537.

42. DiGiovanni C, Reynolds B, Harwell R, Stonecipher EB, Burkle FM. Community reaction to bioterrorism: Prospective study of simulated outbreak. *Emerging Infect Dis.* 2003;9:708–712.

43. Center for Food Safety and Applied Nutrition, Food and Drug Administration. Risk Assessment for Food Terrorism and Other Food Safety Concerns. October 7, 2003. Available at: http://www.cfsan.fda.gov/~dms/rabtact.html. Accessed March 13, 2004.

44. Smith BT, Inglesby TV, O'Toole T. Biodefense R&D: Anticipating future threats, establishing a strategic environment. *Biosecurity and Bioterrorism: Biodefense Strategy, Practice, and Science.* 2003;1:193–202.

45. Chalk, P. *Hitting America's Soft Underbelly: The Potential Threat of Deliberate Biological Attacks Against the U.S. Agricultural and Food Industry.* Santa Monica, Calif: RAND; 2004.

46. Food and Drug Administration. Chemical and Biological Emergency Response Plan. Available at: http://www.fda.gov/oc/ocm/cbplan.html. Accessed May 7, 2004.

47. Federal Emergency Management Agency. Toolkit for Managing the Emergency Consequences of Terrorist Incidents. Appendix A—Biological Weapons. July 2002. Available at: http://www.fema.gov/onp/toolkit.shtm. Accessed August 14, 2003.

48. Centers for Disease Control and Prevention. Emergency Preparedness & Response. Available at: http://www.bt.cdc.gov/agent/agentlist-category.asp. Accessed April 4, 2004.

49. Federal Bureau of Investigations. U.S. Government Interagency Domestic Terrorism Concept of Operations Plan. January 2001. Available at: http://www.fbi.gov/publications/conplan/conplan.pdf. Accessed March 22, 2004.

50. Food and Drug Administration. The Bioterrorism Act of 2002: Title III. Protecting safety and security of food and drug supply. Available at: http://www.fda.gov/oc/bioterrorism/PL107-188.html#title3. Accessed April 19, 2004.

51. U.S. Department of Homeland Security. From the U.S. Department of Homeland Security. Available at: http://www.ready.gov. Accessed May 7, 2004.

52. U.S. Department of Agriculture, Food Safety and Inspection Service. FSIS Safety and Security Guidelines for the Transportation and Distribution of Meat, Poultry, and Egg Products. Available at: http://www.fsis.usda.gov/oa/topics/transportguide_text_aug.pdf. Accessed April 15, 2005.

53. Center for Infectious Disease Research and Policy (CIDRAP) and the Infectious Diseases Society of America. *Anthrax Medical Summary* Available at: http://www.idsociety.org/Content/ContentGroups/Bioterrorism_Resources/Anthrax/Anthrax_Medical_Summary.htm#_Epidemiology:_Weaponized_Anthrax_1. Accessed April 23, 2005.

54. Federal Emergency Management Agency. Toolkit for Managing the Emergency Consequences of Terrorist Incidents. July 2002. Available at: http://www.fema.gov/onp/toolkit.shtm. Accessed August 14, 2003.

55. Centers for Disease Control and Prevention. Emergency Preparedness & Response; Bioterrorism Agents/Diseases. Available at: http://www.bt.cdc.gov/agent/agentlist-category.asp. Accessed April 2, 2004.

56. National Library of Medicine, Specialized Information Services. Biological Warfare. Available at: http://sis.nlm.nih.gov/Tox/biological-warfare.htm. Accessed March 23, 2004.

57. Mead PS, Slutsker L, Dietz V, et al. Food-related illness and death in the United States. *CDC Emerg Infect Dis.* 2000;5. Available at: http://www.cdc.gov/ncidod/eid/vol5no5/mead.htm. Accessed April 12, 2005.

58. Centers for Disease Control and Prevention. Fact Sheet: Anthrax Information for Healthcare Providers. Available at: http://www.bt.cdc.gov/agent/anthrax/anthrax-hcp-factsheet.asp. Accessed April 23, 2005.

59. Federal Emergency Management Agency. Toolkit for Managing the Emergency Consequences of Terrorist Incidents. July 2002. Available at: http://www.fema.gov/onp/toolkit.shtm. Accessed August 14, 2003.

60. Centers for Disease Control and Prevention. Botulism, General Information. Available at: http://www.cdc.gov/ncidod/dbmd/diseaseinfo/botulism_g.htm. Accessed April 2, 2004.

61. Centers for Disease Control and Prevention. Anthrax: Diagnosis/Evaluation (Signs and Symptoms). Available at: http://www.bt.cdc.gov/agent/anthrax/diagnosis/index.asp. Accessed April 2, 2004.

62. Center for Infectious Disease Research and Policy. Initial Assessment of Food System Biosecurity Threats. Available at: http://www.cidrap.umn.edu/cidrap/content/biosecurity/food-biosec/threats/assess.html. Accessed March 22, 2004.

63. Centers for Disease Control and Prevention. Questions and Answers About Plague. Available at: http://www.cdc.gov/ncidod/dvbid/plague/qa.htm. Accessed April 2, 2004.

64. National Library of Medicine, Specialized Information Services. Biological Warfare. Available at: http://sis.nlm.nih.gov/Tox/biological-warfare.htm. Accessed March 23, 2004.

65. Centers for Disease Control and Prevention. Tularemia, Frequently Asked Questions About Tularemia. Available at: http://www.bt.cdc.gov/agent/tularemia/faq.asp. Accessed April 23, 2005.

66. Federal Emergency Management Agency. Toolkit for Managing the Emergency Consequences of Terrorist Incidents. July 2002. Available at: http://www.fema.gov/onp/toolkit.shtm. Accessed August 14, 2003.

67. National Library of Medicine, Specialized Information Services. Biological Warfare. Available at: http://sis.nlm.nih.gov/Tox/biological-warfare.htm. Accessed March 23, 2004.

68. Centers for Disease Control and Prevention. Brucellosis, Technical Information. Available at: http://www.cdc.gov/ncidod/dbmd/disease-info/brucellosis_t.htm. Accessed April 2, 2004.

69. Center for Infectious Disease Research and Policy. Initial Assessment of Food System Biosecurity Threats. Available at: http://www.cidrap.umn.edu/cidrap/content/biosecurity/food-biosec/threats/assess.html. Accessed March 22, 2004.

70. Centers for Disease Control and Prevention. Salmonellosis, General Information. Available at: http://www.cdc.gov/ncidod/dbmd/diseaseinfo/salmonellosis_g.htm. Accessed April 2, 2004.

71. Centers for Disease Control and Prevention. Escherichia Coli O157:H7, General Information. Available at: http://www.cdc.gov/ncidod/dbmd/diseaseinfo/escherichiacoli_g.htm. Accessed April 2, 2004.

72. Centers for Disease Control and Prevention. Shigellosis, General Information. Available at: http://www.cdc.gov/ncidod/dbmd/diseaseinfo/shigellosis_g.htm. Accessed April 2, 2004.

73. Federal Emergency Management Agency. Toolkit for Managing the Emergency Consequences of Terrorist Incidents. July 2002. Available at: http://www.fema.gov/onp/toolkit.shtm. Accessed August 14, 2003.

74. National Library of Medicine, Specialized Information Services. Biological Warfare. Available at: http://sis.nlm.nih.gov/Tox/ biologicalwarfare.htm. Accessed March 23, 2004.

75. Center for Infectious Disease Research and Policy. Initial Assessment of Food System Biosecurity Threats. Available at: http://www.cidrap.umn.edu/cidrap/content/biosecurity/food-biosec/ threats/assess.html. Accessed March 22, 2004.

76. Mead PS, Slutsker L, Dietz V, et al. Food-related illness and death in the United States. *CDC Emerg Infect Dis.* 2000;5. Available at: http:// www.cdc.gov/ncidod/eid/vol5no5/mead.htm. Accessed April 13, 2005.

77. Federal Emergency Management Agency. Toolkit for Managing the Emergency Consequences of Terrorist Incidents. July 2002. Available at: http://www.fema.gov/onp/toolkit.shtm. Accessed August 14, 2003.

78. U.S. Department of Agriculture, Food Safety and Inspection Service. Protecting America's Meat, Poultry, and Egg Products: A Report to the Secretary on the Food Security Accomplishments of the Food Safety and Inspection Service, 2003. April 2004. Available at: http://www.fsis.usda.gov. Accessed May 7, 2004.

79. U.S. Department of Homeland Security. Ready.gov. Available at: http://www.ready.gov. Accessed May 7, 2004.

80. Federal Emergency Management Agency. Food and Water in an Emergency. Available at: http://www.fema.gov/rrr/foodwtr.shtm. Accessed May 7, 2004.

81. Federal Emergency Management Agency. Your Family Disaster Supplies Kit. Available at: http://www.fema.gov/library/diskit.shtm. Accessed April 23, 2005.

82. Center for Food Safety and Applied Nutrition, Food and Drug Administration. Food Tampering: An Extra Ounce of Caution. Available at: http://www.cfsan.fda.gov/~dms/fstamper.html. Accessed December 22, 2003.

83. Food Safety and Inspection Service, U.S. Department of Agriculture. Food Safety and Food Security: What Consumers Need to Know. Available at: http://www.usda.gov. Accessed March 27, 2004.

PART VI

MANAGING THE SYSTEM

Chapter 19 Planning and Evaluating
Nutrition Services for the Community
Julie M. Moreschi, MS, RD, LDN

Chapter 20 Managing Data
Elizabeth Barden, PhD

Chapter 21 Managing Money
Katherine Cairns, MPH, MBA, RD

Part VI provides the reader with fundamental information about public health nutrition funding. Chapter 19 details how nutrition services are planned and evaluated so that effective programs can be implemented to result in positive performance and financial outcomes. In order to evaluate the effectiveness and cost of a program, data must be collected and managed appropriately, as discussed in Chapter 20. Finally, Chapter 21 contains a discussion about how money is managed, which will help the reader take public health nutrition from funding to appropriations.

PLANNING AND EVALUATING NUTRITION SERVICES FOR THE COMMUNITY

Julie M. Moreschi, MS, RD, LDN

Reader Objectives

After studying this chapter and reflecting on the contents, you should be able to:

1. Define planning.
2. List the types of planning.
3. Discuss the need for and advantages of planning.
4. Discuss the history of health education planning models.
5. Understand the steps of planning using a variety of models.
6. Understand the elements of program implementation.
7. List the value of a planning group, and identify the potential membership.
8. Describe why program evaluation is essential.
9. Discuss program impact evaluation.
10. Discuss cost-effectiveness evaluation.

What Is Planning?

What is planning? Why is planning of tremendous relevance to a public health nutritionist's success? This chapter will help you expand your ability to answer these questions, and you will be able to use the concepts presented here to enhance your work performance in this essential management area.

Planning refers to the management function that involves setting goals and deciding the best route for achieving them. In essence, planning deals with the what, where, when, and how of management. It focuses on solving problems and planning for events in the future. Planning is continuous. It involves following certain steps, and proceeding with these steps in a logical, preset manner. (See Figure 19-1.) When planning, an organization considers several options before choosing the final route to reaching its desired outcomes.

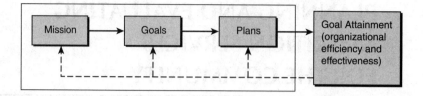

FIGURE 19-1   The Planning Process
Source: Reprinted with permission from Bartol, K. M. & Martin, D. C. 1994.
Management (1st CPCU ed.). McGraw-Hill, Inc. North America.

Types of Planning

There are three main types of planning in public health: strategic, long-term (planning that addresses an organization's overall goals and usually encompasses 3–5 years), and operational (short-term, and deals with the activities required to meet the organization's goals).

A public health nutritionist is involved in all three of the types of planning listed here. Of the three types of planning, the nutrition professional in public health is most often involved in program/project management. Program/project management can occur in any of the three types of planning listed previously. Thus, the majority of this chapter will focus on the planning, implementation, and evaluation aspects of this form of planning.

A great deal of data are available regarding the health status of the U.S. population. Many of the health issues affecting this population can be significantly improved by nutrition and lifestyle changes; thus, the public health nutritionist may find him- or herself creating and implementing programs to impact these relevant and profound health concerns.

For example, in 2001 the three leading causes of death in the United States, as reported by the National Center for Health Statistics, were diseases of the heart, malignant neoplasm, and cerebrovascular diseases, as discussed in previous chapters. The top three risk factors that contribute to the leading causes of death in the United States are smoking, alcohol consumption, and poor nutrition/diet (Timmereck, 2003). Therefore, health promotion and disease prevention activities could substantially impact on unnecessary illness and death. In addition, a public health nutritionist could be involved in implementing programs relevant to achieving the objectives of Healthy People 2010. Planning is essential in the implementation of programs that answer the call to reduce or eliminate these particular healthcare problems.

As discussed in Chapter 3, when conducting a needs assessment in the community, a public health nutritionist may discover certain nutritional issues that trigger the need for program planning. The following are some program planning tasks:

- Assess the needs of the target population
- Identify the problem(s)
- Develop appropriate goals and objectives
- Create an intervention that is likely to achieve desired results
- Implement the intervention
- Evaluate the results

The process of program planning can provide several advantages to an organization. Some of these advantages include:

- Consensus and prioritization regarding organizational goals
- Identification of key membership relative to the project
- Development of specific, measurable objectives
- Identification of steps necessary to reach the established goals
- Sharing task completion among all project members
- Setting specific target dates for task completion
- Focusing on outcomes that will impact the population being served

In conclusion, planning focuses on approaching work in an organized and defined manner. This results in positive outcomes for employees, managers, and the members of the community that are served.

History in Health Education Planning

When approaching public health planning, organizations have no shortage of available models to consider as resources and for potential adoption into their facilities. This fact is illustrated in a 1995 article written by Carol Campbell of the Mississippi Cooperative Extension Service. In her article, titled "Health Education Planning Models—A Review of the Literature, Part II," Campbell shares models that have been used in a variety of settings and that have resulted in some degree of success. Campbell also suggests a generic set of tasks that are necessary to planning, regardless of the model selected or designed (Campbell, 1995) (see Table 19-1).

A discussion of all of the models that Campbell reviews is beyond the scope of this chapter. However, two models, PRECEDE-PROCEED and APEXPH/PATCH, will be briefly reviewed in the following sections.

TABLE 19-1   Health Education Planning Models

Planning Model	Author	Year Developed
Comprehensive Health Education Model	Sullivan	1973
Model of Health Education Planning	Ross & Mico	1980
The PRECEDE Framework	Green, et al.	1980
Model for Health Education Planning and Resource Development	Bates & Winder	1984
Generic Health/Fitness Delivery System	Patton, Corry, Gettman, & Graf	1986
Community Wellness Model	Jenkins	1991
The PRECEDE-PROCEED Model	Green & Keuter	1991
The PEN-3 MODEL	Airhihenbuwa	1992
APEXPH and PATCH	Centers for Disease Control & Prevention	1993
Formative Evaluation, Consultation, and Systems Technique	Goodman & Wandersman	1994

Source: Compiled by author from Campbell, C. 1995. *Health Education Planning Models—A Review of the Literature, Part II.* Mississippi Cooperative Extension Service.

PRECEDE-PROCEED

PRECEDE-PROCEED is a nine-phase planning model designed by Lawrence Green and Marshall Kreuter (see Figure 19-2). Green and Kreuter's overriding principle in this model is that most lasting health behavior change is voluntary in nature and must include input from the individual. This principle is reflected in a methodical planning process, which empowers individuals with understanding, motivation, skills, and active engagement in community affairs to improve their quality of life. The model begins with the end or final consequence and works back to the causes. PRECEDE is the diagnostic and needs assessment phase; the acronym stands for *Predisposing, Reinforcing, and Enabling Constructs in Educational/Environmental Diagnosis and Evaluation.* The PROCEED element of this model refers to the developmental stage of planning and begins the implementation and evaluation process. The acronym PROCEED stands for *Policy, Regulatory, and Organizational Constructs in Educational and Environmental Development.*

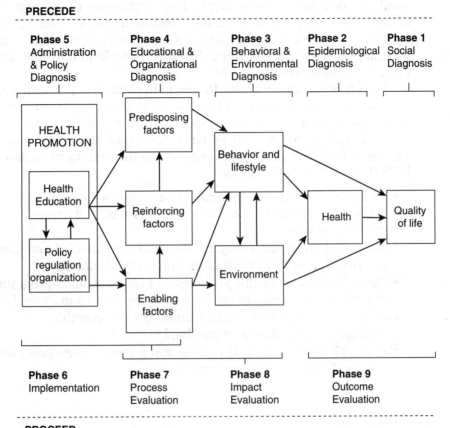

FIGURE 19-2 PRECEDE-PROCEED Planning Model
Source: Reprinted with permission from Robert S. Gold, PhD, DrPH, MACRO International, Inc.; Lawrence W. Green, DrPH, University of British Columbia; & Marshall W. Kreuter. 1998. *EMPOWER: Enabling Methods of Planning and Organizing Within Everyone's Reach.* Sudbury, MA: Jones & Bartlett Publishers.

APEXPH and PATCH

Assessment Protocol for Excellence in Public Health (APEXPH) and Planned Approach To Community Health (PATCH) are two planning processes developed by the Centers for Disease Control (CDC). APEXPH was designed for use by local public health departments, and a workbook is available to assist in implementing the program. The program consists of three major parts:

- *Part I:* Organizational capacity assessment
- *Part II:* The community process
- *Part III:* Completing the cycle

In Part I, the public health department conducts a self-assessment and determines the strengths and weaknesses of the organization in meeting the community's health needs. In Part II, the community health needs are assessed and health status goals and program objectives are defined. In Part III, basic monitoring and evaluation tools are established.

PATCH is a model intended for use in implementing chronic disease prevention and health promotion programs. PATCH was originally established in the mid-1980s with good results; in 1993, APEXPH was introduced to enhance the existing PATCH model. Similar to PRECEDE, the model begins with the individual in mind. PATCH incorporates five phases:

- *Phase I:* Mobilize the community—a group is formed to define the community, address health issues, and create working groups.
- *Phase II:* Collect and analyze data—data are collected and used to determine health priorities and program planning.
- *Phase III:* Choose health priorities and target groups—program objectives and goals are established using data from Phase II.
- *Phase IV:* Choose and conduct interventions—health interventions are designed and implemented.
- *Phase V:* Evaluate PATCH process and interventions—programs and the PATCH process are evaluated.

Planning Models

Public health nutritionists may wish to have a variety of planning models to choose from when implementing public health programs. A variety of models may be needed due to the nature of the project, or a nutritionist and/or the project team may embrace the concepts of one model over another. Four models will be shared in this chapter. These four models provide a starting framework from which you can begin to enhance your planning capabilities.

The 10-Step Planning Model

The first model that will be reviewed is the 10-step planning model, developed by Thomas C. Timmreck, PhD, in his book *Planning, Program Development, and Evaluation.* This chapter will provide a brief overview of the 10-step model, but you will find additional detailed suggestions and guidance by reviewing Timmreck's entire text.

Step 1 focuses on the development of the mission statement, or the information that details the overall direction and purpose of the organization. You can write a strong mission statement by considering the following elements: purpose, function, structure, legitimacy, and tangibility.

Step 2 encompasses the completion of an organization and community assessment. In this step, the organization must collect and evaluate data regarding internal and external factors, resources, regulations, and policies that might affect the feasibility and success of the program being considered for development.

Step 3 and Step 6 focus on the development of program goals and objectives. Step 3 establishes the goals and objectives for needs assessment and feasibility studies, and Step 6 focuses on the project goal and objective development. Goals are defined as a quantified statement of a desired future state or condition; they are generally long-term and have no deadline associated with them. Objectives are defined as any statement of short-term, measurable, specific activity having a specific time limit or timeline for completion. To attain objectives, you must develop a plan of action. Action steps lead to objective accomplishments, which lead to goal attainment. Precision and focus in writing high-quality goals and objectives can make the difference between a program that succeeds and one that fails.

Step 4 deals with the completion of a community needs assessment. The needs assessment must focus on collecting data regarding an established target population. Important decisions to be made when conducting Step 4 include what data to collect, what tool to use to collect the data, and how the data will be analyzed. Revisit Chapter 3 to refresh your memory about needs assessments.

Once data are collected and analyzed, Step 5 focuses on methods to assist in setting priorities. There are multiple factors in the community that influence prioritization decisions, such as people, politics, and finances. A public health nutritionist can use a variety of decision-making tools and techniques to assist in making sound prioritization decisions.

Step 7 helps determine the activities and procedures that need to be performed in order to implement the programs. Factors that need to be considered are the actions that need to take place and the order in which they should occur. Pilot projects to test certain actions may be warranted prior to large-scale implementation. Managerial elements, such as financial and marketing strategies, need to be considered and planned. Once activities are established in this step, timelines are assigned to each item in Step 8.

Step 9 and Step 10 deal with implementation and evaluation, respectively. These planning elements will be discussed in detail later in the chapter.

The P Process Model

The second planning model to be discussed is Johns Hopkins University Center for Communication Program's P Process. (See Figure 19-3.) The P Process provides a framework for the development of strategic health communication programs. The process was developed in 1982 and was used to help design effective communication projects for behavior change. The P Process can be used when developing:

- Project and program design
- Workshops and classes
- Brochures, reports, manuals, posters, presentations, and publications

The five steps in the P Process are described in further detail in the following sections.

Step 1: Analysis

Two types of analysis should be considered: situation and audience/communication. Situation analysis refers to determining the severity and causes of problems, identifying factors inhibiting or facilitating desired changes, developing a problem statement, and carrying out formation research that takes the learners' needs and priorities into consideration. Audience/communication analysis focuses on conducting a participation analysis to identify partners, audiences, and field workers for the project, carrying out a social and behavioral analysis at the community and individual level, and assessing communication and training needs.

Step 2: Strategic Design

Step 2 deals with developing a strategic design for the project. Elements of this step include establishing clear objectives, developing program approaches, determining marketing channels, and creating implementation and evaluation plans.

Step 3: Development and Testing

The development and testing phase is where the actual program or project is developed. It is then revised as needed before full implementation. This step should not only consider the technical and scientific accuracy of the products, but also must include an element of creativity in order to better reach and engage the participants.

Step 4: Implementation and Monitoring

Implementation and monitoring deals with taking the product and disseminating it throughout the target population's community. This phase may incorporate some training or development of personnel delivering the program. The program must be monitored and changes made as necessary to assure a high-quality product.

Step 5: Evaluation and Replanning

The final step in the P Process is the evaluation and replanning phase. During this step, outcomes are measured and future needs are assessed. Programs are redesigned and revised as needed based on data collected during this phase. Outcomes during this phase may warrant that the project begin again at Step 1, the analysis phase.

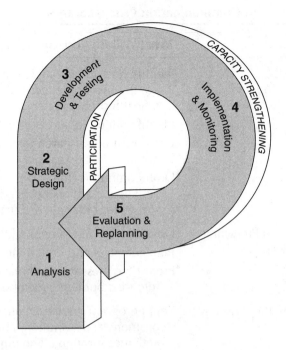

FIGURE 19-3 The P Process
Source: Reprinted with permission from *Health Communication*, Piotrow et al. Praeger, 1997, p. 27, and Health Communication Partnership (December 2003), Johns Hopkins Bloomberg School of Public Health. Available at: http://www.jhuccp.org/training/scope/Pprocess.htm.

The Health Communication Process

The Health Communication Process is a planning model developed by the U.S. Department of Health & Human Services, the National Institutes for Health (NIH), and the National Cancer Institute (NCI). The model was first designed in 1985, and for almost 25 years an ongoing evaluation of the communication programs has confirmed the value of using specific communication strategies to promote health and prevent disease. A reader can obtain a copy of the 250+ page *Making Health Communication Programs Work* by visiting NCI on the Web at http://cancer.gov/pinkbook/ or calling NCI's Cancer Information Service.

The Health Communication Process has four stages. Upon completion of each stage, the planners can expect to accomplish the goals shown in Table 19-2.

The Action for Healthy Kids Planning Process

Action for Healthy Kids (AFHK) is a nationwide initiative focused on improving the nutrition and fitness levels of children in the United States. A complete planning guide for AFHK state team members is available online at http://www.actionforhealthykids.org

TABLE 19-2   Health Communication Process Stages

Stage	What Will Be Accomplished?
1. Planning and Strategy Development	Identify how the organization can use communication effectively to address a health problem.
	Identify intended audiences.
	Use consumer research to create a communication strategy and objectives.
	Draft communication plans, including activities, partnerships, and baseline survey for outcome evaluation.
2. Developing and Pretesting Concepts, Messages, and Materials	Develop relevant, meaningful messages.
	Plan activities and draft materials.
	Pretest the messages and materials with intended audience members.
3. Implementing the Program	Begin program implementation, maintaining promotion, distribution, and other activities through all channels.
	Conduct process evaluation via tracking intended audience exposure and reaction to the program. Determine whether adjustments are needed.
	Periodically review all program elements and make revisions as needed.
4. Assessing Effectiveness and Making Refinements	Assess your health communication program.
	Identify refinements that would increase the effectiveness of future programs.

Source: Compiled by the author.

for use in the development of statewide action plans focused on improving children's health and well-being.

The AFHK planning process, used in the development of its programs, consists of nine components (see Figure 19-4). The planning guide provides a public health nutritionist with guidance and tools to progress through each step of the process. The nine components and a brief description of each are as follows:

1. Understanding the commitment to change:
   - Teams should discuss the commitment to change that should occur during team membership and what it means to the individuals and organization represented in the group.

- Teams should understand that their task is to establish goals that will advance two or more of the AFHK initiatives.
- Teams should understand that their task is to establish goals that will make an impact in the areas of nutrition and fitness.

2. Team members and orientation:

Recruitment

- Teams should decide if their teams are complete, or whether they should develop and implement an outreach strategy to identify and recruit additional members.
- Teams should identify a member who will take responsibility for ensuring that new members are incorporated into the team.

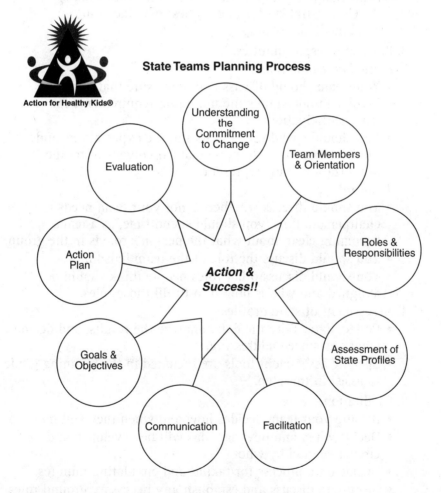

FIGURE 19-4   AFHK State Teams Planning Process
Source: Reprinted from www.ActionForHealthyKids.org.

Individual motivations

- Team members should discuss their personal goals/reasons for participating on the team.
- Team members should discuss their organizations' goals/reasons for having them participate on the team.

Individual contributions

- Team members should discuss what personal contributions they hope to make to the team.
- Team members should discuss what contributions each of their respective organizations could potentially make to the team and working in/alongside other coalitions.
- You should have a discussion about what other groups, if any, in your state are already doing this type of work.
- If an existing group is identified, your team should develop a strategy for how to best manage your combined relationship.

3. Roles and responsibilities:

Individual commitment

- Your team should discuss and make sure that everyone involved understands the minimum requirements for team participation.
- You should spend time discussing the expectations and limits placed on each individual's involvement by the organizations they represent.

Team roles

- You should discuss whether or not your team needs a chairperson. If so, you should spend time, as a team, becoming clear about what the person's role is in the group.
- You should discuss the role of the team liaison.
- You should discuss other roles people think should be assigned and who is poised to fulfill those roles.

4. Assessment of state profiles:

- Collect data. Tally the data, analyze the results, and decide what areas need addressing.
- Specific assessment tools are included in the planning guide to assist in this step.

5. Facilitation:

- Be sure your team decides how and when they will meet.
- Decide when and how agendas will be developed and circulated, and by whom.
- Decide on a process for taking and circulating minutes.
- Be sure to discuss and establish any necessary ground rules for meetings.
- Spend time discussing and choosing a decision-making process that works for your group.

  - Identify a person who will periodically help the team evaluate its meetings. Ask what works and what does not work at meetings.

6. Communication:
   - Be sure to exchange contact information.
   - Have your team identify a member who will maintain all contact information, and make sure it is available to all team members.
   - Be sure to have someone assume responsibility for making a phone tree or listserv of your team members.
   - Decide as a group the way in which team members should report on the progress of the assigned tasks.

7. Goals and objectives:
   - The planning guide provides tools to assist in identifying and prioritizing goals and methods for creating objectives.
   - Spend time discussing and ensuring that all team members have the same understanding and interpretation of the stated goals.
   - Write goals in a detailed, specific manner. One method of doing this is writing SMART (Specific, Measurable, Appropriate, Realistic, and Time-specific) goals.

8. Action plan:
   - Create action plans for each objective.
   - Identify an individual who will monitor progress on the action plans, and report back to the team regarding the status.

9. Evaluation:
   Task
   - A tool for evaluating action plans is included in the planning guide. Identify ways you can evaluate whether or not you are meeting your objectives.
   - Identify a person to monitor progress on action plans, and report back to the team.
   Team
   - Spend time discussing how your team process/team dynamics are functioning. Discuss strengths, and identify ways that you could work more effectively to achieve your goal.

Program Implementation

Program implementation can be defined as the process of putting a project, service, or program into full effect. It is the management of the execution of the project. Program implementation is a critical part of the planning process and requires the creation of an implementation action plan.

Eight factors that can be considered when developing an implementation plan are as follows:

1. *Why:* The effect of the objectives to be achieved
2. *What:* The activities required to achieve the objectives
3. *Who:* The individuals responsible for each activity
4. *When:* A chronological sequence of activities and timing in relation to project implementation activities or organization events
5. *How:* The materials, supplies, technology, devices, methods, media approaches, flow of activities, or techniques to be used
6. *Where:* Which activities will take place at what locations in the community—at the health promotion site, facility, office, clinic, and center
7. *Cost:* An estimate of expenses for materials, personnel, facilities, and time
8. *Feedback:* When and how to tell if the activities are happening as they should be and if adjustments are needed; use timelines

With all of these elements to consider, it can be helpful to create a written implementation plan. Even with the best-laid plans, things can go wrong and barriers may present themselves. It is best to think ahead, anticipate potential problems, and visualize viable solutions, thus making program implementation as smooth and seamless as possible.

An easy method to apply when writing an implementation process is to create action plans or task tables. If a dietitian is managing a project, she can take elements from the eight implementation factors listed above and create detailed action plans. The use of an action plan helps to assure that all necessary elements are included and that deadlines are established to assist in meeting implementation goals.

A sample action plan follows in Figure 19-5.

Project Name & Location:

Objective 1:

The effect of this objective is:

Activity	Responsible Person(s)	Start Date	End Date	Materials, etc. Required?	Cost	Feedback Required

FIGURE 19-5   Sample Action Plan—ABC Corporation

Determining Team Membership

An important component of any planning project is working effectively through joint efforts. Working together as a team has several benefits, such as providing the group with a variety of viewpoints and backgrounds, pooling resources to get work accomplished, satisfying personal and professional needs of the team members, and gaining community support for your initiative. However, development of team membership procedures is not always easy or without cause for concern. Some difficult situations that can arise when coordinating teams are a large group with slow progress on action plans or decision making, difficulty in obtaining volunteer membership due to busy schedules, and conflicts of interest of membership, particularly for members working in for-profit venues.

The *Making Health Communication Programs Work* book provides several tools to assist planning groups in establishing their membership. A partnership planning worksheet is available, which asks questions regarding potential partners, partner roles and tasks, benefits to partners when they participate on the team, as well as many other considerations. This guide also provides an excellent resource entitled *Steps for Involving Partners in the Program* that teams can use when determining membership. (See Table 19-3.)

Xavier de Souza Briggs, from Harvard University, presented an original approach to looking at planning participation in his article, "Planning Together: How (and How Not) to Engage Stakeholders in Charting a Course," available at http://www.community-problem-solving.net/CMS/viewpage.cfm/ pageId=200. Briggs suggests that when making project participation decisions, groups often focus on the how-to elements relative to participation tactics and techniques. He goes on to suggest that we focus more on "Why? Who? What? And How?" A synopsis of his suggestions can be reviewed in Table 19-4.

The AFHK planning guide provides some guidance in its appendix regarding creating a team. It suggests that the team should be broadly representative of interested groups, particularly in the areas of education and health. (See Figure 19-6.) The planning guide also provides teams with a table to use when identifying and contacting potential representatives, an invitation letter for potential members, and a format for keeping in touch with the membership. A factor that is stressed in the AFHK organization is keeping up to date regarding member needs. Leadership of the team should check in with members to make sure that the members' needs are being met, as this can significantly impact member retention.

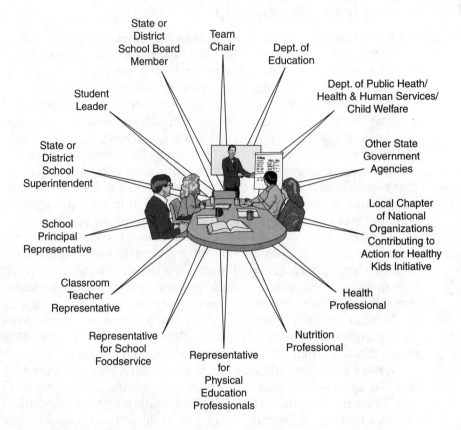

FIGURE 19-6   AFHK Team Membership Diagram
Source: Reprinted from www.ActionforHealthyKids.org.

Health Program Evaluation

The Benefits of Evaluation

Evaluation of health programs is essential in order to assure that objectives are being met. Health programs aim to result in efficient, effective, and quality outcomes, and the goal of an evaluation process is to prove that these aims are being realized. Evaluations focus on proving that programs are cost-effective, that managerial practices are accountable, and that the programs are contributing to improvements in the community's health.

Types of Evaluations

Several types of evaluation can be conducted, and definitions for some of them will be provided here. A *formative evaluation* assesses whether a problem is occurring in a program, the extent of the problem, and if corrective action is necessary. *Summative evaluation* focuses on program impact and program effectiveness. *Program impact* assesses if interventions are producing desired outcomes, and

TABLE 19-3 Steps for Involving Partners in the Program

1. Choose organizations, agencies, or individuals (e.g., physicians) that can bring the resources, expertise, or credibility your program needs.
2. Consider which roles partners might play to best support the program.
3. Involve representatives of the organizations you want to work with as early as appropriate in program planning.
4. Give partners the program rationale, strategies, and messages (in ready-to-use form). Remember that strategic planning, creative messages, and quality production are the most difficult aspects of a communication program to develop and may be the most valuable product you can offer to a community organization.
5. Give partners advance notice so that they can build their part of the program into their schedule, and negotiate what will be expected of them.
6. Allow partners to personalize and adapt program materials to fit their circumstances and give them a feeling of ownership, but don't let them stray from the strategy.
7. Ask partners what they need to implement their part of the program. Beyond the question of funding, consider other assistance, training, information, or tools that would enable them to function successfully.
8. Provide partners with new local/regional/national contacts or linkages that they will perceive as valuable for their ongoing activities.
9. Give partners an appropriate amount of work. Give them a series of small, tangible, short-term responsibilities, as well as a feedback/tracking mechanism.
10. Gently remind partners that they are responsible for their activities; help them complete tasks, but don't complete tasks for them.
11. Assess progress through the feedback/tracking mechanism and help make adjustments to respond to the organization's needs and to keep the program on track.
12. Provide moral support by frequently saying "thank you" and by providing other rewards (e.g., letter or certificate of appreciation).
13. Give partners a final report of what was accomplished and meet to discuss follow-up activities and resources they might find useful. Make sure that they feel they are a part of the program's success.
14. Share one final tremendous "Thank you for a job well done."

Source: Reprinted from *Making Health Communication Programs Work: Planner's Guide,* U.S. Department of Health & Human Services, National Institutes of Health, National Cancer Institute. Available at: www.cancer.gov/pinkbook.

program effectiveness determines if outcomes could be achieved at a lower cost, and deals specifically with cost-benefit and cost-effectiveness analysis. *Process evaluation* assesses the effectiveness of administrative activities and program implementation.

TABLE 19-4   Effective Participation Strategies

Strategic Question	Decision Issues	Caveats
1. Why should we engage stakeholders? Participatory work can serve a variety of overall purposes, such as creating a wider democratic mandate to act, better substantive ideas to drive action, and feelings of psychological "ownership" and investment in collective work.	Are we looking to define a broad issue agenda on which some group or community can plan and act? To set strategies for action on a predefined set of issues? To design a specific project or program, given strategies in place?	Institutions (or an alliance of them) often send confusing signals about why planning is happening; why now; and exactly what the benefits, costs, and limits of participation are likely to be.
2. Who should be involved and in what roles? Effective participation requires setting boundaries that define participants' roles and responsibilities to each other, not as a matter of imposing control but so trust and coordination can develop in place of chaos or "process paralysis."	Who are the primary stakeholders of the decision, project, or policy at issue? Who else might be consulted, or educated, in a broader "public"? Who should organize and sponsor planning events? Facilitate events? Who can observe, and who should make decisions?	Failure to sort out roles can lead to a "circus-tent" approach, in which "more" (players, ideas, events) is assumed to mean "better." Systematic process designs can help—or create the illusion of order, impossible roles, and linear steps that may need to evolve over time.
3. What is the proper scope of our planning process? Few projects or institutions contemplate constant participation in every aspect of decision making, so setting boundaries around the targets of participation—the issues and decisions up for discussion, the authority to decide—is key.	Does our work require broad boundaries so that new issues and interests can constantly be put forward? Are we to generate advice for decision makers, or are we empowered to decide ourselves? How do we relate to those who make everyday (routine) decisions?	Confusion over the scope of participation can quickly undermine the legitimacy and effectiveness of a planning process. Sharp conflicts often emerge when the players have different, and perhaps unstated, assumptions about the appropriate scope of participation.

Strategic Question	Decision Issues	Caveats
4. How should we put our participation strategy to work? Smart tactics, well implemented, put a strategy to work. But tactics should encompass a variety of phases and dimensions of planning, evolving as the project or process evolves.	How should we identify, organize, and convene stakeholders? Build a common knowledge base around the issues we will address? Present information and get feedback? Improve deliberation and shared decision making itself?	Much how-to advice deals piecemeal with creating effective meetings or using information technologies to support decision making. Beware of getting lost in an overload of information, with too few useful ideas and legitimate decisions.

Source: Reprinted with permission from Xavier de Souza Briggs, The Art and Science of Community Problem-Solving Project at Harvard University, 2003. Retrieved from http://www.comminit.com/planningmodels/pmodels/planningmodels-64.html.

Impact outcomes look at outcomes correlated with resources and cost. The PRECEDE model reviewed earlier in the chapter includes an element of impact outcome. This model includes evaluation elements through the use of intermediate objectives applied to the phases of the model. Program intervention models also look at the impact of outcomes. An example of such a model is based on the acronym RASOGO. The acronym stands for:

R   Resources lead to activities.
A   Activities lead to subobjectives.
S   Sub-objectives lead to objectives.
O   Objectives lead to goals.
G   Goals produce outcomes.
O   Outcomes.

Evaluation as a Three-Act Play

In his book, *The Practice of Health Program Evaluation*, David Grembowksi describes program evaluation as a three-act play (see Table 19-5).

In the second act of his model, Grembowski discusses program impact and cost-effectiveness evaluation in great detail. Several designs can be used to measure the impact of programs, each having its own strengths and weaknesses. Designs can be pre-experimental, experimental, or quasi-experimental. Examples of designs in each category are shown in Table 19-6.

The design that is chosen to measure program impact should be feasible; fit well with logistical, political, budgetary, and other constraints of the program; and be able to produce reliable results.

TABLE 19-5   Evaluation as a Three-Act Play

ACT I: Asking the Question

Scene I: Development of a policy question.

Scene II: Translation of the policy question into an evaluation question.

ACT II: Answering the Question

Scene I: Development of an evaluation design to answer the question.

Scene II: Development of the methods to carry out the design.

Scene III: Conducting the evaluation.

ACT III: Using the Answers in Decision Making

Scene I: Translation of evaluation answers back into policy language.

Scene II: Development of a dissemination plan for evaluation answers.

Scene III: Use of the answers in decision making and the policy cycle.

Source: Reprinted with permission from Grembowski, D. 2001. *The Practice of Health Program Evaluation.* SAGE Publications, p. 17.

TABLE 19-6   Types of Program Designs*

Design Type	Subtypes
Pre-experimental	One-group posttest-only design
	One-group pretest-posttest design
	Posttest-only comparison group design
Experimental	Pretest-posttest control group design
	Posttest-only control group design
Quasi-experimental	Single time series design
	Multiple time series design
	Repeated treatment design
	Pretest-posttest nonequivalent comparison group design
	Recurrent institutional cycle design
	Regression discontinuity design

*Refer to statistical resources for further explanations of these designs.

Cost-Effectiveness Analysis

There are three types of *cost-effectiveness analysis* (CEA) that can be conducted for a program. These types are as follows:

- *Cost-benefit analysis:* A method of economic evaluation where all benefits and costs of a program are measured in dollars. Programs have value when their benefits are equal to or exceed their costs, or the ratio of $benefits/$costs is equal to or greater than 1.0, or when the benefit/cost ratio of Program A is equal to or greater than 1.0 and exceeds the benefit/cost ratio of Program B.

- *Cost-minimization analysis:* A type of CEA where Program A and Program B have identical benefit outcomes, and the goal of the analysis is to determine which program has the lower cost.

- *Cost-utility analysis:* A type of CEA in which the outcomes of Program A and Program B are weighted by their value, or quality, and measured with a common metric, such as "quality-adjusted life years." The goal of the analysis is to determine which program produces the most quality-adjusted life years at lower cost.

There are 10 basic steps to conducting a CEA:

1. Define the problem and objectives.
2. Identify alternatives.
3. Describe production relationships, or the CEA's conceptual model.
4. Define the perspective of the CEA.
5. Identify, measure, and value costs.
6. Identify and measure effectiveness.
7. Discount future costs and effectiveness.
8. Perform a sensitivity analysis.
9. Address equity issues.
10. Use CEA in decision making.

A CEA can be an intense and complicated evaluation endeavor. If a planning team has minimal experience with this concept, it may find it necessary to partner with individuals with skill and experience in conducting CEA evaluation processes.

The CDC's Evaluation Process

The CDC also has developed a program evaluation process (see Figure 19-7). The purpose of the CDC evaluation wheel is to help an organization summarize and organize the essential elements of program evaluation, provide a common frame of reference for conducting evaluations, clarify the steps in program evaluation, review the standards of effective program evaluation, and address misconceptions about the purposes and methods of the program evaluation.

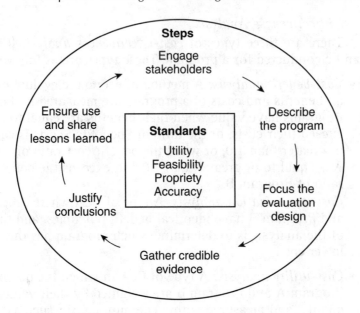

FIGURE 19-7   CDC Evaluation Wheel
Source: Reprinted from Centers for Disease Control. *Framework for Program Evaluation in Public Health.* Available at: http://www.cdc.gov/epo/mmwr/preview/mmwrhtml/rr4811a1.htm.

A summary of the evaluation model's steps is as follows:

Steps in Evaluation Practice
1. *Engage stakeholders:* Those involved, those affected, primary intended users
2. *Describe the program:* Need, expected effects, activities, resources, stage, context, logic model
3. *Focus the evaluation design:* Purpose, users, uses, questions, methods, agreements
4 *Gather credible evidence:* Indicators, sources, quality, quantity, and logistics
5. *Justify conclusions:* Standards, analysis/synthesis, interpretation, judgment, recommendations
6. *Ensure use and share lessons learned:* Design, preparation, feedback, follow-up, and dissemination

Standards of "Effective" Evaluation
1. *Utility:* Serve the information needs of intended users.
2. *Feasibility:* Be realistic, prudent, diplomatic, and frugal.
3. *Propriety:* Behave legally, ethically, and with due regard for the welfare of those involved and those affected.
4. *Accuracy:* Reveal and convey technically accurate information.

The Health Communication Planning Guide's
Outcome Evaluation Process

The *Health Communication Planning Guide* also provides an outcome evaluation process. Results of the evaluation should be used to help identify areas of the program that should be changed, deleted, or augmented. The outcome evaluation process has nine steps, as follows:

1. Determine what information the evaluation must provide.
2. Define the data to collect.
3. Decide on data collection methods.
4. Develop and pretest data collection instruments.
5. Collect data.
6. Process data.
7 Analyze data to answer the evaluation questions.
8. Write an evaluation report.
9. Disseminate the evaluation report.

To summarize, evaluation is an essential element in the planning process. When developing plans, groups need to consider what types of evaluation they wish to conduct. Most evaluation plans will include several elements and will deal with analysis of both the outcome and the effectiveness of programs. Several models and references are available for teams when they are developing plans for evaluation components of programs.

Conclusion

Proper planning, implementation, and evaluation of programs are important managerial functions for the public health nutritionist. A great deal of information, both online and in book format, are available for reference and support when taking on this critical community health program function. Several models are available for both planning and evaluation. The decision of which prototype to use will depend on the nature of the planning task and the team assembled to complete the work. Spending time planning before approaching an endeavor will be rewarded by a resulting product or program that impacts the community's health, thus contributing to professional success for the public health nutritionist and the planning team.

Issues for Discussion

1. Is planning an important skill for a public health nutritionist to possess and justify spending time on? Why or why not? Explain your answer.

2. A public health nutritionist can potentially be involved in three types of planning. What types of work situations may cause a public health nutritionist to apply skills in strategic planning? Long-term planning? Operational planning?

3. You are working in a public health department and are assigned to implement a weight management program for the community. Choose a planning model presented in this chapter, and discuss how to apply the model to the assigned project.

4. Discuss how you would make decisions regarding what team members to include in a public health project.

5. You are continuing work on your community weight management program. Discuss what types of data you would collect in order to evaluate the program.

References

Action for Healthy Kids. 2002. Action Planning Guide. Retrieved May18, 2005 from http://www.ActionForHealthyKids.org.

American Public Health Association. Community Strategies for Health: Fitting in the Pieces. Retrieved April 18, 2005, from: http://www.apha.org/ppp/science/csh.htm.

American Public Health Association. 2004. The Guide to Implementing Model Standards. Retrieved April 18, 2005, from http://www.apha.org/ppp/science/theguide.htm.

Bartol, K. M. & Martin, D. C. 1994. *Management* (1st CPCU ed.). New York: McGraw-Hill.

Boyle, M. A. 2003. *Community Nutrition in Action: An Entrepreneurial Approach* (3rd ed.). Belmont, CA: Wadsworth/Thomson Learning.

Briggs, X. S. 2003. *The Art and Science of Community Problem-Solving Project.* Cambridge, MA: Harvard University.

Campbell, C. 1995. *Health Education Planning Models—A Review of the Literature, Part II.* Mississippi State: Mississippi Cooperative Extension Service.

Centers for Disease Control. 1999. Framework for Program Evaluation in Public Health. Retrieved fromhttp://www.cdc.gov/epo/mmwr/preview/mmwrhtml/rr4811al.htm.

Grembowski, D. 2001. *The Practice of Health Program Evaluation.* Thousand Oaks, CA: Sage.

Health Communication Partnership (December, 2003), John Hopkins Bloomberg School of Public Health. Retrieved June 6, 2005 from http://www.jhuccp.org/training/scope/Pprocess.htm.

Livengood, J. R. 1996. *PATCH: Planned Approach to Community Health Program Summary.* Centers for Disease Control. Retrieved June 6, 2005 from http://www.cdc.gov/nccdphp/patch/00binaries/PATCHCh1.pdf.

National Cancer Institute. Pink Book-Making Health Communication Programs Work Retrieved May 18, 2005 from http://www.cancer.gov/pinkbook/page1.

National Institutes of Health, National Cancer Institute (1995). Theory at a Glance: A Guide for Health Promotion Practice (NIH Publication No. 97-3896). National Cancer Institute. Bethesda, MD. Retrieved June 6, 2005 from http://www.cancer.gov/aboutnci/oc/theory-at-a-glance.

Piotrow, P.T., Kincaid, D.L., Rimon, J.G II, & Rinehart, W. (1997). *Health Communication: Lessons from Family Planning and Reproductive Health*. Westport, CT: Praeger.

Timmreck, T. C. 2003. *Planning, Program Development, and Evaluation: A Handbook for Health Promotion, Aging, and Health Services* (2nd ed.). Sudbury, MA: Jones and Bartlett.

U.S. Department of Health & Human Services, Office of Disease Prevention and Health Promotion. September 1997. Development Objectives for Healthy People 2010. Retrieved from http://www.healthypeople.gov/default.htm.

CHAPTER 20

MANAGING DATA

Elizabeth Barden, PhD

Reader Objectives

After studying this chapter and reflecting on the contents, you should be able to:

1. List the purposes for which data are needed by nutrition professionals.
2. Identify how to use data from various sources to develop a community profile and identify major health problems for that community.
3. Identify how to triangulate data from different sources to gain a more complete picture of a community's health needs, constituents, and resources.
4. Recognize sources of useful data.
5. List the steps in developing a new data collection, analysis, and reporting system.

Given the pervasiveness of personal computing and the widespread availability of original data files on the Internet, the current context of nutrition practice requires all professionals to have a basic competence with the acquisition, analysis, and interpretation of diverse types of data from various sources. Mastering the skills necessary for dealing with data is essential for any nutrition professional who wants to be able to rely on his or her own interpretation of the facts, and not just someone else's or those of "experts." This is particularly important in the current climate, where divergent agendas in combination with shrinking resources at times lead to contradictory interpretations of the same data, or at least to differing outlooks on the relative importance of competing priorities.

Learning to manage regularly released statistical reports and other available data sources can be a tremendous advantage for any professional looking to plan relevant, meaningful, and effective nutrition programs. In addition, nutrition professionals today are not just users but also are consumers of data; that is, not only do nutritionists utilize and generate data themselves in the course of designing and evaluating their own programs, but they also stay current in their field and operate in a team setting by appraising the work of others. Competence with data management, analysis, and interpretation allows one to evaluate the positions others put forth, assess the quality of recommendations that are received, and evaluate the reasonableness of published research findings and public health reports.

Data may be defined broadly as information, especially information organized for analysis and decision making (Morris, 1982). Data include, but are not confined to, statistics, which is the branch of mathematics dealing with the collection, analysis, interpretation, and presentation of numerical data (Spicer & Kaufman, 1990). Objective, statistical data (e.g., a community's leading cause of death, the percentage change in the prevalence of teen pregnancy, or per capita healthcare costs for obesity-related illness) certainly are useful for quantifying and comparing the size of need, degree of achievement, and costs in relation to accomplishment. However, additional types of data, including subjective information such as a community's perceived needs, also are important in accurately characterizing a population and its health service requirements. The definition of what constitutes relevant public health nutrition data has expanded as the availability of information on all facets of life has become easily accessible. For instance, census data about the presence of a telephone in the household at first glance may not appear to be relevant nutrition data. However, it is a pertinent factor to know for a nutritionist who is planning a telephone survey in a given neighborhood, where he or she needs to obtain a representative sample of residents, or for a nutritionist who is planning services that include follow-up telephone counseling.

Data are used in many different contexts within nutrition practice. There are at least four dimensions from which data management for nutrition practice can be considered: 1) using data to plan work (program planning and needs assessment); 2) using data to demonstrate the effectiveness of work (program evaluation); 3) using data to monitor a population (nutrition surveillance), define health objectives and associated benchmarks (e.g., Healthy People 2010), and monitor progress towards meeting those objectives; and 4) collecting and managing new data. This chapter will address each of these dimensions, to give an overview of some of the major issues and processes involved in managing data in a public health nutrition context.

Data in Program Planning and Needs Assessment

An effective nutrition program plan is achieved by following a conscientious planning process that justifies its need, identifies relevant goals and objectives, defines tasks and activities to accomplish those goals, inventories resources available, and explains how results will be evaluated and disseminated (Probert, 1996). Data are used during every phase of the program planning process to achieve the following outcomes:

- To identify the need for new services or initiatives
- To recognize the need for changes in service delivery
- To identify the most appropriate at-risk target population
- To define goals and objectives
- To better target limited resources
- To describe program performance expectations
- To justify a program's budget and to develop grant proposals to secure additional funding when necessary

Needs assessment is the portion of the planning process during which a community and its particular health needs are defined. Overall, the needs assessment phase of the program planning process aims to understand the nutrition requirements of the community, prioritize their identified needs, and target resources accordingly. Chapter 3 discusses the topic of needs assessment in great detail.

Identifying a specific population with specific health and nutritional status challenges and identifying gaps in existing service delivery is accomplished through close examination of both quantitative and qualitative data. A quantitative assessment includes examination of demographic, socioeconomic, health status, and risk indicators. Data for this assessment comes from a review of both regularly published public health reports and scientific research literature that are relevant to the health problem and/or the community. Qualitative methods, such as key informant interviews, focus groups, and informal conversations, derive information from health professionals and community members regarding the community's perceived needs and demands for nutrition-related services. The more subjective information obtained from these sources is necessary to balance the more objective, statistics-driven information that comes from the quantitative assessment; both provide an important piece of the big picture. The needs assessment methodology also includes the compilation of an inventory of existing health and nutrition resources in the community and any major duplication or gaps in available services, as well as service delivery and resource utilization data. A final piece is an assessment by the program planner of the host organization's (usually his or her employer's) mission and willingness to support a proposed nutrition program, both financially and institutionally.

Typically, objective, quantitative data are used in nutrition program planning to address four questions:

1. What are the health problems facing a community? (issues)
2. Where are the problems? (place)

3. Who is at risk? (person)
4. When: Which problems are increasing or declining over time? (time period)

Issues

Planning often begins with an examination of which health issues affect a community. An inventory of the leading causes of morbidity and mortality, the most prevalent chronic diseases, and the leading causes of hospitalization can give a broad overview of the health concerns of the community. This type of data typically is found in regularly published public health reports, such as state or national vital statistics reports, and surveillance system reports. As an example of this type of data, Table 20-1 presents the leading causes of death among U.S. females in 2001. From the table, it is clear that deaths from heart disease and cancer are far more common than deaths from diabetes or kidney disease, for example.

Place

Place describes geographic units, such as the nation, state, county, clinic, or region. Examination of data by place helps to ascertain the geographic extent of the health problem. Maps are an effective way to show differences in health status data by geographical area. For example, Figure 20-1 illustrates regional differences in the prevalence of obesity across the United States, with the central and southern part of the country having a much greater prevalence of obesity than the western part.

TABLE 20-1   Leading Causes of Death, Females—United States, 2001

All Races, Females	Percent*
1. Heart disease	29.3
2. Cancer	21.6
3. Stroke	8.1
4. Chronic lower respiratory diseases	5.1
5. Diabetes	3.1
6. Alzheimer's disease	3.1
7. Unintentional injuries	2.9
8. Influenza and pneumonia	2.8
9. Kidney disease	1.7
10. Septicemia	1.5

*Percent of total deaths due to the cause indicated.

Source: From the Centers for Disease Control and Prevention, http://www.cdc.gov/od/spotlight/nwhw/lcod.htm; accessed April 7, 2004.

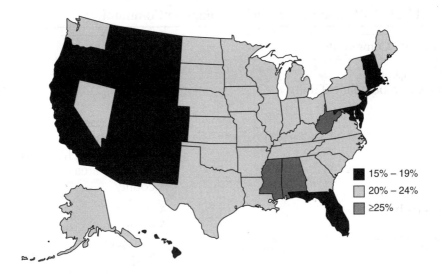

FIGURE 20-1   U.S. Obseity Map, 2002: BMI ≥ 30
Source: From the Centers for Disease Control and Prevention, BRFSS.
http://www.cdc.gov/nccdphp/dnpa/obesity/trend/maps/index.htm; accessed 4/4/04.

Person

Person may be described in many different ways. The words "population" and "community" are sometimes used interchangeably. Most often, though, population refers to all of the inhabitants of a given region (e.g., the U.S. population, or the population of the state of Maine). Community, on the other hand, is usually a subset of a larger population that is defined on the basis of geographic boundaries, political boundaries, or demographic characteristics (Aspen Reference Group, 1997). Another way that communities are defined for planning purposes is on the basis of place of residence, occupation, or other shared personal characteristics; membership in a particular institutional setting; or the clientele of a service-delivery organization. Table 20-2 presents some examples of different ways a community unit may be conceptualized. For instance, a demographically defined community may be described on the basis of age (e.g., preschoolers or senior citizens), gender, ethnicity, income bracket, occupation, or neighborhood (e.g., residents of Center City, Philadelphia, or San Francisco's Chinatown). More commonly, some combination of factors is used to further aggregate individuals by characteristics that may be associated with some known risk (Cole, 1991), such as defining a community of teenage mothers who have not graduated from high school and who live in a particular state, or a community of housebound elderly Asian American immigrants living in Baltimore. A clear, specific definition of the community early in the planning process facilitates data collection and program design.

TABLE 20-2   Different Ways of Defining the Community

Basis of "Community"	Examples
Geographical (may also be political unit)	A town A city A state A housing complex A school district A village or neighborhood A ZIP code area A county
Setting-based	A school A community group A workplace A hospital A university A church A YMCA
Occupational or personal characteristics	Dentists Vegans Nuns Marathon runners

Service delivery-based	Patients in a private medical
	    practice
	Patients in a community
	    health center
	VNA clients
	Meals-on-Wheels clients
	WIC participants

Source: Compiled by the author.

Time

Time frequently is indicated by the use of trend charts. Trends are annual rates reported over a period of time, usually in terms of years. Interpretation of trends involves examination of similarities and differences among various parameters. For instance, an investigator may initially examine the pattern of change over time to see whether a problem is increasing or decreasing. More refined analyses may include comparison of one time period to another, a comparison of time series trends in different geographic areas or among different populations, or a comparison of trends among high-risk groups relative to the general population. Often, trend charts concisely present several aspects of data that allow for multiple interpretations. For example, Figure 20-2 demonstrates that between 1980 and 2000, the prevalence of diagnosed diabetes increased

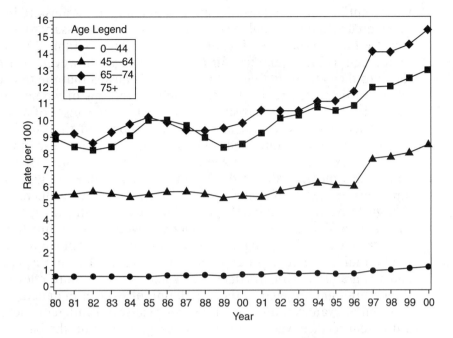

FIGURE 20-2   Prevalence of Diagnosed Diabetes by Age, United States, 1980–2000
Source: From the Centers for Disease Control and Prevention. http://www.cdc.gov/
diabetes/statistics/prev/national/figbyage.htm; accessed April 4, 2004.

among all age groups. This figure also demonstrates that throughout the time period shown (1980–2000), people aged 65–74 years
had the highest prevalence of diagnosed diabetes, followed by people aged 75 or older, people aged 45–64 years, and people less than
45 years of age. Since 1996, the prevalence of diagnosed diabetes
increased considerably among persons greater than 44 years of age,
and much less so among persons less than 45 years of age.

Analysis of Quantitative Data

It is the analysis of the relationship between the parameters of issue, place, person, and time that allows the program planner to
draw conclusions about which priority issue should be addressed
with which community. Different data elements should be used in
combination to more fully characterize the big picture, and to help
narrow down a target audience for intervention. In Table 20-1, data
on the leading cause of death among U.S. women was presented as
an example of how important health issues can be identified. However, that information by itself is not enough for program planning,
unless the program planner is going to tackle one of the top two
leading causes of death with the entire U.S. female population as
the target community! Almost always, the scope of such a project

would not be remotely feasible; more commonly, programs are implemented on a much smaller scale. Therefore, it is necessary to narrow the focus. Table 20-3 includes the same data as Table 20-1 in its far right column (marked *All Races Combined*); however, it also includes the data disaggregated by race. This means that the top 10 causes of death are also listed separately for groups of women on the basis of race. A comparison of how the leading causes of death are ranked within each racial group, as opposed to the rank for women of all races combined, illustrates that there are discrepancies. For example, the prevalence of diabetes among Hispanic American women is almost double that of U.S. women in general, and the prevalence of diabetes for African American women, although lower than among Hispanic Americans, is still far greater than among Caucasian or Asian American women. To a nutritionist interested in designing a diabetes prevention campaign, this might indicate that a program targeted specifically to Hispanic American and/or African American women may be more relevant than a program targeted to the population of women in general.

Similarly, an examination of the same cause of death data yields a different picture when the data are disaggregated on the basis of age (see Table 20-4). As Table 20-1 demonstrated, the leading cause of death for women of all ages is heart disease. However, among women younger than 35 years, the leading cause of death is unintentional injury; among women 35 to 64 years, the leading cause of death is cancer. One potential conclusion for a nutritionist working with preschool children and their parents is that a program aimed to educate kids about a diet that promotes cardiovascular health will be valuable to them in the future; however, this nutritionist recognizes evaluation of the program's effectiveness in reducing deaths from heart disease could not commence for more than 60 years!

Another way of using objective data is to compare them to national health targets, such as Healthy People (HP) 2010 (described further later in this chapter), and/or to compare them to data for a reference population, such as the total U.S. population. In Table 20-5, hypothetical data regarding the prevalence of anemia, short stature, and low birth weight for a community are presented next to the HP 2010 Objectives (U.S. Department of Health and Human Services [DHHS], 2000), the prevalence of the same health issues in the national population, and a national population of low-to-moderate income children (Polhamus et al., 2004).

The data in this table can be interpreted a number of ways. First, a comparison of the sample community data for short stature, anemia, and low birth weight (LBW) to the national target objectives illustrates that the community's health performance, with respect to short stature, actually exceeds national health expectations (3.9% compared to 5%). In contrast, the prevalence of anemia and LBW in the community are more than double the national objectives for

Table 20-3 Comparison of Leading Causes of Death by Race— U.S. Females, 2001

Females, All Ages	Percent[a]				
	Caucasian	African American[b]	Asian/ Pacific Islander American[c]	Hispanic American[d]	All Races Combined
1. Heart disease	29.5	28.7	24.8	25.7	29.3
2. Cancer	21.7	20.8	27.0	21.1	21.6
3. Stroke	8.1	7.8	10.9	6.9	8.1
4. Chronic lower respiratory diseases	5.5	2.4	2.5	2.7	5.1
5. Diabetes	2.8	5.1	3.7	6.1	3.1
6. Alzheimer's disease	3.3	n/a	1.1	n/a	3.1
7. Unintentional injuries	2.9	2.8	3.6	4.7	2.9
8. Influenza and pneumonia	2.9	2.1	3.2	2.8	2.8
9. Kidney disease	1.5	2.9	1.8	1.9	1.7
10. Septicemia	1.4	2.3	n/a	n/a	1.5

[a]Percent of total deaths due to the cause indicated.

[b]Among African American women, Alzheimer's disease was not one of the top 10 causes of death; HIV was 6th, at 1.8%.

[c]Among Asian/Pacific Islander American women, septicemia was not one of the top 10 causes of death; hypertension was 10th, at 1.4%.

[d]Among Hispanic American women, Alzheimer's disease and septicemia were not among the top 10 causes of death; perinatal conditions were 6th at 1.9%, and chronic liver disease was 10th, at 1.8%.

Source: From the Centers for Disease Control and Prevention, http://www.cdc.gov/od/ spotlight/nwhw/lcod.htm; accessed April 7, 2004.

Table 20-4 Leading Cause of Death by Age, All Races—U.S. Females, 2001

Age Range	Leading Cause of Death
1 to 34 years	Unintentional injuries
35 to 64 years	Cancer
65+ years	Heart disease
All ages	Heart disease

Source: Adapted with permission from the Centers for Disease Control and Prevention, http://www.cdc.gov/od/spotlight/nwhw/lcod/01all.pdf; accessed 4/7/04.

TABLE 20-5   Comparison of Selected Health Indicators to Benchmark Target, National Prevalence, and Prevalence Among Low-to-Moderate Income Children

Health Indicator	Age, in years	Sample Data, Hypothetical Community, %	Healthy People 2010 Objective, %	Prevalence among U.S. Population, %	Prevalence among U.S. Low-to-Moderate Income Population %
Short stature	Birth to 5	3.9	5	2.3	6.3
Anemia	Birth to 5	12.0	5	2.8	13.1
Low birth weight	≤ 1	10.8	5	7.8	8.9

Source: Reprinted with permission from Polhamus, B., Dalenius, K., Thompson, D., Scanlon, K., Borland, E., Smith, B., & Grummer-Strawn, L. 2004. *Pediatric Nutrition Surveillance 2002 Report.* Atlanta, GA: U.S. Department of Health and Human Services, Centers for Disease Control and Prevention.

those indicators (12% versus 5% and 10.8% versus 5%, respectively). The data also may be compared to national data (see Table 20-7 and related text later in this chapter for more detail regarding the comparison of local or state to national data). This type of comparison is strengthened by knowing more about the community. For the purposes of the example, assume that a review of census data showed that the community had a median household income well below its state average. Therefore, a comparison between the sample community data and the data presented for national low-to-moderate income children may be more appropriate than simply a comparison to the general U.S. population. For instance, the prevalence of anemia in the sample community is 12%, well above the national prevalence of 2.8%. However, it is actually slightly lower than the prevalence of anemia among the national low-to-moderate income population (13.1%). On the other hand, the prevalence of LBW in the sample community (10.8%) exceeds both the national prevalence (7.8%) and the prevalence among the low-to-moderate income population (8.9%). Health planners may look at the data from all of these angles and decide that efforts to reduce LBW are more of a priority than efforts to reduce anemia, and that little, if any, resources will be allocated to reducing short stature.

Several cautions apply when working with published data. (For an excellent overview of errors and remedies associated with using published data for research purposes, see Jacob, 1984.) First, before making any comparisons, pay close attention to factors such as the time period represented by the data, the definition of the population (e.g., does the data represent the total U.S. population, or just women, or just persons of a specific ethnicity and age, etc.?), how data indicators are defined (e.g., does LBW refer to all births < 2,500 grams, or just to births between 1,500 and 2,500 grams, with very low birth weight a separate indicator for < 1,500-gram births?), and the original data source. High-quality data reports always include this information, and other caveats or definitions are often presented as footnotes. One indicator that is particularly fraught with difficulty is race/ethnicity categories, which are defined in various ways by different data systems. To make valid comparisons, planners must ascertain that the populations being compared are analogous, or at least they must recognize and disclose cases where comparisons are made on the basis of data that differ in some important aspects. This last situation occurs when limited data are available, and inexact comparisons are made knowingly to get a preliminary, overall sense of whether discrepancies exist.

Additionally, it is important to bear in mind that percentages can be deceiving with respect to magnitude; for instance, a mortal event that occurs only 1.5% of the time initially may not give the impression of being common, yet when the population is composed of 1 million people, that small percentage actually reflects 15,000 deaths. Program planners must keep the denominators from which the percentages are computed in mind when making decisions about priorities. It is also important not to look at data in isolation, but to consider relationships between different indicators. For example, when considering the proportion of LBW births, a planner should also consider the total birth rate. A community with 5 births per year may have a LBW prevalence of 20%, if one baby is born at less than 2,500 grams. In contrast, a neighboring community with 500 births per year would have a LBW prevalence of only 5% if 25 babies were born at less than 2,500 grams (a similar prevalence of 20% in this community would represent 100 LBW births!). This example is meant to illustrate that a planner cannot just use the largest numbers to determine the community with the greatest need.

Prioritizing Health Needs

The process of using a range of methods and integrating multiple sources of data to gain a more complete picture of relevant health issues and potential solutions is known as triangulation (Owen, Splett, & Owen, 1999). The analysis of health data that is used to derive a list of priority issues for a given community, in order to select a focus of intervention, is based on many factors. It is a subjective process to rank the issues based on data collected from the quantitative health assessment, the literature review, and the qualitative sources such as key informant interviews and focus groups. The process also is tempered by the constraints of staff, money, time, and political feasibility; it is because of these factors that resources need to be identified early in the planning process, so that realistic and achievable priorities can be established. For example, a publicly funded community health center, with one nutritionist and a limited budget, would likely prioritize local health issues for its program planning differently than would a well-endowed private charitable trust, with a charter to focus exclusively on perinatal health. Analysis of published figures is important, but it is equally important to recognize how things work in the real world. What makes sense theoretically (based on how things look on paper) needs to be balanced with how things work in practice.

For this reason, when planning a public health nutrition program, it is essential to consider other sources of information than just the results of a demographic, socioeconomic, and health risk assessment analysis. It is crucial to speak with key informants to learn their perspectives on where critical needs lie, and on what types of programming might be acceptable to, and be effective with, the chosen target audience. Key informants usually include a combination of the following: subject area experts, such as local providers (e.g., physicians, nurses, WIC nutritionists, nutrition extension service staff); academics; voluntary health association and professional association spokespeople (e.g., the American Dietetic Association, the March of Dimes, the American Academy of Pediatrics); community leaders (e.g., elected officials, clergy, venerated elders, school officials); and the constituents themselves, in order to learn what their values and health expectations are. It is important to directly hear the voice of the intended target audience, as their perceived needs and interests may or may not converge with the prioritized needs identified during the quantitative health assessment analysis. In order to ensure a receptive audience, information regarding acceptability, appropriateness, and usefulness of planned interventions is a must. Sometimes a community will accept a health program for which there is little community demand (but a quantitatively demonstrated need) when it dovetails with something that is highly desired. For instance, WIC nutrition educators in California discovered during their planning process that the greatest perceived need among their intended target audience, non-English-speaking WIC participants, was learning English, not receiving nutrition and health education. They designed a creative program that established an English as a Second Language (ESL) program, using nutrition concepts as the subject matter. In that way, the target audience received a highly desired product, and the nutritionists were able to convey their education messages simultaneously (Wurzbach, 2002).

To enhance decision making when prioritizing health needs, objective and subjective data provide the explicit informational criteria upon which the decisions are based. Sample criteria for decision making include the number of persons affected, disease severity, public perception of the seriousness or changeability of a problem, available resources (including funding, personnel, and redundancy), the political feasibility of intervention, legal mandates, community acceptability, and indicators of organizational support.

Criteria should be clearly stated, understood, and agreed upon by those involved in the decision-making process. Assurances should be made that each alternative will be assessed consistently.

The development of grant applications to secure funds for current or future programming is achieved through a similar examination of data and consideration of priorities and interventions as the process just described. A successful grant proposal (or project proposal) demonstrates health disparities among a particular target audience that are amenable to change through the proposed intervention, so that funders are convinced of the need for action as well as the likelihood that the proposed intervention can meet its stated goals. Please see Appendix G for guidance on preparing grant proposals.

Data in Program Management and Evaluation

Evaluation is a core function within program management. The primary purposes of evaluation are to guide program managers and staff members in deciding whether to change or continue a program or specific activities within a program, allow program managers to assess the outcomes of the program on clients' health, and demonstrate to funding sources that their money is being used efficiently and effectively. In the context of program evaluation, data may be used for clinical quality assurance; evaluation of specific initiatives; monitoring of statewide or national data for trends; measurement of progress towards meeting goals and objectives; and assessment of the impact of conditions on birth outcomes, morbidity, and mortality (CDC, 1988, 1999).

Once a priority health issue and a target community have been selected, the next phase in the program planning process is the selection of interventions appropriate to the target audience, health problem, and setting; development of appropriate intervention goals and objectives; and development of an evaluation plan. Goals and objectives provide direction for a program's work and the standards by which its performance is evaluated. Goals are broad statements of purpose and direction, and need not be quantifiable and time-limited. Objectives, on the other hand, are the framework for program planning, implementation, management, and evaluation. Objectives must be quantifiable and time-limited. Guidelines for writing objectives include the following data categories:

- *Action:* What activities will be undertaken, or what specific changes are desired?
- *Target population:* Who will benefit from these activities?

- *Measurement:* How will success be evaluated?
- *Timeline:* Over what period of time will objectives be met?

Well-written objectives always contain statements that express a quantified result expected within a stated timeframe. For example, a physical activity promotion program at a local hospital could have the following objective: "By June 2006, 45% (up from 20% in January 2004) of County Hospital employees will engage in light to moderate activity for at least 30 minutes per day." In this sample objective, the action is 30 minutes of engagement in light to moderate physical activity; the target population is County Hospital employees; the measurement refers to the percentage of employees who engage in physical activity (expected to be 45%); and this result is expected by June 2006. The figure of 20% in January 2004 provides the baseline against which change will be measured.

Thoughtful definition of goals and objectives greatly facilitates the development of an evaluation plan, which also is done during the planning stage. Because objectives are measurable statements of what the program intends to achieve, for whom, and by when, evaluation statements are complementary in that they state the extent to which change actually occurred within the given time frame, relative to what was expected. In order to evaluate and monitor the *process* of implementation (especially targeting), data must be collected to illustrate whether the program is being delivered as planned to the intended target group. Data also must be collected to monitor program *outcomes* using appropriate, measurable indicators, to assess the impact of the program, and to answer whether the gross outcome was acceptable (Mason et al., 1984). In the case of the sample objective provided above, in June 2006, data would be collected regarding how many hospital employees engage in light to moderate physical activity for at least 30 minutes per day. The percentage of employees who actually met the physical activity objective would be compared to the expected percentage of 45%; if the percentage was 45% or greater, the program could be considered a success. If the percentage was less than 45%, planners could pursue the analysis of additional information collected during program implementation to investigate areas for program improvement, or decide to discontinue program efforts.

The evaluation process is integrally dependent on quality data that is collected as part of program operations. It is necessary to decide during the planning stage what elements of the program will be evaluated (such as, how many client visits were scheduled? When were they scheduled? Who did what activities? At what cost were the activities delivered? What changes occurred among individuals?). This ensures that the appropriate data will be collected during program implementation, provides ongoing management feedback about how the program is being administered, and allows for outcome assessment once the program has ended (or at some regular interval). If evaluation is not considered until after a program has ended, it is unlikely that the required data will be available. For example, consider an 8-week nutrition education lecture series for elderly adults planned at a local community center. Planning, with something as simple as a weekly sign-in sheet, would allow the nutritionist to be able to monitor attendance as the course proceeds (which may show whether interest is increasing or decreasing) and demonstrate, at the course's completion, how many persons were served. Collecting additional information on the sheet (such as gender or age) would provide additional information about who attended for comparison to the expected target audience's characteristics. If the actual participants differed from the expected target audience (for instance, if the majority of attendees were less than 65 years old), the evaluation process would have illustrated that the needs of the intended target audience were not being met by the program as currently designed, even if the number of participants met the number expected.

Data collected through the course of program evaluation also may be used for program advocacy. In this instance, the data are used to highlight the need for services and to promote visibility for specific aspects of services and for the program as a whole. In addition, data regarding the number of clients served and achievements in meeting goals and objectives often are used to positively reflect on a program and justify requests for future funding and other types of support.

Nutrition Monitoring and Surveillance

Nutrition monitoring refers to the ongoing description of nutrition conditions in the population, especially among high-risk groups, for the purposes of planning and evaluation (Briefel, 2001). Nutrition monitoring includes ongoing nutrition surveillance systems, as well as periodic nutrition surveys. Both are used to monitor trends and patterns among key indicators of nutritional status, with the goals of identifying existing and emerging needs, targeting and developing appropriate nutrition interventions, and determining public policies. Surveillance refers to the continuous, systematic collection of data, as well as its timely interpretation regarding the current and changing condition of the population, and the dissemination of those results to those in a position to act on them (Birkhead & Maylahn, 2000). Common characteristics of public health surveillance systems are shown in Table 20-6.

The definition of "population" varies according to the specific aims of a given surveillance system; often, nutrition surveillance activities are designed to document the status of nutritionally vulnerable groups, particularly where data are lacking. Then, the data

Table 20-6   Characteristics of Public Health Surveillance Systems

Purpose	To identify, describe, monitor
Data Collection	Relatively small amount of data per case; continuous; through established mechanisms
Data Analysis	Simple and descriptive
Dissemination	Timely and regular; target public health agencies and others who may use the information
Significance	Identify problems; estimate magnitude of a problem; trigger interventions

Source: Adapted with permission from Teutsch, S. M. 2000. Considerations in planning a surveillance system. In S. M. Teutsch and R. E. Churchill (eds.), *Principles and Practice of Public Health Surveillance* (2nd ed.). New York: Oxford University Press.

can be used to assess the unmet needs of these groups (such as the homeless, the elderly, pregnant women, and children).

Nutrition monitoring also includes periodic observation and measurement of the population, commonly using surveys. A nutrition survey refers to the examination of a population's dietary behavior and nutrient intake, often at single point in time. Major historical examples of nutrition monitoring surveys include the three National Health and Nutrition Examination Surveys (NHANES: NHANES I in 1971–1975; NHANES II in 1976–1980; and NHANES III, conducted in two phases between 1988 and 1994), administered through the Department of Health and Human Services (DHHS), National Center for Health Statistics (NCHS). An additional survey, Hispanic HANES was conducted from 1982 to 1984 to gather comprehensive data on Mexican, Cuban, and Puerto Rican Americans. Since 1999, NHANES has become a continuous annual survey program. The U.S. Department of Agriculture (USDA) has conducted surveys for more than 70 years to obtain information about food use and food consumption patterns; the surveys include the Nationwide Food Consumption Survey (NFCS; 1977–1978), the Continuing Survey of Food Intakes by Individuals (CSFII; 1994–1996 and 1998), and the Diet and Health Knowledge Survey (DHKS; 1994–1996). As a result of the National Nutrition Monitoring and Related Research Act of 1990's goal to improve coordination of nutrition monitoring across agencies, CSFII and NHANES have been integrated. The result is that the common dietary intake methodology and processing system utilized by CSFII has been incorporated into the sample and data collection capability of NHANES. This integrated survey is referred to as *What We Eat in America–NHANES* and includes data collection regarding food intake, dietary supplement intake, food program participation, and other diet-related data from 5,000 respondents per year (Dwyer, Picciano, & Raiten, 2003).

Common nutrition-monitoring data elements include nutritional status indicators for pregnant women, infants, children, school-aged children, or elderly adults. These may include food and nutrient consumption data; knowledge, attitude, and behavior assessments; nutrition service utilization, service delivery, and access to care information; and food supply and food access indicators, in order to address issues such as food security and hunger. For instance, key indicators of childhood nutritional status include height, weight, anemia, birth weight, and breastfeeding history.

Data collected by nutrition surveillance systems are used for many purposes, including:

- To describe, monitor, and document nutritional status, especially for high-risk subgroups
- To provide early warning data and trend data on the extent of malnutrition and nutrition-related health problems
- To support effective programming, planning, evaluation, and policy making
- To enable departments of public health to provide information on nutrition-related problems to legislators and administrators

In the context of nutrition program planning, various nutrition surveillance elements may be relevant to define target population characteristics or to demonstrate a health need. In addition, program-specific data can be assessed for monitoring progress toward goals, relative to surveillance data, as a benchmark.

Two valuable sources of data regarding the health and nutrition status of women and children are the national Pediatric and Pregnancy Nutrition Surveillance Systems. The Centers for Disease Control and Prevention (CDC) began working with five U.S. states in 1973 to develop a system for continuously monitoring the growth and nutritional status of low-income children who participated in federally funded maternal and child health and nutrition programs. By 2002, the Pediatric Nutrition Surveillance System (PedNSS) had expanded to include 38 states, the District of Columbia, Puerto Rico, and six tribal governments (Polhamus et al., 2004). PedNSS aggregates data on demographic characteristics, birth weight characteristics, indicators of nutritional status, and infant-feeding practices for children from birth to age 18. All data submitted to the national PedNSS originate from the clinical service records of participating programs. PedNSS data are not representative of the total population of U.S. children because participation in the programs that originally collect the data is dependent upon income, nutrition risk criteria, or other eligibility requirements. Nationally, in 2002, approximately 83% of PedNSS data records were submitted from the clinical service records of the Special Supplemental Nutrition Program for Women, Infants and Children (WIC), and the majority of the remaining data were submitted from the Early Periodic Screening Diagnosis and Treatment program (EPSDT), the Title V Maternal and Child Health Program, Head Start, and other programs. WIC provides supplemental nutritious foods and nutrition education and counseling to moderate- to low-income pregnant and postpartum women and children up to 5 years of age who are at nutritional risk.

The Pregnancy Nutrition Surveillance System (PNSS) is a national surveillance system implemented in 1979 by the CDC to identify and reduce pregnancy-related health risks. PNSS collects nutrition-related data regarding the medical and behavioral risk factors associated with poor pregnancy outcomes, including weight gain during pregnancy, anemia, timing of initiation of prenatal care, alcohol use, and tobacco use before, during, and after pregnancy. Selected data related to the infant include birth outcome, birth weight, and infant feeding behavior. Data are program-based, primarily obtained from WIC and prenatal clinics funded by Maternal and Child Health Program Block Grants. The states and intertribal organizations that participate in PNSS have varied since its inception.

Comparison of data from a smaller community to data from a larger unit, such as a state or the nation, can identify areas where health improvement efforts may be warranted. For example, comparison of state-level PNSS data to national PNSS data is informative regarding the health and nutritional status of low- to moderate-income women and children in that state, relative to individuals in similar economic circumstances across the nation. Such a comparison could assist that state's WIC program in identifying specific risk factors and needs among its participant population; in planning, implementing, and evaluating nutrition interventions; and in developing and implementing quality assurance protocols. At a more local level, data reports that present data by local program and for the state overall could be produced to enhance targeting of services, provide managerial insights, and facilitate individual local program evaluation. Table 20-7 provides a sample format for comparing demographic, socioeconomic, and health status indicators from smaller to larger data collection units. For a complete series of worksheets that include nutritional status indicators, see Probert (1997). As described earlier, interpretation stems from analysis of similarities and differences between the smaller population of interest and the broader population. Recognize that, at times, data will not be available for every indicator at both levels of the comparison. Additionally, data may need to be obtained from multiple sources (e.g., if the community of interest is not geographically based, U.S. census data will not be available, but perhaps the relevant data would be available from a community source, such as client service records or membership profiles).

Data also may be used for comparison to health performance objectives. In this instance, existing surveillance data are used to provide a baseline for current conditions and to develop target

Table 20-7   Sample Format for Comparing Selected Data Indicators

	Smaller Unit (community, town, or state)	Larger Unit (national data source such as PedNSS)	Potential Data Source
Demographic Characteristics			
Age: • Proportion that are children • Proportion that are elderly	% less than 5 y % less than 18 y % more than 65 y	% less than 5 y % less than 18 y % more than 65 y	U.S. Census
Gender	% male % female	% male % female	U.S. Census
Ethnicity*			U.S. Census
Marital status	% single % married % widowed % divorced	% single % married % widowed % divorced	U.S. Census
Educational attainment	% adults who completed high school or college	% adults who completed high school or college	U.S. Census
Geographic description	% rural % urban % suburban	% rural % urban % suburban	U.S. Census
Socioeconomic Status			
Unemployment rate			U.S. Census, Current Population Survey, state unemployment data
Per capita income			U.S. Census

	Number	Percent	Number	Percent	
Household income • Mean or median per household • With no children under 18 years old • No husband present with children under 6 years old					U.S. Census
Population at or below poverty level • By type of household • By age					U.S. Census

(Continues)

Table 20-7　Sample Format for Comparing Selected Data Indicators (Continued)

	Smaller Unit (community, town, or state)		Larger Unit (national data source such as PedNSS)		Potential Data Source
	Number	Percent	Number	Percent	
Medicaid recipients					Centers for Medicare and Medicaid Services
Recipients of Temporary Assistance to Needy Families (TANF)					U.S. DHHS Administration for Children and Families
Supplemental Security Income (SSI) participation					Social Security Administration
Food Stamp recipients					USDA Food and Nutrition Service
WIC participation					USDA Food and Nutrition Service, state WIC program
Homelessness					U.S. Department of Housing and Urban Development
Community Health Status					
Leading causes of death	**List top five**		**List top five**		National Vital Statistics System, NCHS; state vital statistics registry
Years of potential life lost • Infant mortality • Death rate by age, disease, race, and gender					National Vital Statistics System, NCHS; state vital statistics registry
Most prevalent diseases • Prevalence by age, gender, ethnicity					State department of public health
Leading causes of hospitalization					National Hospital Discharge Survey (NHDS; from NCHS), local hospital discharge data

*Categories vary. It is often useful to collect data using the categorical definitions from the source the data will be compared with. See Office of Management and Budget, *Revisions to the Standards for the Classification of Federal Data on Race and Ethnicity* (commonly known as OMB 15) for federal directives regarding classifying race and ethnicity. Available at: http://www.whitehouse.gov/omb/fedreg/ombdir15.html.

Source: Compiled in part with permission from Probert, K. L. 1997. *Moving to the future: Developing community-based nutrition services (workbook & training manual).* Washington, DC: Association of State and Territorial Public Health Nutrition Directors.

goals for the future, and ongoing surveillance is used for comparison to the target and to assess progress toward meeting those goals. In 2000, the U.S. DHHS published a national agenda, called Healthy People (HP) 2010 (U.S. DHHS, 2000). These national guidelines outlined a federal disease prevention and health promotion agenda to be achieved by the year 2010. HP 2010 contains objectives in multiple health-related areas, including nutritional status. Areas of particular relevance to nutrition include the three major categories: Nutrition and Overweight; Physical Activity and Fitness; and Maternal, Infant, and Child Health. HP 2010 defines a federally determined target and the recommended state-level data source for comparison to the target, such as the Behavioral Risk Factor Surveillance System (BRFSS), PNSS, PedNSS, and NHANES. However, there are gaps and limitations in the current public health nutrition surveillance infrastructure, and HP 2010 identifies priority areas where no current national data sources are available. These are areas that need to be addressed in the development of future surveillance systems, and they illustrate cases where a program planner may need to collect original data to demonstrate need or progress in meeting objectives.

Data Compilation

Data Requirements, Collection, and Management

The recent expansion in data accessibility at the federal, state, and local levels allows nutrition professionals to be more specific in their planning, which increases the likelihood that a true health need will be addressed by nutrition programming and that such efforts will result in a positive change in nutritional status and health for their intended target audience. However, because of the plethora of available data, it is more important than ever to carefully plan for data requirements prior to data retrieval and/or initiation of data collection. Failure to do so can result in a nutritionist becoming mired in data that do not contribute to the primary purpose of the data collection, whether it is for a community profile, program evaluation, or grant development.

The most important step when working with data is to define what you need to know. This process has two main facets: 1) identifying the goal for data collection, and 2) making procedural plans for the data's acquisition, storage, manipulation, and reporting. First, before collecting a single data point, a nutrition program planner needs to know the answers to the following questions relative to goal identification:

- Why collect original data at all?
- What type of data will be collected?

- What method will be used to collect the data?
- What do I need to learn from data analysis?
- What will be done with the information?
- How will the information acquired help in meeting client and organizational needs?

For instance, prior to designing a new questionnaire, a program planner should know what problem he or she is trying to solve, what new information he or she must have to solve it, and who the target population is for the survey. By specifying exactly what he or she needs to know, the planner will limit the questionnaire to only critical fields and eliminate the collection of potentially interesting but unusable information (and thereby will reduce response burden, cost, and processing time). Often, existing monitoring and surveillance systems already may collect the desired information. If the nutrition program planner does not know what he or she is looking for, it is necessary to stop and reconsider why a data collection process is being considered in the first place. It is never good practice to collect data on myriad topics and hope that something useful and informative will emerge.

Second, planning for the data collection procedure begins with a thoughtful self-evaluation of the nutrition program planner's personal and organizational capacity so that data are obtained in a format that can be utilized. For instance, a nutritionist or data analyst who is proficient working with large, complex data files and sophisticated data analysis software may be comfortable obtaining large raw data files from a government website and extracting what he or she requires. Others, who lack those types of skills or who do not have the computer hardware and software (and associated technical support) to use, may be better off working from summary statistics in published reports or from third-party summary data sources.

The next step in procedural planning is to consider the analytic plan. The nutrition program planner must define exactly what he or she hopes to learn prior to data collection to ensure that the appropriate data for the type of analysis desired are obtained. It is an all-too-common scenario that oversights in data collection result in the inability to process data for preferred results, which ends in much frustration and a lot of wasted effort on the part of subjects, data collectors, and data analysts. For instance, if a nutritionist is interested in learning more about nutritional status (in terms of weight-for-age, height-for-age, and weight-for-height) among school-aged children, the failure to include gender as a data collection field on the form during the data collection stage ultimately will result in the inability to generate meaningful results during the analysis stage, even if each child's age, height, and weight are collected. It cannot be emphasized strongly enough that the best results occur when an analysis plan is defined in advance of data collection. This method ensures that all required variables will be identified prior to data collection.

If it is determined that the required data are nonexistent for a given population and a new questionnaire must be implemented, it can be extremely valuable to borrow questions from existing questionnaires. There are at least two advantages to this approach: 1) the data collected locally can be compared to data collected by the original investigators from a larger population (or a population that differs in some other respect, such as income or education); and 2) the existing questionnaire may have been formally validated. The choice of whether to use existing data or to collect new data also is dependent upon the anticipated survey sample size and the method of survey administration (telephone survey, face-to-face interview, mailed survey, etc.).

Final data collection procedural issues to consider include planning for data processing and database management, and deciding when and how results will be presented and disseminated. Although the nutrition program planner may not perform all of these functions, he or she needs to be familiar with them in order to provide managerial oversight.

Bourque and Clark (1992) describe an expanded definition of data processing that goes beyond just data coding, data entry, and verification. In their definition, data processing begins with the selection of a data collection strategy and ends with the completion of data transformations. The process they describe includes:

- Developing response categories during the development of the data collection instrument so that categories for precoded and open-ended questions are defined prior to data collection
- Collecting the data
- Creating data files that are compatible with statistical packages (i.e., Statistical Analysis Software [SAS] or Statistical Package for the Social Sciences [SPSS])
- Transforming data into analytically meaningful variables
- Documenting in writing all aspects of the system

This broad definition is extremely useful as it highlights the multistage process of converting verbal or written information into meaningful data that can be analyzed electronically. Developing operational definitions up front is important so that it is clear exactly what each indicator being collected refers to. This is particularly important when comparison to published data (e.g., from a surveillance system or the U.S. Census) is anticipated, so that similar categorical responses are used, when appropriate. Attention to this process will likely increase success as decisions about data content and format will be addressed at the beginning, decreasing the likelihood that acquired data will not be useable. It also will increase data quality and improve reliability and validity.

Table 20-8 provides a brief overview of some of the considerations involved in the conception and maintenance of an electronic database management system. Note that written documentation of the system should include information about the data content (such as operational definitions, cleaning rules, and transformation decisions) as well as details regarding the maintenance and security of the system itself.

The decision of how results will be presented (particularly with respect to content) can save a lot of time during data analysis by preventing superfluous data analyses or unnecessary formatting of results that are not intended to be used. For instance, if data will be used only for internal purposes, perhaps output that contains all analyses printed straight from the analytic software will be acceptable. If results are intended for publication, perhaps a more polished document with summary results and interpretation highlighted will be prepared.

TABLE 20-8   Selected Database Management Concerns

Personnel
1. Who will enter the data? Who is this person's backup?
2. What credentials do they require?
3. Who will update records?
4. Who will back up the computer file?
5. Are staff adequately trained and supervised?

Data Entry Process
1. Will data be entered on an as-received basis or according to an established schedule?
2. Does the data-entry screen replicate the paper form from which data are to be entered?
3. Does the data need to be coded prior to entry? If so, who will code the data?
4. Are double-entry systems used for quality assurance?

Data Entry Computer Program
1. Does the data-entry program allow for certain data items to be entered automatically on subsequent screens until the data recorder makes a change (e.g., repetition of clinic number on multiple records to facilitate batch entry)?
2. Does the data-entry program effectively validate the data being entered for completeness, use of "must-enter" fields, and "look-up" files?
3. Does the data entry program have the ability to do range checking on values entered? If so, does the system allow for acceptable ranges to change, reflecting values entered in the database over time?
4. Is there a logic audit procedure in the system to locate such errors as misspelled names or addresses, or incorrectly coded race, gender, or disease?
5. Is the system flexible enough to allow variables to be modified as prescribed by changes in state regulations and national recommendations?
6. Are production reports automatically generated for quality assurance of data entry?

Data Security

1. At what level (state or local) will records be changed or deleted?
2. Who owns the data records?
3. If the database is distributed to other users as an electronic file, are there safeguards to prevent overwriting another user's data?
4. Are there safeguards against computer viruses?
5. How and with what frequency are data copied and stored for back-up purposes?
6. Are paper copies maintained (in the event of computer failure)?
7. Do data storage and transfer procedures (whether electronic or paper) meet HIPAA* confidentiality requirements?
8. Are there written policies on data management, quality control, access, release, and security?

---

*The Health Insurance Portability and Accountability Act of 1996 (HIPAA) provide national standards to protect the privacy of personal health information. For details, see http://www.os.dhhs.gov/ocr/hipaa/.

Source: Adapted with permission from Groseclose, S. L., Sullivan, K. M., Gibbs, N. P., & Knowles, C. M. (2000). Management of the surveillance information system and quality control of data. In S. M. Teutsch and R. E. Churchill (eds.), *Principles and Practice of Public Health Surveillance* (2nd ed.). New York: Oxford University Press.

Accessing Existing Data Sources

There are many different sources for quantitative community-level and population-based data on a wide variety of topics. Which types of data and which sources will be used is a matter of strategic choice. Some possible sources include, but are not limited to, population data (e.g., U.S. Census or NHANES), program data (e.g., the WIC program or Head Start), trend data, national objectives (e.g., HP 2010), and cost data. Frequently, national surveillance data also are available at the state level, either from the national agency that operates the system or from the state department that submits the data to the national system.

All of the data sources that are available online are too numerous to mention. FedStats, described on its web page as "the gateway to statistics from over 100 U.S. Federal agencies," is a good place to start finding pertinent sources. In addition, Table 20-9 describes other selected sources of data from federal agencies that are easily accessible and that cover a broad range of data types and content. Other sources may be readily located using a web browser search engine. Many online

> FedStats is available at http://www.fedstats.gov.

data sources offer the options of viewing predefined reports or generating custom tables with data obtained through searches and queries of summary and microdata files. Websites should be visited frequently, because many are constantly in the process of adding new or updated material.

TABLE 20-9   Selected Tools That Provide Access to Federal Sources of Data

Agency	Tool Name	Web Address
DataFERRETT (Federal Electronic Research, Review, & Extraction Tool)*	Ferret	http://ferret.bls.census.gov/
U.S. Census Bureau	Data Access Tools	http://www.census.gov/main/www/access.html
Bureau of Economic Analysis	Gross State Product (GSP)	http://www.bea.gov/bea/regional/gsp/
	National Income and Product Accounts (NIPA)	http://www.bea.gov/bea/dn/nipaweb/index.asp
	State Quarterly Personal Income	http://www.bea.gov/bea/regional/sqpi
	Annual State Personal Income	http://www.bea.gov/bea/regional/spi/
Bureau of Labor Statistics	Most Requested Series	http://www.bls.gov/data/top20.htm
Environmental Protection Agency	EPA Databases and Software	http://www.epa.gov/epahome/Data.html
National Agricultural Statistics Service	Quick Stats: Agricultural Statistics Data Base	http://www.nass.usda.gov:81/ipedb/
National Center for Health Statistics	CDC Wonder	http://wonder.cdc.gov/
National Science Foundation	SESTAT	http://srsstats.sbe.nsf.gov/
Division of Science Resources Statistics	WebCASPAR	http://caspar.nsf.gov/cgi-bin/WebIC.exe?template=nsf/srs/webcasp/start.wi

*This is a multiagency tool that provides access to datasets from two or more federal statistical agencies, such as the U.S. Census Bureau, Bureau of Labor Statistics, and National Center for Health Statistics.

There also are a wide variety of state-level sources of data. Some state departments of public health have created online information services, such as MassCHIP (Massachusetts Community Health Information Profile), where users can obtain community-level data to assess health needs, monitor health status indicators, and evaluate health programs in those states. Other available data sources are hosted by private foundations, such as the Kaiser Family Foundation's State Health Facts, a resource that contains state-level data on demographics, health, and health policy, including health coverage, access, financing, and state legislation, or the Annie E. Casey

Foundation's The Right Start Online, in which data reflecting measures of child well-being are available as profiles, line graphs, national maps, rankings, and raw data for the nation's 50 largest cities and all 50 states.

> MassCHIP is available at http://masschip.state.ma.us. The Kaiser Family Foundation's State Health Facts is available at http://statehealthfacts.kff.org. The Annie E. Casey Foundation's The Right Start Online is available at http://www.aecf.org/kidscount/rightstart/.

It is important to pay close attention to the data source attribution when using a secondary data source (i.e., a data source that is presenting information that the researchers did not collect). For instance, the U.S. Census Bureau is a primary data source because it publishes data collected only by that agency. The Right Start Online, on the other hand, is based on birth certificate data compiled by the National Center for Health Statistics, making it a secondary data source. Another example of a secondary data source is the PeriStats Interactive Perinatal Data Resource, developed by the March of Dimes. This tool is focused on providing perinatal statistics at the state and county levels. PeriStats data are compiled from the CDC, including the National Center for Health Statistics (NCHS), the National Center for Chronic Disease Prevention and Health Promotion, and the National Center for HIV, STD, and TB Prevention; the Centers for Medicare & Medicaid Services (CMS); the Health Resources Services Administration (HRSA); the Substance Abuse and Mental Health Services Administration (SAMHSA); the U.S. Census Bureau; the National Governors Association (NGA); the USDA; and the March of Dimes. Failure to note data's point of origin could result in

> The PeriStats Interactive Perinatal Data Resource is available at http://www.marchofdimes.com/professionals/680_1922.asp.

a program planner collecting data from multiple sources that actually are duplicative rather than complimentary. As indicated previously, it is also critical to note the time period represented by the data, as well as operational definitions for all measures and technical terms used.

Conclusion

A nutrition program plan to address a specific health issue is strengthened by data that demonstrate a community's health and nutritional status (based on demographic, socioeconomic, and health status data), the community's perceived needs (gathered through qualitative methods), and any major duplication and/or gaps in available community services. The use of data in the needs assessment process assures that resources and activities are directed toward a defined target audience with a prioritized health need.

Accurate, timely information is absolutely critical for decision makers, who need to understand a problem's scope as well as its causes and consequences prior to taking action (such as whether to revise a program or initiate something new). Such understanding is achieved through the processes of assessment, analysis, and action. Assessment refers to the detection of the existence of a problem. Analysis is the mechanism by which causes and solutions are identified. Action involves the communication of results to those responsible for initiating action to solve the problem. In addition, related information is essential to monitor and evaluate how well (or poorly) their actions have affected the problem.

The utility of nutrition data is far reaching, as it can be used to improve an agency's capacity to assess, analyze, and design resource-relevant actions; improve organizational and public perception and knowledge; increase effective demand for nutrition-relevant information; and ensure adequate resources for action. This is what is meant by "translating data" into public health action.

Issues for Discussion

1. What is the role of data in the justification for an intervention among a given target audience?
2. What are the skills that a nutritionist requires in order to demonstrate a facility with data management and interpretation?
3. What resources should be allocated to collecting, analyzing, and reporting data for program planning and evaluation?
4. When utilizing a secondary data source versus collecting original data, what are the benefits and tradeoffs in terms of simplicity, time, comprehensiveness, and flexibility?

Acknowledgments

The valuable input of Jan Kallio, Stephanie Lambou, and Rachel Colchamiro is greatly appreciated.

References

Aspen Reference Group. 1997. *Community health education and promotion: A guide to program design and evaluation.* Gaithersburg, MD: Aspen.

Birkhead, G. S. & Maylahn, C. M. 2000. State and local public health surveillance. In S. M. Teutsch and R. E. Churchill (eds.), *Principles and Practice of Public Health Surveillance* (2nd ed.) (pp. 253–286). New York: Oxford University Press.

Bourque, L. B. & Clark, V. A. 1992. *Processing data: The survey example.* Newbury Park, CA: Sage.

Briefel, R. R. 2001. Nutrition monitoring in the United States. In B. Bowman and R. M. Russell. (eds.), *Present Knowledge in Nutrition* (8th ed.) (pp. 617-635). Washington, DC: International Life Sciences Institute.

Centers for Disease Control and Prevention. 1988. Guidelines for evaluating surveillance systems. *Morbidity and Mortality Weekly Report,* 37(S-5 pp. 1-18).

Centers for Disease Control and Prevention. 1999. Framework for program evaluation in public health. *Morbidity and Mortality Weekly Report,* 48(RR-11, pp. 1-40).

Cole, T. J. 1991. Sampling, study size, and power. In B. M. Margetts and M. Nelson (eds.), *Design Concepts in Nutritional Epidemiology* (pp. 53-78). New York: Oxford University Press.

Dwyer, J., Picciano, M. F., Raiten, D. J., & Members of the Steering Committee. 2003. Collection of food and dietary supplement intake data: What We Eat in America–NHANES. *Journal of Nutrition,* 133, 590S-600S.

Groseclose, S. L., Sullivan, K. M., Gibbs, N. P., & Knowles, C. M. 2000. Management of the surveillance information system and quality control of data. In S. M. Teutsch and R. E. Churchill (eds.), *Principles and Practice of Public Health Surveillance* (2nd ed.) (pp. 95-111). New York: Oxford University Press.

Jacob, H. 1984. *Using published data: Errors and remedies.* Newbury Park, CA: Sage.

Mason, J. B., Habicht, J. P., Tabatabai, H., & Valverdi, V. 1984. Nutritional surveillance for programme management and evaluation. In *Nutritional Surveillance* (pp. 140-175). Geneva: World Health Organization.

Morris, W. (ed.). 1982. *The American heritage dictionary of the English language.* Boston: Houghton Mifflin.

Owen, A. L., Splett, P. L., & Owen, G. M. 1999. *Nutrition in the community: The art and science of delivering services* (4th ed.). Boston: McGraw Hill.

Polhamus, B., Dalenius, K., Thompson, D., Scanlon, K., Borland, E., Smith, B., & Grummer-Strawn, L. 2004. *Pediatric nutrition surveillance 2002 report.* Atlanta: U.S. Department of Health and Human Services, Centers for Disease Control and Prevention.

Probert, K. L. (ed.). 1996. *Moving to the future: Developing community-based nutrition services.* Washington, DC: Association of State and Territorial Public Health Nutrition Directors.

Probert, K. L. 1997. *Moving to the future: Developing community-based nutrition services (workbook & training manual).* Washington, DC: Association of State and Territorial Public Health Nutrition Directors.

Spicer, D. A. & Kaufman, M. 1990. Managing data. In M. Kaufman (ed.), *Nutrition in Public Health: A Handbook for Developing Programs and Services* (pp. 312-341). Rockville, MD: Aspen.

Teutsch, S. M. 2000. Considerations in planning a surveillance system. In S. M. Teutsch and R. E. Churchill (eds.), *Principles and Practice of Public Health Surveillance* (2nd ed.) (pp. 17-29). New York: Oxford University Press.

U.S. Department of Health and Human Services. 2000. *Healthy People 2010* (conference edition in 2 vols). Washington, DC.

Wurzbach, M. E. (ed.). 2002. *Community health education and promotion: A guide to program design and evaluation* (2nd ed.). Gaithersburg, MD: Aspen.

CHAPTER 21

MANAGING MONEY

Katherine Cairns, MPH, MBA, RD

Reader Objectives

After studying this chapter and reflecting on the contents, you should be able to:

1. Discuss the nutritionist's responsibilities for managing money.
2. Identify collaborators in the agency budgeting process.
3. Discuss justifications for each budgeted proposal.
4. Describe the major sources for funding public health nutrition services.
5. List and describe major categories for a nutrition program budget.
6. Specify major items in a grant application.
7. Describe major sources of third-party reimbursement for public health nutrition services.

Financing Public Health Nutrition Programs and Services

Providing the community with public health nutrition programs that residents need and want requires that the agency allocate dollars to pay personnel salaries, reimburse their travel, buy equipment and supplies, provide for continuing education of nutrition personnel, and purchase other goods needed to deliver services. Every nutritionist who manages a program, service, or project must take responsibility for requesting, justifying, and negotiating a budget and controlling expenditures within the funds allocated. Fiscal management means understanding the financing and budgeting process while working closely with the following key people in an organization:

- *Agency administrator and board members* who set the agency's fiscal policy and determine how the agency's budget will be distributed to programs and overhead.

- *Finance/fiscal officer or business manager* who maintains accounts, controls expenditures, and can provide advice on the organization's written and unwritten fiscal policies and procedures.
- *Other program directors* who request and manage budgets for programs that should utilize nutrition services. These directors may be convinced to collaborate in funding nutrition services through their internal funding sources or by writing grants for external funding.

Tighter federal, state, and local government agency budgets require nutritionists to compete for the money they need if they want to turn plans for comprehensive nutrition services into action. Convincing a governmental unit or foundation to invest money and become a stakeholder in nutrition services requires that the value of each proposal be justified. Business planning and compelling answers to the following questions will prepare a nutrition administrator for the competitive public and private funding environment.

1. Is there really a need for the service?
2. What are the competing options for the available and new money? The plan, budget, service, product, and their evaluation must stand out from the competition.
3. Can cost-effectiveness data be provided for the type of nutrition service proposed?
4. What stakeholder support and contributions are there for the proposal?
5. What additional community support and media attention can be generated prior to, during, and following the funding decisions?
6. What support does the competition have for the same funding?
7. Are there federal, state, or local requirements/mandates for components of the proposed nutrition service?
8. What potential does the proposed service have to generate income for the agency?
9. Are there federal or foundation grants available to establish and maintain the service into the future?

Competitive proposals for spending new or ongoing money must show evidence of support from individuals and organizations in the community who will benefit from the product or service. They can demonstrate their support by paying fees for services; making in-kind contributions of staff, volunteer time, or space in offices or clinics; writing letters of support; presenting testimony; lobbying proactively; and donating equipment, materials, or cash contributions.

Interdisciplinary teamwork and networking to increase the number of stakeholders in nutrition programs are discussed in other chapters. Financers prefer to fund a service that responds to a demonstrated need that can be met cost effectively. A well-conceived budget for a new service or product details the cost per unit. Services with high start-up costs should show a reasonable cost per unit after the start-up and within the first 6 months of operation. Fiscal managers will ask these questions:

- Will the proposed service or product have a reasonable cost-to-benefit ratio? Funders compare the costs and outcomes of varying types of service delivery options.
- Will the service be carried out with the most cost-effective intervention? For example, will reducing anemia in 80% of a population group within 6 months of diagnosis be less costly if nutrition counseling is provided by a trained and supervised paraprofessional rather than by a nutritionist? Although the outcome may be the same, the costs of different intervention models may vary.

These and additional questions can be used as a checklist in preparing to request the funds needed to initiate the service.

Funds for nutrition services may be secured from a variety of sources. The more diversified the funding base, the more stable the program. The more funding sources used to maintain a public health nutrition program, the less dependent the program is on any one. However, maintaining accountability for too many small funding sources (< $10,000) may be counterproductive.

General Revenue

State governments generate funds through state income taxes, sales taxes, various types of business taxes, and taxes on such products as alcoholic beverages and cigarettes. In recent years, several states have begun to use lotteries and lawsuit settlement proceeds as revenue for public services. Local government units have the authority to tax property owners for municipal services, such as police and fire departments, schools, recreation, and public health. Tax levies are set annually based on the services needed, the priorities of policy makers, the demands of the taxpayers, and outside interests.

Most city, county, or state public health departments derive a portion of their income from general revenue. Public health agencies generally seek their fair share of general revenue as a cornerstone of their base income. Usually, there is keen competition for these funds in a health agency because they generally offer programs funding stability. If there is no general revenue in the budget for nutrition services, nutritionists need to discuss this funding source with agency administrators and business managers to prepare their request for the next budget cycle. Nutritionists may need to be persistent and assertive over several years to succeed.

Acquiring some funding that is not restricted to a specific target population provides flexibility to plan more comprehensive, community-responsive programs.

Grants

Federal Grants

A variety of federal funds are used by state, local, and non-governmental organizations (NGO) to operate food and nutrition programs. Federal agencies that fund major food/nutrition programs and demonstration projects to over 80 million Americans include:

- The Food and Nutrition Service of the U.S. Department of Agriculture (USDA)
- Centers for Medicare and Medicaid Services (CMS) of the U.S. Department of Health and Human Services
- Centers for Disease Control and Prevention of the U.S. Department of Health and Human Services
- Specific health block grant funds from the U.S. Department of Health and Human Services

Requests for Proposals (RFPs)— Invitations to suppliers to bid on supplying products or services that are difficult to describe for a company, or in this example, a public agency.

Personal contacts within each of the major federal or state agencies are useful to obtain advance notice of Requests for Proposals (RFPs) and special project funding.

State Grants

State departments of health, health and human services, agriculture, and education usually provide some funds for nutrition services. The state funds may support selected statewide and/or local services. In many states, a per capita or preestablished formula is used for allocating state and federal funds to local health agencies. State agencies may have special legislated funding for nutrition programs. State agencies also serve as the conduits for federal funds earmarked for local program implementation. Specific federal project funds that state governmental agencies administer through a grants process include:

- Special Supplemental Food Program for Women, Infants and Children (WIC)
- Other supplemental food programs for targeted groups (Farmer's Market, Senior Food Program, Summer Food Programs, Special Milk Programs, Daycare Programs, School Lunch/Breakfast Programs, Congregate Dining)
- Nutrition education special projects
- Maternal and child health special projects
- Health promotion special projects

- Chronic disease intervention/reduction special projects
- Targeted agricultural marketing special projects

Each state's grant application procedure has special requirements that need to be determined by consulting the local agency administrator, state agency, or regional/central office nutrition consultants.

Local Grants or Contracts

Local human or social service agencies, home health agencies, area agencies on aging, mental health agencies, developmental disabilities councils, school districts, jails, community colleges, and other governmental units frequently need nutrition services or have special initiatives or ongoing projects that require nutrition expertise. When agencies do not employ a full-time nutritionist on their own staff, they will often contract for these services as the most efficient method for getting the short-term or long-term services they need. Those local agencies that need part-time nutrition services frequently maintain lists or files of available contractors and their specialists. It is important to cultivate contacts within the local agencies who can advise on their needs, availability of funding, and interest in developing contracts.

Local voluntary health agencies such as the American Heart Association, American Diabetes Association, American Cancer Society, Cystic Fibrosis Association, or March of Dimes chapter or affiliate offices also may need and contract for nutrition services or offer small competitive project grants. For short-term community projects, funds may be obtained from local businesses, banks, civic organizations, or churches.

Foundation Grants

Millions of dollars of private foundation projects are funded annually for foundation-specific priorities. The Internet and the public library are the most valuable resources for identifying these foundation funders. Foundation and grant information centers maintain information on:

- Names and contact persons for local, state, regional, or national foundations
- Information on past funding priorities and projects funded
- Dollar amount of awards for foundation projects
- Criteria and format for submitting funding requests
- Timeline for review of grant requests

Priorities of foundations may change annually. Thus, putting a new twist on an old idea or need may be required for the foundation to consider the proposal. Some foundations prefer that proposals be submitted on behalf of a nongovernmental, nonprofit agency. Nutritionists working in a governmental agency who seek a foundation grant might collaborate with a nonprofit agency that will submit the proposal and subcontract the nutrition work to the public health agency. A sample guide for submitting a grant proposal is located in Appendix G.

Fee for Services

A fee-for-service adjusted for each target population is a useful method for recovering program costs. A basic market analysis is required to determine the range of fees appropriate to charge the various target populations. Fees must be based on actual costs, not guesswork. Making a fee-for-service plan more acceptable to clients of a public health service is a second task, after calculating actual costs. In presenting a plan to establish fees to administrators, government officials, the public, and coworkers, three alternatives might be offered:

1. *Sliding scale fee-for-service:* The fee is based on the client's ability to pay, with the maximum fee being the actual cost of the service; this can be used for all basic public health services.

2. *Actual cost fee-for-service:* The actual cost of providing a service is calculated and revised annually. It is charged for public health services where there are other private and nonprofit providers of the services within a community. These service charges are not put on a sliding scale because of the potential legal issues of unfair competition by a governmental provider. A public agency will by design have few of these services because of need-based planning.

3. *Cost plus fee-for-service:* This pricing model permits a nonprofit agency to recover the actual cost of a service in addition to a profit, which is then used to subsidize another service within the agency. These "cash cows" may include innovative services or products (healthy cooking demonstrations, diet and fitness classes, customized nutrition services for community organizations) or long-standing, fully capitalized services (laboratory tests).

These "price" versus "cost" strategies are dependent on an accurate cost determination and are discussed later in this chapter.

Third-Party Reimbursement

Third-party reimbursement income is received by billing insurance carriers, such as governmental healthcare programs (Medicaid, Medicare), workers' compensation, health maintenance organizations (HMOs)/managed care organizations (MCOs), and/or other special health insurance pools (catastrophic health, state-sponsored alternative care pools, organized employer groups). Each health carrier has its own billing procedures that the agency accounting office must determine and continuously keep updated. It is most cost effective for the agency accounting department to select the three or four third-party reimbursement sources that cover the majority of the agency's clients and bill these carriers. Clients not covered by those carriers would be treated as fee-for-service clients and advised to collect reimbursement from their own carrier. Some organizations contract with healthcare reimbursement firms that require an assignment of benefits from all clients and handle all agency billing for a predetermined fee.

Emerging opportunities for income generation are developing in the area of third-party reimbursement. Nutrition services are increasingly being reimbursed for chronic and acute care interventions. Nutrition and health programs are identifying ways to protect revenue raised from third-party reimbursements to allow a carryover of these funds between fiscal years for program-specific initiatives.

Preparing Budgets and Determining Program Costs

Generating the funds to cover the cost of delivering a nutrition service is an important part of fiscal management. Determining the real cost of a product or service is crucial to setting fees, collecting reimbursements, and writing grants. Preparing a budget for an array of services and then breaking it down into the actual cost of each product/service is the next step.

The budget defines what services can be implemented with the amount of funding available. An annotated budget, as shown in Table 21-1, is one way to walk through the process.

> **Annotated budget**—A budget supplied with critical or explanatory notes.

The Budget Summary

Controlling the budget requires a monthly comparison of projected income to actual expenses and encumbrances (items purchased but not yet paid for). The agency's accounting section should provide a monthly financial summary listing the current status of expenditures compared to the amounts budgeted. Table 21-2 displays an example of this analysis. The program manager must monitor this carefully so that all budgeted resources are wisely used. The monthly financial summary also enables the manager to determine when the income flow is inadequate compared to projections. Fund transfers between program accounts may be needed to balance the budget.

TABLE 21-1   The Annotated Program Budget

Income

A diversified income base is critical to a strong nutrition program. The only "fudge factors" are client fees and reimbursements that are projected based on past income-generating experience.

Grant A		$ XXX
Grant B		$ XXX
Client fees		$ XXX
Program A	$ XXX	
Program B	$ XXX	
Third-party reimbursement		$ XXX
General revenue (local tax levy support)	$ XXX	
State grant/allocation		$ XXX

Total income:		**$ XXXX**

(This should equal or exceed
total expenses.)

Expenses

Salaries		$ XXX
Full-time (specify FTEs)	$ XXX	
Part-time (specify FTEs)	$ XXX	
Fringe benefits		$ XXX
Mileage for local travel		$ XXX
Other travel		$ XXX
Telephone: local, long-distance		$ XXX
Internet connection, allocation		$ XXX
Postage		$ XXX
Film/video reproduction		$ XXX
Printing		$ XXX
Supplies		$ XXX
Office		$ XXX
Food for demonstrations/clients	$ XXX	
Books		$ XXX
Subscriptions		$ XXX
Other educational materials		$ XXX
Software		$ XXX
Space, rental/allocation		$ XXX
Equipment rental/allocation[1]		$ XXX
Copy machines	$ XXX	
Computers	$ XXX	
Telephones	$ XXX	
Video	$ XXX	
Equipment, purchase[2]		$ XXX
Computer/other hardware	$ XXX	
Other office equipment	$ XXX	

Utilities, actual/allocation		$ XXX
Staff training and continuing education		$ XXX
Out-of-town travel	$ XXX	
Lodging	$ XXX	
Registration fees	$ XXX	
Registrations, local	$ XXX	
Memberships	$ XXX	
Other		$ XXX
Indirect costs[3]		$ XXX
Central service charge[4]		$ XXX
Consultant fees[5]		$ XXX
Student stipends[6]		$ XXX
Equipment maintenance fee[7]		$ XXX
Contingent reserve fund[8]		$ XXX

Total expenses	**$ XXXX**

(Total expenses should be
less than total income.)

1. Carefully evaluate the rent vs. buy decision on all equipment.
2. It is important to plan for life-cycle replacement of equipment in each annual budget.
3. There may be an administrative overhead charge included as a percentage of each budget for overall agency indirect costs.
4. Additional overhead may be charged by the county/city/state to cover the costs of attorneys, accountants, executive directors, and central purchasing that provide service but are outside of the nutrition or health department.
5. Include fees for graphic consultants, contract professional/technical assistance, external evaluation specialists, and auditor fees for federal funds received. Contract physician fees for grants/third-party reimbursement requirements, especially if third-party reimbursement will cover the costs and result in nutrition reimbursement.
6. Try to build in student stipends for internships if quality supervision can be provided for the students.
7. Fees are generally charged for some equipment rental based on volume/intensity of use for major equipment repair-only contracts if there is a good payback for high use/frequently broken equipment.
8. A carryover fund for emergencies, reimbursed initiatives.

Source: Compiled by the author.

The monthly budget summary should be used to determine when there is a need to:

- Communicate with staff about the program's financial position
- Trim discretionary costs (supplies, printing, etc.) or increase spending on consumable supplies
- Increase or decrease staffing (overtime/voluntary reduction of hours/layoffs)
- Generate more income (find out why some health carriers are slower to pay or slow down the agency billing process)

A computer spreadsheet is a clear, timesaving tool for preparing the budget summary. There are many fine financial software packages available. Most governmental agencies will require their departments to use their purchased financial software.

Table 21-2   Monthly Financial Summary

	Month		Year-to-Date (YTD)		
	Actual Income	Budgeted Income	YTD Received	YTD Budgeted	YTD (Previous Year)
Income (List all sources)					
Total Income:					

	Actual Expenses	Budgeted Expenses	YTD Expenses	YTD Budgeted Expenses	YTD Expenses (Previous Year)
Expenses (List All Expense Categories)					
Total Expenses					
Variance From Projections					

Source: Compiled by the author.

Determining Costs for Each Service

Determining the costs for each specific service or product requires a slightly different adaptation of the program budget. The program manager must know the approximate utilization of staff and resources directed to each service. Staff time is the largest expense in any service. Time studies or tracking of billable hours are frequently used to assess the amount of staff time each product or service requires. If a time study is not feasible for a variety of reasons (lack of time, staff issues, etc.), a quick, less precise method can be used to approximate the amount of staff time spent in each specific service area. This method is displayed in Table 21-3. Note that administrative time is factored into each service category.

The next step is to cost out staff, supplies, equipment, and other resources for each service area (Table 21-4), then divide the total cost by the number of clients or client visits (or relative value units, a productivity measuring unit used by some programs) expected to be served during the year. This yields a cost-per-contact, or the actual cost to provide each unit of service.

Starting from the program budget, this cost determination analysis takes approximately 2 hours to calculate for each service. A program manager could devote about 2 hours per month to identifying the actual costs of one program per month and make needed adjustments in charges. More complicated systems of cost determination exist, especially for federally funded programs. These can be developed with the guidance of the agency's business manager or accountant. Public health programs have been able to increase their operating income after doing this type of analysis. Health screening programs, therapeutic counseling, and group educational programs are examples of programs for which this cost determination would be useful to document actual costs compared to reimbursed costs. The goal is to move reimbursed costs closer to the actual costs of the public health nutrition service.

Divide total cost by number of clients or client visits (or relative value units used by some programs) expected to be served this year. This gives a cost per contact or encounter, which is the actual cost to the program to provide each unit of this service. This can also be analyzed by the actual number of clients served in the most recent reporting period.

TABLE 21-3   Staff Allocation by Service/Cost Center for Cost Determination

Staff Member Name	Total FTE	WIC	Diabetes Clinic	Home Visits	Education Group	Newspaper Column	Weight Reduction Class
Clerical							
Amy Jones	1.0	0.9	0.0	0.0	0.0	0.0	0.1
Jean Brown	0.8	0.1	0.1	0.3	0.2	0.1	0.0
Nutrition Assistants							
Tom Smith	1.0	1.0	0.0	0.0	0.0	0.0	0.0
Betty White	0.8	0.8	0.0	0.0	0.0	0.0	0.0
Pam Johnson	0.7	0.7	0.0	0.0	0.0	0.0	0.0
Terry Jones	1.0	0.5	0.0	0.5	0.0	0.0	0.0
Nutritionists							
Mary Stokes	0.8	0.8	0.0	0.0	0.0	0.0	0.0
Sue Austin	1.0	0.0	0.0	0.1	0.3	0.1	0.5
Steve Doe	1.0	0.0	0.0	0.1	0.3	0.1	0.5
Kate Conner	1.0	0.2	0.1	0.1	0.4	0.1	0.1
Total	**9.1**	**5.0**	**0.2**	**1.1**	**1.2**	**0.4**	**1.2**

FTE = Full-Time Equivalent

Source: Compiled by the author.

Service Productivity Analysis

A second stage of analysis for program managers concerned about the high cost of a given service is a service productivity analysis. A simple analysis of service productivity levels involves multiplying the total FTEs allocated to each service by 2,080 (paid hours) or 1,800 (billable hours) for each full-time equivalent position and dividing by the number of clients or contact visits. See Figure 21-1 for an example.

Cost-Effectiveness and Cost-Benefit Analysis of Services

The third and final challenge of fiscal management is to evaluate the service/product once the costs and providers have been identified. Cost-benefit analysis and cost-effectiveness analysis are most commonly utilized for evaluations. A cost-benefit analysis is used

TABLE 21-4   Cost Determination for a Nutrition Service

Service: Nutrition counseling in-home visits
Date of cost determination: 12-21-05

Salaries		Comments
Jean Brown, .3 FTE	$ XXX	Full-time equivalent (FTE) by salary
Terry Jones, .5 FTE	XXX	
Sue Austin, .1 FTE	XXX	
Steve Doe, .1 FTE	XXX	
Kate Conner, .1 FTE	XXX	
Fringe benefit allocation	XXX	Based on required allocation
Mileage for home visits	XXX	Allocated or actual use
Telephone	XXX	Allocated on estimated/actual use
Postage	XXX	Allocated on estimated/actual use
Duplicating	XXX	Allocated on estimated/actual use
Supplies	XXX	Allocated on estimated/actual use
Office rental	XXX	Allocated based on space occupied
Equipment	XXX	Allocated based on use
Training/education	XXX	Allocated
Other	XXX	
Subtotal	XXX	
Indirect cost rate (___%)	XXX	Apply to subtotal
Total cost of service	**$ XXX**	

Source: Compiled by the author.

in the planning process to decide if a program/service should be undertaken. A cost-effectiveness analysis is undertaken in planning to determine the least costly way to provide the service or program.

Through the application of these analysis tools, the nutritionist can make services generate income and become increasingly self-supporting. There is great risk in taking an innovative service idea, guessing at a charge for the service, providing the service, and later questioning why the staff time commitment is so excessive in relation to the financial return. An analysis of the project, including the documented need, the population to be served, favorable pricing, and realistic income expectations could turn the innovation into a source of income.

Developing Skills in Grant Writing

Most nutritionists need to become grant writers so that they can obtain outside income to support innovative services, reach new populations, develop and test interventions, and initiate special projects; any or all of these may then turn into long-term, income-producing services. Several hints for grant writing are as follows:

- Maintain a grant idea folder in which to file innovative ideas that would require external funding. These can be ideas with a one-paragraph description as contributed by staff members. The community needs assessment will help produce some ideas for needed community services.
- Foster staff development by conducting an internal seed grant program within the section or agency. Allocate a small amount of money each year to this research and development (R&D) fund.
- Find several grant writers and reviewers within the agency with whom to brainstorm ideas and advice on writing grant proposals.
- Reduce all grant proposals to one-page worksheets as an initial step. A sample worksheet is shown in Figure 21-2.
- Maintain a large network of project collaborators to work with on grant proposals of mutual interest.
- Identify reliable people and organizations that can be counted on to write support letters, even on short notice. Some of these individuals/agencies may prefer that the support letter be written for their signature.
- Plan on writing grants that will generate three to four times the dollar amount from the grant as the program is committing.
- Practice writing concisely. If the idea cannot be conveyed in two double-spaced pages, including needs statement, methods, objectives, budget, and collaborators, grant writing will be too time-consuming.

Service: Nutrition counseling in-home visits
Date of cost determination: 7-21-05

1. How long should it take to provide one unit (visit) of this service?

2 hours (includes direct service time, travel time, charting, case conference, and administration)

2. How long does it take to provide each unit (visit) of this service?

Agencies may calculate this based on:

- **2,080 hours** (1.0 FTE paid with vacation/sick days included) or
- **1,800 billable hours** (1.0 FTE excluding vacation/sick/holiday hours)

Total FTEs: 1.1 × hours = 1,980 billable hours or 2,288 hours

Total service units: 650 home visits

1,980 divided by 650 budgeted home visits = **3.5 hours per home visit**

2,288 divided by 650 budgeted home visits = **3.52 hours per home visit**

3. Explain the difference between the answers to 1 and 2.

- 3.5 (or 3.52) hours per visit (actual) compared to 2.0 hours per visit (estimate) is significant. Thus, staff take almost twice as long to complete the home visit service as what they estimated during the budget cycle *or* too many staff are assigned to this activity.

- Suggest that staff adjust expectation to 2.5 hours per visit and expect 792 home visits this year, or reduce staff to 0.92 FTEs to provide 650 visits. In order to break even financially for this service, staff productivity must increase or staff must be reassigned/reduced.

- The budget for home visit service is based on an actual reimbursed cost of $65.00 per home visit. If the number of home visits can be increased from 650 to 792 with the existing staff, the program will generate an additional $9,230 this year. Healthcare payers will not reimburse more than $65.00 per visit this year. Suggest that staff initiate a quality improvement audit of existing clients to document outcomes. Bring results with actual higher costs to health plans for negotiated reimbursement increases for serving high-risk Medicaid/Medicare population in the next year.

FIGURE 21-1   Service Productivity Analysis
Source: Compiled by the author.

- Maintain a file of agency information that can be pulled for grant attachments. Items such as Agency Internal Revenue Tax Exemption 501(c)(3) statements, audited budgets, lists of board members, agency descriptions, federal identification numbers for the agency, and personnel curriculum vitae should be in this file.
- Maintain a file of copies of grants submitted previously.

- Use word processing and spreadsheet software to write the narrative and prepare the budget spreadsheet. This makes it easier to revise the proposal without introducing errors.
- Get on the mailing lists of every agency and foundation that announces related grant/contract RFPs that can be identified.

Conclusion

These hints for grant writing will undoubtedly be added to and shared with other people. Sharing the work and the glory when a new grant comes to the agency is the mark of a true professional. Researching grant funds and writing proposals takes time. Alas, well-written proposals are not always funded. Even experienced grant writers receive rejections. It takes persistence. If a proposal is rejected, ask for a copy of the grant evaluation sheet and try again, and again.

Issues for Discussion

1. Given the staffing patterns described in Table 21-4 and Figure 21-1, is the nutrition program using the best mix of staff and allocation of staff time to result in the desired outcomes? What additional information would be useful? What productivity-enhancing strategies would be useful for the nutrition staff involved in the home visiting service?
2. Suggest a grant application idea to increase financial resources for the home visiting service. Complete a Grant Application Internal Worksheet (Figure 21-2) for your idea and discuss.
3. How should fees for nutrition services be established, and how should this income be most effectively allocated?
4. Explore the healthcare billing/coding references for your state Medicaid program and identify two potential billing codes for public health nutrition services. Identify the state and federal requirements (documentation, supervision, service provider, eligibility) for use of these billing codes. Medicaid reimbursement rates paid by the state Medicaid agency should be public information. Request the reimbursement rate for the billing codes you identified for different healthcare providers. Discuss your findings.

Project Title (5 to 7 words):
_____

Amount Requested: _____

Total Project Cost: _____

Project Collaborators:

Project Summary:

Statement of specific problem or need:

Target population:

Objectives: Measurable and Time-Specific	Methods	Evaluation: Tied to Objectives
_____	_____	_____
_____	_____	_____
_____	_____	_____

Budget, including in-kind contributions:

Letters of support to be sought:

FIGURE 21-2   Sample Grant Application Internal Worksheet
Source: Compiled by the author.

References

Baker, J. 1999. *Cost accounting for healthcare organizations: Utilizing information and technology for effective decision making.* New York: McGraw-Hill Professional.

Baker, J. & Baker, R. W. 2003. *Healthcare finance: Basic tools for non-financial managers.* Boston: Jones & Bartlett.

Conklin, M. T. & Simko, M. D. 1983. Cost-benefit and cost-effectiveness analyses of nutrition programs. *Quality Review Bulletin*, 9, 166–168.

Dever, G. E.A.1997. *Improving outcomes in public health practice: Strategies and methods.* Gaithersburg, MD: Aspen.

Disbrow, D. 1989. The costs and benefits of nutrition services: A literature review. *Journal of the American Dietetic Association, Suppl. 89*(4), S4–S63.

Gapenski, L. 2001. *Healthcare finance: An introduction to accounting and financial management* (2nd ed.). Chicago: Health Administration Press.

Lighter, D. & Fair, D. 2000. *Principles and methods of quality management in healthcare.* Gaithersburg, MD: Aspen.

Omachonu, V. 1991. *Total quality and productivity management in healthcare organizations.* Norcross, GA: Institute of Industrial Engineers.

Schramm, W. F. 1985. WIC prenatal participation and its relationship to newborn Medicaid costs in Missouri: A cost/benefit analysis. *American Journal of Public Health*, 75(8), 851–857.

"Nutrition Services in Managed Care—An ADA Position Paper" *Journal of The American Dietetic Association*, 102 (2002): 1471–1478. Retrieved on May 18, 2005 from: http://www.eatright.org/Public/Other/index_adar1002a.cfm.

Warren, C., Reeve, J., & Fess, P. 2001. *Accounting.* Cincinnati, OH: South-Western College Publishers.

Special Note

Katherine Cairns, MPH, MBA, RD, was an original author from the first edition of Mildred Kaufman's *Nutrition in Public Health* (1990). Portions of this chapter are reprinted with permission from the publisher.

PART VII

MOBILIZING PERSONNEL

In Part VII, Chapter 22 reviews the core functions of the professionals who make up the public health nutrition team and designate job responsibilities needed to carry out the programs and services. In addition, Chapter 23 educates the reader on effective management skills that enable the public health nutrition profession to perform necessary services, including public health nutrition education, which is discussed in Chapter 24. Education is the final result of all the program planning, scientific data collection and findings, nutrition policy, money appropriation, and safeguarding and distribution of food for the American public.

CHAPTER 22

STAFFING PUBLIC HEALTH NUTRITION PROGRAMS AND SERVICES

Cynthia Taft Bayerl, MS, RD, LDN

Reader Objectives

After studying this chapter and reflecting on the contents, you should be able to:

1. Discuss changing trends that impact public health nutritionists' job functions.
2. Compare and contrast the job functions of nutrition personnel who work in public health and community settings.
3. Describe the educational requirements for nutritionists who work in public health settings and how those qualifications might be obtained.
4. Discuss how job satisfaction and salary impact staffing.
5. List various work settings for public health nutrition positions.

A working knowledge of current and emerging trends in public health is important to appreciate more fully the roles and responsibilities of staffing in public health nutrition programs. Healthcare trends greatly influence the public health nutritionist's scope of practice and thus the roles and functions she or he assumes in the healthcare arena. Recent consumer trends indicate that there is an increased interest in both personal health and health information to be provided by qualified providers, including nutrition personnel.[1, 2] This trend may be attributed, in part, to major changes that have occurred in the healthcare environment, as well as more media coverage of relevant consumer-focused research findings. These changes have begun to impact how nutrition personnel work to provide more effective public health services. Some of these changes include:

- Socioeconomic and demographic changes, including ethnic diversification within the U.S. population[3]
- Changes in eating habits and food preparation, resulting in more obesity[4]

- New advances in food technology and biochemical and molecular research, which have changed what types of food we eat, how we eat it, and who prepares it
- Adverse economic factors that affect food supply and demand as well as health and nutritional status

To understand and to meet the challenges associated with these emerging trends, public health agencies must hire and train staff with the knowledge and skills to provide effective services beyond the traditional model of direct-care nutrition counselors.[5] In order to understand the role and function of today's public health nutrition personnel, an understanding of the definition, role, and responsibilities of these providers is important.

Staffing Trends

Public health nutritionists in community agencies are responsible for nutrition and physical activity programs, which focus on community-wide health promotion and disease prevention. The term *public health nutritionist* is used for the professional who has completed academic course work in biostatistics, epidemiology, environmental studies, health program planning and evaluation, and advanced nutrition. Historically, public health nutritionists are differentiated from the dietitian on the basis of providing community care, rather than direct care, to individual patients/clients.

In many agencies, both dietitians and public nutritionists perform similar job functions and can be classified in similar job categories.[6] Public health nutrition services, including those at federal, state, and local levels, are described in detail by Kaufman and colleagues within the Association of State and Territorial Public Health Nutrition Directors (ASTPHND).[7] The landmark publication *Personnel in Public Health Nutrition for the 1990's* provides an excellent basis for defining job titles of professional and paraprofessional staff and their roles, responsibilities, and function within state and local programs.[8] Within the field of public health nutrition, the 2003 survey by the ASTPHND serves as the common definition for most current job descriptions and functions for public health staff.[6]

Current trends, which have shifted the focus of the public health system from an individual to a population-based system, is described best by the Institute of Medicine (IOM) in *The Future of Public Health*[9] and *The Future of the Public's Health in the 21st Century*.[10] The IOM further describes trends in the public health system, detailing the roles and responsibilities of public health personnel, including those within the Maternal and Child Health (MCH) programs, one of the largest employers of nutritionists through the Special Supplemental Nutrition Program for Women, Infants and Children (WIC). IOM definitions are based on a detailed study of public health systems and include strong recommendations on the purpose, function, and mission of public health as a system to assure conditions in which people can be healthy. The IOM used this detailed study to act as a catalyst to inform the public about the improvements in Americans' health, which have prevented countless deaths and improved the quality of life. These improvements, in many instances, are due to the successes of public health systems. The IOM also used its study to address a concern that the nation has lost sight of its public health goals and has allowed the public health system to fall into disrepair. The study has been used to communicate a sense of urgency about the need to maintain current preventative efforts to sustain the capability of existing public health programs and to meet future public health needs. The IOM recommends that public health staff will need to focus on the following three core functions in order to transition from the current client-focused system to a population-based approach:

1. *Community assessment:* The IOM recommends that every public health agency collect, assemble, analyze, and document information on the health of the community on a regular and systematic basis. Community assessment includes ongoing data collection and dissemination of statistics on the community's health status and needs. Systemized studies would result from these assessments, and would include population health trends and controlled epidemiological studies of community health problems. Nutrition assessment and the study of the nutrition profile of the population will provide the basis for developing new, population-focused nutrition programs. As the IOM has specified, the state public health agency

---

Epidemiological studies—
Research that is derived from data compiled from a population. Some different types of epidemiological studies include:

- *Correlational studies—* Comparison of the frequency of events between two populations, which do not have to be at a specific time.

- *Cross-sectional studies—* Comparison of the frequency of events between two populations at the same specific time.

- *Cohort or incidence studies—* A population is followed over time to assess data incidences.

- *Case-control studies—*Subjects with specified characteristics are followed and compared to other subjects who don't have those characteristics.

- *Controlled trials—*Usually the study of subjects, using randomized selection and a double-blind method (both researcher and test subject are not privy to study group assignment), to evaluate a hypothesis.

Review more about nutritional studies in Chapter 2.

bears the responsibility for leadership in the development and implementation of nutrition assessment at the state level. At both the state and local community levels, staff responsibilities for the assessment function would include monitoring and surveillance of nutritional status and population needs, as well as resource identification and collection and interpretation of data. Identifying community needs using multiple data sources, forecasting trends, ensuring a safe supply of food and water, and evaluating outcomes are important components to an effective state-of-the-art public health nutrition program. In order to successfully accomplish community nutrition assessment, personnel must have the skills necessary to evaluate how interrelated systems such as health, education, human services, food supply, and financial and insurance systems are interconnected, as well as how these systems are interdependent. Interactions among these arenas and between nutrition and the public health system as a whole will need to be assessed.

2. *Policy development:* The IOM advocates the use of scientific knowledge in decision making (see Chapter 2). Public health agencies should lead in the development of public health policies that take a strategic approach to public health and use a democratic process (see Chapters 7 and 8). For example, policies and programs that address the highest perceived needs of the community will need to include nutrition and health policy. Policy development also includes:
   - Setting priorities
   - Development, implementation, and evaluation of community plans
   - Assumption of leadership, where overall goals include nutrition programs

3. *Public health assurance:* The IOM places the public health agency in the leadership role to assure the community that the services necessary to achieve agreed-upon goals will be provided. Policy can be implemented by encouraging actions by other entities (in both the private and public sector) through regulation and/or by direct-care service. The public health agency would invite key policy makers and the general public to collaborate in determining community-wide health policies, which would govern every member of that community including those who are unable to afford it. Public policy assurance also includes a wide scope of functions, which are described by Probert.[12] In her book, *Moving to the Future*, the author indicates that the following public health policy functions should exist:

- Implementation of effective nutrition strategies
- Access to services and quality in the implementation of public health and community nutrition plans
- Ensuring safety, access, and adequacy of the food supply to promote and maintain the health of the population
- Responding to food and nutrition crises
- Support for monitoring and surveillance systems
- Provision of population-based and culturally competent nutrition education
- Provision of nutrition services to high-risk, underserved, and culturally diverse populations
- Nutrition counseling to persons with health conditions related to poor nutritional status (e.g., diabetes, cardiovascular disease, hypertension)
- Planning for emergency preparedness
- Marketing
- Providing nutrition information to the public
- Encouraging public and private sector collaborations
- Mobilizing nutrition resources
- Setting standards for various levels of nutrition staff, including maintaining accountability to the community through setting goals and measuring progress towards those goals

In order for nutrition personnel to carry out these core functions, they will need to be supported by strong administrative and managerial leadership, which is essential to provide a successful transition from direct-care services to those that include all three of these core functions.

Core Functions in Nutrition Service Systems

Generally, the state public health agency is recognized as the lead agency to develop and implement systems that will assess, monitor, and evaluate the nutritional status of the entire state.[9] Personnel, at both the state and local levels, need to have the necessary skills to participate in the planning, implementation, and evaluation of nutrition service systems. Qualified personnel will enable the community to identify and procure funding and resources from local, state, and federal agencies to provide services that focus on nutrition and physical activity. Community public health programs include services to low-income populations (e.g., school breakfast and lunch programs, Food Stamps, and WIC) as well as services targeted to promote the health of the general public.[5]

In 2002, the ASTPHND surveyed public health personnel and reported that more than 78.7% of the public health nutrition workforce indicated that their primary area of practice was in direct client services or the *assurance* core function. Approximately 9% indicated that *management/administration* of these programs was their primary area of focus; 5.3% reported focusing on *assessment*; and 2.4% indicated *public policy* including *population interventions* (e.g., community organization, advocacy and policy development) as their primary area of focus. Over 90% of the public health nutrition workforce works in the WIC program. WIC remains the largest public health nutrition program in the United States.[6-8]

Core Public Health Functions Interrelated with Essential Public Health Functions

Core public health functions and essential public health functions are interrelated. Creation of public health programs, which are based on both core and essential public health functions, are important in providing comprehensive, standard community-based programs. In work funded by the Department of Health and Human Services, titled *Public Health in America* (illustrated in Figure 22-1), the essential functions and interrelationship of the core public health functions are described.[13] This information is supported by research in community settings, which is based on science as well as the practice of public health.

Historically, the work of public health nutritionists has been studied by and supported through collaborations with colleagues in academia. The collaboration has been essential to understanding the issues from both the research perspective and in practice. The lessons learned have been used to effectively teach emerging and seasoned nutritionists public health solutions to nutrition issues. For example, Haughton and Keir propose using the IOM studies on public health systems, including core functions, to develop curriculum and continuing education. This includes providing distance and on-campus education to prepare the workforce with the knowledge and skills necessary to understand and practice core public health functions.[5, 6]

Integration of core and essential public health services will move the health of the nation closer to the objectives outlined in Healthy People (HP) 2010, which are highlighted in Figure 22-1. The success of HP 2010 will depend in part on how healthcare professionals, including nutritionists, integrate the core functions and essential health functions into their portfolio of skills.

Essential Public Health Services

Nutrition services and the recruitment and hiring of effective personnel to staff these nutrition services depend on a thorough under-

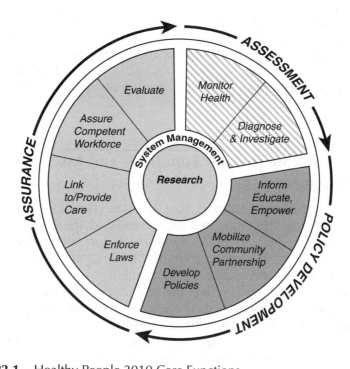

FIGURE 22-1   Healthy People 2010 Core Functions
Source: Department of Health and Human Services from *Public Health in America.*[13]

standing of the relationship between core public health functions and subsequent public health programming. Probert, in *Moving to the Future*[12], described the following essential public health services:

- Monitor health status to identify community health problems.
- Diagnose and investigate health problems and health hazards in the community.
- Inform, educate, and empower people about health issues.
- Mobilize community partnerships to identify and solve health problems.
- Develop policies and plans that support individual and community health efforts.
- Enforce laws and regulations that protect health and ensure safety.
- Link people to needed personal health services and assure the provision of healthcare when otherwise unavailable.
- Assure a competent public health and personal healthcare workforce.
- Evaluate effectiveness, accessibility, and quality of personal and population-based health services.
- Research for new insights and innovative solutions to health problems.

If public health programs are to provide both core and essential functions, then staffing will need to reflect training, expertise, and time spent in delivery of both of these services. This recommendation supports thinking that the functions of nutrition personnel have not undergone the recommended systematic changes as outlined by the IOM.[7, 8]

Nutritionists' Role in Core Functions and Essential Public Health Services

Current thinking indicates that the core functions and essential public health functions can be addressed at the federal, state, and local levels. Probert, in *Moving to the Future*, describes the importance of nutrition services as part of a comprehensive public health system in addressing the mission of public health, as outlined by the IOM.[12] Current trends reflect the importance and need for nutrition personnel at all levels to be aware of the essential public health services, as they are the foundation for their scope of practice. The essentials and core functions are the drivers of change from the traditional model of assurance to the inclusion of assessment and public policy in current public health models.

According to Probert, the essential public health nutrition services are:

- Assessing the nutritional status of specific populations or geographic areas
- Identifying target populations that may be at nutritional risk
- Initiating and participating in nutrition data collection
- Providing leadership in the development of and planning for health and nutrition policies
- Recommending and providing specific training and programs to meet identified nutrition needs
- Raising awareness among key policy makers about the potential impact of nutrition and food regulations and budget decisions on the health of the community
- Acting as an advocate for target populations on food and nutrition issues
- Planning for nutrition services in conjunction with other health services, based on information obtained from an adequate and ongoing database focused on health outcomes
- Identifying and/or assisting in development of accurate, up-to-date nutrition education materials
- Ensuring the availability of quality nutrition services to target populations, including nutrition screening, assessment, education, counseling, referral for food assistance, and follow-up

- Participating in nutrition research and demonstration and evaluation projects
- Providing expert nutrition consultation to the community
- Providing community health promotion and disease prevention activities that are population based
- Providing quality assurance guidelines for personnel dealing with food and nutrition issues
- Facilitating coordination with other providers of health and nutrition services within the community
- Evaluating the impact of the health status of populations who receive public health nutrition services

Healthy People 2010 and Leading Health Indicators

The HP 2010 objectives were developed by the U.S. Department of Health and Human Services and released in 2000. HP 2010 is a set of health objectives for the nation to achieve over the first decade of the new century. Many different people, states, communities, professional organizations, and others use these objectives to help develop programs to improve healthcare. The report contains approximately 400 goals, of which 66 are directly related to nutrition, with 21 specifically related to improving the nutritional status and eating habits of Americans. HP 2010 builds on initiatives pursued over the past two decades. The 1979 Surgeon General's report, *Healthy People*[15], along with *Healthy People 2000: National Health Promotion and Disease Prevention Objectives*[16], established national health objectives and served as the basis for the development of state and community plans. Like its predecessors,

> Read about Healthy People 2010 at http://www.healthypeople.gov.

the HP 2010 objectives support the broad goals of the Surgeon General's report by increasing the quality and years of healthy life and eliminating health disparities among different segments of the population. Healthy indicators, which are a way to categorize the health objectives, are used for the first time in the HP 2010.

Several of the leading health indicators are relevant to the field of nutrition/dietetics. These include overweight and obesity, physical activity, and access to healthcare. These health indicators are focal areas for many public health providers, including nutritionists. In order to effectively work with clients, these providers require a variety of skills.[18] The effectiveness of nutrition personnel working within their communities helps determine the success of the community in meeting the targeted public health outcomes.[18]

Emerging Trends That Impact Staffing

The Bureau of Labor Statistics (BLS)[1] and The American Dietetic Association (ADA)[11] have recently reported on trend data, which include projections on the impact of the economy and other factors on staffing. The BLS publishes information biennially in the *Occupational Outlook Handbook*. The handbook utilizes employment and census data to predict the growth in employment for specific occupations, including nutrition services. However, it does not differentiate between the commonly used terms *registered dietitian*, *dietitian*, and *nutritionist*. This lack of differentiation among the job descriptions makes it difficult to clearly identify which types of nutrition personnel or specific staffing will benefit from the projection figures. In the ADA study, Kornblum utilized the BLS data to report the projected number of jobs for various nutrition positions and services into the year 2005, and in which sectors of the job market they would occur.[11] This report indicates that the demand for dietetics professionals will increase as the demand for food service expertise and nutrition counseling increases in a variety of settings, including hospitals, nursing homes, schools, prisons, community health programs, and health clubs.[22] The following areas of public health interest have generated the increase:

> Read about The Bureau of Labor Statistics' *Occupational Outlook Handbook* at http://www.bls.gov/oco/home.htm.

- The public's interest in nutrition and the emphasis on health education and prudent lifestyles will add to the present demand for credentialed and highly skilled nutrition personnel to provide the service.
- As life expectancy increases and the elderly live are more commonly living to 100+, community-based settings such as nursing homes will need the services of skilled nutrition providers to assist the geriatric population with emerging health- and nutrition-related issues.
- Contract food services, as found in residential care facilities and other social service agencies, will require qualified nutrition personnel to oversee compliance as well as provide therapeutic programs to residents.

Within these sectors, the greatest growth in the number of nutrition personnel needed is projected to be in physicians' offices (54%), offices of other health practitioners (63%), personal services such as Diet Workshop (60%), childcare services (64%), home healthcare (91%), and residential care (129%). Third-party reimbursement and the aging of the population are projected to play a role in demand. Industries projected to have a lower growth rate for nutrition personnel include hospitals (7%), education (16%), and government (0.5%).[11]

As part of its membership database study, an ADA survey of 59,198 eligible members reviewed a range of topics, including demographics, professional information (e.g., years in service), education background, and employment.[22] The study, which covered the period from 1991 to 1999, reported that employment in hospitals had declined by 8.4%, while employment in other health-related settings (clinics or ambulatory care centers, extended care facilities, health maintenance organizations, and with physicians and other care providers) had increased by 5.3%. Employment in community/public health programs also had increased by 2.5%. Employment in all levels of government had decreased by 2.7%, even though employment in all levels of government accounted for nearly one-quarter of all past jobs held by registered dietitians. The salary of nutrition personnel in both full- and part-time jobs remained virtually unchanged.[22]

The ADA collected data in 2002 to identify trends, issues, and events that were likely to influence the dietetics field and the ADA as a professional organization.[4] Broad trends, such as shifts in demographics of the U.S. population and in the number of college students entering the field of dietetics, were examined. The report discussed new opportunities for personnel and concluded that opportunities exist in the following major areas:

- Nutrition counseling, which has a greater interest in diet/nutrition for the public at large
- Nutrition, as it relates to the growth in the U.S. population
- Nutrition and healthcare, as it relates to the increasing cultural and ethnic diversity of the U.S. population
- Illness prevention, in particular food safety and functional foods, which have been linked to health promotion

The report also discusses the fact that competing sources of nutrition information from the Internet, the food industry, alternative nutrition, and medicinal providers are a potential threat to qualified nutrition personnel.[4] A new publication by the ADA, *Achieving Excellence: Clinical Staffing for Today and Tomorrow*, outlines parameters for clinical nutrition staffing for registered dietitians and dietetic technicians in both inpatient and outpatient settings.[23] The author acknowledges various challenges, including that there is no universally accepted method for staffing, and that budget constraints are the lead factor negatively impacting staffing ratios. This is further hindered by the fact that the service model is being used, rather than focusing on desired patient outcomes or benchmarking reports.

A wide range of nutrition care procedures are used by practitioners and facilities to meet various standards including those of the Joint Commission on Accreditation of Healthcare Organizations (JCAHO), as discussed in Chapter 15. JCAHO standards, which in the past were mainly used by hospitals or by dietitians in clinical settings, are now used by many community-based healthcare facilities. The ADA reports authors propose the use of staffing in any setting to correlate with desired patient outcomes. A variety of strategies, based on the performance improvement model, should be used to monitor clinical indicators and outcomes. A performance-based model measures performance indicators using measurable characteristics of products, such as processes, services, and systems used to track and improve performance. One of the tools with the model is called a "dashboard," which consists of the indicator, the actual performance, a performance benchmark, an indicator value, a data source, a benchmark source, trends, and comments. Information is collected and reported on a quarterly basis. The authors discuss a system of nutrition care based on evidence-based practice using a host of tools, including data and validated measures and procedures, on which to base performance and management.[23]

> Read about the Joint Commission on Accreditation of Healthcare Organizations (JCAHO) at www.jcaho.org.

Other Tools to Assess Nutrition Services and Staffing

Tools such as *Moving to the Future: Developing Community-Based Nutrition Services*[12] and the *Bright Futures* series, which includes publications on nutrition[24], oral health[25], and physical activity[26], have been developed for healthcare providers and nutritionists to expand their skills. These and other tools provide effective communication vehicles to help deliver clear, focused messages to motivate healthy behavior changes to meet the goals established within the HP 2010 objectives.

The American Dietetic Association Definition of Nutrition Personnel

The ADA is the nation's largest organization of food and nutrition professionals, with nearly 70,000 members.[27] Approximately 75% of the ADA's members are registered dietitians (RDs), and 4% of its members are registered dietetic technicians (DTRs). Other members include clinical and community dietetics professionals, consultants, food service managers, educators, researchers, and students. ADA members represent a range of practice areas and interests including public health; sports nutrition; medical nutrition therapy; diet counseling; cholesterol reduction; diabetes; heart and kidney disease; vegetarianism; food service management in business, hospitals, restaurants, long-term care facilities, and education systems; education of other healthcare professionals; and scientific research. The following are ADA definitions of qualified personnel:[28]

- *Registered dietitian (RD):* The RD must pass a national examination administered by the Commission on Dietetic Registration and complete continuing professional educational requirements to maintain registration. Some RDs hold additional certifications in specialized areas of practice, such as pediatric or renal nutrition, nutrition support, and diabetes education. Most RDs work at hospitals and medical centers, in private practice, or at other healthcare facilities. Many work in community and public health settings, academia, and research. A growing number work with the food and nutrition industry and business, journalism, sports nutrition, corporate wellness programs, and in other nontraditional settings. Nearly half of all ADA members hold advanced academic degrees.

- *Dietetic technician, registered (DTR):* A registered dietetic technician is a food and nutrition practitioner, often working in conjunction with a registered dietitian, who has met the minimum academic and professional requirements to qualify for the credential "DTR." In addition to DTR credentialing, some states have regulatory laws for registered dietetic technicians. Like RDs, DTRs must complete professional educational requirements to maintain their registration. DTRs work in hospices, home healthcare programs, food service operations, and government and community programs such as Meals on Wheels. DTRs must complete at least a 2-year associate's degree in an approved dietetics technology program from an accredited U.S. college or university. Besides the 2-year degree, DTRs also must have supervised practice experience in community programs, healthcare, and food service facilities. They must pass a nationwide examination and continuing education courses throughout their careers. The ADA has proposed that the designation "DTR" be changed to "DT" (Dietetic Technician).

- *Public health nutritionist:* The title "Public Health Nutritionist" is reserved for positions that require dietetic registration status and a graduate-level science degree that includes environmental sciences, health program planning, management, and evaluation. The term is usually used for an individual with a master's degree in public health nutrition.

- *Community nutritionist/dietitian:* A community nutritionist/ dietitian is an individual with a baccalaureate degree who is a registered dietitian or registration-eligible dietitian.

- *Community nutrition educator:* A community nutrition educator is an individual with a baccalaureate degree with a minimum of 15 hours of course work in nutrition from a regionally accredited college or university.

It is important to understand the academic preparation guidelines so that nutritionists/dietitians can more fully understand a host of factors including various job functions, skills, employee performance, job expectations, recruitment and retention issues, and job satisfaction.

Academic Preparation of the Nutrition Staff

Academic preparation of the nutrition staff can vary significantly depending upon the job function. Information from the ASTPHND workforce survey indicates that more than half of public health staff had at least a bachelor's degree with a focus on nutrition or dietetics. Among the WIC workforce, 53.7% had a degree in nutrition or dietetics, whereas 69.5% from the non-WIC workforce had a similar degree.[6] The WIC workforce has a higher number of bachelor's degrees in public health

> See the ADA website at http://www.eatright.org/public/7782_13280.cfm for current nutrition/dietetics programs.

(2.3%) or community nutrition as compared to their non-WIC counterparts (1.8%). The non-WIC workforce had a higher percentage of advanced degrees (28%), such as a master's degree in nutrition/dietetics, versus 14% with a master's degree in public health.[6] For information on which nutrition/dietetic programs have been approved by the American Dietetic Association, refer to the ADA website[25], which also lists additional references to public health programs having a nutrition program.

In addition to definitions of job classifications, the ADA has established a definition of nutrition services for Medicare-eligible clients, which is referred to as medical nutrition therapy (MNT).[29] MNT includes nutritional diagnostic, therapeutic, and counseling services provided by a registered dietitian and can effectively treat and manage disease conditions. MNT can:

- Reduce or eliminate the need for prescription drug use
- Help reduce complications in patients with disease
- Improve patients' overall health and quality of life

The academic preparation for registered dietitians and other nutrition personnel who work in public health/community settings must include MNT training as a part of direct-care services to individuals.[29]

Opportunities in Government Employment

Federal Government

The federal government is the largest employer of public health nutrition personnel, and it funds many nutrition programs through state and local community agencies. The United States Department of Agriculture (USDA) is one branch of the federal government that administers primary food assistance programs, which include the Food Stamp Program, the National School Lunch Program, and WIC. These three programs accounted for the majority of the $34.1 billion spent on USDA food assistance in 2001. In addition, the USDA funds other public health nutrition programs and the staffing of food assistance programs, including the Cooperative Extension and the Center for Nutrition Policy and Promotion, which coordinates government efforts to review and publish the Dietary Guidelines for Americans (in coordination with the Department of Health and Human Services).[35] Local agencies also contribute to the funding of public health nutritionist staffing, but the amount varies from state to state.[36]

The federal government is the largest single funding source of nutrition programs to state and local government agencies. Nearly 68% of public health personnel work for state or local government health agencies.

The WIC program is the major employer of public health nutrition staff. This program alone funds 78% of the full-time-equivalent public health nutritionists.[37] The results of the 2000 ASTPHND survey indicated that 90% of respondents worked in WIC, as compared to 85.4% in 1994.[6] The WIC program provides nutritious foods, nutrition education, and healthcare referrals to meet the special nutrition needs of low-income pregnant, postpartum,

> Read more about the WIC program at http://www.fns.usda.gov/wic/.

and breast-feeding women, and their infants and children up to 5 years of age, who are at nutritional risk.[38] Because WIC is the largest employer of public health nutritionists in the country, it is important to understand the goals and current challenges of the program[37], as well as the personnel issues, such as recruitment and retention.[39] Information on the roles of personnel and the WIC service standards are outlined in the WIC Nutrition Services Standards.[40]

Administrative Staff

Personnel in Public Health Nutrition for the 1990's[8] identifies three professional job classifications with management and budgetary responsibility: the public health nutrition director, the assistance public health nutrition director, and the public health nutrition supervisor. In the 2000 ASTPHND survey, the degree to which the job descriptions match the public health nutrition workforce was quite high. Ninety-three percent of the workforce were public health nutrition directors, 79% were assistant directors, and 95% were public health nutrition supervisors. In addition to supervising personnel, 65.7% of directors responded that they had responsibility for the agency's entire nutrition budget, while 26.3% of directors and 40.1% of assistant directors had responsibility for a more limited budget.[6] Other areas issues that nutrition personnel need to consider when developing and implementing effective nutrition service systems and hiring qualified providers include the following:

- Number of providers versus the number of clients
- Cultural and ethnic diversity of services and staffing
- Training needs
- Effective use of resources
- Salary
- Job satisfaction
- Reimbursement by third-party payers for nutrition services

Staffing Ratios

Personnel in Public Health Nutrition for the 1990s proposed a mathematical formula to estimate the ratio of nutrition personnel to clients.[8] In another publication, the author proposed a recommended staffing ratio of one public health nutritionist to 50,000 people. Haughton and colleagues estimated the number of public health nutritionists from the 1990 census data for all states and territories to be approximately 4,379, which was an 83% increase from the those levels identified in prior ASTPHND surveys.[5] In the more recent articles describing the roles and responsibilities of the nutrition workforce, it is hypothesized that the roles and responsibilities of the workforce are expected to shift to population-based services and to add the two core functions of public policy and community assessment. It is difficult to estimate whether these calculations remain pertinent. No other study to date has been identified that provides information on staffing ratios in public health settings.

Diversity

One of the two major goals of HP 2010 is to eliminate ethnic and class disparities in the workforce. The development of a culturally competent health service workforce is one strategy that will help accomplish this goal. HP objective 1-8 specifically addresses the goal of increased representation of ethnic minorities in the health professions.[14] In 2000, Greenwald and Davis[39] surveyed newly credentialed RDs, DTRs, and education program directors to better understand why males and minorities were underrepresented in the field of nutrition. RDs and DTRs primarily attributed the underrepresentation of minorities to the limited visibility of the field; they attributed the underrepresentation of men to the traditional association of the field of nutrition to women, an association typically characterized by low salaries. Educators, in contrast, attributed the minority underrepresentation to a disadvantage in education, particularly in science. Proposed solutions included flexible time lines for completion of programs, outreach to elementary and lower-division college students, tutoring, mentoring, encouragement by program faculty, scholarships, and the creation of professional networks to identify potential new minority entrants into the field.

In the ASTPHND survey, professionals and paraprofessionals were asked to rank their top-10 training needs when communicating with their clients; responses included dealing with low-literacy populations (6%) and cultural competency (3.9%).[6] Although low literacy and cultural competency were not ranked high under communication needs, nutritionists did not identify the need to improve their own skills in this area. However, the lack of diversity in the public health nutrition workforce was evidenced in several parameters within other areas of survey results. Over 95% of the ASTPHN survey respondents were female. Ethnic diversity was greater among the WIC workforce as compared to non-WIC staff: Latino/Hispanic Americans made up 20.8% of the WIC workforce versus 5.8% of the non-WIC workforce; African Americans were 11.5% versus 7.4%, and Asian Americans were 6.6% versus 5%. Although the diversity of the WIC workforce was more representative of the population than the non-WIC workforce, it was not considered representative of the WIC participants themselves, which is an important component if culturally and linguistically diverse nutrition services are to be effective.[40] Eighty-three percent of the ASTPHND respondents reported English as their primary language (non-WIC 91% vs. WIC 83%), which does not demonstrate linguistic diversity.[4]

New initiatives, such as the American Public Health Association's (APHA) initiative, have been established to help public health nutritionists increase the diversity of the workforce. To assist current and emerging nutrition programs, two organizations have developed initiatives to address diversity issues. The ADA has developed a model to help practitioners develop multicultural competencies as well as learn to identify how the profession can more effectively work with diversity issues of practitioners and clients.[40,41] The APHA's initiative targets undergraduates to enhance educational opportunities in public health nutrition.[42]

Staff Training Needs

Nutrition personnel who responded to the 2000 ASTPHND survey identified the following practice areas where they could use more training for their current work:

- Diet/nutrition to prevent chronic disease
- Low breast-feeding rates
- Low birth weight
- Iron-deficiency anemia
- Obesity/overweight

The focus on maternal and child health areas for training was surprising because a large number of respondents who work in public health nutrition programs work in the WIC program.[6] The authors hypothesized that if official health agencies were to shift to performing public health core functions, as recommended by the

IOM, they would need to obtain the knowledge and skills necessary to practice assessment and evaluation in order to be more knowledgeable to meet the nutrition objectives in HP 2010. The ASTPHND report proposed that continuing education interventions should be offered by professional organizations (i.e., ASTPHND, ADA, and APHA). Distance and on-campus educational opportunities should

Read more about the ADA's list of nutrition and dietetics training programs at http://www.eatright.org/public/careers/94.cfm.

be offered through approved public health nutrition programs so that more staff will have access to educational opportunities to enhance their skills. As an adjunct to existing funding, nutrition personnel will need to advocate for new funding streams to provide training in areas focused on public health core functions. These include cultural diversity and linguistic competency training, so public health staff can communicate more effectively with their clients and more fully understand the needs of their community.

Staff Resources

Many resources and tools are available to expand the skill level of nutritionists working in public health or community settings. Multiple websites from federal and state agencies, such as the CDC and USDA, provide tool kits and best practices. In addition, resources such as the ADA's *Guidelines for Community Nutrition Supervised Experiences*[20] were developed for various levels of personnel (e.g., registered dietitians, associate-level diet technicians, and bachelor's degree nutritionists) to help expand their skills. The tool, available in Appendix D, was developed to assist those who lack the training or supervised experiences in community nutrition and who work in nutrition positions that are based on the traditional client-focused model (assurance) but need to transition to a practice that will be more population/systems focused (public policy and assessment). The knowledge and skills of nutrition personnel need to be consistent with the mission of public health, which is to assure conditions in which people are healthy. Cutting-edge tools and training, as well as mentoring programs, are needed to guide emerging practitioners and mid-career change candidates who want to enhance their skills and be prepared for the future. Other resources/tools to enhance staff knowledge and skills include the position papers of professional associations, such as the ADA, the American Academy of Pediatrics, and the National Association of WIC Directors. Position papers can be used to support public policies, which guide the practice of nutritionists.

Position papers are derived from the latest available research and focus on such issues as promotion of breast-feeding, child and adolescent nutrition programs, food technology and safety, effectiveness of medical nutrition therapy, and elderly nutrition. These papers, in addition to including relevant data in a practice area, also discuss implications on practice and staffing of nutrition programs. One of the more recent papers, titled *The Role of Dietetics Professionals in Health Promotion and Disease Prevention*[41], supports the hypothesis that diet plays an important role in health promotion and disease prevention. Therefore, nutrition personnel should be trained in primary prevention in addition to the more traditional role in clinical settings (secondary and tertiary prevention), which focuses more on a disease management model. This position paper is provided for the reader in Appendix C. Other ADA position statements are available at its website, http://www.eatright.org/Public/index_7705.cfm.[42] Position papers can also be used with policy makers and community leaders to provide evidence that healthy eating habits, coupled with other healthy lifestyle behaviors, have the potential to reduce the risk of chronic disease. Nutritionists and dietitians can use the information as part of the public policy core functions used to shape safe and supportive environments, build community coalitions, and redirect health services to include health promotion as a primary approach to delivering healthcare.

Job Satisfaction

A study of public health personnel in the Virginia[43] and North Carolina[45] WIC programs found that associations exist between employee job satisfaction and consumer satisfaction. These associations translate to improved program participation rates. WIC benefits, namely food vouchers and nutrition education, were found to be insufficient incentives for the participants to continue to return on a regular basis to the program. The burden of other considerations, such as transportation to the clinic, wait time to obtain an appointment, and/or food vouchers, were deterrents to program participation. A negative correlation among low pay, low visibility, and limited resources has been associated with giving a poor image of the nutrition profession, which has been shown to lead to some job dissatisfaction. The negative effects identified by participants in public health nutrition programs (e.g., long wait, language and transportation barriers, limited culturally diverse food options, limited cost of food package) were also thought to be inversely tied to the job dissatisfaction felt by many nutrition personnel working directly with these clients, making job retention a challenge.[6,43]

Reimbursement Impacts Staffing

Changes in the healthcare system, including fee-for-service and other methods such as prepaid capitated and managed care, have had a profound effect on the number and types of jobs available to dietetics professionals, the settings in which they work, and their roles and responsibilities. Although health promotion and prevention activities that include screenings and health education should be a top priority for healthcare providers and organizations, the value of these activities still is under debate. Many managed care organizations offer preventative services (e.g., health education workshops, discounts at fitness centers) for their enrolled populations. Population-based prevention activities (such as changes in the community environment to promote health) have not been considered the responsibility of private healthcare organizations. Studies by the ADA on the cost effectiveness of MNT are in progress and are expected to support the hypothesis that prevention and control of chronic illness would save healthcare costs. A finding consistent with this theory would both support and justify third-party payers providing nutrition services as part of subscribers' healthcare benefits, as it would be a cost-effective way for both the insurer and the client to save precious healthcare dollars.[44]

State and Local Governments

At the local level, nutrition personnel are staffed through federally funded programs in departments of education, public health, and public assistance, with some states providing additional staffing funds.

Conclusions

Staffing public health programs with qualified people to meet the challenges of the rapidly changing environment and emerging research is an exciting opportunity for public health nutritionists. Trend data support the concept that nutrition positions are increasing at the same rate as other healthcare provider jobs. These same studies also demonstrate that consumers have an increased awareness of and interest in nutrition and health. The expanding cultural and ethnic diversity of the U.S. population offers opportunities to advocate for nutrition services for populations who are interested in good healthcare as part of the American dream. The types of job settings are expanding, thanks to heightened interest in nutrition and the aging and diversification of the population. While this is occurring, the public health system is transitioning from a traditional model of directcare services (assurance) to one that focuses on population-based health promotion and disease prevention that includes public policy and assessment of core functions.

To meet these new challenges, low-cost, accessible, and flexible training opportunities need to be available so that public health staff can expand their skills while working to support themselves and their families. Training opportunities coupled with competitive salaries will enhance recruitment and retention of qualified personnel.

Nutrition services, including MNT, offer exciting new opportunities to qualified nutrition care providers, which include registered dietitians, nutritionists, registered dietetic technicians, and other nutrition personnel, both professional and paraprofessional. Reducing challenges to securing third-party reimbursement for MNT, as part of public health intervention to prevent such conditions as obesity, will go a long way to expand the horizons beyond disease-based intervention.

Additional research is needed to measure outcomes of nutrition intervention as they relate to decreasing chronic illness. Securing government funding for research in combination with additional research monies from industry is critical to support best practices and intervention protocols. These studies are necessary to demonstrate the cost effectiveness and efficacy of nutrition services, which also includes the cost associated with staffing.

Staffing public health nutrition programs is a continuing challenge. The ever-changing healthcare landscape, diversity issues, and the rising cost of doing business in the United States continue to challenge the already burdened healthcare system. In spite of rapidly rising healthcare costs, consumers continue to demonstrate an increased interest in nutrition. The population wants quick access to information and qualified professionals. Simultaneously, nutritionists are interested in achieving gains in several areas, including:

- Increased recognition by consumers and the profession
- Training opportunities to enhance their skills
- Equitable income

To improve job satisfaction, employers must provide a wide range of educational opportunities for public health nutritionists. Continuing flexible educational opportunities is a step in the right direction towards improving job satisfaction. Distance and web-based learning programs offer flexibility for employers to continue to support the continuing education needs of our profession.

The impending retirement of long-time WIC staff will affect the number of qualified personnel ready and able to assume a seamless transition to management of WIC programs. In order to prepare for a projected shortage of nutrition personnel by 2005, the profession will need to develop outreach programs to potential nutrition students from diverse cultural and linguistic populations, as well as address the issues of income parity, job satisfaction, and continuing education.

Issues for Discussion

1. *Shortage of personnel:* The traditional model of public health nutrition services is one-to-one and group counseling. Discuss two ways that nutrition assessment and public policy could enhance the role of nutritionists and improve nutrition services on the local, state and federal level.

2. *Funding:* The federal government has historically funded public health nutrition services. With increased constraints on federal budgets, discuss two or three potential ways that nutritionists can use their new skills in assessment and public policy to advocate for an increased level of nutrition services budgets.

3. *Job satisfaction:* Discuss how the publics' participation and satisfaction with public health nutrition services impacts staff recruitment and retention both positively and negatively.

4. *Aging of providers:* How would you propose to recruit and retain new staff to meet the challenge of the upcoming wave of retirement of public health nutritionists?

5. *Training opportunities:* In the present healthcare system, it is difficult for public health nutritionists who work full time to enhance and expand their skills when most higher education programs are full time, costly, and held during work hours. What types of programs would you suggest to academic institutions and other interested partners so that ethnically and culturally diverse nutrition staff can move up the career ladder and provide much-needed services to a culturally diverse U.S. population?

6. *Job functions of nutrition staff:* Compare and contrast the various major job functions of nutrition personnel who work in public health and community settings.

7. *Recruitment and retention of staff:* Encouraging people to enter and stay in public health positions is problematic due to dissatisfaction with low salary and benefits. What are some ideas you could suggest that might help retain and recruit nutrition personnel?

References

1. U.S. Department of Labor. Occupational Outlook Handbook, 2004–05 edition. Available at: http://www.bls.gov/oco/. Accessed April 26, 2005.

2. United States Census 2000. U.S. Census Bureau. Available at: http://www.census.gov/main/www/cen2000.html. Accessed May 20, 2005.

3. The Institute for the Future. *Health and Healthcare in 2010.* San Francisco, Calif.: Jossey-Bass; 2000.

4. Jarratt J, Mahaffie JM. Trends affecting the dietetics profession and the American Dietetic Association. *J Am Dietetic Assoc.* 2002;102(12):1821.

5. Haughton B, Story M, Keir B. Profile of public health personnel: Challenges for population/system-focused roles and state-level monitoring. *J Am Diet Assoc.* 1998;98:664–670.

6. McCall M. *Survey of Public Health Nutrition Workforce: 1999–2000.* Washington, DC: USDA, FNS; January 2003.

7. Kaufman M. *Nutrition in Public Health: A Handbook for Developing Programs and Services.* Rockville, Md.: Aspen; 1990.

8. Dodds JM, Kaufman M. *Personnel in Public Health Nutrition for the 1990's.* Washington, DC: The Public Health Foundation; 1991.

9. Institute of Medicine, Committee for the Study of the Future of Public Health, Division of Health Care Services. *The Future of Public Health.* Washington, DC: National Academy Press; 1988.

10. Institute of Medicine, Committee on Assuring the Health of the Public in the 21st Century. *The Future of the Public's Health in the 21st Century.* Washington, DC: National Academy Press; 2002.

11. Kornblum, TH. Professional demands for dietitians and nutritionists in the year 2005. *J Am Diet Assoc.* 1994;94:212–222.

12. Probert, KL. Moving to the Future: Developing Community-Based Nutrition Services. Washington, DC: Association of State and Territorial Public Health Nutrition Directors; 2003: 87–88.

13. U.S. Department of Health and Human Services. Public Health in America. Available at: http://www.Health.gov/phfunctions/public.htm. Accessed April 26, 2005.

14. U.S. Department of Health and Human Services. *Healthy People 2010: Understanding and Improving Health.* 2nd ed. Washington, DC: U.S. Government Printing Office; November 2000. Available at: http://www.health.gov/healthypeople.

15. Public Health Service, Office of the Surgeon General of the United States, Department of Health and Human Services, Nutrition Policy Board. The Surgeon General's Report on Nutrition and Health 1998. Publication No. 88-50210. Available at: http://profiles.nlm.nih.gov/NN/B/C/Q/G/.

16. U.S. Department of Health and Human Services. *Healthy People 2000: National Health Promotion and Disease Prevention Objectives.* DHHS Publication No. 91-50212. Washington, DC: U.S. Government Printing Office; 1991.

17. Dodd JL, Bayerl CT. Nutrition in the community. In: Saunders Mahan K and Escott-Stump S, eds, *Krause's Food, Nutrition, and Diet Therapy.* 11th ed. Philadelphia; 2004:340–362.

18. U.S. Department of Health and Human Services. What Are the Leading Health Indicators? Available at: http://www.health.gov/healthypeople/LHI/lhiwhat.htm. Accessed April 26, 2005.

19. U.S. Department of Agriculture. Marketing and Regulatory Programs (MRP) Mission Area Strategic Plan 1999-2002. Available at: http://www.ams.usda.gov. Accessed April 4, 2004.

20. Mixon H, Dodds J, Haughton B. *Guidelines for Community Nutrition Supervised Experiences.* 2nd ed. Public Health/Community Nutrition Practice Group, American Dietetic Association; 2003. Available at http://www.phcnpg.org. Accessed February 2004.

21. Bayerl CT, Ries J. *Early Start: Nutrition Services in Early Intervention Program.* Boston, Mass.: Department of Public Health; 1995.

22. Bryk JA, Kornblum T. Report on the 1999 membership database of the American Dietetic Association. *J Am Diet Assoc.* 2001;101:947–953.

23. Biesemeier, C. *Achieving Excellence: Clinical Staffing for Today and Tomorrow.* Chicago, Ill.: American Dietetic Association; 2004.

24. Story M, Holt K, Sofka D. eds. *Bright Futures in Practice: Nutrition.* 2nd ed. Arlington, VA: National Center for Education in Maternal and Child Health; 2002. Available at: http://www.brightfutures.org/ nutrition/resources.html. Accessed April 26, 2005.

25. Casamassimo, P. ed. *Bright Futures in Practice: Oral Health.* Arlington, VA: National Center for Education in Maternal and Child Health; 1996. Available at: http://www.brightfutures.org/oralhealth/pdf/ index.html. Accessed April 26, 2005.

26. Holt K, Sofka D. eds. *Bright Futures in Practice: Physical Activity.* Arlington, VA: National Center for Education in Maternal and Child Health; 2001. Available at: http://www.brightfutures.org/physicalactivity. Accessed April 26, 2005.

27. The American Dietetic Association. Available at: http://eatright.org/ public/index_13038.cfm. Accessed April 26, 2005.

28. The American Dietetic Association. Accredited or Approved Education Plans. Available at: http://eatright.org/public/7782_13280.cfm. Accessed April 26, 2005.

29. American Dietetic Association. Evidence Mounts on the Effectiveness of Medical Nutrition Therapy. Available at: http://www.eatright.org/Public/ GovernmentAffairs/98_evidence2000.cfm. Accessed April 26, 2005.

30. American Dietetic Association. http://www.eatright.org/ GovernmentAffairs/98_8723.cfm. Accessed April 4, 2004.

31. Carey M, Gillespie S. Cost effectiveness of medical nutrition therapy. J Am Diet Assoc. 1995;95:88–91. Available at: http://www.eatright.org/ Public/Governmentaffairs/92_accost-effective. Accessed April 4, 2004.

32. Economic Research Service. Briefing Room: Food and Nutrition Assistance Programs. Available at: http://www.ers.usda.gov/briefing/ foodnutritionassistance. Accessed April 26, 2005.

33. U.S. Department of Agriculture. WIC Farmers' Market Nutrition Program. Available at: http://www.fns.usda.gov/wic/FMNP/FMNPfaqs.htm. Accessed April 26, 2005.

34. Anderson JC, Bybee DI, Brown R, McLean DF, Garcia EM, Breer ML, Schillo BA. 5-A-Day fruit and vegetable interventions improve consumption in a low-income population. *J Am Diet Assoc.* 2001;101:195–202.

35. U.S. Department of Agriculture. Revitalizing Quality Nutrition Services in WIC. Available at: http://www.fns.usda.gov/wic/CONTENT/RNQS/ RNQS.htm. Accessed April 4, 2004.

36. U.S. Department of Agriculture, Food and Nutrition Services. *Recruitment Strategies for Public Health/Community Nutritionists. Final Report.* Alexandria, VA: USDA; 1995.

37. U.S. Department of Agriculture, Food and Nutrition Service. WIC Nutrition Service Standards. Available at: http://www.fns.usda.gov/wic/. Accessed April 4, 2004.

38. Harris-Davis E, Haughton, B. Model for multicultural nutrition counseling competencies. *J Am Diet Assoc.* 2000;100:1178–1185.

39. Greenwald HP, Davis RA. Minority recruitment and retention in dietetics: Issues and interventions. *J Am Diet Assoc.* 2000;100(8):961–966.

40. Food and nutrition section exposes students to public health careers. *The Nation's Health.* 2002;XXXII. Available at: http://www.apha.org/ tnh/. Accessed March 29, 2004.

41. Hampl J, Anderson J, Mullis R. The role of dietetics professionals in health promotion and diseases prevention. *J Am Diet Assoc.* 2002;102(11): 1680–1688. Available at: http://www.eatright.org. Accessed March 29, 2004.

42. American Dietetic Association. ADA Position Papers. Available at: http://www.eatright.org/public/index_7705.cfm. Accessed April 26, 2005.

43. Chance KG, Green CG. The effect of employee job satisfaction on program participation rates in the Virginia WIC program. *J Public Health Manage Pract.* 2001;7(1):10–20.

44. Olecko WA, Blacconiere MJ. Job satisfaction in public health: a comparative analysis of five occupational groups. *J Royal Soc Health.* 1995;115:386–390.

45. Green, CG, Harrison H, Henderson K, Lenihan A. Total quality management in the delivery of public health services: A focus on North Carolina WIC programs. *J Public Health Manage Pract.* 1998;4:72–82.

Other References

ASTPHND. Guidelines for Comprehensive Programs to Promote Healthy Eating and Physical Activity. Nutrition and Physical Activity Work Group. Available at: http://www.fns.usda.gov/oane/menu/nuteducation.htm.

ASTPHND. *Strategies for Success: Curriculum Guide.* 2nd ed. Association of Graduate Programs in Public Health Nutrition, Inc.; 2002. Available at: http://nutrition.Utk.edu/resources/StrategiesForSuccess.pdf. Accessed April 26, 2005.

Hatner-Eaton C. Public health departments and the quality movement: A natural partnership. *Clin Performance and Quality Healthcare.* 1995;3:35–40.

Hess AMN, Haughton B. Continuing education needs for public health nutritionists. *J Am Diet Assoc.* 1996;96:716–718.

Johnson DB, Easton DL, Wahl PW, Gleason C. Public health nutrition practice in the United States. *J Am Diet Assoc.* 2001;101:529–534.

Owen, AL, Splett PL, Owen GM. *Nutrition in the Community: The Art and Science of Delivering Services.* 4th ed. Boston, Mass.: WCB/McGraw-Hill; 1999.

Starbaugh, C. ed. Call to Action. *Better Nutrition for Mothers, Children, and Families.* Washington, DC: National Center for Education in Maternal and Child Health; 1990.

Tuttle CR, Derrick B, Tagtow A. A new vision for health promotion and nutrition education. *Am J Health Promotion.* 2003;18(2):186–191.

U.S. Department of Health and Human Services, Public Health Service. *The Public Health Workforce: An Agenda for the 21st Century.* Washington, DC: APHA; 2000.

Wellness Councils of America. Steps to a healthier U.S.: Joining forces: health promotion takes the hill. *Absolute Advantage.* 2004;3(6). Available at: http://www.eatright.org.

CHAPTER 23

MANAGING PUBLIC HEALTH NUTRITION PERSONNEL

Esther Okeiyi, PhD, RD, LDN

Reader Objectives

After studying this chapter and reflecting on the contents, you should be able to:

1. List at least 10 responsibilities of a public health nutrition director or manager.
2. Describe the five major management functions involved in managing nutrition personnel in the nutrition division of public health.
3. Explain the "six M's" of management.
4. Explain at least three activities performed under each of the five major functions of a director.
5. Differentiate between strategic planning and operational planning, as well as between a job description and a job specification.
6. Describe the relationships among the following: job analysis, job description, and job specification.
7. Distinguish between the characteristics of a manager and the characteristics of a leader.
8. Discuss the characteristics of a good performance appraisal.
9. List the advantages of a performance appraisal.
10. Compare the goals and objectives, job descriptions, and mission statements of the nutritional division of the two types of public health divisions represented in this chapter.
11. Compare the job description for the directors of the two nutrition divisions discussed in this chapter.
12. Develop a mission statement for the two types of public health nutrition divisions discussed in this chapter.
13. Define the following terms: planning, organizing, delegating, controlling, and Behavioral Anchored Rating Scale.

Today's public health nutrition managers recognize the need for a clear understanding and effective application of management principles in day-to-day operations. However, sometimes they may feel overwhelmed by the various terms applied in the field of scientific management. Therefore, public health nutrition directors or managers need to become familiar with these terms and principles, because no unit in the public health department will provide a greater opportunity for applying these management skills. Mackenzie (1969), building on the works of Fayol, illustrated the elements, continuous and sequential functions, and activities of managers.

Mackenzie indicated that the elements that today's managers are faced with are ideas, things, and people. These are considered the main components of an organization. Thus, the manager's task related to *ideas* is to think conceptually about issues or matters that need to be resolved. The tasks relating to *things* are to administer or manage the details of the director's affairs. The task relating to *people* is to exercise leadership and influence people so that they accomplish desired goals.

The Role of a Public Health Nutrition Director/Manager

A public health manager, also referred to as a director of nutrition services, wears many hats as a leader in his or her department. The responsibilities of a public health manager or director may include, but are not limited to:

- Providing leadership in all areas of a nutrition division of a public health department
- Recruiting, orienting, and training nutritionists in the nutrition division
- Supervising nutritionists and their work
- Motivating employees, conducting performance appraisals, and disciplining employees when necessary
- Maintaining good communication between the nutritionists and staff, and between the director and employees
- Handling concerns and grievances
- Planning, implementing, and evaluating program and service outcomes
- Organizing the nutrition division
- Planning the budget and controlling costs
- Interacting and working with other divisions in the public health department
- Representing the health department as an expert in the area of nutrition within and outside the public health department

- Ensuring esprit de corps among the nutritionists
- Generating income by soliciting grants and writing grant proposals for funding programs and employee positions in the division
- Networking and partnering with the community
- Keeping abreast of laws, changes in the community, community needs, and health needs

The major role of a public health nutrition director or manager can be divided into five areas: planning, staffing, organizing, leading, and controlling. The director utilizes available resources to accomplish the organizational goals. There are six main resources available to the director, which are known as the "six M's" of management: manpower, market, machine, method, material, and money. *Manpower* represents the employees. *Market* represents the clients and the community that the nutrition division serves. *Machines* include the equipment used in producing services, such as assessment tools, the computer, and storage cabinets. *Materials* represent the supplies, software, and training and promotion materials needed to run the programs. *Methods* represent the processes, policies, procedures, and guidelines stipulated by the division, government, and funding agencies. *Money* represents the financial aspect of the operation. The following sections take a closer look at the major roles of the nutrition director in a health department.

Planning

Planning is the establishment of a mission statement, goals, and objectives, and the determination of strategies to accomplish the goals and objectives. A mission statement is the first step in planning; it represents the philosophy or purpose that drives an organization. The division's mission statement must be derived from the overall mission of the public health department and provides an overall direction for the organization. Although goals are stated in general terms, objectives are specific and must be stated in measurable terms related to actions or activities. The following are examples of short-range objectives and goals pertaining to personnel:

GOALS:
1. The nutrition division will reduce the employee turnover rate annually.
2. To make employees successful.

OBJECTIVES:
1. The nutrition division will reduce the employee turnover rate from 50% to 25% by the end of 2005.
2. The number of employees indicating satisfaction with their productivity will increase by 25% the first year and 50% the second and third years.
3. All employees will participate in at least two professional conferences annually.

The three types of planning are the *strategic plan*, the *intermediate plan*, and the *operational plan*. The strategic plan involves making decisions about the future, forecasting for the future, and making decisions based on the environment and the current and anticipated available resources. A strategic plan serves for 3 to 15 years and should be reviewed regularly. Managers at the top of the organizational structure develop the strategic plan. In strategic planning, strengths and weaknesses of the organization or the unit are analyzed. The strategic plan document serves as a foundation for an intermediate plan, which covers a 1- to 3-year period. Middle level managers or supervisors may develop an intermediate plan. It is through the intermediate plan that policies are developed. Finally, the operational plan describes a day-to-day action plan. It dictates the plan for a period of one year or less.

There are three major levels of managers, each of whom is responsible for a different level of planning. The *top managers* function at the policy-making level of the organization. They are responsible for broad, comprehensive planning involving strategic planning and long-range goals. The *middle-level managers* are responsible for developing policies; and *first-line managers*, at the technical or operational level, are responsible for developing procedures and methods.

The level of managers involved in developing any plan may be based on the size of the organization/unit and the levels of management in that unit. It is clear from the job descriptions in Figures 23-2 through 23-4 that directors in different nutrition divisions in the public health department may perform different responsibilities, based on the division's size, levels of management, and how that particular organization is structured. For example, the director of nutrition at Durham County Health Department delegates most of the first-line and middle management functions to her team leaders. These team leaders plan, orient, train, and provide direct supervision to their area employees. The nutrition manager or director works with other division managers internally, planning and coordinating efforts relating to the public health department, and representing the division by providing expertise in matters relating to nutrition. An example of a public health department issue that can affect all divisions is bioterrorism. The nutrition director may contribute ideas regarding how the nutrition division may handle such matters in terms of managing food sanitation and safety. Externally, the manager or director represents the public health department, negotiating for community partnerships, contracts, funding, and projects. In addition, the manager implements nutrition programs and works with other stakeholders, such as government agencies and community key players.

A good plan is vital to a successful organization. It determines how well and smoothly an operation performs. In the long run, a good plan prevents many problems for both the director and the division as a whole. Planning increases effectiveness and efficiency. *Effectiveness* refers to an operation's ability to accomplish its goals and objectives. *Efficiency* refers to an operation's ability to achieve maximum results with minimum input. It is important that employees are involved in the planning. It keeps everyone knowledgeable of what is going on in the unit. In addition, employees are more likely to buy into the plan if they are part of the planning team.

Staffing and Employee Evaluation

Directors are responsible for hiring the right people for the positions in their divisions. Once employees are hired, they are introduced to the job and organization during a formal orientation program, and subsequently are given an organized training period in preparation for their job. The orientation process may take 3 to 5 days. The amount and length of training are dependent upon each employee's previous training and experience. Over time, the employees are evaluated periodically, typically after the first 90 days on the job and annually by the manager to inform them of how well they are doing. This is referred to as a *performance appraisal.* A performance appraisal is a formal method of providing constructive feedback to an employee regarding how well or poorly the employee is performing his or her job. The objectives are to positively influence, motivate, strengthen, and enhance the employee's work performance. The performance appraisals must be job related.

Performance appraisals have many advantages, including:

- Aiding employees in defining future goals and providing an objective set of criteria to measure job performance
- Providing a basis for modifying poor work habits
- Providing a means of gathering employees' suggestions for improving performance, methods, and morale
- Demonstrating a source of documentation in the event of litigation
- Providing a basis on which to determine promotions and wage increases
- Providing a means to seek an alternative to termination
- Helping to pinpoint personal weaknesses and how to improve them

Overall, a performance appraisal is an effective motivational tool. The appraisal should not be used as a punishment or as an opportunity for vindictiveness. Also, it must not be a one-way process, but should be a mutual discussion between an employee and the manager. For the evaluation to be effective, the employee must be informed about the process prior to starting work and a week or two before the actual evaluation. A performance appraisal must be conducted in a private environment.

Employees are entitled to be informed about how they are progressing in regards to their jobs. Every employee is also entitled to be informed about the criteria being used for their evaluation. These criteria can be covered during orientation, training, or in-house meetings. Opportunities should be given to the employees to ask questions about information that is not clear to them. Although there are many evaluation tools available, the Behavioral Anchored Rating Scale (BARS), as documented by Payne-Palacio and Theis (2001), is generally considered the best and most effective tool for employees' performance appraisals. This tool identifies specific behaviors for each performance level in each task and job category and provides a scale with which to rate employees. The Management by Objectives (MBO) system is another performance evaluation tool managers can use. With this tool, both the manager and the employee agree on performance objectives, and the employee is evaluated on how well the objectives are accomplished.

Discipline is used when all other measures have failed to bring the employee up to standard regarding desired work performance. Any disciplinary action against an employee should be legally defensible. It may be advisable to double check with the legal office of the department before taking disciplinary action. Disciplinary actions should be immediate, consistent, and impersonally based, and the evaluation criteria must be known in advance. The work rules must be clear, fair, and reasonable, and they must be reviewed regularly.

A manager must be alert to signs of grievances in employees, whether verbal or nonverbal, and should have a plan to deal with these. Some of the signs may include indifference toward the job or toward other employees, excessive tardiness and absences, decline in quality of work, and excessive complaints. The first line of action by a manager may be to have a face-to-face, private discussion with the employee. The manager may point out changes observed and concern for the employee's progress. Discussion of the problem may lead to brainstorming strategies between the employee and the manager for solving the problem. If the problem persists, documentation and a Grievance Action Form may be completed and serve as a warning to the employee. A Grievance Action Form is a form for written record of a grievance and action taken. Grievance proceedings usually follow three to four steps after discussion: verbal warning, written warning, second written warning, and final warning, followed by termination, if the employee has been ruled against.

Organizing

In order for the goals and objectives of a nutrition division to be accomplished, the manager must organize the resources in an orderly fashion. *Organizing* is the act of carefully grouping the organization's resources and activities, including human resources, by type of tasks performed. The organizing process establishes relationships among all functions of management. How the public health nutrition division is organized is based on its mission, goals and objectives, and areas of nutrition services provided to the community. For example, whereas some nutrition divisions of public health departments focus on providing nutrition services to women, infants, and children through the WIC program, others focus on preventing and reducing disabilities among individuals or groups, such as the elderly, children, and home-bound individuals. Convalescents and the poor in the community, both of whom are at nutritional risk, also can be provided nutrition-related services. The nutrition division also may serve those who come to a clinic for another health reasons, but are identified as candidates at high nutritional risk. In each case, the service areas of a public health nutrition division will be easily discernable on the unit's organizational chart. See Figure 23-1 for a typical example of an organizational chart for a public health nutrition division.

The following steps are used in developing an organizational structure:

1. Define organizational goals and objectives.
2. Analyze and classify work to be done.
3. Describe in detail the work or activity in terms of the employees.
4. Determine and specify relationships of the jobs to each other and to management.
5. Organize the employees by tasks and activities and show their relationship to each other and to management.
6. Clearly delineate staff and line positions. *Line positions* are in the direct chain of command that are responsible for the achievement of organizational goals (Griffin, 1999). *Staff positions*, in contrast, provide expertise, advice, and support for the line positions. Examples of staff positions are the advisory board, consultants, and secretaries. In an organizational chart, line positions are shown with solid unbroken lines, whereas staff positions are shown with broken lines or dotted lines. The lines depict lines of communication and control. *Scalar principle* indicates that a clear and unbroken line of authority flow from the bottom position to the top position in the organization.
7. Organizational charts should be reviewed and updated periodically as positions change. An interview with the directors of the nutrition division of Durham County and Wake County Public Health Departments (Rebecca Freeman MPH, RD, LDN and Miriam Peterson, MPH, RD, LDN) revealed that they are currently in the process of reviewing and realigning the department's job description and, therefore, the organizational charts. Proper organization of employees requires that managers be assigned a number of employees

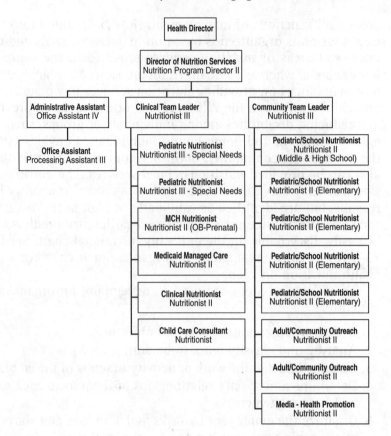

FIGURE 23-1   Organizational Chart for Durham County Public Health Department Nutrition Division
Source: Reprinted with the permission of the Director of the Nutrition Division of Durham County Health Department, Durham, North Carolina, 2004.

that they are capable of managing. This is known as span of control. According to the principle of unity of command, under no circumstance should an employee report to more than one supervisor or manager.

The tools for structuring an organization include job descriptions, job specifications, job breakdowns or analyses, and job design. A *job description* is an organized list of duties, skills, and responsibilities required in a specific position. A *job specification* is a written statement of minimum standards that must be met by an applicant for a particular job. It covers duties involved in the job, working conditions specific to the job, and personal qualifications required to carry out the responsibilities successfully. A *job analysis* or *breakdown* is written documentation of a study conducted on all aspects of a specific job. It provides information used in developing job descriptions. Figures 23-2 through 23-4 show examples of job descriptions for a managerial position and two nutritionists' positions in two different types of public health nutrition divisions with different missions. A *job design*, developed from job analysis, is concerned with structuring jobs to improve organization efficiency and employee satisfaction. Jobs are divided into manageable units based on employees' expertise.

Leading

Leadership and management are not the same, although the words are sometimes used interchangeably (Bittle & Newstrom, 1990; Tamel & Reynolds, 1981). Characteristics of managers and leaders are outlined in the book *Executive Leadership* by Tamel and Reynolds. Leadership is the activity of influencing other people's behavior toward the achievement of desired objects. It involves influencing others without coercion to achieve the organization's goals and objectives. Simply stated, it is getting people to do what you want them to because they want to do it. Management, on the other hand, is the function of running an organization by effectively integrating and coordinating resources in order to achieve desired objectives. Managing a nutrition division should be combined with leadership qualities and activities. A director leads the human resources in an organization while managing the nonhuman resources used in operating the division.

Leaders share decision making, information, authority, reward, trust, drive, motivation, and vision with their employees. They work well with employees and demonstrate respect, concern, and empathy. They honor differences in employees. The leader takes risks for the benefit of a work group. On the other hand, a good manager may effectively plan, organize, and control finances and productivity, but have less success in dealing with employees (Hudson, 2000).

A common characteristic of a leader is native intelligence. This means he or she has the ability to acquire and retain knowledge, and respond quickly and productively to a new situation. Leaders have drive, which they need in order to achieve and feel successful. They have integrity and self-confidence, and are experts in what they do. George and Jones (2002) summarized the traits that correlate strongly with leadership. Leadership skills are partly innate and partly learned (Boyle & Morris, 2002). Leaders have strong personal mastery that impels them to struggle for change in an organization. They seek out risks, dislike mundane tasks, are concerned about people, and strive to achieve personal goals. They derive power from personal relationships and relate with people in intuitive ways. They question established procedures and create new concepts. They are concerned with results (Tamel & Reynolds, 1981, p. 59). There is a high correlation between leadership and the ability to relate, influence, motivate, coordinate, delegate, and communicate (Hudson, 2000).

McGregor's X and Y Theories— Different ways in which managers view employees. There are two theories: Theory X and Theory Y.

Theory X—Managers believe that workers are motivated by only one thing: money. They are selfish, lazy, and hate work. The manager believes that workers need to be closely controlled and directed.

Theory Y—Managers believe that workers are motivated by many different factors apart from money. They enjoy their work. The manager believes that employees will happily take on responsibility and make decisions for the business.

Contingency Theory—The belief that performance is a result of interaction between two factors: leadership style and situational favorableness.

Maslow's Theory—The hierarchy of human needs theory. The needs of an individual exist in a logical order (physiological, safety, belonging, esteem, and self-actualization); the basic root needs must be satisfied first.

Hertzberg's Theory—A theory regarding motivation; also called the two-factor theory. Work characteristics causing dissatisfaction (i.e., work conditions, pay, and interpersonal relationships) are quite different from those causing satisfaction (i.e., achievement, recognition, and opportunity for growth).

McClelland's Theory—An individual's motivation and effectiveness in certain job functions are influenced by three needs: achievement, affiliation, and power.

Leading and Influencing

In leading, the manager and subordinate's relationship is critical. McGregor's *X and Y Theories* of leadership are based on the fact that a leader's attitudes toward employees influence their job performances. The *Contingency Theory* of leadership promotes the idea that the type of leadership provided should be contingent on the type of employees and the situation in which the organization exists (Fielder & Garcia, 1987; McGregor, 1985).

Motivating

Another aspect of leading is creating an environment in which subordinates can be motivated and excited to perform their job well. A leader must understand the concepts of human motivation. To accomplish the goals and objectives of the division, the people who produce the products and services need to be well led and motivated. Interaction between a leader and his or her subordinates will result in the leader being able to elicit what motivates the employees. There is no one method to create conditions that will motivate employees. Maslow (1943), Hertzberg (1966), McClelland (1985), and Vroom (1994) all developed theories on how employees are motivated in a work environment. An experienced leader may employ Abraham Maslow's *Hierarchy of Needs Theory* by first determining the point of motivation need for each subordinate. Hertzberg's two-factor theory, which is similar to Maslow's needs theory, identified two major factors, job satisfiers and job dissatisfiers, that can motivate or dissatisfy employees, respectively. Job satisfiers are motivators and include achievement, recognition, responsibility, advancement, the work itself, and potential for growth. The job dissatisfiers are known as maintenance or hygiene factors and must be present for job satisfaction to occur. They include pay, supervision, job security, working conditions, organizational policies, and interpersonal relationships on the job. McClelland's *Motivation Theory* supported Maslow's theory and emphasized that employees are usually at different levels of need, which can be high or low.

An employee will respond positively to motivation if the degree of need is high. Vroom's Expectancy Theory stipulates that employees will be motivated if they can link the job performance to the expected reward. For example, if they expect a better reward for better performance, then they will be motivated to perform. Motivators can range from a simple pat on the back, affirming work well done, to public recognition of the employee in a meeting, publishing an employee's accomplishments, offering incentives, or rewarding an employee by delegating managerial tasks.

> **Vroom's Theory**—Assumes that behavior results from conscious choices among alternatives whose purpose is to maximize pleasure and minimize pain. The key elements to this theory are referred to as *expectancy, instrumentality,* and *valence.*

Coordinating

A director must coordinate all aspects of the various parts of employees' work so that they flow smoothly. The public health nutrition division director can accomplish this through departmentalization or specialization by functions, clients, geographic areas, number of persons, or time. Figure 23-5 shows an example of a leader's way of organizing nutritionists' job tasks by area and delegating *team leaders* to supervise the subordinates. Some tasks may be delegated to free the director's time to do other tasks. *Delegating* is essential in distributing workloads. It enriches and enlarges employees' jobs and contributes to employees' improved job knowledge, job motivation, professional development, and job accomplishment. When job responsibilities are delegated, authority must accompany them. The manager must guide the employee to understand the limits of the authority, and what decisions and actions can be made without consultation. Delegating, developing, and motivating employees are all acts of leading.

Communicating

Effective leadership depends on the ability of the leader to communicate with his or her subordinates. Communication includes being able to transmit ideas and goals, receive messages from internal environments, listen, network, interact with others, and manage both formal and informal organizations. A true leader must resist the temptation of showing favoritism among employees.

Director Position Description
Present Title: Program Manager I   Proposed Title: Program Manager II

The primary duties of this position are to direct the Women, Infants and Children's Nutrition Program and to lead a cross-agency initiative to develop an integrated, consumer-friendly system for access and entry to the combined Human Services agency.

50%   Women, Infants and Children's (WIC) Nutrition Program
Planning
Assesses needs of the WIC Program's client population and establishes long- and short-range program goals and objectives to meet those needs. Sets program priorities.

Develops the annual budget for the WIC Program and allocates funds within the program to achieve goals. Identifies and secures new resources to support program goals.

Establishes collaborative linkages within the agency and with external agencies to facilitate needed services.

Directing
Manages the WIC Program budget and provides accountability for program revenues. Oversees the management of projects funded through grants as well as projects subcontracted to other organizations. Prepares periodic reports for grant-funded projects.

Establishes policies, procedures, and work standards. Determines staffing patterns. Oversees the development of job descriptions for WIC Program staff.

Hires WIC Program staff and conducts performance reviews. Delegates selection of administrative support staff to administrative support supervisor.

Provides direction and feedback to supervisory and advanced practice staff regarding program operation. Oversees changes in the program's computer system.

Oversees the monitoring of the 120 supermarkets and grocery stores throughout the county that serve as vendors for the program. Assures high-quality vendor services to program participants. Oversees identification and investigation of program integrity issues.

Oversees the development of nutrition education materials. Issues and presents informational material through the media. Presents information to community groups and at professional conferences and meetings.

Represents the WIC Program in agency administrative meetings. Assumes leadership roles in relevant professional organizations.

Establishes and maintains cooperative relations with civic, educational, governmental, medical care, and other agencies concerned with food and nutrition in order to strengthen and promote program activities.

Evaluating
Evaluates program information to assess outcomes and improve operations. Oversees quality assurance activities of the WIC Program. Involves staff in analysis of program-specific data and in formulation of new strategies.

FIGURE 23-2   Wake County Human Services; Family and Youth Success
Source: The reproduction of this information is with permission of Rebecca Freeman, MPH, RD, LDN, Director of the Nutrition Division of the Durham County Health Department, 2004.

40% Access and Entry

Planning

Within Human Services, works with Outcome Group Leaders and other staff throughout the agency to identify areas in which client access to services needs improvement. Establishes long and short-term goals and objectives for improving these services.

Investigates targeted areas of access to service to determine underlying causes of problems. Uses a variety of strategies, including surveys of the public and agency staff and technical studies, to assess problem areas.

Analyzes results of investigation to develop methods and systems to improve access to services. Develops strategies and time lines to implement needed change.

Directing

Directs needed change through a variety of activities, as needed, including the following:

- Promotes and facilitates the establishment of collaborative linkages within and outside of the agency to support new methods of accessing services
- Establishes new positions, hires staff, and moves staff within the agency
- Oversees renovations to work areas
- Identifies and secures needed equipment and software
- Assures necessary training for appropriate staff
- Develops project budgets
- Oversees management of new units until they are well established
- Communicates changes to agency staff and to the public

Evaluating

Uses benchmark and follow-up studies to assess change in case of access to services.

Uses results of follow-up studies to refine approaches to improving access to services.

10% Other Duties

Facilitates and coordinates activities of School Health Program nutritionists. Supervises nutritionist serving the Women's/Adolescent Health Program. Performs related duties as requested.

Required knowledge, skills and abilities: Mastery of the field of public health nutrition with broad knowledge of principles, theories, and practice of public health nutrition; working knowledge of accounting principles, of methods of financing health services including grant preparation, of reimbursement systems, of method of control revenues and expenditures with considerable skill in forecasting fiscal needs and preparing budget justifications, and in applying cost benefit/cost effectiveness analysis; working knowledge of epidemiological and biostatistical principles and the principles of computer-based data collection and analysis. Ability to communicate effectively, orally and in writing, and to make public presentations.

FIGURE 23-2   (Continued)

Women, Infants, and Children Nutrition Program
Position Description
Nutritionist

Assesses WIC program applicants' or participants' nutritional needs based on anthropometric, biochemical, clinical, and dietary data. Develops plan of care, provides individualized nutrition counseling, documents in the medical record, and makes appropriate referrals. May also provide nutrition education to groups of participants.

85%   Patient Care: Provides direct assessment of WIC Program applicants' or participants' (pregnant women, breast-feeding women, postpartum women, infants, and children 1–5 years) nutritional needs based on anthropometric, biochemical, clinical, dietary, and socioeconomic data; develops a plan of care including medical nutrition therapy, if indicated, based on assessment; determines appropriate food prescription; provides individualized nutrition counseling based on needs and resources identified in the assessment; determines required nutrition follow-up; refers clients to appropriate healthcare, social, and/or community service resources; documents above information in medical record according to state and federal WIC guidelines.

Provides individualized nutritional assessment and counseling for those individuals identified as high risk with conditions including, but not limited to, prematurity, failure to thrive, bronchopulmonary dysplasia, congenital heart disease, gastroesophageal reflux, dysphasia, chronic renal failure, hypercholesterolemia, hypernatremia, obesity, diabetes, hypertension, eating disorders, and/or mental conditions affecting nutritional status that require specialized dietary modifications in nutrients, calories, fluid, or texture for achievement of therapeutic nutrition goals.

Interprets nutritional assessment and recommendations for physicians, nurses, developmental disability specialists, social workers, psychologists, and other members of patient care team; utilizes multidisciplinary team approach to provide coordinated patient care.

Provides individualized follow-up nutrition counseling for high-risk participants and/or caretakers.

5%   Professional Consultation: Confers with and provide consultation to physicians, nurses, social workers, psychologists, and other healthcare providers regarding high-risk patients or those with special needs in order to coordinate optimal patient care.

Serves as liaison with other community health professionals for questions about special programs and updates on new policies.

Participates in the planning for and supervision of the public health field experience for medical students and graduate nutrition students.

Consults with industry representatives regarding new products and literature pertaining to nutrition.

FIGURE 23-3   Job Description for a Nutritionist in the Nutrition Division at Wake County Human Services Department
Source: The reproduction of this information is with permission of Rebecca Freeman, MPH, RD, LDN, Director of the Nutrition Division of the Durham County Health Department, 2004.

10% Other Duties: Serves as a nutrition information and education specialist for the community.

Area of focus: Assumes responsibility for oversight of one area of client care for the program: nutrition education classes; educational materials development and procurement; tracking and follow-up of elevated blood lead levels; vitamin supplementation for infants; breast-feeding support (including in-home project); and special formulas and nutritional products.

Attends in-services and workshops on nutrition-related issues to meet minimum standards of 15 hours continuing education per year as required by the Commission on Dietetic Registration.

Participates in the development of the WIC Program plan and the WIC Program policy and procedure manual.

Performs various other related duties as requested by the nutritionist supervisor.

Minimum Education and Experience Requirements:

Master's degree in nutrition and dietetics or related field; one year of experience in the field of nutrition. Appropriate licensure (Registered Dietitian or Registered Dietitian Eligible) required.

FIGURE 23-3 (Continued)

The director represents both the employees and management. The employees look up to the director as representative of management. The director, therefore, must be able to: 1) interpret the mission, goals, objectives, and policies of the organization to the employees in a way that garners their cooperation and confidence; 2) motivate and guide the employees with their job; 3) assist in employees' professional development; 4) listen to and empathize with employees as needed; 5) provide training to both individuals and groups; and 6) evaluate employees and implement discipline when needed.

Leading and directing are synonymous. Directing requires continuous decision making, conveying these decisions to subordinates, and ensuring appropriate actions. Also, it requires coordinating

Democratic—This style is also called participative, because it encourages employee participation in decision making. The manager checks with the employees before making a decision and can act as a coach or problem solver for the group.

Autocratic—A leadership style that does not encourage employee input. The manager makes all decisions. Employees are expected to obey management decisions without asking any questions.

Laissez-faire—A leadership style also known as the "hands-off" style. The manager provides little or no direction and gives employees as much freedom as possible. All authority or power is given to the employees, and they must determine goals, make decisions, and resolve problems on their own.

1. Present Classification Title
   of Position
   <u>Nutritionist II</u>

2. Usual Working Title of Position
   <u>Public Health Nutritionist</u>

3. Requested Classification of
   Position
   <u>N/A</u>

4. Name of Immediate Supervisor

5. Supervisor's Position Title
   & Position Number

6. Name of Employee

7. Pres 15 Digit BOSUN. Prop

8. Dept., University, Commission,
   or Agency

9. Institution and Division
   <u>Nutrition Division</u>

10. Section and Unit—Nutrition
    Division

11. Street Address, City,
    and County

12. Location of Workplace, Bldg.,
    & Room No.

I. A. PRIMARY PURPOSE OF ORGANIZATIONAL UNIT:

The Nutrition Division is one of seven Health Department Divisions. The Division provides a multifaceted public health nutrition program that is based on a comprehensive community assessment and is integrated into the medical and educational services and organizational mission of the Health Department. The program focuses on disease prevention and the reduction of disability through health promotion, restoration, and/or management of disease.

Registered dietitians/nutritionists provide medical nutrition therapy services to patients with medical/nutrition problems and/or programming in coordination with the following Health Department services:

All clinics (nutrition, adult, STD, HIV+/AIDS, family planning, obstetric, prevention)

In-home services (home health)

School health

Health promotion program

Child, maternity, and pre-inter-conceptional care coordination.

Nutrition management and support for acute or chronically ill and handicapping conditions

Nutritionists conduct community/population assessments, and plan, implement, and evaluate community interventions. Through agreements and contractual arrangements, nutritionists provide services in schools, area medical centers, the county social services department, and the area mental health program.

FIGURE 23-4   Job Description for a Nutritionist in the Nutrition Division at Durham Public Health Department
Source: The reproduction of this information is with permission of Rebecca Freeman, MPH, RD, LDN, Director of the Nutrition Division of the Durham County Health Department, 2004.

B. PRIMARY PURPOSE OF POSITION:

To plan, initiate, coordinate, and/or facilitate nutrition programming, prevention strategies, and nutrition interventions for preschool through elementary age children and their families in Durham County including developing ongoing relationships with other department personnel and community agencies, providing leadership in promoting and instructing optimal nutrition and health habits to elementary children and their families; providing consultation on programming/curriculum development; and participating on interdisciplinary boards and committees.

C. WORK SCHEDULE:

Monday–Friday, 75 hours bi-weekly. Evening and weekend hours are often required.

II. A. DESCRIPTION OF RESPONSIBILITIES AND DUTIES:

(Method Used: Order of Importance)

45% PRESCHOOL AND ELEMENTARY (PRE-K–5) SERVICES DELIVERY

Develop and conduct nutrition interventions aimed at screening/assessment results.

Coordinate and/or participate in assessment of known child populations with common health/nutrition problems/goals, and identify new populations as new research indicates.

Forward referrals from school nurses and educators to the clinical nutrition team.

Refer to and coordinate with other services for which the child is eligible or needs, including school food service, educators, other therapists, and health practitioners.

Instruct classes on nutrition and physical activity related topics.

45% PRESCHOOL AND ELEMENTARY (Pre-K–5) WELLNESS CONSULTATION

Participate on intra- and inter-departmental planning teams to focus on elementary health and nutrition interventions in the schools and the community.

Develop/maintain relationships with community leaders, school administrators, nurses and educators, food service system, and state/federal campaign initiatives to:

Initiate nutrition and health-related projects and interventions targeting population-based and individual nutrition health problems and wellness issues of preschool and elementary children.

Plan and present in-service training and education to leaders, educators, and health and food service personnel.

Provide consultation on school nutrition curriculum and resources.

Develop/procure materials on maintenance of normal and at-risk nutrition practices, while providing consistent and current information.

Participate in community/association/school boards/committees that have an elementary and/or wellness focus, as well as government bodies affecting child nutrition legislation.

(Continues)

10% PROGRAM DEVELOPMENT

Use media opportunities to increase awareness of and interest in nutrition and health issues of preschool/elementary children and their families.

Seek grant funding for special projects promoting normal nutrition and targeting special needs children.

Plan and participate in field training of master's level nutrition students.

Develop/revise policies and procedures and standards of care for elementary nutrition services as nutrition sciences advance.

Develop and conduct staff development sessions for health professionals.

Evaluate and/or develop educational materials and models.

Attend continuing education courses on specialized topics pertaining to position responsibilities and to meet the continuing education requirements for the Commission on Dietetic Registration or the state Nutrition/Dietetics Licensing Board.

Develop a yearly work plan with objectives, time frames, and quarterly assessments of accomplishments.

Disaster Relief—Participate in disaster relief activities as needed/assigned.

Other—Participate in other activities (including bio-terrorism response) as assigned by the department or supervisor.

II. B. OTHER POSITION CHARACTERISTICS:

1. Accuracy Required in Work:

Accurate and current knowledge of medical nutrition therapy, social sciences, and medical diagnosis is required to customize nutrition assessment and counseling.

Accurate and current knowledge of wellness issues and medical conditions relating to nutrition, including but not limited to diabetes mellitus, blood lipid levels, obesity, dental problems, and anemia as they affect preschool and elementary children is important for the nutritionist to function effectively and confidently in the community setting.

2. Consequence of Error:

Negligence (error) in determining need for and identifying dietary lack of nutrients needed by preschoolers and elementary children for growth and maintenance or promoting misinformation can result in health risk or problems in children.

3. Instructions Provided to Employee:

Community team leader orients nutritionist to county, department, and nutrition division policies and procedures and to department and division services and program concepts and role of this employee in reaching department and division objectives. Annual work plan developed by nutritionist and approved by community team leader serves as guide on which the nutritionist plans strategies/activities. Nutritionist uses own knowledge base and clinical judgment and ability to research medical/nutrition resources in providing services developing wellness initiatives.

FIGURE 23-4   Job Description for a Nutritionist in the Nutrition Division at Durham Public Health Department (Continued)

4. Guides, Regulations, Policies, and Reference Used by Employee:

Uses medical, nutrition, and drug reference books and journals, reports of the National Academy of Science and the U.S. Surgeon General, other national association reports, and population descriptions and community assessments and analyses. Additional references include the health department and nutrition division's policies and procedures.

5. Supervision Received by Employee:

The nutritionist is responsible for planning daily activities to accomplish work plan. He or she submits an activity report daily for statistics and a monthly report with a summary of accomplishments and goals for the next month. The Community Team Leader reviews nutritionist's activities and plans at least monthly. The Community Team Leader conducts an annual performance review with the nutritionist.

6. Variety and Purpose of Personal Contacts:

Consults with and makes recommendations to public health nurses, social workers, and educators regarding child health issues. Contacts with nutritionists, nurses, health educators, community and school leaders, program administrators, media, state program consultants in health and education departments, and university professors regarding nutrition issues and programming for preschool and elementary children.

7. Physical Effort:

Requires a physically and emotionally stable person who can transport portable display boards, models, and audio-visual equipment.

8. Work Environment and Conditions:

The health department is located in a high-crime inner city area. Travel around the county in unsafe neighborhoods is required.

9. Machines, Tools, Instruments, Equipment, and Materials Used:

Automobile for transportation.

Computer for PowerPoint presentations, nutrient analysis, spreadsheets, database, and word processing. Brochures and other selected media for age/grade-level appropriate instruction, for consultations with interdisciplinary team, and for group presentations.

Models of foods and the human body for individual and group instruction.

Audiovisual equipment for documentation and presentations.

Digital camera for capturing educational events.

10. Visual Attention, Mental Concentration, and Manipulative Skills:

Mental concentration is required in researching, understanding, and planning interactive programs for children and parents that will have a positive impact. Visual attention and mental concentration are vital in conducting classes, committee meetings, and group meetings. Frequent reading of technical resources, editing written reports, and the use of computers require close visual attention.

(Continues)

11. Safety for Others:

Confidentiality of identity or information of individual children is observed at all times.

12. Dynamics of Work:

New research findings and public health concerns regarding health and dietary wellness factors require the nutritionist to constantly review nutrition and medical journals for the latest findings and implications for programming. New findings also dictate the need to change standards of practice, and make adjustments in childhood interventions. New funding sources and changes in reimbursement programs may result in changes in programming and priorities in providing nutrition services, which may affect this nutritionist's responsibilities.

III. KNOWLEDGE, SKILLS, & ABILITIES, AND TRAINING & EXPERIENCE REQUIREMENTS:

A. Knowledge, Skills, and Abilities:

Considerable knowledge of principles of normal and therapeutic nutrition and drug and nutrient interaction at all stages of life is necessary. Thorough knowledge of wellness theories, components, and practices is needed as well as thorough knowledge of preschool and elementary school health issues; considerable knowledge of disease pathophysiology (normal and abnormal) and how nutrition relates to all separately and together; considerable knowledge and skill in nutrition and dietary assessment techniques, specifically as they apply to children with medical problems; knowledge of human behavior and techniques for affecting behavior change; highly skilled in public communications and ability to relate to children, local and state administrators, groups, and the media; skill in forming committees and conducting meetings; skill in interviewing and counseling; ability to appreciate various socioeconomic levels and lifestyles with respect for individual differences; skill in monitoring and maintaining quality standards of nutrition using current standards of practice; skill in organization and management of time and resources; skill in application of education methodologies and principles; skill in program planning; considerable skill in written and oral communication for the public and professionals.

B. Required Minimum Training:

A bachelor of science degree in foods and nutrition, public health nutrition, or dietetics, and one year of nutrition experience. American Dietetic Association Commission on Dietetic Registration certification or licensed to practice dietetics/nutrition by the State of North Carolina. Master's degree in nutrition or public health.

FIGURE 23-4 Job Description for a Nutritionist in the Nutrition Division at Durham Public Health Department (Continued)

and directing the work of employees to accomplish organizational goals. The director as a leader organizes and fits the right employees to jobs based on their abilities, assists in the orientation and training of employees, listens to and handles grievances, solves problems, and makes decisions in a timely and logical manner. She or he schedules and conducts employee meetings regularly. As a leader, she or he must keep abreast of the legal ramifications regarding public health nutrition. There is no one best style of leadership; rather, style must be adapted to fit the situation. Leaders can use different styles of leadership—democratic or participative, laissez-faire, or autocratic—depending on the employees they lead. The leader must accept leading responsibilities as well as earn the employees' trust. The quality and the amount of supervision may determine the success or failure of the organization in accomplishing its goals and its ability to attract government funds to stay afloat.

Managers of today's employees must understand that good communication is essential in managing cultural, ethnic, and racial diversity. As the ethnic composition of the workforce continues to become increasingly more diverse, good communication will become essential. A good leader must understand and accept ethnic pluralism. *Ethnic pluralism* is the coexistence of ethnic and racial groups. For example, it is okay to be both Cuban and American. Individuals do not have to shun or deny their Cuban ethnicity to be Americans or vice versa because they have dual ethnic identities and are bicultural (Tanke, 1990). The leader must correct misconceptions, misunderstandings, biases, and stereotyping within and outside the unit. It is the leader's responsibility to help employees to understand and respect their own and each other's culture as well as work better with each other. Knowledge of ethnicity is fundamental to being an effective multicultural manager.

Conflicts between employees and between employees and management do occur from time to time. A leader must not ignore conflicts that exist in the work environment or allow them to linger for a long period of time. They affect team morale, efforts, and productivity. The leader must facilitate conflict resolutions by attempting to influence behavior change among the individuals involved.

The work plan in Figure 23-6 is an example of an explicit communication document developed between a director and nutritionists, spelling out what their annual goals are, what is expected of them, and what it means to exceed expectations. This is an example of effective leadership in which employees are not left to guess what is expected of them. Employees are guided and evaluated by the content of this document, and nutritionists may self-evaluate themselves using this tool.

COMMUNITY NUTRITION/WELLNESS SERVICES

Focus: Adolescent nutrition/wellness in middle schools, high schools, and the community

Nutritionist #1   RD, LDN

Focus: Child nutrition/wellness in elementary school and the community

Nutritionist #2   RD, LDN
Nutritionist #3   MPH, RD, LDN
Nutritionist #4   MPH, RD, LDN
Nutritionist #5   MPH, RD

Focus: Health promotion/wellness for adults and families, community outreach

Nutritionist #6   RD, LDN
Nutritionist #7   MPH, RD, LDN

Focus: Health promotion/wellness, media

Nutritionist #8   MPH, RD, LDN

Community Team Leader: Organizing and staffing for community nutrition/wellness services

Nutritionist #9   MPH, RD, LDN

CLINICAL NUTRITION SERVICES

Focus: Infants and children with special health needs

Nutritionist #10   MPH, RD, LDN
Nutritionist #11   MAT, RD, LDN

Focus: Pregnant and breast-feeding women

Nutritionist #12 MPH, RD, LDN

Focus: Medicaid managed care/Durham community health network patients

Nutritionist #13 MS, RD, LDN

Focus: Health department clinics and referrals from the community

Nutritionist #14 MS, RD, LDN

Focus: Child care consultation

Nutritionist #15 MS, RD, LDN

Clinical Team Leader: Organizing and staffing for medical nutrition therapy services

Processing Assistant

Staff #1

Office Assistant

Staff #2

Director of Nutrition Services

FIGURE 23-5   Durham County Health Department Organization of Nutrition Services by Area
Source: The reproduction of this information is with permission of Rebecca Freeman, MPH, RD, LDN, Director of the Nutrition Division of the Durham County Health Department, 2004.

Controlling

Controlling is a mechanism to ensure that resources, quality of services, and client satisfaction are regulated appropriately and adequately. It also involves regulating the activities of employees in the division to ensure that they meet the established standards and goals. Control functions require the director to determine which activities need control, such as establishing and communicating standards to employees, measuring performance, and correcting deviations. This means staffing positions with the right qualified employees, developing and retaining them, and ensuring quality in programs and services provided to the clients. It also means making sure that clients indicate satisfaction with services provided, and ensuring that funding partners are satisfied with how their funds are managed. All of these are control functions. Additionally, managing the budget, costs, and information is considered a control function. The ability to reallocate personnel or realign the budget when facing financial constraints and still accomplishing objectives is control.

Studies by Snead, Burnell, and Anderson (1992) and Rogers and Broadhurst (2002) revealed that control management is a major aspect of a manager's responsibility in nutrition and dietetics. Budgeting includes both planning and controlling functions. Managers must be able to prepare and report financial analyses, control program costs, generate income, detect irregularities in client services or cost overruns, and handle complex projects and programs. The American Dietetic Association (ADA) role delineation study of 1998 agreed that managers or directors in public health are responsible for preparing financial analyses and financial reports, controlling program costs, monitoring program financial performance, documenting program operations, and making decisions regarding capital expenditure. The nutrition division usually undergoes periodic review or audits of its accounts. The directors must be able to manage and report the status of the thousands of dollars entrusted into their care.

Therefore, the public health nutrition director must have basic knowledge of accounting, preparing a budget, interpreting financial documents, and preparing financial reports for all income and expenses generated in the unit. It is important that as the director, he or she must know how to write for grants, develop the budget for grants, justify the reasons for requesting the amount being sought, and manage programs. Usually, the amount funded is dependent on how well the justification is written.

Managers and directors must regularly and continuously monitor productivity of their employees. Quality control, quality assurance, continuous quality improvement, and total quality management are all related concepts and can serve as tools for accomplishing this managerial function. *Quality control* is defined as determining if the products or services being provided meet the minimum standards of acceptability. *Quality assurance* is defined as a process of identifying "problem areas" within a unit and taking action to correct them. The results are monitored over time to see if the problems have been resolved and remain resolved. Quality assurance monitoring may necessitate a development of policies and procedures in patient (client) care protocols, thereby ensuring consistency from practitioner to practitioner. For example, a typical problem may be timeliness in screening to identify high-risk patients. Another example may be inconsistent methods for determining desirable body weight. Quality assurance must be ongoing, using a method such as *continuous quality improvement* (CQI), which helps identify areas that can be strengthened, and working to make those areas better. When all the departments or areas of the organization are studied to determine problem areas and work to correct them, it is called *total quality management* (TQM).

For a nutrition unit in a public health department, quality assurance is a most applicable tool. The Nutrition Division of the Durham County Health Department uses weekly and monthly meetings as a quality assurance strategy. The team leaders of each focus area (Figure 23-6) meet weekly with their employees and discuss the week's events and challenges. The team leaders, in turn, meet with the director weekly to apprise her of their work productivity, issues, and challenges from their individual areas. During the monthly meeting of the division, each of the focus area team leaders give a progress report presentation to all employees (Freeman, 2004, personal interview). Controlling, therefore, provides a process of making sure that established objectives and plans are being accomplished.

Employee Name: Start of Review Period

WORK OBJECTIVE 1: Education Programming
Plan and present school and community nutrition education programs.
(Health Department Objective 1)   Priority (HP)

PERFORMANCE EXPECTATIONS:
(Outline major tasks, activities, benchmarks necessary to complete the work objective. Also, list measures of effectiveness to assess the completion of the work objectives such as quantity, quality, target dates, or costs.)
- Plan and provide a nutrition education class in after-school programs in each of two schools once per year.
- Plan and provide three nutrition education classes in elementary schools during summer school by August 2004.

FIGURE 23-6   Annual Work Plan for a Nutritionist, Durham County Health Department Nutrition Division
Source: The reproduction of this information is with permission of Rebecca Freeman, MPH, RD, LDN, Director of the Nutrition Division of the Durham County Health Department, 2004.

- Conduct 50 taste-test sessions each academic year. Taste tests can accompany a nutrition education class.
- Plan and conduct at least one nutrition promotion in three elementary schools each academic year.
- Plan and provide nutrition education classes (135 classes divided between 3 schools per academic year).
- Contribute one nutrition article, newsletter, or staff bulletin to two target schools reaching students, parents, or staff. Articles can be the same at each school.
- Provide parent handouts with four of the nutrition lessons during the school year.
- Create one bulletin board theme for display in each school by the close of academic year 2004.

CONDITIONS:

(Identify resources WITHOUT which the objective cannot be met. Some possible conditions are equipment, training, budget, staffing. Conditions are usually associated with new projects or programs.)

Changes in the environment, which diminish participation.

Requests from schools/communities are not made for materials, equipment, and presentations.

Lack of student, staff, parent, or health professional involvement and interest in participating through the established support structure.

EXCEEDS:

Participates in more than one PTA or other parent involvement session.

Participates in a community/school health fair.

Participates in more than one promotion per school year.

Writes more than one newsletter article per school year at one of the two target schools reaching students, parents, or staff.

Provides more than 135 classes divided among 3 target schools during the academic year.

Creates more than one bulletin board theme for display in each school by the close of academic year 2004.

WORK OBJECTIVE 2: Program Development

- Needs assessment, planning, and collaboration of two selected target elementary schools and/or community groups to increase the health of food stamp recipients or eligible children and families.

(Health Department Objective 1)   Priority (MP)

PERFORMANCE EXPECTATIONS:

(Outline major tasks, activities, benchmarks necessary to complete the work objective. Also, list measures of effectiveness to assess the completion of the work objectives such as quantity, quality, target dates, or costs.)

- By August 30, 2004, notify principals at target schools for return of program.
- Revise or create three lessons for the 2004-2005 school year.

(Continues)

- Obtain enrollment documentation for each classroom in which programming occurs.
- Develop new materials and/or review and evaluate materials, tools, and equipment used in elementary nutrition education as needed.
- Develop new questions and revise last year's screening tool based on needs expressed by team members and results from 2003-2004.

CONDITIONS:

(Identify resources WITHOUT which the objective cannot be met. Some possible conditions are equipment, training, budget, staffing. Conditions are usually associated with new projects or programs.)

Changes in the environment or barriers to programming realized.

Lack of support for nutrition programs from target schools, school support services, community, and social entities or parent involvement.

EXCEEDS:

Create or revise more than three lessons.

Create three or more new forms or materials for the program.

WORK OBJECTIVE 3: Program Evaluation

Evaluation of two selected target elementary schools and/or community groups to increase the health of food stamp recipients or eligible children and families.

(Health Department Objective 1)   Priority (MP)

PERFORMANCE EXPECTATIONS:

(Outline major tasks, activities, benchmarks necessary to complete the work objective. Also, list measures of effectiveness to assess the completion of the work objectives such as quantity, quality, target dates, or costs.)

- Assess the needs of the school environment/complete the environmental checklist by May 31, 2004.
- Assess nutrition, food safety, and physical activity knowledge and behavior of selected classes after intervention. Final evaluations completed by May 21, 2004.
- Conduct ongoing evaluations and revisions of program priorities, services, and projects as needed.

CONDITIONS:

(Identify resources WITHOUT which the objective cannot be met. Some possible conditions are equipment, training, budget, staffing. Conditions are usually associated with new projects or programs.)

Changes in the environment or barriers to programming realized.

Lack of support for nutrition programs from target schools, school support services, community, and social entities or parent involvement.

EXCEEDS:

Screenings/surveys completed ahead of schedule.

Complete environmental evaluation ahead of schedule.

FIGURE 23-6   Annual Work Plan for a Nutritionist, Durham County Health Department Nutrition Division (Continued)

WORK OBJECTIVE 4: Consultation and Training

(List major area of responsibility/key accountability in your position.)

Provide consultation, training, technical assistance, and/or information guidance on health promotion as appropriate.

(Health Department Objective 1)   Priority (LP)

PERFORMANCE EXPECTATIONS:

(Outline major tasks, activities, benchmarks necessary to complete the work objective. Also, list measures of effectiveness to assess the completion of the work objectives such as quantity, quality, target dates, or costs.)

- Provide consultation with school nurses, cafeteria managers, and staff and teachers regarding nutritional questions and concerns pertaining to students as requested.
- Provide and evaluate nutritional materials and equipment to be used in teaching nutrition.
- Train and orient new employees and/or students and interns individually or as groups.
- Conduct training sessions to educate and assist school personnel in making changes in the environment.
- Serve on Health Department (Employee Recognition, School Health Team) and Nutrition Division committees (Social, Strategic Planning) as assigned or volunteered.
- Represent viewpoint of Nutrition Division and provide updates of committee activities to division staff.
- Involve Division staff in work of committee as appropriate.
- Solicit feedback from Division staff to take to committee.
- Actively participate in the work of the committee.
- Attend all meetings unless excused by supervisor.
- Let committee chair know if unable to attend meeting after being excused by supervisor.

CONDITIONS:

(Identify resources WITHOUT which the objective cannot be met. Some possible conditions are equipment, training, budget, staffing. Conditions are usually associated with new projects or programs.)

Requests for training or consultation not received.

No committee available to join.

EXCEEDS:

Provides nutrition education/training for DPS staff and/or other community agencies.

WORK OBJECTIVE 5: Career Development

Increase knowledge through continuing education opportunities.

(Health Department Objective 1)   Priority (MP)

(Continues)

PERFORMANCE EXPECTATIONS:

(Outline major tasks, activities, benchmarks necessary to complete the work objective. Also, list measures of effectiveness to assess the completion of the work objectives such as quantity, quality, target dates, or costs.)

- Increase knowledge through continuing education on school health and school-age children as they relate to nutrition and general health.
- Complete an average of 15 hours yearly (75 hours in 5 years) of continuing education certified by the Commission on Dietetic Registration.
- Attend other career development training as needed or required.
- Participate in professional organizations pertaining to the fields of nutrition and health.

CONDITIONS:

(Identify resources WITHOUT which the objective cannot be met. Some possible conditions are equipment, training, budget, staffing. Conditions are usually associated with new projects or programs.)

Funding available and permission granted to attend continuing education opportunities.

No scheduling conflicts.

EXCEEDS:

Greater than 15 hours of continuing education yearly.

Takes initiative in identifying continuing education opportunities.

PERFORMANCE FACTORS:

JOB KNOWLEDGE/APPLICATION:

Measures understanding of assignments and application of special knowledge, training, skills and ability required to perform position assignments.

Priority (MP)

PERFORMANCE EXPECTATIONS:

(Outline major tasks, activities, benchmarks necessary to complete the work objective. Also, list measures of effectiveness to assess the completion of the work objectives such as quantity, quality, target dates, or costs.)

- Knowledge of nutrition as it relates to elementary ages.
- Increase knowledge of nutrition as it relates to children through continuing education opportunities.
- Increase knowledge of primary/elementary education techniques through continuing education opportunities.
- Increase knowledge of the Spanish language through continuing education opportunities.
- Abide by state, county, departmental, and professional ethics.
- Maintain dietetic registration with the Commission on Dietetic Registration, American Dietetic Association by completing an average of 15 hours of approved continuing education yearly.

FIGURE 23-6 Annual Work Plan for a Nutritionist, Durham County Health Department Nutrition Division (Continued)

- Participate in all nutrition division staff meetings, community team meetings, and school health team meetings when scheduled to work.
- Participate in the local dietetic association.

CONDITIONS:

Conflict of meetings with planned community or school activities or with days scheduled to be considered as time off from work.

Funding not available or permission not granted to attend continuing education event.

EXCEEDS:

Greater than 15 hours of approved continuing education yearly with emphasis on nutrition as it relates to children.

PERFORMANCE FACTORS:

CUSTOMER SERVICE:

Measures the effectiveness of working with others in the organization (internal customers) and offering assistance or delivering service to external customers. Priority (HP)

PERFORMANCE EXPECTATIONS:

(Outline major tasks, activities, benchmarks necessary to complete the work objective. Also, list measures of effectiveness to assess the completion of the work objectives such as quantity, quality, target dates, or costs.)

- Returns phone calls and e-mails within agreed upon time frame. Leaves message if person is unavailable.
- Responds to requests in the mutually agreed time frame.
- Distributes CQI tool as indicated by Division Director and Supervisor.
- Communicates in a sensitive, courteous manner and observes confidentiality as needed.
- Communicates with others in a constructive manner.
- Provides Community and Clinical Team members, health educators, school nurses, etc. with information received pertaining to their program area and routes newsletters, printed materials as appropriate.

EXCEEDS:

Receives an average score of good or excellent on greater than 90% of DINE customer service evaluations.

Programs are followed up with a letter to the contact person.

Consistently completes tasks within the time frame or ahead of schedule.

PERFORMANCE FACTORS:

QUANTITY/QUALITY OF WORK:

Measures the degree of accuracy, thoroughness, and appearance of completed work. Priority (HP)

(Continues)

PERFORMANCE EXPECTATIONS:

(Outline major tasks, activities, benchmarks necessary to complete the work objective. Also, list measures of effectiveness to assess the completion of the work objectives such as quantity, quality, target dates, or costs.)

- Materials, letters, and other correspondence will appear professional with no grammatical or spelling errors.
- Time sheets and other legal documents will be accurate.
- Fewer than two monthly reports will be turned in late.

EXCEEDS:

One or no late monthly reports.

PERFORMANCE FACTORS:

WORK HABITS:

Measures the person's compliance with county policies (i.e., attendance, leave, lunch) and norms set by the supervisor.   Priority (MP)

PERFORMANCE EXPECTATIONS:

(Outline major tasks, activities, benchmarks necessary to complete the work objective. Also, list measures of effectiveness to assess the completion of the work objectives such as quantity, quality, target dates, or costs.)

- Follows work schedule as agreed upon with supervisor.
- Fewer than six late reporting occurrences to the work station during a 12-month period.
- Completes accurate monthly reports and submits to supervisor by the next working day after the end of the month.
- Requests leave time from supervisor prior to taking annual leave or planned sick leave.
- Works alternate hours from regular work schedule with prior approval.
- Arranges with supervisor any alternate work hours prior to working alternate hours.

EXCEEDS:

Builds in efficiency by actively supporting team efforts to plan and conduct and evaluate program objectives.

No more than one late reporting occurrence to the work station during a 12-month period.

FIGURE 23-6   Annual Work Plan for a Nutritionist, Durham County Health Department Nutrition Division (Continued)s

Conclusions

This chapter discussed how employees in a nutrition division of a public health department are managed. The manager or director must combine management and leadership skills in managing the resources (the six M's of management) in his or her unit. The five main functions in directing the activities of the employees work in tandem to accomplish the goals and objectives of the nutrition division.

Issues for Discussion

1. Why is it important to have job descriptions? How is having appropriate job descriptions a win-win for both the employee and the manager?

2. Discuss some problems you have experienced at your workplace. How could these have been avoided if a good manager was in place? What disciplinary actions should have occurred?

References

American Dietetic Association. (1998). The American Dietetic Association standards of professional practice for dietetics professionals. *Journal of the American Dietetics Association, 98* (1), 83–87.

Boyle, M. A. & Morris, D. H. (2002). *Community nutrition in action: An entrepreneurial approach.* Belmont, CA: Wadsworth, Thompson Learning.

Bittle, L. R. & Newstrom, J. W. (1990). *What every supervisor should know.* 6th ed. New York: McGraw-Hill, 189–190.

Fielder, F. E. & Garcia, J. E. (1987). *New approaches to effective leadership.* New York: John Wiley & Sons.

George, J. M. & Jones, G. R. (2002). *Organizational behavior.* 3rd ed. Upper Saddle River, NJ: Prentice Hall.

Griffin, R. W. (1999). *Management.* 2nd ed. Upper Saddle River, NJ: Prentice Hall.

Herzberg, F. (1966). *Work and nature of man.* Cleveland, OH: World.

Hudson, N. (2000). *Management practice in dietetics.* Belmont, CA: Wadsworth, Thompson Learning, 53–87.

Kane M. T., Estes C. A., Colton D. A., & Eltoft C. S.(1990). Role delineation for registered dietitians and entry-level dietetic technicians. *Journal of the American Dietetics Association, 90(8)*, 1124–1133.

Leslie, J. B., Dalton, M., Ernest, C., & Deal, J. (2002) Managerial effectiveness in a global context: Center for creative leadership report. Retrieved May 24, 2005 from http://www.ccl.org/CCLCommerce/pdf/publications/ccl_managerialeffectiveness.pdf.

Mackenzie, A. (1979). The management process in 3-D. A diagram showing the activities, functions and basic elements of the executive's job. *Journal Nursing Administration* (11):30–33. Retrieved May 26, 2005, from http://www.ncbi.nih.gov/entrez.

Maslow, A. H. (1943). A theory of human motivation. *Psychology Review, 50,* 370–396.

McClelland, D. C. (1985). *The achievement society.* New York: Free Press.

McGregor, D. (1985). *The human side of enterprise.* New York: McGraw Hill.

Metzger, N. (1982). *The healthcare supervisor's handbook.* 2nd ed. Rockville, MD: Aspen.

Payne-Palacio, J. & Theis, M. (2001). *West and Wood's introduction to food service.* 12th ed. Upper Saddle River, New Jersey: Merrill Prentice-Hall.

Rogers, D., Leonberg, B. L., & Broadhurst, C. B. (2002). 2000 Commission on dietetic registration, dietetics practice audit. *Journal of the American Dietetic Association, 102*(2), 270–292.

Snead, J., Burnell, E. C., & Anderson, M. (1992). Development of financial management competencies for entry level dietitian. *Journal of the American Dietetic Association, 92,* 1223–1229.

Tamel, M. E. & Reynolds, H. (1981). *Executive leadership.* Englewood Cliffs, NJ: Prentice Hall, 59.

Tanke, M. L. (1990). *Human resources management for hospitality.* Albany, NY: Delmar.

Vroom, V. H. (1994). *Work and motivation.* San Francisco: Jossey Bass.

Witte, S. S., Escott-Stump, S., Fairchild, M. M., & Papp, J. (1997). Standard of practice criteria for clinical nutrition managers. *Journal of the American Dietetics Association, 97*(6), 673–678.

CHAPTER 24

LEVERAGING NUTRITION EDUCATION THROUGH THE PUBLIC HEALTH TEAM

Deepa Arora, PhD

Reader Objectives

After studying this chapter and reflecting on the contents, you should be able to:

1. Discuss how a nutritionally balanced diet can prevent the onset and development of several diet-related, preventable, chronic diseases.
2. Explain why education is an important tool for modifying diet-related behavior.
3. Describe how nutrition education campaigns provide a low-cost method for encouraging and sustaining healthy food habits.
4. Discuss the challenges nutrition educators routinely face, including noncompliance with their recommendations and providing services that are culturally and linguistically sensitive.
5. Clarify why nutrition education is best provided by a team of qualified public health professionals.
6. Explain why continuing education programs and in-service programs are vital for sharing recent developments in the field of nutrition with all members of the nutrition education team.
7. Explain why the members of the nutrition education team must adhere to the principles of effective teamwork and group development in order to establish an effective nutrition education program.

Why Is Nutrition Important?

Lifestyle choices, such as nutrition, smoking, drinking, physical activity, and psychological stress, have the greatest impact on health and longevity. Innumerable studies in the literature show the detrimental effect of poor dietary habits on health and on the development of disease.[1] Dietary factors have been shown to be linked to 4 of the 10 leading causes of death: coronary heart disease, stroke, some types of cancer, and type 2 diabetes.[1] It has been shown, for

691

example, that obesity and/or being overweight significantly increases the risk of developing diabetes, heart disease, stroke, and hypertension.[1] According to the report titled *The Surgeon General's Call to Action to Prevent and Decrease Overweight and Obesity,* released in December 2001, approximately 300,000 deaths in the United States each year are linked to obesity and overweight. In the year 2000, obesity- and overweight-linked medical problems cost the U.S. economy $117 billion.[2] Thus, early intervention to encourage weight loss before an individual becomes overweight or obese may be the desired course of action. Public health personnel can encourage changes in dietary choices to help reduce the incidence of preventive disorders in those populations most susceptible to them.

> Read about The Surgeon General's Call to Action to Prevent and Decrease Overweight and Obesity at http://www.surgeongeneral.gov/topics/obesity/calltoaction/CalltoAction.pdf.

Many studies have effectively shown that changes in people's dietary patterns can reduce the incidence of chronic diseases such as heart disease and cancer. In the past 35 years, deaths due to heart disease have declined by 45%, although it is still the leading cause of death in the United States.[3] This reduction is attributed to a decrease in the intake of animal fat and cholesterol, as well as a decline in smoking. In 2001, the U.S. Department of Health and Human Services released the findings from the Diabetes Prevention Program.[4] This program was a major clinical trial that compared the effects of dietary modifications and exercise with the effects of an anti-diabetes drug in combating the development of type 2 diabetes in individuals with an impaired glucose tolerance test and who were at risk for developing the disease. The results were dramatic in that the risk of developing type 2 diabetes decreased by 58% in participants who exercised and followed the suggested diet, as compared to 31% in those that took the anti-diabetes drug. Thus, introducing dietary modifications to meet the Dietary Guidelines for Americans can significantly impact the health of an individual and society.

> You can read more about the 2005 Dietary Guidelines for Americans at http://www.nal.usda.gov/fnic/dga/.

Modifying Nutrition-Related Behavior

As discussed in previous chapters, the U.S. Public Health Service, along with public and private organizations, has developed a set of public health objectives called *Healthy People* (HP). The goals of the HP initiative include helping individuals of all ages increase life expectancy and improve their quality of life.[1] These goals are to be met through a variety of approaches that aim to improve the nutritional status of the population by improving access to comprehen-

sive, high-quality healthcare services; increasing the availability and
effectiveness of educational and
community-based health promotion programs designed to prevent

You can read more about the
Healthy People Initiative at
http://www.healthypeople.gov.

disease and improve health and quality of life; and improving core
competencies in health providers' training.

Health-related behaviors show a strong correlation with education. People who are better educated make healthier choices and
show better health-related behaviors. Public health practitioners
can use the medium of education to promote healthy behaviors and
healthy lifestyles. A big challenge for public health professionals is
to develop educational programs and initiatives for nutrition education and health promotion in communities that are characterized
by a lower socioeconomic status and low levels of education.

Definition of Nutrition Education

Nutrition education is a process of learning that influences the
knowledge, beliefs, attitudes, and behavior of an individual or a
community and allows them to make more intelligent decisions regarding dietary choices in order to improve health and reduce the
risk of developing chronic diet-related disorders, such as obesity,
diabetes, heart disease, hypertension, and osteoporosis. A group of
public health professionals can provide nutrition education by
studying nutrition-related health problems and then planning, developing, organizing, and implementing educational programs to
address some of the frequently occurring health concerns.

Impact of Nutrition Education

Education can impact the behavior of families and communities in
a very strong and powerful manner. Individuals gain knowledge of
the world and their surroundings, helping them build certain skills
and capabilities that, in turn, boost their self-confidence and self-
esteem.[5] As the family and the community develop, there is an improvement in health and health resources, reduced exposure to
environmental health hazards, gains in socioeconomic status, and,
thus, additional purchasing power for buying health care and medical care. Along this road to development, public health professionals can play a very important role in improving the nutritional
status of communities by imparting nutrition education with a message of "managed lives/healthy lives." Nutrition education can be
provided in hospitals, health agencies, schools, churches, work-
places, and recreational facilities. Thus, public health professionals
have a diverse array of venues where they can reach their target

populations. Target populations can include individuals, families, organization leaders, community leaders, and influential people who could make a greater impact on the community to facilitate voluntary actions conducive to a nutritionally balanced and healthy diet.

How Effective Are Nutrition Education Campaigns?

Millions of dollars are spent on marketing and advertising for high-profit foods, including those rich in refined carbohydrates and fats. Regrettably, not enough money is available for nutrition education campaigns that promote healthy food choices. As an example, the food industry and the National Cancer Institute have at most contributed $2 million towards the *5 A Day for Better Health* campaign, which encourages the consumption of fruits and vegetables. In contrast, the advertising budget for junk foods could be as high as $100–$500 million.[6] In a recent report, the Kaiser Family Foundation stated that the media contributes significantly towards childhood obesity by airing advertisements worth billions of dollars showing candy, cereal, and fast food. This has contributed significantly to the increased incidence of obesity in children aged 6–11 years, which has risen from 4.2% in 1963–1970 to 15.3% in 1999–2000.[7] Thus, there lies an ever-widening gap between the funds available for advertising for fast foods and those available for promoting healthy food choices. A suggestion was made to generate funds for public health campaigns[6] by imposing a small tax on fast foods and junk foods. This could generate significant revenue, which could be added to the pool of funds available for nutrition education to promote healthy food choices. The question, however, remains as to whether advertising and marketing strategies can lead to an improvement in the dietary choices made by individuals. Bill Reger and colleagues[8] studied the impact of different health promotion strategies, such as paid advertising, public relations, and community education, on inducing people to switch from consuming high-fat milk to consuming low-fat milk. They reported that these low-cost measures did result in a change in the type of milk consumed and that these changes were sustained. In a study reported from Finland, an educational campaign to reduce heart disease incidence in affected communities was highly effective in improving dietary habits, reducing the risk factors for heart disease, and lowering the incidence of disease and death.[6] Since the funds for nutrition education campaigns are limited, it is essential to design and implement low-cost programs that use multiple strategies, have a simple and clear message, involve the family, and are repeated over a long time period. Such programs will be effective in encouraging and sustaining improved dietary habits in communities.

Challenges Faced by Nutrition Educators

By providing nutrition education programs to communities at risk of developing nutrition-linked chronic diseases, nutrition educators hope to provide information, skills, and reinforcements in order to encourage people to introduce modifications into their dietary patterns to protect or improve their health. However, it is easy to impart knowledge related to nutrition to the target population, but difficult to actually introduce changes in the dietary pattern because those changes are not inherently rewarding or satisfying.[5]

Thus, providing nutrition education involves not just dispensing knowledge and information, but also supplying ways and means to change attitudes and behavior. The challenge is for people to retain and follow the recommended changes in dietary practices. Noncompliance can result from a number of factors, including: 1) communication is ineffective; 2) the client is not paying attention; and 3) the message is misinterpreted.[9] Thus, the whole concept of nutrition education needs to be viewed differently. It is just not enough to design programs and deliver information to the public in a one-time interaction.[10] In order to bring about any significant change in the lifestyle of individuals or communities and impact health in a positive manner, the process of imparting knowledge and encouraging changes has to be continued over a period of time. The approach has to be slow, but consistent. Nutrition educators must understand that most individuals know what they need to do in order to remain healthy, but strongly resist making any modifications in their daily habits. Thus, individuals and communities have to be motivated to change; the individual must be taught that he or she is responsible for his or her own health decisions and is in full control over his or her own well-being, particularly as it relates to food and nutrition.

It is much more challenging to introduce behavioral changes through educational programs that depend entirely on mass media and have little interpersonal contact. While designing programs that target nutrition education, public health professionals must realize the value of one-on-one communication with individuals. Developing a good relationship and maintaining close contact with the target population is an integral component of a successful nutrition education program.

In order to produce a strong desire to change and an intense motivation to incorporate changes into their dietary patterns, people need more than just knowledge transfer, information availability, and attitude change. Skills and adequate resources must be available to support the motivated individual. Social support and rewards for the behavioral change are necessary if the changes are to be incorporated and sustained over time. Public health professionals must therefore train individuals, families, employers, community leaders, and influential people in the community to provide support for recommended changes in their dietary habits.

A major barrier faced by nutrition educators is the lack of linguistically and culturally appropriate services.[11] There is a dearth of translated materials in different languages for audiences that are not adequately proficient in English. Such individuals have trouble understanding even basic information related to nutrition, health, and healthcare services. This problem is further compounded by the fact that the number of bilingual providers and trained interpreters is limited. The public health team must be cognizant of this issue and have appropriate training procedures prepared for communities that are Hispanic American, Asian American, or non-English speaking. Thus, in order to convey the message of sound nutrition and help audiences imbibe the principles of nutrition in health and in different disease states, public health personnel must bridge the language gap. Another challenge along similar lines is that dietary habits are culturally sensitive. Health promotion programs that emphasize nutrition will have to be designed specifically, or be "custom-made," for the target communities, keeping in mind their dietary food habits, regional food choices and selection, food preferences, and cultural limitations. Any recommendation that is not culturally appropriate will not be easily acceptable to the public. In a policy adopted in 2001, the American Public Health Association advocated that federal agencies use resources that are culturally sensitive and linguistically relevant, along with translators.[12] The association also encouraged healthcare providers to collaborate with federal agencies to provide culturally and linguistically appropriate services.

> See the American Public Health Association's website at http://www.apha.org.

It is also imperative that public health professionals consider gender differences in designing nutrition education programs. Women in several societies have a tendency to take a back seat in their own healthcare decisions and neglect their own health. Those resources available at home are used to take care of the health requirements of other family members at the expense of their own health. Clearly, improvements in health via nutrition education have to be targeted towards all family members. Women must be encouraged to view themselves as important members of their family and the community, with a great responsibility towards themselves, their family, and the community. They must recognize that they are a powerful tool to bring about change in society, including societal values and thinking.

The public health team also must recognize the need to remove cultural barriers that impede the progress of healthy change in communities. Along with outreach programs for health promotion and nutrition education, additional programs must address the problem of cultural and social barriers to change.

It is also important to keep in mind that if nutrition education and health promotion programs are to be successful, they should be imparted not only at the level of the individual, but also at the level of the community. Public health professionals in community health centers and community-based organizations can reach communities that are otherwise disenfranchised. They can target their programs towards specific populations so the message can be delivered more effectively, and be better retained and implemented. Community-based organizations are important because many of them arise out of personal experiences and thus better understand the pulse of the community.[11]

Who Should Provide Nutrition Education?

To prevent the spread of nutrition misinformation, consumers must have access to trained/qualified nutrition professionals and other health and allied health professionals who have received sound training in nutrition. The providers of nutrition information must be registered or licensed nutritionists who have fulfilled the requirements and standards established by state and national regulations. However, it has been noted that to improve the acceptance and inclusion of suggested dietary modifications, as well as compliance, the desired dietary patterns must be emphasized repeatedly. A client/patient must meet with several health professionals during his or her care, so it is important that every member of a person's medical care team be well-trained and well-versed in the principles of nutrition. Repeated emphasis on improving dietary habits and remaining healthy will have a greater impact than counseling by a single individual. Thus, if the message of managed lives/healthy lives is to be delivered, it must entail a combined strong effort by a group of individuals (the nutrition education team) who can shape public health efforts to promote health in communities. It is the responsibility of the public health nutrition education team to spread the message of nutrition, particularly in communities where the risk for developing preventable chronic disorders like diabetes and heart disease are high.

The Nutrition Education Team

Many professionals in public health disciplines are involved in providing total care of the individual. Some of these can be important members of the nutrition education team, which can include public health nutritionists/dietitians, dietetic technicians, physicians, nurses, pharmacists, social workers, psychologists, health educators, medical educators, and physical and occupational therapists, among others.[13,14] Each of these professionals can contribute his or her expertise towards the nutritional care of the community as a whole or to an individual client. Activities that these professionals can provide at a healthcare facility include assessing the nutritional status of the patient and prescribing an appropriate diet, indicating possible food-drug interactions, planning modified diets and menus, supervising food services, assisting the patient with meal selection, helping those unable to feed themselves, recording data on food allergies and acceptance, providing nutrition counseling, and making arrangements for financial assistance and home services. The following section discuss the responsibilities of each member of the nutrition education team.[13,14]

Nutritionists/Dietitians and Dietetic Technicians

The nutritionists/dietitians and dietetic technicians play a very important role in providing comprehensive nutrition care to the client. They are an integral part of the professional staff working in hospitals, health clinics, well-baby clinics, nursing homes, schools, and daycare centers. In hospitals, health clinics, and nursing homes, dietitians assess the nutritional status of patients, provide dietary counseling, prescribe diets, plan menus, and supervise food services. In addition, dietetic technicians assist patients in menu selection, and record daily dietary intake and data on food acceptance. In schools and daycare centers, nutritionists are responsible for planning nutritionally balanced meals for children, providing a variety of foods that meet the Dietary Reference Intakes for different nutrients.

In hospitals and medical settings, nutritionists must also be actively involved in client case discussions and exchange information with the physicians and the nursing staff on the patient's dietary intake. While providing nutrition care to the patient, they must actively educate the patient about the nutrition modifications necessary for controlling his or her medical disorder and preventing any further deterioration. This close interaction with the other members of the team allows for reinforcement of the information delivered to the patient, fills in any gaps in information, and prevents any contradictory message from reaching the patient. Thus, in order to reinforce the message of nutrition education, it is imperative that nutritionists, physicians, nurses, and other professionals involved in the care of the patient collaborate closely in the screening, diagnosis, treatment, and follow-up. Each professional should be cognizant of the important role played by others, respect their professional qualifications, and leave room for all to contribute to the nutrition care of the patient.

As a member of the public health team, another responsibility of the nutritionist is to provide updated nutrition information to the other members of the team. Recent developments related to nutrition in children or adults that focus on normal or therapeutic nutrition, as well as recently published articles from refereed scientific publications or journals, should be shared with the other members of the nutrition education team. This would ensure that all of the public health professionals are on top of new developments in the field of nutrition and can provide appropriate education to their clients. Nutritionists can also invite the other members of the team to some of their nutrition counseling sessions to observe their interaction with the client and learn some effective approaches for conveying dietary information. Special sessions could be arranged by the nutritionist to reinforce the principles of nutrition in a state of health or disease for the other members of the patient care team. This would also strengthen the ability of other team members to provide nutrition education to clients in the absence of the nutritionist.

In addition to group sessions, nutritionists can consult on individual cases with the other members of the nutrition education public health team. The responsible physician, nurse, pharmacist, and nutritionist can have a conference to discuss the medical records of the client, family history, the medical treatment prescribed, and the nutrition approaches involved in caring for the patient. The team can also discuss the most effective strategies that can be employed for the dietary care of the patient. The progress made by the client should be evaluated on a regular basis to ensure compliance with the dietary recommendations.

Physicians

Medical doctors obtain anthropometric, clinical, biochemical, and general dietary intake data from their patients to diagnose disease and assess the health and nutritional status of the patient. Following the diagnosis, they recommend the type and course of treatment in order to control the disease and prevent further health deterioration. As part of treatment, as well as disease prevention and health promotion, physicians suggest the appropriate diet for the patient. In the case of patients with disease conditions that need extensive dietary modifications, most physicians will provide a referral to a qualified nutritionist for detailed assessment, planning, and patient counseling concerning the preparation of the diet. It is very important at this stage that the physician maintain a positive and encouraging attitude toward the dietary modifications recommended. They should be able to convince their patients as to why the dietary change is essential and how it will help treat the disease and prevent any further damage to their health. This positive attitude is developed only if physicians themselves are convinced of the importance of sound nutrition; this can be achieved only through proper training in their medical curricula. Physicians who fail to emphasize the importance of nutrition at this stage and do not encourage changes in dietary habits deter the patient from following any diet-related advice provided by another member of the nutrition team.

Nurses and Nursing Assistants

Nurses interact with the patient frequently and assist the patient in menu selection, help those unable to feed themselves, record data on food intake and acceptance, and counsel patients on health and nutrition promotion. Nurses can also educate their patients using standard educational materials available in health clinics and hospitals. They can provide overall dietary guidance for different diet-related disorders and refer the patient to the nutritionist for more detailed and specific information on the dietary modifications recommended. They can motivate and reinforce the dietary recommendations to their patients for an extended period of time and thus serve as very valuable sources of nutrition education.

It is very important that the members of the nutrition team interact with each other to discuss the progress made by the patient in following the suggested dietary recommendations. Frequent dialogue with a patient allows nurses to know more personal information about the patient than the other members of the team. In particular, nurses that pay home visits recognize the physical, emotional, and financial limitations of the patient. Sharing their experiences with the other members of the team can also pave the way for making additional suggestions and changes in the prescribed diet to better fit the environmental, social, physical, and financial circumstances of the patient.

Pharmacists

In some scenarios, the role of the pharmacist is to provide information to the patient on possible interactions between different drugs and food. Additionally, pharmacists form an integral part of the medical team that will screen and treat the patient. Thus, close interaction among the pharmacist, physician, nutritionist, nurse, and patient allows the pharmacist to explain any food-drug interactions to the patient and prevent complications.

Social Workers

Social workers help those patients who are in need of placement services. They are able to assess the physical, emotional, financial, and social stresses encountered by the patient that would prevent him or her from following the recommended medical and dietary advice. Social workers provide guidance and suggestions to patients to allow them to face challenges and find workable solutions, and thus prepare them to follow the recommended medical and dietary advice. Because they interact with the patient on a more personal level, social workers can serve as an important vehicle for the delivery of nutrition information, help the family with meal budgeting and meal planning, and thus be an active contributor to the process of nutrition education.

Psychologists

The role of the psychologist is to counsel clients on their mental health condition and suggest treatment. They study the emotional, financial, and social constraints faced by the patient in following the desired treatment, help the patient to deal with emotional stresses, and strengthen him or her psychologically to accept and follow the recommendations. Psychologists provide emotional security and support to patients in need, enabling their patients to think clearly and make the right eating and drinking choices.

Physical and Occupational Therapists

Physical and occupational therapists interact closely and for an extended period of time with clients in need of therapy. Patients who have difficulty eating or swallowing need help from these therapists to overcome their handicap to function more efficiently. Therapists must work closely with the nutritionist to decide which foods will be appropriate for the patient, as well as provide the desired nutrition. Subsequently, they interact with the family and the client to train them as to appropriate feeding procedures and regimen. During each session, these therapists could prove invaluable in transferring nutrition-related information to the client. Patients usually receive therapy over a period of time, which may extend into weeks or even months in some cases, so adequately trained physical/occupational therapists could serve as a vehicle for slow dispersal of knowledge to the patient. Because nutrition education is an ongoing endeavor, these professionals can play an invaluable role as a member of the nutrition education team.

Dentists and Dental Hygienists

Promoting oral hygiene and preventing the development of cavities and tooth-related disorders is the function of the dentist. Dentists and dental hygienists, in their interaction with the client, discourage the use of high-sugar food items and encourage the use of nutritive foods. In other words, these professionals also contribute significantly to improving the nutritional status of their clients.

Health/Medical Educators

In public health departments, health clinics, and hospitals, health/medical educators play a very important role as members of the nutrition education team. Being education specialists, they design, implement, and assess educational activities that involve all the other professionals of the public health nutrition team. They can develop and revise the curriculum, select appropriate methods and materials, and also train the staff effectively. Health educators must be able to develop good relationships with the public so that they can identify the needs and problems of the community and then develop programs to address these concerns. The health educator can also market educational campaigns to the target audience.

Veterinarians

The American Public Health Association recognized the need for veterinarians in public health services, in every health department and health clinic.[12] They recommended that schools of public health and applied public health programs provide facilities for continuing education and recruitment outreach to veterinarians. Veterinarians play an important role in promoting food safety, especially pathogen control, and in the surveillance of food-borne diseases.[12]

The Public

Public health should not be limited to only experts who advise the public on what to do and what not to do. There are not enough public health educators available to interact with the public. Therefore, the onus of improving the diet and health of communities also lies on the public itself. More active participation is required of the public.[15] Each individual must recognize his or her own responsibility towards maintaining good health. Each individual must consider his or her own actions to understand what needs to be changed to improve nutritional status and maintain good health.

It would be ideal if each trained professional could associate with a community-based organization for enough time to train some members of the organization. This responsibility could thereafter be taken up by these members to train others in the organization. The organization could then expand its educational activities to other organizations. Thus, a chain reaction would follow whereby one individual would educate another until the whole community was informed. "Each one, educate one." Such would be the motto of all community organizations to achieve good nutrition and health for all.

Are These Professionals Adequately Trained in the Discipline of Nutrition?

Clearly, if the members of the nutrition education team have a responsibility to provide advice that impacts dietary choices, they must have adequate training in the discipline of nutrition. Registered dietitians are trained nutritionists with national accreditation; licensed or certified dietitians are also qualified nutritionists with state accreditation; and some professionals have academic degrees in nutrition from an accredited institution.[16] These individuals possess, in addition to satisfactory training in the principles of nutrition, membership in relevant professional societies like the American Dietetic Association, the American Society for Clinical Nutrition, the Society for Nutrition Education, and the Institute of Food Technologists to keep them informed of recent advances in the field of food and nutrition. In order to maintain their professional status, registered dietitians must take a certain number of continuing education credit hours every 5 years to update their skills and knowledge. The American Dietetic Association holds registered dietitians to high standards, so these individuals are reliable and trustworthy sources of nutrition information.[16]

> American Dietetic Association: http://www.eatright.org.
>
> American Society for Clinical Nutrition: http://www.ascn.org.
>
> Society for Nutrition Education: http://www.sne.org.
>
> Institute of Food Technologists: http://www.ift.org.

In 1985, the Committee on Nutrition in Medical Education, a part of the Food and Nutrition Board of the National Research Council, identified the lack of adequate training for medical students in the United States and recommended that nutrition be added to the curriculum as a required course.[17] The National Nutritional Monitoring and Related Research Act was passed in 1990 to ensure that medical students and practicing physicians in the United States have adequate training in the field of nutrition and how it relates to human health. However, despite efforts to improve training for medical students and physicians in the discipline of nutrition, the curriculum offered at many U.S. medical schools still does not adequately concentrate on this discipline. Physicians provide very limited nutrition education during patient care and in clinical practice. Physicians routinely fail to underscore the importance of diet in the treatment of nutrition-related diseases like diabetes, heart disease, obesity, osteoporosis, and anemia, among others. In 1993, it was reported that annually 300,000 to 800,000 preventable deaths in the United States were linked to nutrition.[18]

For the treatment of major public health disorders such as obesity, diabetes, and atherosclerosis, pharmaceutical and technological approaches are preferred over nutritional interventions. The Nutrition Academic Award program was developed in 1997 by the National Heart, Lung and Blood Institute to improve nutrition-related knowledge and skills among medical school students, residents, fellows, faculty, and practicing physicians. This initiative is intended to improve the application of nutrition principles in patient care and clinical practice. It should reinforce the existing efforts to improve the qualifications and training of physicians in the science of nutrition. In addition to training medical students, some recipients of the Nutrition Academic Award also provide training to students of other health professional schools, such as dental programs, dietetic programs, nursing schools, pharmacy schools, physician assistant programs, public health programs, exercise physiology programs, physical education programs, and health ecology programs.

Education Programs

Continuing Education Programs

Accrediting agencies provide continuing education programs for health professionals, including physicians, nurses, pharmacists, and nutritionists, to provide an avenue to the most updated and recent information about innovative clinical intervention strategies, clinical trials, and medical success stories. Such continuing education programs can be planned for all health professionals, regardless of whether they work in private practice, healthcare facilities, community health centers, public health departments/agencies, or educational institutions.[14] Medical and health professional schools can also plan these continuing education programs for health professionals, because they provide both knowledge and practical training tips for successful clinical practice.

In-Service Education Programs

In-service education programs can be planned in hospitals and public health agencies for their public health personnel. A committee of medical educators, physicians, nurses, nutritionists, pharmacists, social workers, and psychologists can plan the program in order to address the most common medical concerns.[14] This would be a good platform for sharing recent developments in the scientific literature, exchanging ideas, asking questions, and sharing critical thinking. Any challenges and concerns can be addressed, and constructive suggestions can be made. Such educational programs could also provide an avenue for reinforcing the existing information related to suggested dietary practices in a state of health or disease. The team can discuss the existing nutrition care for different medical conditions, any new modifications to be introduced, any existing drawbacks, and new suggestions for overcoming some of them. The dietitian can demonstrate the planning of modified diets to the group so they can share these ideas with their clients.

As with any educational program, program assessment should form an integral part of the educational effort. Participants should evaluate the program to see if learning occurred. Any suggestions for improvement should be taken into consideration while planning the next in-service education program. The nutrition department in healthcare facilities and public health nutritionists can provide a monthly newsletter highlighting new findings for the benefit of the other members of the public health team. Collectively, all these measures may ensure that the nutrition knowledge of healthcare professionals meets the professional standards set by accrediting agencies.

National Initiatives to Promote Nutrition Education

The Team Nutrition Initiative

The Food and Nutrition Service of the U.S. Department of Agriculture developed the Team Nutrition Initiative in order to improve the nutritional quality of meals served to schoolchildren and to encourage foods that reflect the dietary guidelines and are low in fat and sodium.[19] As part of its activities, Team Nutrition has developed messages and educational materials linked to nutrition that can be used in schools throughout the country. Team Nutrition

> See the Team Nutrition Initiative at http://www.fns.usda.gov/tn/.

provides training to food service professionals in schools to help them prepare and serve meals that both meet the nutrition requirements of children and appear appetizing. This initiative also provides nutrition education for parents as well as children to help them make healthy food choices and improve their health. For additional support of this activity, Team Nutrition involves school administrators and community leaders who can reinforce the message effectively. Team Nutrition spreads its message using different communication strategies, such as food service interventions, activities in the classroom, schoolwide events, promoting healthy actions at home, programs in the community, media events, and media coverage. The effectiveness of Team Nutrition depends on successful partnerships among federal, state, and local agencies. The Team Nutrition initiative shows that school administrators, teachers, community leaders, and agencies at the local, state, and federal levels can all play a very important role in spreading the message of nutrition education to families and communities.

Action for Healthy Kids

As discussed in previous chapters, the U.S. Department of Agriculture, the U.S. Department of Education, and the Centers for Disease Control and Prevention have partnered with other organizations to establish Action for Healthy Kids.[20] The main objective of Action for Healthy Kids is to improve the health of schoolchildren by encouraging the consumption of nutritionally balanced meals and promoting physical activity. Schoolchildren are faced with serious diet-related health problems, and this organization, which works at the local level, can make a significant impact by disseminating nutrition information to address these concerns.

Teamwork

Strategies for Developing an Effective Public Health Team

A team consists of a group of individuals working together to achieve a shared goal.[14] In an ideal team, members function synergistically, leading to increased efficiency and productivity. The emphasis is seldom placed on individual team members; rather, the team as a total entity is always paramount. To achieve the shared goal, team members are involved in activities that are interdependent instead of independent. With different individuals contributing their skills and knowledge to the team, each member of the team learns about the important role and position of different professional contributors on the team. They learn to respect each other's expertise and also appreciate how all the disciplines come together to address a common goal. In the public health arena, teamwork is very crucial because the efforts of the physician, nutritionists/dietitians, dietetic technicians, nurses, pharmacists, social workers, psychologists, health educators, medical educators, and physical and occupational therapists contribute tremendously towards improving the health and nutritional status of the individual, family, or community. As discussed earlier, such integrated efforts are necessary to address the physical, emotional, social, economic, cultural, and personal issues linked to the individual, family, or community. Not only can these professionals address the problem from different perspectives, but they also can reinforce the message of health and nutrition education to bridge the gap between knowledge and practice. Thus, teamwork can prove to be an economical way of addressing the health and nutrition needs of an individual, family, or community.

Teams can serve a patient group or a population, and their membership is fluid depending on the needs of the people served. Team functions can include planning, program delivery, and case discussions and conferences. A nutrition education team can assess the needs of its client population, identify areas that need emphasis, design and develop programs to address those needs, and set up conferences for clients with complex and chronic problems. Subgroups may form within a team to provide special services. In a team, leadership roles are clearly defined and assigned.

Strategies and Characteristics of a Properly Functioning and Effective Team

For a team to function in the most productive and efficient manner, team members have to be focused on the objectives, share leadership roles, and be accountable for their actions. Some of the defining features of a successful team are the following[20]:

- *Zero in on the objectives:* Any team should, at the onset, be aware of the goals to be achieved. Each member of the team should be very clear about the goals and objectives of the project. Additionally, the team members should be in agreement regarding the specific outcomes and parameters to be used to assess whether the goals have been adequately reached.

- *Accentuate a participatory style:* In a team as diverse as a public health team, different ideas are bound to arise because members originate from different disciplines. Members must be encouraged to listen and acknowledge alternate points of view in order to obtain a view of the "big picture."[21] As team members begin to respect each other, recognize each other's contributions, and trust each other, they can address the health issue more appropriately. While some members look at the broader picture, others look at small details; while some address the physical aspect, others deal with emotional issues; while others stress the economic aspect, some will focus on social influences. This is perhaps one of the best ways of finding solutions together.

- *Increase the sense of belonging and connectedness:* The work of any team is considerably enhanced if the members have a strong sense of connection with other team members and with the objectives of the team. All members of the team should have a sense of belonging and a strong desire to meet the defined goals and objectives.

- *Organize the team:* The specific responsibilities for the team should be mutually agreed upon by all team members. Because a public health team is inherently multifaceted, as are the problems it intends to address, clear leadership roles should be defined for different team activities.[21] Team members should be identified by discipline, knowledge, skills, specialization, experience, and interests.

- *Promote team responsibility:* Given the interdependent nature of any team, members of the team must be encouraged to take responsibility for completing individual duties in a timely manner.[21] When necessary, team members should also assist one another to collectively achieve the objectives of the team.

- *Encourage equal influence:* The team must be built on the premise that the viewpoints and contributions of all members are of equal value, and therefore all members must be willing to yield influence on all issues facing the team. Each member of the team must recognize and respect the contributions made by the other members of the team. Members must pay close attention to the suggestions made by others and then collectively arrive at one decision.

- *Establish a time line for the work to be done and commit to allotting time to do the work:* After the activities necessary to achieve the desired goals and objectives are planned and explained to all the members of the team, every member must then assume responsibility for the activities and make the necessary time commitment to work towards them.

- *Define measurable outcomes and work products:* As per the commitment of each team member, at the end of the time period designated for the activity, tangible work products should be visible. Each person on the team must show his or her contribution towards attaining the planned goals and objectives of the team. The resources available to the team must be shared equally by all the members; there should be no competition or turf guarding. Team members come from different disciplines, so there should be complete understanding between all the members about the role and responsibilities of each member. Cooperation with each other along with administrative support will allow the team to function efficiently and effectively.

- *Discuss and resolve all problems together:* As each member of the team undertakes activities to move in the planned direction, some problems and challenges may arise. For smooth resolution of all such problems, the team members must communicate on a regular basis to discuss and formulate solutions. Thus, all challenges must be faced by the team collectively and solutions finalized with mutual consent.

Team Leader

All teams must be led by a team leader. This individual must have the skills of a manager to lead the team smoothly in the planned direction. The leader is selected from the team itself not just for professional expertise, but also for possessing management skills to keep the team cohesive. The team leader must understand very clearly the mission of the team and communicate this mission to all members. It is the responsibility of the team leader to charge the team and orient all the members with the goals and objectives of the team. The leader must be involved in the selection of the team members and be able to delineate the roles and responsibilities of each one.[14] After setting the direction of the team, the leader must follow up the progress of the team on a regular basis, encourage cooperation and collaboration among the team members, and peacefully resolve any conflicts that may occur. The team leader must have the skills to deal with differences of opinion and power struggles within the team.[22] The leader plans for regular team meetings to monitor progress, share any achievements, discuss concerns and challenges, and encourage exchange of ideas and suggestions. The leader encourages participation by all team members to facilitate close interaction among all members of the team and promote an atmosphere of openness and trust. The leader must guide the discussion during each meeting to promote effective decision making, and also ensure that the focus remains on the topic under consideration.[22] Thus, in order to develop a productive team, selection of an efficient and effective leader is very important. To function as an effective leader, an understanding of the process of group development is of paramount importance.

Group Development

A group can face different issues as it matures, including interpersonal relationships, group behavior, and leadership. To address issues of interest, groups can be organized on a temporary or permanent basis.[22] Groups can be small or large, formal or informal, and with membership that may remain constant over a period of time or undergo frequent changes. A group must develop a sense of cohesiveness so that even group members who originate from different backgrounds view the interests of the group over the interests of the individual. Some strategies for successful group development are highlighted in Table 24-1.

TABLE 24-1   Strategies for Successful Group Development

Strategy	Activity/Advantage/Outcome
Shared leadership	Responsibility for group facilitation should be given to all group members. Several leadership roles are necessary; they need not be performed by one person.
Clearly stated goals and objectives	Group members must reach a consensus on the group's goals and objectives; the group's mission should be periodically reexamined and amended, if necessary.
Ground rules established	Acceptance of rules and procedures adds to the cohesiveness of the group.
Acceptance of conflicts and disagreements	Group members must recognize that conflicts and disagreements are inevitable. All decisions cannot be unanimous; groups should work hard to reach a consensus.
Members are effective listeners	Group members should listen to alternate points of view to improve the quality of decision making; all members should be encouraged to participate to make the group a successful "learning team."
Group meetings are constructive	Although group decisions should not be rushed or forced, discussions should not continue indefinitely. All group sessions should be wrapped up meaningfully.

Source: Compiled by the author.

Stages of Group Development

Table 24-2 highlights the feelings and behavior of group members as they progress through the different stages of group development. These stages are discussed further in the following sections.

Stage 1: Forming

Group members get to know each other in Stage 1, which is called *forming*. They form impressions about the different members of the group and recognize similarities and differences. An atmosphere that is informal, not intimidating, and encourages conversation is a good start for the first stage of group development.[22,24,25] The group leader is looked to for orientation, guidance, and direction.[14] The reason for the existence of the group—the group's charge—is indicated clearly by the leader to the members of the group.[22,24,25] Members become acquainted with the goals and objectives of the team—in short, the mission of the team. They discuss the activities to be undertaken to accomplish the goals and objectives, and the ground rules are well established and understood.[24,25] Any controversial issues are avoided during the discussion. No one wants to get into conflicts; every member wants to feel a part of the group and has the desire to belong and be accepted by the group.

Stage 2: Storming

In the next stage, called *storming*, group members plan and organize the activities for the task. At this point, conflicts may arise between the members and also between the members and their leader.[23,24,25] Controversies arise over leadership, structure of the group, the power of each member, and who is in charge. The responsibility of each member, the rules and regulations, the rewards associated with performance, and the criteria for evaluation are constant issues of debate. There is an underlying competition between the team members as all tend to evaluate each other, and this generates hostilities.[14,23,24,25] Some members tend to dominate over others and try to gain influence and support, whereas others remain completely silent. Subgroups may form as a result of this internal conflict and may even challenge the leader of the group.[14] No problem solving occurs at this stage.

Stage 3: Norming

In Stage 3, called *norming*, group members begin to respect each other and support each other.[14] This makes the group more cohesive and close-knit. Group members begin to acknowledge and accept the knowledge, skills, and expertise of different professionals in the group.[24,25] As the group members begin to know and trust each other, they change their preconceived ideas or notions about each other and work together to resolve group issues.[23,24,25] The group becomes more cohesive and productive. Members develop a sense of belonging to the group and begin to exchange ideas and thoughts. This stage is, therefore, characterized by high creativity.

TABLE 24-2   Stages of Group Development: Member Feelings and Behaviors

Stage	Member Feelings	Member Behavior
Forming	Apprehension; excitement; desire to belong	Form impressions about other group members; try to understand the goals and objectives of the group; try to define activities; avoid conflicts and disagreements.
Storming	Resistance; resentment; jealousy	Arguments over group structure, leadership, ground rules, and responsibilities; competition between the team members.
Norming	Acceptance; respect; trust; sense of belonging	Work together towards the goal; group more creative and cohesive; resources pooled together for maximum efficiency.
Performing	Ease; comfort; acceptance; encouragement; unity; confidence; interdependence	Team is highly productive; members respect the contributions of all others on the team; team is focused and united in problem solving.
Adjourning (Deforming, Mourning)	Relief; pride; happiness	Members discuss the group's achievements and future projects and collaborations.

Source: Compiled by the author.

Stage 4: Performing

Stage 4 is referred to as *performing*. In this stage, the team is most productive. All team members are fully cognizant and fully accepting of the contributions and roles of the other members of the team.[14] Team members are at ease with each other in problem solving and working towards the planned objectives.[24,25] They can work comfortably as a group, as a subgroup, or individually. Initiatives and suggestions made by different members are accepted by all others; members encourage feedback from each other.[14] Members are highly focused on task functions and obtaining the desired goals and objectives. The group is very united in its efforts; group morale and confidence are very high.[23,24,25]

At this stage, the performance and the productivity of the group "peak." The pitfalls that might have troubled the group until this stage are avoided, and the group forges ahead with a renewed sense of accomplishment. And accomplish the group does, with self-assuredness. The group members concentrate on finding optimal solutions to problems at hand. Interdependence among the group members reaches an all-time high, with no need to seek validation from the other members. Because the members identify very strongly with each other at this stage, group loyalty reaches a new crest. Further, members refuse to let themselves be pigeonholed into specific categories and roles, and regularly switch gears from being independent members to being members of a subgroup to being a complete unit. The "means" at this stage is hard work, and the "end" is greater productivity.

Stage 5: Adjourning

This stage is also referred to as "deforming or mourning." Rather than viewing this stage as an extension of the above four stages, one can look at this stage as an adjunct. Clearly, this stage is not critical to the overall functioning of the team. Rather, the focus is solely on the emotions of the people who had made up the team until now.[24,25] In this stage, after the group has accomplished its task, it is effectively disbanded. The group members could reiterate their support of the steps they have taken together to achieve results. They could also discuss whether they would consider working together again. Members highlight individual and collective accomplishments and make decisions regarding future collaborative efforts. They may also feel opposing emotions at this stage: on one hand, some pain of farewell could be felt; on the other hand, there could be considerable relief that the project is finally over.[24,25]

Although five stages have been identified in the process of group development, not all groups will pass through them. Some groups may not be successful in overcoming the challenges associated with the earlier stages and never get past them. Groups that are able to negotiate all the stages eventually prove to be the most productive and efficient.

Conclusion

In this chapter you learned that the significance of nutrition in preventing the onset of disease and controlling the progression of chronic diseases cannot be underscored. However, the benefits associated with a healthy diet can be achieved only if the public is aware of the principles of nutrition in a state of health and in a state of disease. It is the responsibility of public health professionals like nutritionists, physicians, nurses, pharmacists, social workers, psychologists, and others to make conscious efforts individually and collectively to provide nutrition education for the benefit of the community.

Issues for Discussion

1. What are some of the criteria that can be used to assess the impact and effectiveness of a nutrition education program?
2. What strategies can be adopted to emphasize the importance of nutrition to professionals in the health and allied-health disciplines involved in providing complete care to the patient?
3. What level of training in the field of nutrition is considered to be "adequate" for medical school students?
4. What measures can be taken to reduce the challenges faced by nutrition educators?
5. Is nutrition education the responsibility of nutritionists alone?
6. How can the effectiveness of in-service education programs be enhanced?

References

1. U.S. Department of Health and Human Services. *Healthy People 2010: Understanding and Improving Health.* 2nd ed. Washington, DC: U.S. Government Printing Office; November 2000.
2. U.S. Department of Health and Human Services. *The Surgeon General's Call to Action to Prevent and Decrease Overweight and Obesity.* Washington, DC: U.S. Government Printing Office; December 2001.
3. Ernst ND, Sempos CT, et al. Consistency between U.S. dietary fat intakes and fetal serum cholesterol concentrations. *Am J Clin Nutr.* 1997;66(suppl):965S–972S.
4. National Institute of Diabetes and Digestive and Kidney Diseases, National Institutes of Health. *Diet and Exercise Delay Diabetes and Normalize Blood Glucose,* NIH publication No. 04-5099, May 2004. Accessed on June 7, 2005 from http://diabetes.niddk.nih.gov/dm/pubs/preventionprogram.
5. Green LW, Potvin L. Education, health promotion, and social, and lifestyle determinants of health and disease. In: Detels R, McEwen J, Beaglehole R, Tanaka H, eds. *Oxford Textbook of Public Health. The Scope of Public Health,* 4th edition, Volume 1. New York, NY: Oxford University Press Inc.; 2002:113–130.
6. Nestle M, Dixon LB. Do education campaigns induce communities to change their diets and improve health? In: Nestle M, Dixon LB, eds. *Taking Sides. Clashing Views on Controversial Issues in Food and Nutrition.* Guilford, CT: McGraw-Hill/Dushkin; 2004:174–175.
7. The Henry J. Kaiser Family Foundation. *The Role of Media in Childhood Obesity.* Program for the Study of Entertainment Media and Health. Publication Number 7030; February 2004. Accessed on June 7, 2005 from www.kff.org.
8. Reger B, Wootan MG, Booth-Butterfield S. A comparison of different approaches to promote community-wide dietary change. *Am J Prev Med.* 2000;18(4):271–275.

9. Tones K. Health promotion, health education, and the public health. In: Detels R, McEwen J, Beaglehole R, Tanaka H, eds. *Oxford Textbook of Public Health. The Methods of Public Health, 4th edition, Volume 2.* New York, NY: Oxford University Press Inc.; 2002:829–831.

10. Breckon DJ, Harvey JR, Lancaster RB. Current perspectives of practice and professional preparation. In: *Community Health Education—Settings, Roles and Skills for the 21st Century.* Gaithersburg, MD: Aspen Publication, 1998.

11. Ro M. Moving forward: Addressing the health of Asian American and Pacific Islander women. *Am J Pub Health.* 2002;92(4):516–519.

12. [No author listed]. Policy statements adopted by the governing council of the American Public Health Association, October 24, 2001. *Am J Pub Health.* 2002; 92(3): 468.

13. Weigley ES, Mueller DH, Robinson CH. Food, Nutrition and Health. In: *Robinson's Basic Nutrition and Diet Therapy, 8th edition.* Upper Saddle River, NJ: Merrill Prentice Hall, 1997: 4–5.

14. Joyner G, Kaufman M. Leveraging nutrition education through the public health team. In: Kaufman M, ed. Nutrition in Public Health. Gaithersburg, MD: Aspen Publication; 1990: 420–436.

15. Avery B. Who does the work of public health? *Am J Pub Health.* 2002;92(4):570–575.

16. Leeds MJ Good nutrition for a healthy life. In Leeds MJ (ed.): *Nutrition for Healthy Living.* Boston, MA: WCB McGraw-Hill; 1998:13–15.

17. Pearson TA, Stone EJ, et al. Translation of nutritional sciences into medical education: The Nutrition Academic Award Program. *Am J Clin Nutr.* 2001;74:164–170.

18. McGinnis JM, Foege WH. The actual causes of death in the United States. *JAMA* 1993; 270:2207–2212.

19. Food and Nutrition Information Center, U.S. Department of Agriculture, Agricultural Research Service. *TEAM Nutrition 2004 Action Plan.* Accessed on June 7, 2005 from http://www.fns.usda.gov/tn/ActionPlan/index.htm.

20. U.S. Government Accounting Office. *School Lunch Program: Efforts Needed to Improve Nutrition and Encourage Healthy Eating.* GAO-03-506; May 2003. Accessed June 7, 2005 from http://searching.gao.gov/index.html.

21. Management Sciences for Health and the United Nations Children's Fund. Strategies for Developing an Effective Team. Accessed May 2, 2005 from http://erc.msh.org/quality/ittools/ittipstm.cfm.

22. Breckon DJ, Harvey JR, Lancaster RB. Working with groups in leadership roles. In Breckon DJ, Harvey JR, Lancaster RB: *Community Health Education—Settings, Roles and Skills for the 21st Century, 4th edition.* Gaithersburg, MD: Aspen Publications; 1998: 245–251:1998 .

23. Manion J, Lorimer W, Leander WJ. Building New Teams: A Discipline. In: *Team-based health care organizations: Blueprint for success.* Gaithersburg, MD: Aspen Publications; 1996: 55–84.

24. Tuckman, B. Developmental Sequence in Small Groups. *Psychological Bulletin,* 1965: 63; 384–399.

25. Tuckman, B. & Jensen, M. Stages of Small Group Development. *Group and Organizational Studies,* 1977: 2;419–427.

PART VIII

SURVIVING IN
A COMPETITIVE WORLD

Part VIII discusses many features that are important to any program—networking, marketing, earning internal administrative support, striving for excellence, and envisioning the future. For any program to be successful, these elements must be present, although they continue to be some of public health nutrition's most daunting challenges. In order for programs to work and meet the needs of those targeted to receive help, networking and marketing must be carefully planned. Chapters 25 and 26 give the reader an insight into these tools. Chapter 27 stresses the need for us to also market our nutrition programs *within* the organization of public health to assure survival. Finally, Chapter 28 reminds us all that public health nutrition is a dynamic process that changes constantly. We must be able to anticipate needs and provide for them if we are to be successful.

CHAPTER 25

NETWORKING FOR NUTRITION

Patti S. Landers, PhD, RD/LD

Reader Objectives

After studying this chapter and reflecting on the contents, you should be able to:

1. Define common terms related to networking.
2. Discuss the difference between networks, alliances, and coalitions.
3. Give examples of nutrition issues that might be addressed by networks or coalitions.
4 List the benefits of networking for nutrition.
5. Identify characteristics of a successful nutrition coalition.
6. Describe the responsibilities of a lead agency and steering committee in maintaining a nutrition coalition.
7. Develop your own professional networking plan.

Call it a clan, call it a network, call it a tribe, call it a family. Whatever you call it, whoever you are, you need one.[1]

Think of your network of contacts as a professional family. Networks are important both personally and professionally. The purpose of this chapter is to explore how relationships ranging from a network to coalition building are constructed and nourished. These interactions can benefit you personally. In addition, they are vital to promoting nutrition and making better health available to the individuals and families that we seek to reach and serve. Later in the chapter, you will find tips about how to improve your own networking skills.

Networks, Alliances, Coalitions, and Consortiums

Nutrition experts interact with one another at varying levels of organization. There are many terms used to describe these groups. They are often called networks, alliances, associations, coalitions, consortiums, leagues, or federations. We will discuss a few of these terms that are representative of them all.

In the most informal sense, a *network* is a group of people who form relationships to share ideas, information, and resources. *Alliances* are often semi-official and loosely organized. In alliances, instead of people acting as individuals, the members tend to be made up of representatives from different organizations with similar goals. *Coalitions* are the most structured type of group, and are more formal in nature. Built for a specific purpose, coalitions are often formed to address a particular problem or need in the community. *Consortiums* are similar; they are large groups of organizations, formed to undertake enterprises beyond the resources of any one member.

Networks

We all have links of communication that connect us to other people. For example, most nutrition professionals attend district, state, or national meetings as a means of keeping up with new information and maintaining continuing education requirements. Telephone conference calls and Internet listservs also provide valuable contacts. These types of informal networks can be an excellent way of finding out about employment opportunities and gathering data to be used in program planning and evaluation.

An Internet nutrition website can be used as a community for nutrition students and dietitians. There may be a message board where students exchange information about classwork, explore different academic programs, and discuss internships. A career center part of the website may provide information about writing resumes and examples of which questions to expect at a job interview. It can even tell prospective employees how to negotiate for a better salary. Employers may pay to place listings on the site. Job seekers may sometimes post their resumes for free and view a list of open positions and their locations. A speaker's network may be available, where an organization needing a speaker can view people's credentials. Or, members can enroll in a referral network, if it exists, where others wanting nutrition services can find contact information.[2]

At a higher level, nutrition networking efforts can be encouraged or even mandated by funding agencies. The Food and Nutrition Service (FNS) of the United States Department of Agriculture (USDA) provides matching funds for states and communities to supply Food Stamp Nutrition Education (FSNE) programs. The goal is to increase the likelihood that all Food Stamp recipients will make healthy food choices and engage in active lifestyles consistent with the Dietary Guidelines for Americans and the MyPyramid (formerly the Food Guide Pyramid [FGP]). Because of the tremendous growth in expenditures for the Food Stamp Nutrition Education program, from $661,000 in 1992 to over $192 million in 2003,[3] networking has become very important and is being mandated by the USDA to avoid duplication of services.

The following provides an example of how the USDA promotes networking: If a Cooperative Extension Service or community agency writes an FSNE plan that includes breast-feeding education, the group must document that it is collaborating with WIC (the Special Supplemental Nutrition Program for Women, Infants and Children). Why? Both Food Stamps and WIC are USDA programs and many women participate in both. USDA wants to be sure that the information each woman receives is consistent. Because the WIC program has primary responsibility for breast-feeding education, it takes the lead.[4]

> **Cooperative Extension Service—** A research-based program that provides outreach services and education to consumers.

Alliances

"An alliance is the state of being allied: a bond or connection between families, states, parties, or individuals."[5] Alliances and consortia may be semi-official. For example, the Oklahoma Nutrition Alliance is a loose-knit group of people interested in nutrition education in the Oklahoma City area. Representatives come from the food industry, cooperative extension, public schools, state agencies, Native American tribes, WIC, the regional food bank, university nutrition departments, and other areas. The members were originally a part of a larger group formed in 1996 for another purpose. When that group disbanded, some of the representatives felt they benefited from networking with other agencies and did not want to stop; they formed the Nutrition Alliance. Quarterly meetings continue at rotating sites. The success of this organization is due to the commitment of a key individual who takes the lead in organizing meetings and sending out e-mail reminders.

The following provides an example of how the Alliance has functioned: Nutrition students at the University of Oklahoma Health Sciences Center wanted to give lessons in public schools. Their professor contacted a health educator working with the schools, who arranged for them to teach a series of three classes in each of 20 schools. A dairy industry representative provided copies of a student workbook for a MyPyramid curriculum. A beef industry representative furnished large MyPyramid posters for each school. The collaboration was a tremendous success and the nutrition students reached over 1,100 fourth graders while building their own teaching and presentation skills.

Consortia and Coalitions

"A consortium is a group formed to undertake an enterprise beyond the resources of any one member, while a coalition is defined as a temporary alliance of distinct parties, persons, or states for joint action."[5] Coalition building is considered a formal process where public and private agencies, communities, businesses, and volunteers unite as partners to combine resources and work together toward a common goal. An example is the Georgia Coalition for Physical Activity and Nutrition (GPAN).[6] This group of public and private agencies, nonprofit organizations, industry groups, and businesses has defined its mission as improving the health of all Georgians, particularly those with low incomes, by promoting healthy eating and physical activity. The group developed a campaign with targeted "Take" messages, encouraging the public to:

- Take Action (be physically active).
- Take 5-A-Day (eat five or more servings of fruits and vegetables daily).
- Take Down Fat (eat less fat through smaller portions and changing cooking methods).
- Take Charge of Your Health.

GPAN has over 50 member organizations with a formal set of bylaws. There are elected officers, a board of directors, and an advisory board composed of elected officials and the president of a medical school.

An example of a consortium at the national level is the U.S. Department of Health and Human Services' Healthy People.[7] The initiative promotes partnerships designed to enable diverse groups to work together to improve health. Healthy People has partners from all sectors. Federal agencies serve as coordinators. All state and territorial health departments and more than 400 national membership organizations, including the American Dietetic Association, the American Public Health Association, and the Institute of Food Technologists, belong to the Healthy People Consortium.

"The twenty-first century will be the age of alliances."[8]

By engaging in networks, alliances, coalitions, and consortia, nutritionists can design interventions and services that are more likely to meet community needs and priorities. In order to effectively network, the nutritionist must have community-leader contacts, so it is important to dedicate time to community and professional service. At the heart of an effective network are successful relationships that lead to productive partnerships. Some benefits of networking include:

- Expanding understanding about an issue
- Generating innovative approaches
- Overcoming political, cultural, and bureaucratic barriers
- Reducing duplication of effort
- Bringing together complementary resources
- Sharing risks and limiting liability

Collaborating with Others for Nutrition Networks

When forming a nutrition network, alliance, or coalition, the first step is to bring individuals together to explore an issue and clearly identify their purpose or define a problem. It is vital to come to a consensus about purpose and problem. Where do you find people and organizations that will become good partners? Figure 25-1, from *Moving to the Future: Developing Community-Based Nutrition Services* (Workbook & Training Manual),[9] illustrates potential sectors that may include organizations and businesses that deal with food and nutrition issues.

After you have assembled a group of potential partners, one of the most important features of this stage is relationship building. Therefore, each person must feel that they have had an opportunity to give their perspectives and that others in the group have heard them. This may take several meetings and a significant amount of time.

After a problem or general purpose has been identified, it is helpful if each member of the group tells how his or her organization is related to the problem. As illustrated in Figure 25-2, you may want to use a RACK analysis to inventory partners. This acronym stands for Resources, Access, Constraints, and Knowledge.

Consider the example problem of hunger in a community. The following RACK analysis gives examples of resources, access, constraints, and knowledge that can be provided by members of a community nutrition network. These represent inputs that community agencies make toward the problem or purpose of the network or coalition.

Resources

A primary resource would be food or funds to buy food. Which agencies would you want to enlist who could help with this resource? Examples would include emergency food assistance pantries, a regional food bank, area food markets and food processors, and the local agencies responsible for administering the Food Stamp program and other food distribution programs such as WIC.

Other resources, such as space, furniture, telephones, office equipment, and supplies, would also be needed. The next issue is: Who could provide personnel to take applications from hungry people and send them to the right agencies? This may be solved in the "access" category.

Access

Who has access to people who do not have enough food? Partners who can help in this area may include schools, places of worship, healthcare facilities, childcare centers, and social service agencies. However, even if we know who needs the food, constraints may prevent distribution.

Ensuring a Diverse, Representative Coalition

Goal/Objective:

_____

Nutrition Intervention:

_____

Member's names

Expertise

Public Relations	
Administration	
Financial Management	
Fundraising	
Legal	
Evaluation	
Program	
Health/Nutrition	

Geographic Area

State	
City/County	
Rural	
Suburban	

Fields Represented

Health	
Business/Industry	
Education	
Politics	
Legal Groups	
Information	
Recreation	
Community Groups	
Religious Organizations	
Service/Voluntary Organizations	

Ethnicity

African American	
Asian	
Caucasian	
Hispanic	
Native American	
Other	

Age

16–20	
21–35	
36–50	
51–65	
Over 65	

Gender

Female	
Male	

FIGURE 25-1   Building Coalitions to Address the Nutrition Needs of the Population
Source: Reprinted with permission from Probert K. _Moving to the Future:_
Developing Community-Based Nutrition Services (Workbook & Training Manual).
Washington, DC: Association of State and Territorial Public Health Nutrition
Directors; 1996. Available at: http://www.movingtothefuture.org. Accessed
April 6, 2004.

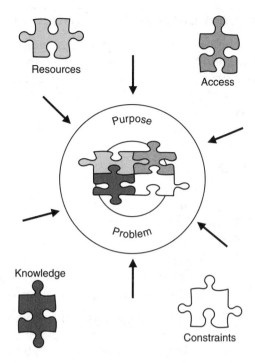

FIGURE 25-2   Elements of a RACK Analysis
Source: Developed by Patti Landers, PhD, RD/LD.

Constraints

Most partners in a network will have constraints of one kind or another. For example, a regional food bank may have plenty of food, but be unable to distribute it directly to hungry people. Local food pantries can perform that role. Other constraints may be cultural or political barriers to service. For example, a community agency may be able to provide office space and telephones, but has no funds to hire personnel who speak languages other than English.

Knowledge

A university may have expertise in research and how to evaluate a program, but lack access to data for analyses. Social service agencies or cooperative extension may employ nutritionists or paraprofessionals who are trained as nutrition education aides to provide instruction about dietary quality, food safety, and food resource management; however, they cannot teach hungry people who are not enrolled in their programs.

Any coalition should engage in frequent evaluation. New problems may be identified and a RACK analysis may prove helpful in identifying which new partner agencies or business the coalition should seek to involve.

Developing a Community-Based Nutrition Network

In *Moving to the Future: Developing Community-Based Nutrition Services* (Workbook & Training Manual),[9] Karen Probert defines a coalition as a structured arrangement for cooperation and collaboration between otherwise unrelated groups or organizations. Each group retains its identity, but all agree to work together toward a common, mutually agreed upon goal. In the handbook, Probert lists seven items that need to be in place for a coalition to succeed:

1. Staff support
2. Focal point of coordination
3. Specified system of communication
4. Actively involved community leaders
5. Strong relationships between private and public sector groups
6. Communication networks within the community
7. A constituency for public health that can advocate for resources and for the attention of elected officials

Probert also provides job descriptions and lists ways for members to participate. These tools may aid in building a successful coalition.

The Community Tool Box[10] provides over 6,000 Internet pages of practical skill-building information on over 250 different topics, including how to build partnerships and coalitions. In his book *Quick Tips: Principles for Coalition Success,*[10] Tom Wolff of AHEC/Community Partners states that a shared mission and goal is vital to a successful coalition. Members must be able to set aside their own self-interest in favor of what will benefit the target audience. Wolff also emphasizes that the coalition membership must be diverse, and should include representatives from business, government, and the clergy, as well as members of neighborhood groups, young people, and the disenfranchised.

> **Community Tool Box—**
> Available at http://ctb.ku.edu.

When forming a nutrition coalition, it is essential to identify a lead agency. This organization should be willing and able to commit personnel and financial resources as well as have some experience in coalition building. If an agency, rather than an individual, is committed to lead the group, the project will continue, even if a personnel vacancy occurs and the individual who was serving as contact person leaves.

Because coalitions are formal and structured, it is important that members write a mission statement, goals, and objectives. Bylaws should be put in place, too. Most coalitions have a steering committee. This subgroup may also be called the executive or coordinating committee. Typically, the steering committee includes the coalition chairperson and a representative from the lead agency. The chair or facilitator is often, but not always, from the lead agency and conducts coalition meetings.[11] Some groups prefer to rotate the position. Although someone must chair the group, leadership should be shared as much as possible, and everyone should feel they have input into decisions through a clear, democratic process. To aid in good communication, the coalition should have regular meetings. The chair or secretary should send out minutes to all members. Successful coalitions have clear short-term and long-term goals. The members plan often, focus efforts, and measure results. They engage in ongoing evaluation at all stages of their work. The coalition should have an annual meeting that includes all of the members. The chair or steering committee should publish and distribute a yearly report. Table 25-1 lists examples of potential issues and partners who might come together in a nutrition coalition.

Professional Networking

Professional organizations provide a support and networking system for public health nutritionists. The American Dietetic Association (ADA) is the nation's largest organization of food and nutrition professionals and serves the public by promoting optimal nutrition, health, and well-being.[12] The ADA has state, district, and student affiliate groups that provide for excellent peer networking through meetings and the annual Food & Nutrition Conference & Expo. ADA members also can choose to participate in the Nationwide Nutrition Network. At the ADA website (www.eatright.org), consumers, doctors and other healthcare professionals, restaurant owners and managers, and food manufacturers and distributors can enter a ZIP code to find local dietetics professionals for individual consultations, program development, workshops and seminars, and special projects. ADA holds an annual Public Policy Workshop in Washington, D.C., where dietitians network and focus on how they can become involved with members of Congress to impact legislative issues key to the profession and the nutritional health of Americans. ADA dietetic practice groups (DPGs) also provide opportunities for networking with others. Of particular interest to public health nutritionists are the following DPGs: Public Health/Community Nutrition, School Nutrition Services, Hunger and Environmental Nutrition, Nutrition Education for the Public, Gerontological Nutritionists, Nutrition Educators of Health Professionals, Pediatric Nutrition, Weight Management, and Women's Health and Reproductive Nutrition.

The American Public Health Association (APHA) is the oldest and largest organization of public health professionals in the world. APHA has been influencing policies and setting priorities in public health for over 125 years. Throughout its history it has been in the forefront of numerous efforts to prevent disease and promote health.[13] The APHA Food and Nutrition section contributes to long-range planning in food, nutrition, and health policy, which may affect the nutritional well-being of the public. Priorities of the

TABLE 25-1   Food and Nutrition Issues and Potential Partners

Issue	Potential Partners	Real-Life Examples
Childhood obesity	Schools, PTAs, teachers, principals "Ys," local Boys and Girls clubs Daycare centers Pediatricians Dietetic association American Alliance for Health, Physical Education, Recreation, and Dance 4-H clubs and cooperative extension State and local health departments (child and maternal nutrition, WIC) Hospital wellness programs	• Coalition for a Healthy and Active America http://www.chaausa.org • Action for Healthy Kids, http://www.actionforhealthykids.org • Center for Weight and Health at UC Berkeley http://nature.berkeley.edu/cwh/ • Georgia Coalition for Physical Activity and Nutrition http://www.g-pan.org • National Coalition for Promoting Physical Activity http://www.ncppa.org
Hunger and homelessness	Human services agencies Social/family agencies Dietetic association Housing authorities Churches/interfaith councils Ministerial associations Food banks Soup kitchens/food pantries Salvation Army College and university students America's Second Harvest Area food processors Grocery stores Restaurants	• Arkansas Hunger Coalition http://www.arkansashunger.org • Los Angeles Coalition to End Hunger and Homelessness http://www.lacehh.org • Alabama Hunger Coalition http://www.achr.com/hunger_coalition.htm • America's Second Harvest http://www.secondharvest.org • Hunger Coalition at California State University, Fullerton http://www.fullerton.edu/deanofstudents/volunteer/hunger.htm • New York City Coalition Against Hunger, http://www.nyccah.org

Source: Reprinted with permission from Cohen L, Baer N, Satterwhite P. *Developing Effective Coalitions: An Eight-Step Guide.* Toronto, ON: Ontario Injury Prevention Resource Centre; 1998.

section include promotion of public health nutrition policy, elimination of racial and ethnic health disparities, education and training for public health workers, and increasing and strengthening membership. An advantage of membership in APHA is the opportunity to interact not only with nutrition professionals, but also with the wider public health community, including physicians, nurses, and health educators.

The Society for Nutrition Education (SNE) is an international organization of nutrition education professionals who are dedicated to promoting healthful, sustainable food choices and who share a vision of healthy people in healthy communities.[14] Members conduct research in education, behavior, and communication; develop and disseminate innovative nutrition education strategies; and communicate information on food, nutrition, and health issues to students, professionals, policy makers, and the public. SNE members share ideas and resources through the *Journal of Nutrition Education and Behavior,* a newsletter, an annual conference, and a members-only e-mail listserv. Divisions offer networking opportunities for members with similar interests and expertise.[14] Groups of special interest may include the Public Health Nutrition and the Social Marketing Networks divisions.

Networking Tips

Developing a strong network requires planning and deliberate action. First, list your personal and professional goals and the contacts you need to make in order to achieve them. The book *The WetFeet Insider Guide to Networking*[15] suggests that your existing and potential contacts are made up of your inner circle, your expanded network, and the network you never knew you had. People who know you well are in your inner circle; these are your family, friends, and current and former colleagues. Your expanded network includes acquaintances with whom you've had brief contact, other members of professional groups, or e-mail correspondents. The network you never knew you had includes "friends, relatives, and colleagues, relatives, and colleagues or friends."[15]

Here are some tips that will help you develop your personal network:

- Cultivate a wide circle of friends and acquaintances in many different venues.
- Stock a good supply of business cards and carry them with you at all times. Every time you meet someone you feel might be a good contact, take out one of your cards. Write a personal note on the back before you give it to them. This will let the person know about your interests and make them more likely to keep up with your contact information. They will usually offer you one of their business cards in return. Immediately write a reminder to yourself on the back. Just a

phrase like "childhood obesity poster in Atlanta" will help you to remember them. Then, when you contact that person later, they will be impressed that you know who they are and what they did.

- Have a date book or PDA, and keep it handy and current.
- Keep an updated resume template on file at all times. You'll want to customize it for each specific situation. For example, your resume needs different emphasis areas depending on the type of position you are seeking. If applying for a job as a clinical dietitian, you would highlight education and work in hospital settings. If you were looking for a position in a nonprofit agency, you would stress your training and experience in collaborating with other people. Listing volunteer activities that show your community involvement would be important. Demonstrating skill with grant writing would be especially impressive.
- Be a member of one or more professional organizations. Always attend local and state meetings. Volunteer to be on committees and help at events. Always do a good job, even with small tasks. Your skills will become known and soon you will be asked to take a leadership role.
- Attend a national conference, at least every other year. If possible, travel with someone in the organization that you do not know well. Getting out of town and having block time to network is very important.
- Immediately follow up on contacts you make with a card, brief phone call, or e-mail message.
- Prepare in advance for follow-up meetings.
- Work to improve social skills. Good social skills are essential to networking. At meetings or parties, be outgoing, even if it is not natural for you. Do not stand in a corner by yourself. Go up to others who look lonely and strike up a conversation, or join a group and introduce yourself. Do not forget your business cards. Keep them handy even at social events. If social occasions are painful, investigate a public speaking group like Toastmasters where you can improve communication skills.
- Be sincere. Help others and they will help you.
- Always remember to say thank you.

Conclusions

It is important to be professionally competent in what you know; however, who you know may be just as vital to accomplishing your objectives in promoting better health and nutrition.

Networking includes relationships built at both personal and professional levels. These associations may range from informal interactions with individuals and groups of people for information, ideas, and resources, to semi-official alliances, and then on to structured coalitions that were purposefully organized to address a particular nutrition problem or need in the community.

When building a coalition, it is important that membership be diverse and representative. You may want to use a RACK analysis to categorize resources, access, constraints, and knowledge of potential coalition member organizations. Write a mission statement, goals, objectives, and bylaws. Choose a steering committee and chair to interact with both coalition members and the lead agency that has committed personnel and financial resources to the coalition.

Networking, allying yourself with others, and coalition building will allow you to maximize resources, increase access to target audiences, minimize or overcome constraints, and use knowledge to benefit yourself and others. Use the tips listed near the end of the chapter to help you develop a strong personal system of contacts.

Issues for Discussion

1. How do the benefits of networking justify your investment of time and effort?
2. How can professional networking relationships benefit you personally?
3. Where do you want to go in your professional career? How can networking help you to achieve that goal?

References

1. Howard J. *Families*. New York, NY: Simon and Schuster; 1978.
2. Hall R, Warner J. Nutritiononestop.com. Available at: http://www.nutritiononestop.com. Accessed April 3, 2004.
3. U.S. Department of Agriculture. Nutrition Program Facts: Food Stamp Nutrition Education. Available at: http://www.fns.usda.gov/fsp/nutrition_education/factsheet.htm. Accessed March 22, 2004.
4. U.S. Department of Agriculture. 2005 Food Stamp Nutrition Education Plan Guidance Highlights from A to Z. Available at: http://www.nal.usda.gov/foodstamp/atoz20052.pdf. Accessed April 3, 2004.
5. Merriam-Webster. Online Dictionary. Available at: http://www.m-w.com. Accessed April 3, 2004.
6. GPAN. Georgia Coalition for Physical Activity and Nutrition. Available at: http://www.g-pan.org. Accessed April 5, 2004.
7. U.S. Department of Health and Human Services. *Healthy People 2010: Understanding and Improving Health*. 2nd ed. Washington, DC: U.S. Government Printing Office; 2000.

8. Austin JE. *The Collaboration Challenge: How Nonprofits and Businesses Succeed through Strategic Alliances.* New York, NY: John Wiley & Sons; 2000.

9. Probert K. *Moving to the Future: Developing Community-Based Nutrition Services* (Workbook & Training Manual). Washington, DC: Association of State and Territorial Public Health Nutrition Directors; 1996. Available at http://www.movingtothefuture.org. Accessed April 6, 2004.

10. Wolff T. Community Tool Box. University of Kansas. Available at: http://ctb.ku.edu. Accessed April 3, 2004.

11. Cohen L, Baer N, Satterwhite P. *Developing Effective Coalitions: An Eight-Step Guide.* Toronto, ON: Ontario Injury Prevention Resource Centre; 1998.

12. American Dietetic Association. Welcome. American Dietetic Association. Available at: http://www.eatright.org. Accessed April 5, 2004.

13. American Public Health Association. About APHA. Available at: http://www.apha.org. Accessed April 5, 2004.

14. Society for Nutrition Education. Identity Statement. Society for Nutrition Education. Available at: http://www.sne.org. Accessed April 5, 2004.

15. WetFeet. *Networking Works.* San Francisco, CA: WetFeet Inc.; 2004.

16. D'Angelo A. *The College Blue Book: A Few Thoughts, Reflections and Reminders on How to Get the Most Out of College and Life.* Granite Bay, CA: The Collegiate EmPowerment Company; 1995.

CHAPTER 26

MARKETING NUTRITION PROGRAMS AND SERVICES

Nancie Herbold, EdD, RD

Paul N. Taylor, PhD

Reader Objectives

After studying this chapter and reflecting on the contents, you will be able to:

1. Compare and contrast simple marketing, business marketing, and social marketing.
2. List and define the four Ps of marketing and some additional Ps of social marketing.
3. Discuss types of market research and how they can be used in preparing a plan for a public health nutrition program.
4. Compare and contrast the ethics of business marketing and social marketing.

Marketing Defined

The opening years of the 21st century clearly indicate that nutritionists must understand the nuances of marketing and how its concepts are used, not only to promote public health through nutrition, but also to counter messages that may not be in the best interests of the public health. Whereas, you would be hard pressed to find My Pyramid explained in a television or newspaper advertisement, it is easy to find examples of marketing for weight-loss supplements, meal replacements, and "low-carb" foods. Relatively recently, healthcare professionals and organizations realized the value of marketing to reach desired objectives. The nutritionist, as an important member of the healthcare team, must understand the power and value of marketing as a tool, and use marketing concepts to inform and educate the public as part of an effective nutrition program.

How, then, does the nutritionist define marketing? The National Public Health Leadership Institute provides this comprehensive definition:

"Marketing" can denote a continuum of efforts and activities ranging from simple "marketing" to the more complex "media advocacy"; each form of marketing involves a relationship and two-way interaction between the marketer and those to whom the marketing is being directed. Simple "marketing" involves targeted communication of information based on audience research. "Social marketing" aims to create attitudinal and/or behavioral change in a target audience by emphasizing relevant benefits to that audience. "Branding" strives to define and establish a positive image or impression for a product via a linked association with a visual or auditory cue that will, when re-experienced, stimulate a quick, almost hard-wired short-cut reminder of the positive value of the product. "Media advocacy" is a strategy designed to bring about a political action and/or policy change through the reframing of issues in mass media.[1]

In this chapter we will focus on simple marketing and social marketing, although other forms of marketing will be mentioned. We will also distinguish between traditional or business marketing and social marketing.

Business Marketing Versus Social Marketing

A practical definition of business marketing is given by Pride and Farrell: "The process of creating, distributing, promoting, and pricing goods, services, and ideas to facilitate satisfying exchange relationships with customers in a dynamic environment."[2] In business marketing, therefore, an exchange of goods or services occurs between a buyer and a seller such that both buyer and seller are satisfied. The dynamic environment in which these exchanges occur consists of uncontrollable forces (consumers, competition, the economy, politics, government, the media, and technology) that affect the marketing mix . Because the marketing environment is dynamic, the most successful marketers continuously evaluate their marketing plans and change them as necessary to ensure that their product is available at the right time, in the right place, and at an acceptable price.

Social marketing, when introduced in 1971, was defined as:

> . . . the design, implementation, and control of programs calculated to influence the acceptability of social ideas and involving considerations of product planning, pricing, communication, distribution, and marketing research.[3]

More recently, Andreasen described social marketing as:

> . . . the application of commercial marketing technologies to the analysis, planning, execution, and evaluation of programs designed to influence the voluntary behavior of target audiences in order to improve their personal welfare and that of their society.[4]

These definitions describe the activities of nutritionists, public health agencies, and other government and private agencies (e.g., the CDC, the Robert Wood Johnson Foundation) who desire to change food choices and eating behaviors among their constituents. Whereas, business marketing focuses on maximizing organizations' profits by fulfilling customers' needs and desires, social marketing focuses on benefiting the target audience and the general society by influencing social behaviors.[5]

Andreasen proposes six benchmarks to identify approaches that could be legitimately called social marketing:[6]

1. Interventions are designed and evaluated using behavior change as a benchmark.
2. For all projects, formative research is conducted to understand the target market, intervention elements are pre-tested before being implemented, and interventions are monitored as they are introduced.
3. Resources are used to maximum efficiency and effectiveness by carefully segmenting target audiences.
4. Influence strategies are designed to create attractive, motivational exchanges with target audiences.
5. All four Ps of the traditional marketing mix are considered in developing strategy: create attractive benefit packages (products); minimize costs (price); make the exchange convenient and easy (place); and communicate powerful messages through media appropriate to the target audiences (promotion).
6. The program strategy anticipates and accounts for the competition likely to be faced by the desired behavior.

In the more than 30 years since the advent of social marketing, two separate lines of thought have emerged regarding its definition. Thus, a nutritionist implementing a program to inform the public about the role of trans-fatty acids in the prevention of heart disease is following the premise of Kotler and Roberto, that social marketing programs are "aimed at increasing the acceptability of a social idea or practice in one or more groups of target adopters."[7] In contrast, the 5-A-Day campaign, a joint venture between the National Cancer Institute (NCI) and the Produce for a Better Health Foundation that encourages the public to eat five servings of fruits and vegetables per day, is following the premise of Andreasen that the ultimate objective should be behavior change in the target population.[6,8]

Whatever definition of social marketing one wishes to adopt (and there are others besides those mentioned[9]), the use of social marketing to develop a nutrition program plan requires commitment from top-level management, adequate funding and personnel, marketing skills, and vision.

As with any nutrition program, the foundation is thorough research, beginning with defining the problem. Once data have been collected and analyzed, recommendations can be made to form the outline of the program and to delineate the marketing plan.

Marketing Research

Marketing research is necessary to plan, develop, and implement a successful social marketing program for an organization. Market research begins with defining the problem and gathering data to understand all aspects, a process that is similar to a nutrition assessment. Data will consist of both objective and subjective information. Marketing research provides information on the knowledge, beliefs, attitudes, wants, and practices of the targeted population necessary to develop strategies for behavioral change.[10] The better the problem is understood, the greater the likelihood of developing a successful plan.

Secondary Data

Secondary data are information collected by other groups and agencies. Health indicators collected by the federal government, such as the National Health and Nutrition Examination Survey (NHANES) data, are one example of secondary data. State Departments of Public Health collect state health statistics, such as infant mortality rate, teen pregnancy rate, and chronic disease incidence and prevalence, which are all are examples of secondary data. There are many helpful websites for data collection (Table 26-1). Private polling data collected by organizations such as AC Nielsen and the Roper Center also may be helpful.

Secondary data collected within an organization are referred to as *internal data*. The number of patients who visit the nutrition cardiac program, the costs of the services, and popular days and times for services are all considered internal secondary data. In contrast, the data collected by an outside entity are regarded as *external secondary data*. It is important to gather as much secondary data as possible to save time, effort, and money.

A review of the professional literature is an important part of collecting information. This review can provide clarity on the problem and uncover successful and unsuccessful approaches to the same or a similar problem. A literature review can also lead to helpful websites. For example, Project LEAN (Leaders Encouraging Activity and Nutrition) and Team Nutrition both address the issue of healthy eating and physical activity in schoolchildren. These groups' websites provide background information and examples of activities used in these programs.[11,12] The literature will discuss details of programs and provide authors' names and affiliations, making it easy to contact someone for additional information. The review of the literature can also uncover food, nutrition, and health trends (e.g., the increase in consumer use of fortified foods,[13] attention to body image prompting adherence to low-fat diets,[14] and increased fish consumption to aid heart disease prevention[15]).

TABLE 26-1   Helpful Websites

www.eatright.org	American Dietetic Association
www.apha.org	American Public Health Association
www.diabetes.org	American Diabetes Association
www.americanheart.org	American Heart Association
www.marketingpower.com	American Marketing Association
www.social-marketing.org	Social Marketing Institute
www.restaurant.org	National Restaurant Association
www.fao.org	Food and Agriculture Organization of the United Nations
www.ift.org	Institute of Food Technologists
www.who.org	World Health Organization
www.cdc.gov	Centers for Disease Control and Prevention
socialmarketing-nutrition.ucdavis.edu	Center for Advanced Studies in Nutrition and Social Marketing
www.cdc.gov/mmwr/	Morbidity and Mortality Weekly Report
www.cdc.gov/nchs/	National Center for Health Statistics
www.census.gov	National Census Bureau
www.phli.org	National Public Health Leadership Institute
www.fda.gov	Food and Drug Administration
www.fedstats.gov	Fedstats
www.hhs.gov	U.S. Department of Health and Human Services
www.usda.gov	U.S. Department of Agriculture
www.healthstats.gov	Healthstats
www.ropercenter.uconn.edu	Roper Center for Public Opinion Research

Source: Compiled by the authors.

Data can also be gathered from trade association research. The National Restaurant Association (NRA) collects information on food eaten away from home and the latest trends on new foods, diners' preferences, and spending patterns. Forty-two percent of the household food dollar is spent on food eaten away from home, and August is the most popular month to eat out, according to information retrieved from the NRA website.[16] *American Demographics* and *Brandweek* are other sources of information on consumer trends and buying practices.[17] *Brandweek*, for instance, reports that women were targeted with an advertising campaign for a new cereal fortified with nutrients and vitamins (Harmony™) that described the product as a "support system for women."[18]

After gathering the secondary data, the nutritionist should assess what is lacking. Once gaps in the collected secondary data are identified, primary data collection should begin.

Primary Data

Primary data is information collected from focus groups, observations, mail or telephone surveys, interviews, and the like. Primary data help to focus the problem and define targeted audiences. For example, after interviewing mothers with young children, it was uncovered that fresh fruit was not being offered to children at home. The parents did not lack knowledge about the health benefits of fruits and vegetables, but the local supermarket had closed recently. Parents now shopped at a local convenience store where only a limited variety of fresh produce was available and was more expensive than what had been available at the supermarket.

Collecting primary data can provide insight on the attitudes, beliefs, and consequent nutrition and health behaviors of a population. For example, if a cultural group (e.g., Chinese American, Indian American, or Latin American) believes in the humoral theory of health, where illnesses are classified as either "hot" or "cold," and remedies and food are classified into the same two categories, a "hot" illness needs to be treated with a "cold" remedy to bring the body into balance.[19] A person ill with a cold might not be willing to consume orange juice because orange juice is classified as a "cold" food by humoral theory health practitioners.[20]

Qualitative and Quantitative Data

Primary information includes qualitative and quantitative data. Qualitative data are usually obtained from small samples of the targeted group; interviewers frequently use open-ended questions in focus-group formats or in-depth interviews with key informants to obtain knowledge about the problem. Key informants are individuals who are knowledgeable about the targeted population and can provide insight and history on the specific problem. Because of the small sample size, the results cannot be generalized to the larger target population. Stakeholders should also be interviewed. They are individuals who are interested in addressing the problem, such as the community health educator, the school nurse, or the area Director on Aging.

Formative evaluation uses qualitative data to help understand attitudes, beliefs, and perceptions. Formative evaluation is undertaken during the development of a social marketing program. It includes pre-testing of ideas and materials, allowing for revisions prior to implementing the full program.[21]

Quantitative data are objective indices from a selected sample where results are expressed in numerical terms. As an example of quantitative data, Yussman reports "17% of adolescents and children reported using herbal remedies."[22] Both qualitative and quantitative data are used in the planning of social marketing strategies.

Market Segmentation

Market segmenting is used to target a social marketing strategy to a particular group. Rather than apply the "average" approach where mean age, income, and education are used to produce an "average American,"[23] market segmenting more narrowly focuses groups (e.g., Latina American women, adolescents, urban dwellers).

Market segmentation is based on:

- *Demographics:* Age, race, sex, income, education
- *Geographics:* Country, state, urban/rural, climate
- *Psychographics:* Attitudes, values, beliefs, personality traits
- *Behavior:* Benefits wanted, usage

To best tailor your marketing strategy, it is important to identify the market segment. Subgroups within populations may be further segmented; for instance, African Americans might be subcategorized into men with hypertension and men without hypertension. Individuals with diabetes might be subcategorized into low-literacy individuals with diabetes and high-literacy individuals with diabetes.

It is important in social marketing to consider the multicultural nature and beliefs of our society (Table 26-2) and the media habits of the various ethnic groups.[24] Even when a marketing campaign is targeted to Asian Americans, you may want to subdivide this market even further. For example, is the population you want to reach Chinese American or Vietnamese American? Both groups share many cultural values, but there are differences as well. Most Asian cultures are rooted in Confucianism, where deferring to the father/husband and holding elders in high esteem is part of the Confucian practice.[25,26] However, the extent to which these behaviors and cultural norms are practiced may be influenced by how long the group has lived in the United States, income level, and education (Table 26-3).

**TABLE 26-2   African-Origin Beliefs Compared with Beliefs
of Other American Subcultures**

African-Origin Beliefs	American Mainstream Beliefs	Latin American–Origin Beliefs	Asian-Origin Beliefs
Spirituality: Powers greater than humans exist and are at work.	Humans can shape their destiny if God is willing.	God shapes our destiny.	Mixed.
Harmony: Humans and their environment are interdependent and connected, as are the parts of their lives.	Humans can shape their environment for humanity's betterment.	Same as American mainstream.	Same as African-origin.
Movement: A rhythmic orientation to life, is manifested in music and dance, behavior, and approach.	Life and time are linear, progress is important.	Resist change, rely on traditions.	Same as African-origin.
Verve: A preference for tuning in to several stimuli rather than a singular orientation; energy and intensity.	Achievement and competition directed; specialized roles; play fair; keep busy.	Preserve relationships over achievement; individual style important.	Preserve group cohesion; self unimportant.
Affect: Emotional expressiveness and sensitivity to emotional cues; feelings and cognition integrated.	Feeling and thinking are separate.	Same as African-origin.	Little emotion expressed.
Communalism: Interdependence of people; a social orientation.	Individualistic orientation.	Same as African-origin.	Same as African-origin.
Expressive individualism: Focus on a person's unique style and spontaneity.	Mixture of social conformity and individual expression.	Social conformity.	Social conformity.

African-Origin Beliefs	American Mainstream Beliefs	Latin American– Origin Beliefs	Asian-Origin Beliefs
Orality: Importance of information learned and transmitted orally; call and response.	Low context, words equal message; direct; superiority of written word.	High context, relationship determines style; indirect.	Same as Latin-origin.
Social time perspective: Time viewed in terms of the event rather than the clock.	Linear concept of time and future orientation.	Social time and past orientation.	Time is circular and social.

Source: Adapted from Willis (1992), Carr-Ruffino (1996), Hammond and Morrison (1996), de Mooij (1998), Hofstede (1997) as printed in Tharp M. *Marketing and Consumer Identity in Multicultural America*, pp.181–182. © 2001 by Sage Publications. Reprinted with permission of Sage Publications, Inc.

TABLE 26-3   Selected Sociodemographic Characteristics of the Population 18 Years and Older by Race/Ethnicity

Race	Income 3-Year Average 2000–2002	Not High School Graduate (Percent)	High School Graduate or Higher (Percent)	Less than Bachelor's Degree/Some College (Percent)	Bachelor's Degree or Higher (Percent)
Caucasian	$47,194	16.3	83.7	75.2	24.8
African American	$29,982	22.4	77.6	85.1	14.9
Hispanic American	$33,946	42.8	57.2	90.6	9.4
Asian/Pacific Islander American	$54,999	12.6	87.4	57.4	42.6

Source: Reprinted with permission. Available at:
http://www.census.gov/hhes/income/income02/3yr_avg_race.html and
http://www.census.gov/population/socdemo/education/ppl-169/tab01a.pdf.

The *¡Salud! campaign* targeted Latino American children and their caregivers to increase knowledge of folic acid's effect on neural tube defects. The campaign was culturally sensitive and included public service announcements (PSAs) in both Spanish and English. Latina celebrities were used in advertisements on billboards, buses, and bus stop shelters, and in magazines and newspapers. Seventy-seven percent of those surveyed responded that they were aware of the ¡Salud! campaign. The number of individuals who knew about the positive association between folic acid and the decrease in neural tube detects, although small, increased by 10%.[27]

Age can also be a factor when segmenting a market. Different generations have different identifying characteristics (Table 26-4). For example, adults over the age of 45 have contributed to an increase in alcohol consumption at dinner because of their exposure to the message that alcohol may decrease heart disease.[28] Children are another segmented market, one with influence on purchasing decisions. For example, 40% of children were considered to have "a lot of influence" on the purchasing of cold cereal.[29] By using market segmenting, a customized plan and strategy can be developed that increases the likelihood of yielding greater success.

The Social Marketing Mix

In traditional business marketing, the specific combination of marketing elements used to achieve objectives and satisfy the target market is known as the marketing mix. Those variables over which an organization has control include the four Ps of marketing: product, place, price, and promotion.[30] Social marketing plans also use the four Ps, and some authors espouse additional Ps for social marketing, such as partnership, policy, politics, positioning, publics and purse strings.[31-33] These additional Ps, with the possible exception of Positioning, usually pertain to the uncontrollable variables of the marketing environment. Alcalay and Bell[33] regard "Positioning" as "a psychological construct that involves the location of the product relative to other products and activities with which it competes." As such, the nutrition program manager must position the product to maximize benefits and minimize costs. For instance, breast-feeding could be repositioned as a way for a family to establish a special relationship with their child from birth, as was done in the National WIC (Special Supplemental Nutrition Program for Women, Infants, and Children) Breast-feeding Promotion Project (described further later in this chapter).[34]

TABLE 26-4   Characteristics to Consider When Planning a Social Marketing Campaign for Different Generations

Veteran Generation (born before 1945)	Baby Boomers (born 1946–1965)	Generation X (born 1966–1976)	Generation Y (born 1977–1994)
Fastest growing group of Internet users is over age 55.	Were socialized to do work; workaholics; married later, had children later.	Environmentally conscious.	Have a lack of future expectation; most multicultural generation.
Military/war background; influential voters.	Think work is recreation; are very competitive.	Humor is critical for communication; loud music; fast moving images.	Computers and the Internet are natural to them; media savvy.
Like gadgets; are patient; conservative; range from fixed income to substantial investments.	Have high levels of expectations; optimistic; idealistic; interested in social causes.	Want the truth directly; cynical.	Will live in smaller families with single parents; 75% have working moms.
Respect teachers because of rank; polite; use proper grammar.	Value education; treat them as though they are young.	Invented casual clothes at work.	Family values are very important; have much in common with their grandparents.
Dislike off-color humor or language.	Have a lot of info but little hands-on experience.	Technology is very important; use minimal written material.	Use hands-on, interactive creativity and games.
Like to interact with people, not machines.	Know how to share.	Demand more visual variety on the page.	There are more of them than there are baby boomers.
Don't like to be put on the spot.	Are obsessive about themselves; "me" generation.	Do not read for pleasure; give short bits of information.	Want to make money and have less stress in life.

Source: Compiled by the author from: Marconi J. *Future Marketing.* Lincolnwood, IL: NTC Business Books, 2001; Stetter L. *Learning with Style.* Boston, MA: Pottruck Technology Resource Center, Simmons College, May 22, 2003; and Tharp M. *Marketing and Consumer Identity in Multicultural America.* Thousand Oaks, CA: Sage Publications, 2001.

Product

In traditional business marketing, the product is either tangible (a good) or intangible (a service or an idea). Public health nutrition products are usually intangible (e.g., distributing weight-control counseling, consulting on developing food service menus). Tangible public health nutrition products might include such things as humanitarian rations distributed to populations in disaster-stricken areas or surplus dry milk powder distributed to low-income populations. In stark contrast to business marketing, the social marketing product may be offered or provided to the customer without considering whether the customer wants or needs the product. For example, a patient diagnosed with diabetes or cardiovascular disease may be automatically referred for nutrition counseling whether or not the service is wanted. To overcome reluctance or outright denial of service benefits, the product must be carefully designed, implemented, and followed up to maximize the probability of the patient's acceptance of a need for the service and eventual beneficial behavior change.

Nutrition Program Product Design

Designing a nutrition program product that will have maximum potential for success requires careful planning. Some factors to consider include:

- Naming the product (establishing a brand)
- Product packaging
- Differentiating the product from its competitors
- Considering product lifetime
- Continually revising to adapt to a changing market environment.

As an example, consider the National WIC Breast-feeding Promotion Project described by the Social Marketing Institute.[34] Started in 1989, the breast-feeding project failed to effect significant behavioral changes in the WIC population. When the product, breast-feeding as a medical health decision, was redefined to emphasize the loving bond the mother would share with her child, breast-feeding rates in the target population rose significantly both in-hospital and at 6 months postpartum.

Read more about the Social Marketing Institute at http://www.social-marketing.org.

In packaging the product, planners considered that focusing on the emotional benefits of breast-feeding would be more appealing to the target audience than focusing solely on the health benefits of breast-feeding. They differentiated the product from its competitor (formula feeding) by positioning the product in the target audience's view in a specific and appealing way (familiar bonding from birth), and also by defining and understanding all aspects of the competition's product, including the competing product's related components of price, place, and promotion.

When developing a nutrition product, include long-range planning to ascertain the probable lifetime of the product. Remember that the marketing environment is dynamic and that today's ideal product may be obsolete in the future due to changes in, for example, technology or public policy. Just as the successful business marketer looks beyond the product being designed to forecast future needs and demands of the consumer, so too does the successful social marketer include strategic planning as part of product development. The National WIC Breast-feeding Promotion Project was succeeded at the U.S. Department of Agriculture (USDA) by the Fathers Supporting Breast-feeding project,[35] targeting African American fathers to positively influence a mother's decision to breast-feed. This change was made as a result of strategic planning coupled with National WIC Breast-feeding Promotion Project evaluation results.

Pre-testing the Nutrition Program Product

Pre-testing the product, using a sample of the target market, will provide useful information on the appropriateness of the product's design. The National WIC Breast-feeding Promotion Project was pre-tested in 10 states from 1996 to 2000.[34] The only state with pre-testing data at this writing is Iowa, which showed an increase in awareness of the breast-feeding messages targeted in the campaign and more positive attitudes on breast-feeding.[36]

Place

"Place" denotes the location where tangible goods are offered and also includes the product's distribution system, that is, the channels through which the product is offered to the target market (including storage, transport, sales, and delivery). For intangible products, place may denote the location where a service is offered, including the channels through which the target market will be reached (e.g., clinics, hospitals, daycare centers, congregate meal sites, shopping malls, agricultural fairs, in-home demonstrations). When considering place, remember to ensure that the product will be accessible to the target market and that product delivery is of high quality.

When place was considered for the National WIC Breast-feeding Promotion Project, the partners focused on identifying the places where mothers and their friends and relatives would seek infant care information: homes, hospitals, and birthing centers. Additional partnerships were formed to develop the distribution channels; hospital environments were made more supportive of breast-feeding mothers; and other breast-feeding promotion organizations and professional associations were called upon to endorse and disseminate the program.[34]

Price

"Price" is perhaps the most critical component of the marketing mix for both traditional business and social marketing, because price is the component most evident to the consumer in the target market. In business marketing, price is often a competitive tool and can assist a business to develop product image.[37] In most cases, business marketers establish a product's price so that the business will profit and the consumer will be happy with the value received. Social marketers, however, are not usually interested in generating a profit. (Remember that the ultimate objective in social marketing is to effect a behavioral change that will benefit the individual, the community, or the society.) In social marketing situations where money is involved as part of the exchange between parties, program managers may want to recover all or a portion of their costs for goods or services. They must then develop a pricing strategy that will not negatively affect participation in the program. Options range from full-cost recovery through sliding-scale fees to "suggested donations." A public fundraising campaign aimed outside the target market might also be employed. For example, too low a price may diminish the consumer's perception of product quality, whereas too high a price might be unaffordable for some consumers. A free product not only might diminish perception of product quality, but also might diminish the consumer's sense of self-esteem.[38]

In social marketing, the price component is often not monetary; rather, it may be based on such intangibles as time, effort, disapproval, or embarrassment. If these costs are thought to outweigh the benefits, then the consumer will perceive the product's value to be low and will be less likely to "buy."[38]

The pricing strategy for the National WIC Breast-feeding Promotion Project aimed to minimize or eliminate the barriers (perceived costs) to breast-feeding for new and prospective mothers. Women who doubted their breast-feeding ability, those who perceived breast-feeding to be embarrassing, and those for whom breast-feeding conflicted with active lifestyles and relationships were targeted. For each group of women, public education materials and a counseling program were developed so that healthcare providers could assist them in identifying and working through the misperceptions.[34]

Promotion

Promotion is the means to introduce the product to the targeted audience. Promotion involves communicating a message through a variety of media to create awareness and promote action. The 5-A-Day campaign, for example, is a promotion to encourage the public to eat five or more servings of fruits and vegetables per day. The campaign is a joint venture between the National Cancer Institute (NCI) and the industry group, Produce for a Better Health Foundation. The 5-A-Day promotion includes a fruit and vegetable of the month with corresponding recipes.[39]

Advertising

Advertising is an important part of a promotional campaign. Advertising can take many different forms, from print to television. Advertising is expensive; therefore, choosing the correct medium is important. *Reach* and *frequency* are important to consider when selecting the advertising medium. Reach refers to the number of people exposed to a message during a given period of time (how many people the message will "reach"). Frequency is the number of times an individual will be exposed to the message.[21] Paying for expensive advertising that does not reach the targeted audience, is a costly mistake. Sometimes, lower-level ad campaigns, such as flyers, are more effective than television advertising. Flyers can saturate a particular neighborhood on bulletin boards, as health fair handouts, on car windshields (check local ordinances), or packed with groceries at a local supermarket. Advertising of any kind needs to be more than a one-time event.

The targeted population must be reminded of the action to take, and reinforcement is needed for behavior change to occur. Advertising, as part of a social marketing campaign, may promote social/nutritional services such as School Breakfast or Meals on Wheels. Table 26-5 outlines a social marketing campaign to increase participation in the School Breakfast program.[40] The Food for Thought campaign uses a cost-effective combination of live delivery, publicity, public relations, and advertising techniques to maximize the potential for exposure and success.

Advertising must be accurate, its message must be clear and consistent, and the main points must be repeated. The message must be relevant to the target population. For example, children are interested in food that tastes good and is "fun," whereas adults are interested in nutritional value.[41] The advertisement should also stress the action to be taken. The National Diabetes Education Program, for example, in a radio public service announcement (PSA) tells listeners to serve more fruits and vegetables, lean cuts of meat, and high fiber foods (Figures 26-1 and 26-2).

An advertisement can be amusing or frightening, provide a testimonial, or use a celebrity spokesperson. Whatever tone the advertisement takes must be acceptable to the targeted population. PSAs are advertisements for a social action or cause. Television and radio stations set aside free airtime for PSAs to meet Federal Communications Commission requirements. However, most PSAs are aired during non-primetime hours, limiting the reach of the PSA.[42]

**TABLE 26-5   Food for Thought Campaign, Phase 1:
School Breakfast Program Theme: "GET A JUMP ON THE DAY!"**

	Students	Parents	Education Professionals
Message to Each Audience	"Breakfast at school is cool."	"Your child needs breakfast."	"Your students will do better if they eat breakfast."
Live Delivery Formats to Launch Campaign	• "Kickoff" assembly • Give out healthy breakfast pack (mini-box cereal, fruit, juice, nutrition tips booklet, bulletin for parents) • Jump rope demo/contest • Health teacher speaks	• PTO meeting • Show samples of healthy breakfast pack • Walk-through nutrition tips & bulletin information • Give out new applications for monetary aid	• Teachers' meeting • School committee meeting • Show samples of healthy breakfast pack • Give out educators' flyer & discuss points therein

Publicity	• Poster:
	  – in schools
	  – in libraries
	  – in civic centers
	  – in city stores
		• Poster:
		  – in supermarkets
		  – in libraries
		  – in civic centers
		  – in city stores
			• Poster
			  – in schools
			  – in libraries
			  – in city stores

Public Relations Activities	• TV PSAs (network & cable) • Radio PSAs • School newspaper articles (where available)	• TV & radio talk shows • TV PSAs (network & cable) • Radio PSAs • Newspaper articles	• TV & radio talk shows • TV PSAs (network & cable) • Radio PSAs • Newspaper articles
Advertising Activities	• :30 TV spot (cable) • :60 radio spot • Print ad in school newspaper	• :30 TV spot (cable) • :60 radio spot • Print ad	• :30 TV spot (cable) • :60 radio spot • Print ad

Source: Reprinted with permission from Massachusetts Department of Education, 1993.

Healthy Celebrations (:60 PSA)

American Indians, here's an important message from the [organization]. As American Indians, we gather for many ceremonies and celebrations. There's nothing harder for family members and friends with diabetes than making healthy food choices at a big feast. Let them know you're on their side. Offer a variety of low-fat, high-fiber foods. That means lots of fruits and vegetables. Cut the fat by serving lean cuts of beef and mutton, fish, and poultry without the skin. Use vegetable oil instead of lard in your cooking. And serve more high-fiber foods, like corn, beans, squash, and whole grain breads. Make your next gathering a celebration of healthy eating for everyone. Make it a time to help your loved ones control their diabetes for life. Call **[organization]** at **[phone number]** to learn more.

FIGURE 26-1 National Diabetes Education Program Indian Campaign: Healthy Celebrations Live-Read Radio Script
Source: Sponsored by the National Diabetes Education Program, a joint program of the National Institutes of Health and the Centers for Disease Control and Prevention.

Websites

How do you get consumers to use Internet websites? Websites can be referenced in your print advertisements or your radio and television PSAs. Consumers should be given the site's Uniform Resource Locator (URL), so that they can log on to the website for more information. If a consumer has not seen your promotional materials but uses the Internet to find information, the nutritionist or health organization needs to make sure that the website is included in the major search engines' referencing systems. A fee will be charged by a search engine for an organization to be included in its database.[43] Also, where a website link appears in a search engine's results is important. Is the website the first one listed, or the fiftieth? How many times a website is visited ("hits") is valuable information and should be tallied using readily available automatic counters.

We suggest the following steps for Internet marketing:

1. Acquire a domain name.
2. Build a website.
3. Put the website on a server.
4. Promote the site.
5. Update the site.[43]

Personal Selling

Personal selling is another tool used in promotional campaigns. Personal selling is achieved through one-to-one counseling, group meetings, roundtable discussions, classes, presentations, telephone conversations, and electronic mail (email). Characteristics of positive personal selling include the following:

Healthy Family Reunion (:30 PSA)

There's nothing harder for a person with diabetes than making healthy food choices at a big family reunion. Let your family members with diabetes know you're on their side. Serve a variety of low-fat, high-fiber foods. That means lots of fruits and vegetables . . . lean meats, fish, and chicken . . . whole grain breads, peas, and beans. Help your family members control their diabetes for life. Call **[organization]** at **[phone number]** to learn more.

FIGURE 26-2   National Diabetes Education Program, African American Campaign: Healthy Reunion Live-Read Script
Source: Sponsored by the National Diabetes Education Program, a joint program of the National Institutes of Health and the Centers for Disease Control and Prevention.

- Initiating positive contacts, not negative situations
- Being reliable, not unavailable
- Making recommendations, not demands
- Using candid, not accommodative language
- Using "we" problem-solving, not "I want" language
- Using easily understood terms or local jargon, not long, scientific explanations
- Showing respect and concern, not disdain, hostility, or indifference
- Being courteous, not abrupt
- Being attentive, not interruptive[44]

Public Relations
Public relations is a means to gather free publicity for your product, business, service, or idea. Public relations is a valuable component of a social marketing campaign. Although publicity is free, time and materials are not. It is important to develop publicity objectives for guidance to advance your social marketing agenda. Examples of public relations that can garner publicity include:

- Health fairs
- Athletic events (walkathons, road races, golf tournaments)
- Cook-offs, cooking demonstrations, and taste testings
- Fruit and vegetable gardening competitions
- Weight loss and physical activity competitions
- Nutrition poster design contests
- Eating clubs

Any of these activities can be sponsored with other like-minded organizations, such as the American Heart Association, the President's Council on Physical Fitness, or the Fruit and Vegetable Grower's Association. An example of a joint public relations activity is the "Milk Run," a 10K road race sponsored by the Massachusetts Dietetic Association in collaboration with the Milk Promotion Board. Activities associated with the event include:

- A carbohydrate-loading dinner available to all race registrants
- A series of nutrition talks
- Booths with nutrition information open to the public the day of the race

By holding the Milk Run a week prior to the Boston Marathon, some world-class athletes were in the city and ran the Milk Run as a warm-up for the marathon. Because elite runners participated in this road race, there was more media coverage of the event than might otherwise have occurred. Press releases, PSAs, and media interviews were a few of the publicity activities that the Dietetic Association's public relations committee provided during the months leading up to the race.

Other means to achieve publicity objectives include:

- Public speaking at community events, schools, and senior centers
- Writing nutrition columns for local newspapers
- Providing short nutrition messages for local radio stations
- Acting as a nutrition resource expert for the media on late-breaking nutrition news

Because this publicity is free, you have limited control over where, when, and how the information will be used. Few professional writers will send you copy of an interview for your approval before publication, although nutritionists have occasionally reviewed copy of an interview for accuracy. A nutrition television spot may end up being cut during editing, so your PSA may be aired at 2 a.m. For successful publicity when working with the media, you must be prepared to:

- Develop a fact sheet on your issues
- Have photographs and other props available for media interviews
- Provide anecdotal information that personalizes your message
- Develop case histories of interesting people who achieved positive health outcomes

Send query letters and press releases, or call local newspapers, television stations, and radio stations to promote your nutrition topic. Discuss why this topic is of interest to audiences. Do not be discouraged if inroads are not made immediately; be persistent. If a reporter or writer needs a quote from a nutrition professional, your name may come to mind. If you receive a call from a media person, be prompt in returning the call; the caller usually has a deadline to meet. If a reporter knows you are prompt with your reply and that you have interesting information, you are more likely to be called again. This starts the building of a media relationship.

Public relations is not only publicity, but also includes providing the following:

- Comfortable and user-friendly environments to obtain nutrition services
- Locations that are accessible
- Operating times that are convenient for customers
- Helpful personnel
- Education materials that are clear and easy to read

All of these qualities can generate goodwill from the customer and positive "word of mouth" publicity to their family and friends.

Evaluation

Important components of any social marketing effort are evaluation and estimating success. Evaluation is an ongoing process and should not be left until the entire project is complete. Evaluation should start with the inception of the idea and the problem to study. The following questions are important to consider at the beginning of the evaluation process:

- How do we define the problem?
- What are our goals and objectives?
- Who is the market we want to reach?
- What information do we have about the problem and the target market?
- What is our message?
- What communication media will we use?
- Will they be cost effective?
- What is the timing?
- How will we measure our goals and objectives?
- How will we evaluate the program?[45]

There are three types of evaluation to consider when assessing your social marketing campaign: *formative evaluation*, *process evaluation*, and *outcome evaluation*.

Formative Evaluation

Formative evaluation begins during the development of the social marketing program. Formative evaluation helps to define the problem and to refine possible interventions. It includes pre-testing of ideas, procedures, and materials, and using focus groups, surveys, and interviews.[21] For example, you may ask, "Did the target market understand the PSA message?" "Was the print material at a readability level appropriate to the audience?" "Was the action requested of the target market realistic?" This type of information allows revisions to be made before the full program is implemented.

Process Evaluation

Process evaluation assesses the implementation of the social marketing program. Did the plan proceed as outlined? Did the PSA air during the appropriate month? Were print materials delivered in adequate quantities to the correct locations? Are activities occurring according to schedule? Did the program reach the target market?[21] Process evaluation uses continuous quality improvement (CQI) to monitor progress. CQI is a tool based on the premise that there is always room for improvement.[46] Customers are asked how satisfied they are with the services, materials, venues, and costs associated with a program. CQI has been used in healthcare, including nutrition services, since the 1990s.[47-50]

Outcome Evaluation

Outcome evaluation (sometimes referred to as *summative evaluation*) determines whether the goals and objectives of the social marketing campaign are met.[21] It is important that the goals and objectives are well defined at the inception of the social marketing process, otherwise it is difficult to measure the success of meeting them. Goals and objectives should be specific in order for them to be evaluated effectively. An example of an objective that can be measured is: "Twenty percent of the target audience/market will increase fruit and vegetable consumption by 1 serving within 3 months of initiating the campaign."

Marketing Ethics

The opening years of the 21st century were marked by several major business scandals in the United States and other countries.[51-54] In this climate, it is important to revisit the topic of business ethics, in general, and of marketing ethics, in particular.

Whether engaging in business or social marketing, the marketer must begin with a strong code of personal ethics. With a good sense of the moral principles and values that govern individual and group behavior within a society, one can reliably choose the right and just action when faced with a moral dilemma. Ethics courses may be found in colleges and universities, and ethics may be incorporated into the curriculum in elementary and high schools. However, the elementary school curriculum is not consistent across the country, and there is debate about the best approach for teaching ethics (AKA "building character"[55]) as well as over where and when ethics can be taught. Many believe that codes of personal ethics are already formed by the time a person enters college,[56] and there is evidence that geographic and cultural variables affect the process.[57,58] Others hold that ethics can be taught at the college level.[59,60] It is evident that the process of ethical development is multifactorial and that some elements of truth may be found in each of the disparate views.

Kerin and colleagues[61] hold that in marketing, ethics are concerned with personal morals and values in juxtaposition with organizational, legal, and societal morals and values. Situations present themselves in an ethical, legal matrix in which technically legal actions could be viewed as unethical, or in which ethical actions may not be seen as legal. In such an environment, the nutritionist must learn to think and plan like a marketer, under the guidance of personal ethics informed by sociocultural, business/industry, and corporate ethical guidelines. (See Chapter 1 for a review of ethical considerations in public health.)

Traditional business ethics in the last century were largely guided by the principle of *caveat emptor*. By the 1990s, consumer interests had overtaken those of business, ushering in an era of "consumer sovereignty."[62] Although exceptions exist, today most traditional business marketing ethics are guided by the principle that the customer's wants and needs are paramount, and profit-generating activities are aimed at customer satisfaction. Social marketers, too, are focused on the customer, but with the ultimate aim of improving their personal welfare and that of their society.[4] Thus, the social marketer faces ethical challenges that are not seen in traditional business marketing, challenges that are only now being identified and studied.[63] As the dimensions of marketing ethics in both traditional business and social marketing contexts are explored and debated, the nutritionist, drawing on a strong personal code of ethics, would do well to follow the guidelines of the American Dietetic Association's Code of Ethics.[64]

Caveat emptor—The principle in commerce that the buyer *alone* is responsible for assessing the quality of a purchase before buying.

Consumer sovereignty—Alludes to the power consumers have in directing market economies because goods and services are produced and exchanged mostly to satisfy consumer desires.

In closing this overview of marketing ethics, we must point out that many of the ethical dilemmas that a public health nutritionist is likely to face will arise from cultural differences between the nutritionist and the client or the population being served. The United States is a multicultural land with minority ethnic populations from most parts of the world. When serving those whose ethnic backgrounds differ from your own, make an effort to understand the societal culture and norms that govern them, as well as those that underlie the prevailing U.S. societal culture and norms. When entering into partnerships with multinational or global organizations, be sure to consider the often-great differences in marketing ethics of the cultures represented.[65-70]

Issues for Discussion

1. How can a nutritionist promote healthful eating practices to people who are convinced that a currently popular diet plan is appropriate for everyone?
2. What opportunities exist for a public health agency to form partnerships to address the need for people to consume water for optimum health while conserving water for protection of the resource?
3. How can and should a nutritionist approach promoting healthful eating practices for children in partnerships with multinational fast food and toy companies?

References

1. National Public Health Leadership Institute. CB #8165, Chapel Hill, NC 27599-8165; http://www.phli.org:9018/. February 11, 2002. Available at: http://www.phli.org:9018/Marketingconference. Accessed June 07, 2004.
2. Pride WM, Ferrell OC. *Marketing: Concepts and Strategies.* 12th ed. Boston, MA: Houghton Mifflin Co.; 2003:4.
3. Kotler P, Zaltman G. Social marketing: An approach to planned social change. *J Marketing.* 1971;35:5.
4. Andreasen AR. *Marketing Social Change: Changing Behavior to Promote Health, Social Development, and the Environment.* San Francisco: Jossey-Bass; 1995:7.
5. Andreasen AR, Kotler P. *Strategic Marketing for Nonprofit Organizations.* 6th ed. Englewood Cliffs, NJ: Prentice-Hall; 2003:15.
6. Andreasen AR. Marketing social marketing in the social change marketplace. *J Public Policy & Marketing.* 2002;21:3.
7. Kotler P, Roberto E. *Social Marketing.* New York: The Free Press; 1989:24.
8. Andreasen AR. Social marketing: Definition and domain. *J Public Policy & Marketing.* 1994;13:108.
9. Maibach EW. Explicating social marketing: What is it, and what isn't it? *Social Marketing Q.* 2002;8:7.
10. Kotler P, Roberto E. *Social Marketing: Strategies for Changing Public Behavior.* New York: The Free Press; 1989:290.
11. California Department of Health Services. California Project LEAN: Leaders Encouraging Activity and Nutrition. Available at: http://www.californiaprojectlean.org/programs. Accessed May 21, 2004.
12. U.S. Department of Agriculture, Food & Nutrition Service. TEAM Nutrition. Available at: http://www.fns.usda.gov/tn. Accessed May 21, 2004.
13. Sloan AE. The top 10 functional food trends: The next generation. *Food Technol.* 2002;56:32.

14. Gruber AJ, Pope Jr. HJ, Lalonde JK, Hudson JI. Why do young women diet? The roles of body fat, body perception, and body ideal. *J Clin Psychiat.* 2001;62:609.

15. Kris-Etherton PM, Harris WS, Appel LJ. American Heart Association Nutrition Committee: Fish consumption, fish oil, omega-3 fatty acids, and cardiovascular disease. *Circulation.* 2002;106:2747.

16. National Restaurant Association. Available at http://www.restaurant.org. Accessed June 8, 2004.

17. Marconi J. *Future Marketing.* Chicago: American Marketing Association, NTC Business Books; 2001:46.

18. Reyes S. Shopping list: Quick, classic, cool for kids. *Brandweek.* June 17, 2002;43:S52.

19. Bogumil C. Humoral theory in cultural food beliefs. June 10, 2002. Available at: http://food.oregonstate.edu/ref/culture/humoral.html. Accessed June 8, 2004.

20. Beijing Medboo Health Center. Traditional Chinese Dietotherapy. Available at: http://www.ontcm.com/healthy/foods.htm. Accessed June 8, 2004.

21. U.S. Department of Health and Human Services. *Making Health Communication Programs Work: A Planner's Guide.* NIH Publication No. 92–1493. Washington, DC: National Cancer Institute; April 1992.

22. Yussman SM, Auinger P, Weitzman M, Ryan SA. Complementary and alternative medicine use in children and adolescents. *J Adolesc Health.* 2002;30:105.

23. Tharp MC. *Marketing and Consumer Identity in Multicultural America.* Thousand Oaks, CA: Sage Publications; 2001:13.

24. Ibid., 113.

25. Ibid., 263.

26. Wong AM. *Target: The U.S. Asian Market.* Palos Verdes, CA: Pacific Heritage; 1997:69.

27. Perez-Escamilla R, Himmelgreen D, et al. Marketing nutrition among urban Latinos: the !Salud! campaign. *J Am Diet Assoc.* 2000;100:698.

28. Whitaker L. A tasty business. *Psych Today.* 1999;32:52.

29. Gurber S, Berry J. *Marketing To and Through Kids.* New York: McGraw-Hill; 1993:21.

30. Kotler P, Turner RE. *Marketing Management: Analysis, Planning, Implementation, and Control.* Canadian 8th ed. Scarborough, ON: Prentice Hall Canada; 1995:96.

31. Weinreich NK. *Hands-On Social Marketing: A Step-by-Step Guide.* Thousand Oaks, CA: Sage Publications; 1999:5.

32. Mississippi Urban Research Center, Jackson State University, Southern Prevention Intervention Center. What is social marketing? Social marketing tools promote health issues. *Adinkra Newsletter.* Fall 2001;2. Available at: http://www.apinonline.org/Pubs/Newsletters/Adinkra.SPIC-Fall2001_Issue2.pdf. Accessed June 8, 2004.

33. Alcalay R, Bell RA. *Promoting Nutrition and Physical Activity through Social Marketing: Current Practices and Recommendations.* Davis, CA: Center for Advanced Studies in Nutrition and Social Marketing, University of California; 2000:3.

34. Social Marketing Institute. Success Stories: National WIC Breast-feeding Promotion Project. Available at: http://www.social-marketing.org/success/cs-nationalwic.html. Accessed June 9, 2004.

35. U.S. Department of Agriculture, Food & Nutrition Service. Fathers Supporting Breast-feeding. Available at: http://www.fns.usda.gov/wic/Fathers/SupportingBreast-feeding.HTM. Accessed June 9, 2004.

36. Szcodronski H, Dobson B, Losch ME, Bryant C. *Iowa's Implementation of the WIC National Breast-feeding Promotion Project. Loving Support Makes Breast-feeding Work. Project Report and Summary of Findings.* Des Moines, IA: Iowa Department of Public Health; May 2002:29.

37. Spears M. *Foodservice Organizations: A Managerial and Systems Approach*, 4th ed. Upper Saddle River, NJ: Prentice-Hall; 2000:98.

38. Weinreich NK. What Is Social Marketing? Weinreich Communications; 2003. Available at: http://www.social-marketing.com/whatis.html. Accessed May 23, 2004.

39. U.S. Department of Health and Human Services, National Cancer Institute. Five a Day Recipe Box. Available at: http://www.5aday.gov. Accessed June 8, 2004.

40. Massachusetts Department of Education. Food for Thought Campaign. "Get a Jump on the Day"; 1993.

41. Baltas G. The effects of nutrition information on consumer choice. *J Advertising Res.* March–April 2001:57.

42. Small Business Association, Women's Business Center. Public Service Announcements. Available at: http://www.onlinewbc.gov/docs/market/mk_psa_pr.html. Accessed June 4, 2004.

43. Marconi J. *Future Marketing.* Chicago: American Marketing Association, NTC Business Books; 2001:204–210.

44. Kaufman M. *Nutrition in Public Health.* Rockville, MD: Aspen; 1990:308.

45. McDonald MH, Keegan WJ. *Marketing Plans That Work.* Boston, MA: Butterworth Heinemann Publishers; 1997:113, 114.

46. Leebov W Ersoz C. *The Healthcare Manager's Guide to Continuous Quality Improvement.* Lincoln, NE: iUniverse, Inc., Authors Choice Press; 2003.

47. McLaughlin CP, Kaluzny AD. *Continuous Quality Improvement in Healthcare: Theory, Implementation and Applications.* 2nd ed. Boston, MA: Jones & Bartlett; 1999.

48. Knapp ML. Applying continuous improvement to community health. Collaborative effort by the American Society for Quality and the Institute for Healthcare Improvement identifies components of model for community health improvement; model is based on quality improvement techniques. *Quality Progress.* 1998;31:43.

49. Behrens RI, Blocker AK. *Continuous Quality Improvement and Nutritional Care Planning: A Manual for Long-Term Care Facilities.* Rockville, MD: Aspen; 1993.

50. Jackson R. *Continuous Quality Improvement for Nutrition Care.* Amelia Island, FL: American Nutri-Tech, Inc.; 1992.

51. *Economist.* Keeping an eye on business. 2004;371:68.

52. Verschoor CC. Unethical workplace is still with us. *Strategic Finance.* 2004;85:15.

53. Tsianiar B, Shannon E. Cooking the books. *Time*. November 17, 2003;162:55.

54. Colvin G. Scandal outrage, part III. *Fortune*. October 28, 2002;146:56.

55. Davis M. What's wrong with character education? *Am J Educ*. 2003;110:32.

56. Carroll AB, Scherer RW. Business ethics in the current environment of fraud and corruption. *Vital Speeches of the Day*. June 15, 2003;69:529.

57. Mayer D. Community, business ethics, and global capitalism. *Am Business Law J*. 2001;38:215.

58. Barker TS, Cobb SL. A survey of ethics and cultural dimensions of MNCs. *Competitiveness Rev*. 2000;10:123.

59. Lawson RA. Is classroom cheating related to business students' propensity to cheat in the "real world"? *J Business Ethics*. 2004;49:189.

60. Alsop R. The top business schools (a special report): Right and wrong: Can business schools teach students to be virtuous? In the wake of all the corporate scandals, they have no choice but to try. *Wall Street Journal*. September 17, 2003; eastern edition:R9.

61. Kerin RA, Berkowitz EN, Hartley SW, Rudelius W. *Marketing*. 7th ed. New York: McGraw Hill; 2003.

62. Smith NC, Lawler III EE, Berndt ER. Marketing strategies for the ethics era. *Sloan Manage Rev*. 1995;36:85.

63. Brenkert GG. Ethical challenges of social marketing. *J Public Policy & Marketing*. 2002;21:14.

64. American Dietetic Association. Code of ethics for the profession of dietetics. *J Am Diet Assoc*. 1999;99:109.

65. Palazzo B. U.S–American and German business ethics: An intercultural comparison. *J Business Ethics*. 2002;41:195.

66. Pitta DA, Fung H-G. Ethical issues across cultures: Managing the differing perspectives of China and the USA. *J Consumer Marketing*. 1999;16:240.

67. Singhapakdi A, Rawwas MYA. A cross-cultural study of consumer perceptions about marketing ethics. *J Consumer Marketing*. 1999;16:257.

68. Taka I. Business ethics in Japan. *J Business Ethics*. 1997;16:1499.

69. Izraeli D. Business ethics in the Middle East. *J Business Ethics*. 1997;16:1555.

70. Stajkovic AD, Luthans F. Business ethics across cultures: A social cognitive model. *J World Business*. 1997;32:17.

CHAPTER 27

EARNING ADMINISTRATIVE SUPPORT

Jeanette Beasley, MPH, RD

Reader Objectives

After studying this chapter and reflecting on the contents, you should be able to:

1. Review environmental factors that influence the administration's priorities.
2. Describe components of the strategic plan that help to provide insight into administrative goals and objectives.
3. Delineate elements of the community needs assessment that are important to highlight to administrators.
4. Discuss strategies for increasing the administrators' perceived value of the nutrition division, including partnering with other divisions within the agency, working with the policy board, and developing positive relations with the media.
5. Identify potential funding sources to bolster support for nutrition services.

Earning the support of the administration within your agency begins with understanding both external and internal forces influencing agency priorities. By remaining current with the agency's focus, the nutrition division can adapt the nutrition plan to meet the changing needs of the agency and survive in the current healthcare environment.

Another important strategy to increase the relevancy of the nutrition division within your organization is to partner with other divisions sharing common goals. Along with developing positive working relationships internally, involvement with the policy board as well as the local media can increase the exposure and value of the nutrition division in the eyes of both the agency administration and the general public.

In networking with the community, gaps in nutrition-related services may be identified and brought to the attention of the administration. If funding is a barrier to developing a new program, identify potential external funding sources and seek administrative support to apply for grant monies.

The Administration's Perspective

Management and delivery of healthcare services is influenced by economic, political, and social forces. In order to promote nutrition services within your organization, it is critical to analyze the dynamics operating within your agency. By doing so, you will better understand the influences and motivations of the administration. Shortell and Kaluzney (2000) identified several key forces impacting healthcare delivery that have implications for management, and for the nutrition department in particular, including the increased focus on evaluation of programs and services, the integration of information technology, the aging of the population, and changing demographics of the United States that are leading to increased cultural diversity.

Understanding the impact of these trends on the healthcare system is important in ensuring that the nutrition division progresses along with the rest of the agency. In this environment of increased accountability, evaluating both the implementation and the effectiveness of existing nutrition programs and services is now routinely expected. Nutrition departments that integrate information technology into daily practices will be more time and cost efficient. Reaching out to elderly populations by implementing programs to improve food security for community members who do not have convenient access to grocery stores is an example of addressing the aging of the population.

> An excellent web-based source for nutrition information in a large number of diverse languages is available at http://ethnomed.org/ethnomed/patient_ed/ and http://www.spiral.tufts.edu.

Consider ethnic and cultural diversity by providing nutrition education materials in languages that are highly prevalent in your community, and provide culturally sensitive recipes and meal plans. Examples such as these illustrate to the administration that the nutrition division is current with issues critical to improving the community's public health infrastructure.

Healthy People (HP) 2010 objectives (as discussed in other chapters) provide a framework for understanding national priority areas for health promotion and disease prevention. The 467 objectives in 28 focus areas offer guidelines for focusing program planning within healthcare organizations. Reviewing the HP 2010 objectives listed in the Nutrition and Overweight focus area, along with focus areas related to nutrition including cancer, chronic kidney disease, and diabetes, can provide the nutrition professional with a better understanding of the healthcare needs of the nation, the government's priorities with respect to funding initiatives, and the administrator's perspective. Furthermore, nutrition-related HP 2010 objectives can be used to build administrative support for initiatives. For example, one of the HP 2010 objectives is to "increase the proportion of persons aged 2 years and older who consume at least two daily servings of fruit." Based on Continuing Survey of Food Intakes by Individuals (CSFII) data, 28% of the population currently meets the goal; the HP 2010 target is to increase the percentage of the population consuming two fruits daily to 75%. Presenting this data to the administration provides justification and support for the fruit and vegetable promotion programs within the nutrition division.

> The HP 2010 Nutrition and Overweight focus area is available at: http://www.healthypeople.gov/Document/HTML/Volume2/19Nutrition.htm.
>
> The Continuing Survey of Food Intakes by Individuals (CSFII) is available at: http://www.barc.usda.gov/bhnrc/foodsurvey/Csfii89.html and http://www.pop.psu.edu/data-archive/daman/csfii.htm.

Presenting state and local data, if available, will increase the relevancy of the problem for decision makers. For example, state-level statistics estimating fruit and vegetable consumption, derived from Behavioral Risk Factor Surveillance System (BRFSS) data, are available from the Centers for Disease Control's 5 A Day website. These data can also be used to explain to administrators why a social marketing program will be targeted to a specific high-risk group, because average fruit and vegetable intake can be grouped by demographics, including age, level of education, race, and income level.

> The Behavioral Risk Factor Surveillance System (BRFSS) is available at: http://www.cdc.gov/brfss/.
>
> The Centers for Disease Control's 5 A Day website is available at: http://www.cdc.gov/5aday.

Understanding the Agency Vision and Strategic Plan

The extent to which each of these environmental factors and HP 2010 objectives influence the vision, goals, and objectives of individual public health agencies may be better understood by reviewing the organization's planning documents, such as the strategic plan, annual report, and budget. By reviewing the agency's strategic plan, the nutrition professional will better understand the underlying philosophy of the agency, as well as the current priorities and perspectives of the administrators. The following are the key components of a strategic plan, along with a description of how they can assist you in identifying areas of interest to the agency administration:

- *Mission statement:* Defines the purpose of the organization, and can often provide a better understanding of the underlying philosophy of the agency.

- *Major objectives:* Highlight the priorities of the organization with realistic, measurable, achievable outcomes.
- *Action plan:* Delineates a method for achieving objectives. This section provides an indication of the agency's approach to finding solutions to current issues of interest.
- *Resources needed:* Includes personnel, funds, equipment, and space required to meet objectives. Identify areas where nutrition-related resources could assist in achieving goals, and bring these to the attention of the administrator.
- *Evaluation system:* Delineates the process for assessing the effectiveness of the plan. A description of the evaluation process can provide insight into ways in which the performance of the administration is measured within the organization.

Synergizing with the Strategic Plan

By reviewing the agency's planning documents in concert with the *community needs assessment* (discussed in Chapter 3), public health nutritionists can evaluate whether their role in the organization is meeting the needs of the public they are serving and is within the framework of the organization's goals. Using components of the community needs assessment can be an effective tool in garnering support for nutrition services from administrators, funding agencies, and the public alike. The following list describes how elements of the community needs assessment can be used to directly increase administrative support for nutrition programs:

- *Assessment:* Composed of copious amounts of data related to community demographics, the health and nutrition of community members, perceived needs, and community assets; this section can be reframed for presentation to decision makers to highlight the need for nutrition services in the community. If your assessment included focus group data regarding the impact of the WIC program on participants, share a direct quote from a participant about ways the program can be improved along with program numbers to support these suggestions. By providing both testimonials from community members and data to support initiatives, you are showing the administration that your department is in touch with the needs of the community.
- *Priorities, goals, and objectives:* Present concise, realistic, measurable objectives to the administrators in order to show that the nutrition department is organized around common goals that are relevant to community needs.

- *Nutrition plan:* Use the nutrition plan to highlight the steps required to achieve the stated objectives. Emphasize the assets of the nutrition department, and also identify gaps along with proposed solutions for addressing barriers to achieving the objectives.
- *Implementation:* Summarize the implementation process to the extent needed to highlight the efficiency, organization, and teamwork of the nutrition division in working toward common goals.
- *Evaluation:* As discussed in Chapter 19, evaluating activities of the nutrition division is important for documenting program impact, as well as identifying areas for continuous quality improvement.

Prior to preparing evaluation results for presentation to the administration, review the agency's annual report for ideas on how to format results. For example, if the report relies heavily on charts and graphs rather than qualitative data, recognize that the administrator is more familiar with reviewing quantitative data within agency documents. In addition to increasing the likelihood the administrator will respond favorably to the activities of the nutrition division, results presented in this manner will be more likely to be included in next year's annual report, thereby increasing exposure of the nutrition division's activities to policy makers and budget reviewers.

Partnering to Achieve Shared Goals

Forging partnerships between the nutrition division and groups sharing common goals and objectives provides the opportunity to capitalize on the benefits of combining resources and avoiding the duplication of services. Although the administration's expectations of the nutrition division may seem ambitious given the limited staff and budget allocated to the department, a review of the responsibilities of other divisions within the organization may provide insight into opportunities for working together on initiatives with common goals.

Effective teams focus on the shared purpose of the collaboration by developing goals and priorities required to fulfill the need. In doing so, the process is directed towards a shared commitment, and members identify skills and contributions required for the effort. Fostering positive relations with team members further integrates the nutrition division into the framework of the healthcare organization and provides the potential to increase the overall productivity of the agency.

Relations with the Policy Board

The Board of Health or Board of Directors, often appointed by elected officials, is responsible for approving policies and programs, appointments of personnel, budgets, and legislative initiatives. Special interests of individual board members may influence policy decisions that directly impact the nutrition department. Representing the nutrition division at board meetings and advocating for nutrition-related programs will increase the likelihood that nutrition services will be viewed as important to improving the public's health, rather than being marginalized as major events shift resources to high priority areas. Therefore, it is important for representatives from the nutrition department to attend meetings and interact with board members in order to remain current with the priorities of the Board.

For example, an outbreak of foodborne illness in the community resulting in hospitalizations and lost productivity provides an opportunity for nutritionists to educate food service workers regarding proper procedures for prevention of further outbreaks. By reaching out to the community when the relevancy of the issue is high, you increase the likelihood that food safety tips will be translated into behavior change. Furthermore, the education campaign increases exposure of the nutrition department to the community as well as policy makers, and will show the administrator that the nutrition division is responsive to high-priority health issues within the community.

Communications with the Media

Another opportunity for strengthening both administrative and community support for nutrition-related initiatives is to build a good rapport with the local media. There are several ways to build a relationship with the media, including inviting the media to cover events sponsored by the nutrition division, providing copy for nutrition-related topics of interest to the public, and answering questions for nutrition-related news stories. Each of these methods can promote positive public relations between the public and the public health agency.

Before communicating with the media, it is important to contact both the public relations division within your agency and your administrator to be certain you understand the rules and regulations associated with media communications. For example, you may need to obtain approval of press releases from the public relations department prior to dissemination to media outlets.

Preparing and Distributing Press Kits

Press kits are packets of information describing an event or program written in a format conducive to dissemination by media outlets. Press kits can include a press release, pictures, program logos, press passes to the event, an invitation to participate in the program, and/or fact sheets related to program activities and time lines. By announcing programs and events in advance, the publicity could result in increased attendance and lead to a more successful intervention.

In order to increase the likelihood that your information will be noticed by various local media organizations, including radio, television, and newspaper outlets, ask the public relations department within your agency for strategies that have worked in the past. There may be a particular person at each organization to whom health information press kits should be directed, or a template that facilitates publicizing the event in the format familiar to each specific organization. If your agency doesn't have a public relations department to assist you, contact a colleague who has worked successfully with the organization in the past, or call the organization directly for assistance. For more information on marketing your message, see Chapter 26, *Marketing Nutrition Programs and Services.*

Promoting Nutrition Messages through Media

Nutrition is in the news daily, hitting the headlines with topics ranging from newly released surveillance statistics and epidemiological evidence associating particular foods with risk for cancer to the latest fad diet book extolling the benefits of a particular dietary regimen. The media seeks credible sources to interpret the implications of research findings on the public's health. Registered dietitians have a responsibility to promote evidence-based recommendations based on sound scientific research, and assisting the media in reporting research findings is another way to provide nutrition education. As an added benefit, the media will credit their source, thereby providing an opportunity to promote the image of the nutrition division within your agency.

Once way to establish positive relationships with the media is to offer to write copy for a particular topic area of interest to the media organization. For example, if new research findings are published on the benefits of cruciferous vegetables for reducing cancer risk, you could suggest writing a piece summarizing the evidence and providing tips for preparing cruciferous vegetables for the newspaper's health section. In your correspondence to the editor, outline a few nutrition-related topics you consider to be newsworthy and would be willing to research in order to write an educational piece for the paper. This provides a service to the media, who are often under pressure to meet deadlines, while promoting the image of the nutrition division within your agency as a credible source for health-related information.

Maintain records of newspaper articles, letters to the editor, public service announcements, and any other correspondence the nutrition division has with the media. Estimate the impact of your message by tracking the reach, such as the circulation of the newspaper or the size of the audience for the radio station. If the message was part of a particular nutrition program or service, include this data when writing up the impact evaluation for the project.

Obtaining Financial Support for Nutrition Programs and Initiatives

As the nutrition division reaches out to the community, it is likely that gaps in the public health infrastructure will be identified that are not addressed in the planning documents of the agency. Possible reasons the problem was not addressed in the strategic plan include lack of awareness, no known solutions, or emergence after the development of the strategic plan. In discussing the problem with the administrator, you may both agree that the problem is important and that a workable solution has been proposed, but the administrator does not have the funds to allocate to the proposed program. Discuss the possibility of applying for grants to address the problem. The administrator will likely support proposal writing as a mechanism to increase revenue and appreciate the initiative

TABLE 27-1   Web Resources for Identifying Grant Opportunities

Name	Source
U.S. Department of Health and Human Services	http://www.grants.gov/
Catalog of Federal Domestic Assistance	http://12.46.245.173/cfda/cfda.html
Food and Nutrition Service: WIC Special Project Grants	http://www.fns.usda.gov/oane/MENU/DemoProjects/WICSPG/WICSPG.htm
National Institutes of Health	http://grants.nih.gov/grants/
American Dietetic Association	http://www.eatright.org/Public/7772.cfm
Foundation Center	http://fdncenter.org/
Robert Wood Johnson Foundation	http://www.rwjf.org/index.jsp

displayed by the nutrition division. Obtaining funding from a range of sources also increases the stability and capacity of the nutrition division to provide programs and services.

The administrator may direct you to funding sources likely to be interested in reviewing your proposal. Potential funding sources include the government, foundations, corporations, or charges for services rendered. Several web-based resources are available to identify funding agencies and provide guidance in preparing applications. Given the time-sensitive nature of requests for proposals, searching online funding databases is often more productive than searching through paper-based directories. Table 27-1 provides a list of available web resources for identifying grant opportunities.

Issues for Discussion

1. Discuss why getting internal support for nutrition programs is as important as controlling external variables.
2. Describe how internal marketing is different from external marketing.
3. What is the competition that public health nutrition faces, and why should public health nutrition be maintained?

References

Centers for Disease Control and Prevention, National Center for Chronic Disease Prevention and Health Promotion. Nutrition and Physical Activity, 5 A Day Data and Statistics. Available at: http://apps.nccd.cdc.gov/5ADaySurveillance/. Accessed May 10, 2005.

Culberson, Elaine B. (1990). Earning administrative support. In M. Kauffman (ed.), *Nutrition in Public Health: A Handbook for Developing Programs and Services* (pp. 455–465). Rockville, MD: Aspen.

Liebler, Joan G. & McConnell, Charles R. (1999). Planning. In Liebler & McConnell (ed.), *Management Principles for Health Professionals* (pp. 114–121). Gaithersburg, MD: Aspen.

Porter-O'Grady, Tim & Kreuger Wilson, Cathleen. (1998). *The Healthcare Team Book.* St. Louis, MS: Mosby, pp. 65–70.

Shortell, Stephen M. & Kaluzny, Arnold D. (eds.). (2000). Organization theory and health services management. In Shortell & Kaluzny, *Healthcare Management: Organization, Design, and Behavior.* 4th ed. Albany, NY: Delmar Thomson Learning, pp. 8–9.

Splett, Patricia L. & Roth-Yousey, Lori. (1999). Managing money: Budgeting and grant writing. In A. L. Owen, P. L. Splett, & G. M. Owen (eds.), *Nutrition in the Community: The Art and Science of Delivering Services.* 4th ed. (pp. 493–507). Boston, MA: McGraw-Hill.

U.S. Department of Health and Human Services. (November 2000). *Healthy People 2010: Understanding and Improving Health.* 2nd ed. Washington, DC: U.S. Government Printing Office.

CHAPTER 28

STRIVING FOR EXCELLENCE AND ENVISIONING THE FUTURE

Marcia Thomas, MS, MPH, RD

Pamella Darby, MS, MPH, RD

Reader Objectives

After studying this chapter and reflecting on the contents, you should be able to:

1. Identify the multidisciplinary roles of the public health nutritionist.
2. Describe the ways in which such roles help to advance public health nutrition efforts.
3. Suggest strategies for successful professional development.
4. Describe future challenges and ethical considerations facing public health nutritionists.

Motivation for Excellence

The public health nutritionist has stepped into a 21st century full of both opportunities and challenges. On the one hand, there is an assortment of innovative technologies at our fingertips, technological advances in medicine, and improved methodologies for implementing and evaluating public health interventions. On the other hand, we live and work in communities struggling with obesity, food insecurity, chronic disease, lack of medical insurance, and health disparities. The current health environment leaves us with no other choice but to challenge ourselves professionally, constantly striving for excellence in the field of public health so that we may meet such challenges and advance our efforts.

The motivation to achieve excellence in our field should stem from an understanding that existing opportunities must be embraced in such a way as to foster collective action toward improving the nutritional status of populations. Such opportunities include utilization of innovative technologies, enhanced modes of communication and education, collaboration, advocacy, professional development, and academic training. Globally, health is on the fore-front of political and social agendas, with an ever-increasing awareness and interest in food and nutrition. This chapter seeks to encourage today's nutritionists to confront with confidence the professional demands that arise, prepared to take on the many challenges of our field.

The Multidisciplinary Roles of the Public Health Nutritionist

Most of us enter the field of public health nutrition with the goal of educating the public about healthy eating to prevent and manage illness and disease. What we find when we begin our work is that there is so much more than just food involved in teaching people how to eat well.

The Institute of Medicine's 2003 report, *The Future of the Public's Health in the 21st Century*, encourages a broad training and practice of public health "because integrated interdisciplinary teaching is important to the preparation of a well-trained workforce that is capable of addressing today's broad array of public health issues. . . ."[1] To be effective leaders in today's dynamic health environment, public health nutritionists must take on multidisciplinary roles, often wearing different hats at the same time. Success in the field, which translates to public health action, requires that nutritionists be ready to serve as educators, researchers, and advocates throughout the course of their careers.

Nutrition Educator

A hat we all wear is that of nutrition educator, even though efforts occur on many levels and the characteristics of communities and population groups may vary. Therefore, needs assessments prove invaluable to community nutrition activities and help to provide a framework for program planning and evaluation. From considering the location of supermarkets to cultural beliefs about food and health, ongoing assessment is necessary to understand how to begin and maintain work within populations and communities.

In a time when such huge health disparities exist, public health nutritionists must take on the role of educating the public about those inequalities and helping to move communities towards healthier behaviors. We know that the public values the role of nutrition in prevention of disease, but making dietary changes has proved difficult.[2] To improve results, nutritionists must be included in the planning, implementation, and evaluation of health promotion and disease prevention programs.[3] Furthermore, nutritionists in public health are in the

> **Evidence-based practice—**
> Utilizing nutritional information that is based on scientific studies from reputable sources.

uniquely qualified position to educate not only the lay public, but also other health professionals, policy makers, the media, and private organizations about evidence-based practice.

Nutrition Researcher

Nutritionists in public health settings should also wear the hat of researcher. Investigation is critical to our understanding of the many nutritional concerns and risk factors facing our communities and vital to the development of effective public health practice and interventions. Through dissemination of research, we can reach a larger audience (via publications, presentations, and media) by sharing findings and recommendations for practice to colleagues, policy makers, and the general public.

Not all nutritionists focus full-time on research or become part of large, multidisciplinary studies, such as working as epidemiologists, in academia, or in research centers. Many are involved in research activities that are intertwined in ongoing work such as program evaluation, assessment of intervention effectiveness, or focus groups to qualitatively assess a population of interest. The information collected from nutritionists working within small, local community programs can be extremely valuable to others working within similar environments and may direct work done within a larger population. Frequently, public health nutritionists collect data, but never share their results with others. Program evaluations, small quality assurance projects, and lessons learned from building partnerships should all be shared with the rest of the field and may be just what is needed to help drive future research. In almost all settings, nutritionists can engage in various levels of research, either independently or collaboratively. Nutritionists are encouraged to collect data, as data directs policy and policy drives action. It is our responsibility as public health nutritionists to ensure that policy favors optimal nutrition for all populations. Evidence-based practice is the cornerstone of all health-related initiatives, and therefore the successful public health nutritionist should look at research as a means to turn obstacles into opportunities.

The hallmark of public health inquiry is community-based participatory research (CBPR). CBPR emerged in the past few decades to become a focus of public health research. CBPR differs from community research in that partnerships are built among multidisciplinary teams, where members of the community are active partners in all aspects of the research and have equal weight in the research process. Partners bring their own expertise and interest to the group and view the health problem from their own perspective. By looking at health problems from the community level, we can focus on the social, cultural, and physical environment and, hopefully, come closer to creating healthy and sustainable communities.[4]

Nutrition Advocate

A third hat worn by nutritionists is that of advocate. Nutritionists have the responsibility to push their ideas forward. For example, nutritionists advocate for the following:

- Elimination of health disparities
- Equal access to nutrition services for all who need them
- Inclusion of nutrition professionals in multidisciplinary teams
- Improved nutrition reimbursement for services
- Increased funding for nutrition programs and community resources

In order for nutritionists to be heard, we need to stand up for our services and ensure that nutrition professionals are in the position of providing necessary information to the public.

Education in Public Health and Nutrition

Given the advances in public health and the complexity of our nutrition environment, a formal education in both nutrition and public health prepares professionals to meet the dynamic challenges presented locally and internationally. Increasingly, community nutrition jobs seek candidates who are registered dietitians (RD) and who possess advanced training in public health. This combination ensures that the professional has a rooted knowledge of nutrition science, expertise in clinical assessment and nutrition education, and can combine such principles with socioeconomic determinants to improve nutrition in community settings. Although degrees in both nutrition and public health are not required to work in the field of public health, such credentials will increase one's credibility in the job market and allow for advancement in the field.

Both schools of public health and programs in public health provide the primary professional degree for nutritionists seeking public health training, the Master of Public Health degree (MPH). The MPH degree trains professionals to approach health problems with an ecological framework, wedding biological risk factors with behavioral, social, and environmental determinants. Although they vary by program, areas of specialization are offered and several programs offer a concentration specifically in public health nutrition. In addition to one's area of specialization and fieldwork, there are five core components of a public health degree: biostatistics, epidemiology, health services administration, environmental health, and social and behavioral sciences. In recognition of the ongoing evolution and complexity of such determinants of health, the Institute of Medicine's (IOM) Committee on Educating Public Health Professionals for the 21st Century has recently identified eight additional areas that will benefit the trained public health workforce:

informatics, genomics, communication, cultural competence, community-based participatory research, policy and law, global health, and ethics.[5] Many programs have already incorporated these new areas of public health into their existing coursework, and it is likely that in the future all public health programs will be required to include these components in their curriculum. (In addition, several other college degree and university programs have been developed that also share the goals of health promotion and public health.) For those wishing to pursue further advanced training in public health research and leadership, doctoral degrees are available (either PhD or DrPH).

Several systems are in place to monitor and assess the quality of public health educational programs. The Council on Education for Public Health (CEPH) was created in 1974 by the American Public Health Association (APHA) and the Association of Schools of Public Health (ASPH) to accredit schools and programs of public health.[6] CEPH is recognized by the U.S. Department of Education and was established to serve the community by ensuring that graduates of public health programs are adequately prepared to serve as leaders in public health.

In response to an increasing need for adequate education of our future public health workforce, the Council on Linkages between Academia and Public Health Practice (composed of public health leaders in the community and academia) developed Core Competencies for Public Health Professionals in 2001.[7] The skill set provides specific competencies in the following eight areas:

1. Analytical assessment
2. Policy development/program planning
3. Communication
4. Cultural competency
5. Community dimensions of practice
6. Basic public health sciences
7. Financial planning and management
8. Leadership and systems thinking

The skill sets are further divided by professional level—front line, senior level, and supervisory/management staff—and have been acknowledged by the Centers for Disease Control and Prevention and the APHA. In addition, the Association of Graduate Programs in Public Health Nutrition, Inc. (AGPPHN) developed the *Strategies for Success: Curriculum Guide* to provide a recommended framework for the content of graduate-level public health nutrition programs.[8] Like the Core Competencies for Public Health Professionals, the Curriculum Guide provides a skill set, but is specific to public health nutrition curriculum, including:

- Knowledge and skills
- Food and nutrition sciences

- Research and evaluation
- Communication and culture
- Management and leadership
- Public health fieldwork

The Importance of Professional Development

Throughout this book, we have discussed the various roles of the nutritionist and the impact that public health efforts can have on improving the health of communities. To ensure that those efforts have a positive and lasting impact, adequate and ongoing training of the public health workforce is essential.[9,10] Advances in research, epidemiology, and technologies have increased our awareness of the prevalence and burden of diseases and associated risk factors. At the same time, progress in intervention and evaluation methodologies, social marketing, and health promotion have allowed us to move forward in affecting positive change within our communities. A combination of public health training and ongoing professional development will equip the nutrition workforce with the tools needed to take an active role in such complex efforts.

Keeping Abreast of Current Knowledge

As with all health professionals, it is imperative that nutritionists working in public health stay abreast of current events, advancements in nutrition knowledge, and ongoing public health activities in order to serve the community effectively. Although nutrition and public health education provides the necessary foundation upon which to build a successful career, the nutritionist is held accountable for maintaining and enhancing professional practice. This involves ongoing continuing education and participation in professional development. For example, the Commission on Dietetic Registration (CDR) requires that all dietitians report continuing professional development activities to maintain registration status. Through individualized self-assessment, dietitians identify ongoing strategies to ensure professional competence. Although there is no parallel monitoring system for MPH credentials, the Continuing Education Program of the APHA was established to "maintain and enhance professional knowledge, to increase technical proficiencies, and to enable members to promote and protect environmental and community health."[11]

Strategies for ongoing professional development include the following.

Membership in Professional Organizations

Membership in professional organizations such as the ADA and the APHA provides public health professionals with numerous opportunities for professional development through:

- Continuing education activities
- Professional committees
- Discussion groups
- Professional meetings
- Scholarly publications
- Professional resources and networks

The ADA supports numerous professional interest groups (dietetic practice groups or DPGs), which allow nutrition professionals to be active in specific areas of nutrition. Several DPGs of the ADA may be of particular interest to public health professionals, including Hunger and Environmental Nutrition, Nutrition Education for the Public, Public Health/Community Nutrition, and School Nutrition Services. APHA members can choose from 25 discipline-based sections and 7 special primary interest groups (SPIGs), including the Food and Nutrition Section of the APHA. In

> View the variety of available DPGs at http://www.eatright.org.

addition to national organizations, there are numerous state and local professional societies, including affiliates of both the ADA and the APHA. Through professional memberships, nutritionists not only stay informed of current events in the field, but also build lasting professional and social networks.

Listservs

Listservs are an efficient and convenient way of keeping up with the latest news and activities surrounding nutrition and public health. They provide information on the latest media news, journal articles, policy actions, and upcoming events in public health. Many international, national, and local agencies allow both professionals and the general public to join distribution lists. Examples of listservs of interest include:

- *Agency for Healthcare Research and Quality:* http://www.ahrq.gov/
- *The American Dietetic Association:* For members only, http://www.eatright.org/
- *The Centers for Disease Control and Prevention:* Includes the *Morbidity and Mortality Weekly Report* and National Health and Nutrition Examination Survey, http://www.cdc.gov/subscribe.html
- *International Food Policy Research Institute:* http://www.ifpri.org
- *National Institutes of Health:* http://list.nih.gov
- *U.S. Department of Health and Human Services:* http://www.usda.gov
- *U.S. Food and Drug Administration:* http://www.fda.gov

- *World Health Organization Weekly Epidemiological Record:* http://www.who.int/wer/en/
- *World Health News, Harvard School of Public Health:* http://www.worldhealthnews.harvard.edu

Obviously, these are just a few examples. To avoid being overwhelmed with e-mails, listserv memberships should be individually prioritized to those that are most useful. Also, many listservs permit members to customize e-mails, allowing you to choose the number and/or content of notifications received.

Conferences, Lectures, and Workshops

Conferences, lectures, and workshops are another way to stay abreast of the latest news and research in the field; gain insight into new, innovative public health interventions and activities; network and build valuable resources; and share best practices among colleagues. In addition to annual meetings of larger organizations, nutritionists should take advantage of the many workshops, meetings, and lectures that take place on a variety of public health topics throughout the year. Listservs, journals, and websites (both the ADA[12] and the APHA[13] provide a calendar of events on their websites) serve as excellent resources for upcoming public health events.

Journals and Public Health Publications

Peer-reviewed articles and other public health publications provide a rich source of knowledge on the latest research, insights, and lessons learned in practice. To engage in interdisciplinary dialogue, nutritionists should embrace a wide variety of topics and be aware of the various perspectives shaping public health systems in the current social, medical, and political environment. Furthermore, by keeping up with recent publications, the nutritionist can help to separate fact from fiction when nutrition information reaches the general public.

Academic Courses and/or Programs

Public health is an evolving discipline with ever-emerging methodologies and practices. When possible, the public health nutritionist should consider strengthening his or her current state of knowledge with additional coursework in public health or nutrition programs. For example, you might enhance your current job performance through additional training in language and culture, computer and Web technologies, communications and media, or research and statistical methodologies. If you do not have formal training in public health as mentioned previously, you should strongly consider advanced training through graduate or certificate public health programs. Formal education in public health prepares the nutrition workforce to meet the challenges of complex health issues facing communities, adds credibility and marketability to professional pursuits, and provides the skills necessary to advance to leadership roles in agencies or organizations.

Maintaining Political Awareness

Much of public health action is influenced by politics, so it is critical that nutritionists stay abreast of current events and the political environment. Although some nutritionists may be directly involved in the political scene through advocacy and grassroots efforts, all nutritionists are affected in some way by political agendas, perhaps through funding, changes in school policies, insurance reimbursement, or community resources. Many professional organizations provide resources through websites and listservs that keep members informed of political action and policy development. Newspapers and political publications should be included in the list of resources for all public health nutritionists.

Utilizing Technology

Technological improvements have made the 21st century an exciting time to practice public health. In addition to new advancements in science and medicine, the public health workforce is witnessing innovations in surveillance, communication, and geographic information systems (GIS). As they become mainstream, utilization of such technologies will be important for all public health professionals in order to fully participate in professional activities. Based on the IOM report on preparing the public health workforce, it is likely that more and more educational programs in public health will require such instruction as part of their curriculum. In the meantime, most colleges and universities as well as government public health agencies provide opportunities for training in computer programs, GIS, statistics, surveillance, and web design.

Collaborations

One of the most significant strategies for professional advancement is through partnerships and collaboration. Collaboration allows for a synergistic approach to public health issues, pulling together the skills and resources of multiple parties to improve the health of populations, which is the ultimate goal of public health professionals. Through professional and community partnerships, nutritionists can augment individual resources, ideas, and political momentum to accomplish a greater good than by acting alone. Such collaborations lead to creative, comprehensive, practical, and transformative thinking.[14] In addition, partnering with the community helps to foster trust and empowerment, thereby allowing for the implementation of community-based interventions that improve health outcomes. As the health of communities improves, especially when the community members themselves actively participate in the process, trust between the health professional and the community is likely to be further strengthened. Thus, the cycle continues, leading to the potential formation of additional collaborations.

To encourage sustainable action, partnerships should exist beyond the professional circle to welcome community participation. Depending on the desired outcome and goal, nutritionists should seek collaborations with community leaders and community-based organizations, school administrators, universities, government officials and policy makers, parent groups, and private organizations and businesses. The more people on the same team, the easier it will be to build trust, and the more consistent the messages to the public.

Future Challenges in Public Health Nutrition

Continuing Issues for Discussion

As we move into the future and find an older, more inactive population, higher rates of chronic disease, and enormous health disparities, nutritionists must serve as authorities on nutrition issues and be ready to jump into the solution of the health problems facing our world today. As we forge ahead with scientific and technological advances in health improvement, ethical issues emerge in many aspects of public health practice. As we decide on a research objective or a treatment/prevention protocol, we must think about the moral values and implications involved in the decisions. We should know the issues, the differing opinions, and where we, and the community, stand on these ethical questions.

According to the University of Pittsburgh's Center for Bioethics and Health Law:

> Technology has changed the very boundaries and possibilities of life. Scientific discoveries have blurred the traditional distinctions among birth, life and death as well as given us a vast array of new treatments to combat pain and suffering.[15]

For example, as we move forward with genomics, what will that mean for nutritional science? Will we no longer need to change our behaviors to prevent disease? Will parents want to test their unborn babies for unwanted chronic diseases?

Many current-day issues, not quite as obvious as the aforementioned questions, provide examples of ethical dilemmas that we face on a regular basis:

1. Who should provide nutrition education to the public—nutrition professionals, the media, government, physician groups, or private industry? What is the responsibility of government in ensuring appropriate nutrition care for the public?
2. Given the increasing rates of childhood obesity, what are the implications for children of food advertising on television? Should the food industry have a role in the prevention of childhood obesity?

3. Despite the rise in obesity, there are still a large number of food insecure households. Who is responsible for ensuring that all Americans have access to enough food?

4. Given technological advances, should genetically modified foods be sold in the marketplace? If so, does the public have the right to know if their food is genetically altered?

5. As we face a new era where the public health workforce is increasingly involved in bioterrorism preparedness, how are public health nutritionists being trained to ensure the safety of our food and water supply?

6. What role does the government play in regulating our food choices? Does the government have an obligation to step in and, if so, how far?

7. In an aging society with rising healthcare costs, are the elderly being forced to choose between adequate nutrition and health care? How are public health nutritionists working as advocates for our seniors?

Public health nutrition is a dynamic and exciting field. Its issues challenge us daily and allow us to grow and develop in ways we may not have imagined when we selected this career path as students. Public health allows us to deal with complex issues, technology, an ever-changing environment, and ethical issues, all of which present new opportunities. In order to meet the demands of the field, we need to be prepared for the associated challenges. Our work places us in a unique position where we are able to inform on food and nutrition policy, advocate for nutrition services, serve as media spokespeople, and help create healthier communities. The rigorous training and life experiences should enable us to survive and thrive in this dynamic field.

References

1. Institute of Medicine. *The Future of the Public's Health in the 21st Century.* Washington, DC: The National Academy Press; 2003:366.

2. O'Sullivan Maillet J, Borra ST, Niedert K, et al. Dietetics in 2017: what does the future hold? *JADA.* 2002;102(10):1404–1406.

3. American Dietetic Association. Position of the American Dietetic Association: the role of dietetics professionals in health promotion and disease prevention. *JADA.* 2002;102(11):1680–1687.

4. Israel BA, Schulz AJ, Parker EA, Becker AB. Review of community-based research: assessing partnership approaches to improve public health. *Annu Rev Public Health.* 1998; 19:173–202.

5. Gebbie E, Rosenstock L, Hernandez LM, eds. *Who Will Keep the Public Healthy? Educating Public Health Professionals for the 21st Century.* Washington, DC: The National Academy Press; 2003.

6. Council on Education for Public Health. About CEPH. Available at: http:// http://www.ceph.org/i4a/pages/index.cfm?pageid=3274. Accessed May 11, 2005.

7. Council on Linkages. Core Competencies Linkages. Available at: http://www.trainingfinder.org/competencies/list.htm. Accessed May 11, 2005.

8. Association of Graduate Programs in Public Health Nutrition, Inc. *Strategies for Success: Curriculum Guide*, 2nd ed. Available at: http://nutrition.he.utk.edu/AGPPHN/mission.htm. Accessed August 14, 2004.

9. U.S. Department of Health and Human Services. The Public Health Workforce: An Agenda for the 21st Century. Available at: http://www.health.gov/phfunctions/pubhlth.pdf. Accessed May 11, 2005.

10. Centers for Disease Control and Prevention. Task Force Report on Public Health Workforce Development. Available at: http://www.phppo.cdc.gov/owpp/workforcedev.asp. Accessed May 18, 2005.

11. American Public Health Association. Continuing Education Program Mission Statement. Available at: http://www.apha.org/education/ce_mission.htm. Accessed May 11, 2005.

12. American Dietetic Association. Calendar of Events. Available at: http://www.eatright.org/Public/ConferencesAndEvents/96_9588.cfm. Accessed May 11, 2005.

13. American Public Health Association. Calendar of Events. Available at: http://www.apha.org/calendar/. Accessed May 11, 2005.

14. Lasker RD, Weiss ES, Miller R. Partnership synergy: a practical framework for studying and strengthening the collaborative advantage. *Millbank Q.* 2001;79:179–205.

15. University of Pittsburgh's Center for Bioethics and Health Law. Overview. Available at: http://www.pitt.edu/~bioethic/overview.htm. Accessed May 11, 2005.

PUBLIC HEALTH NUTRITION: A HISTORICAL PERSPECTIVE

Mary C. Egan, MS, MPH

Abstract

This historical perspective describes important milestones and selected threads of concern in the development of public health nutrition services. Emphasis is given to nutrition service for mothers, children, and families from the mid-1800s through the 20th century. Efforts in the 1800s were primarily directed to building the foundation for public health nutrition services: organizing state health departments and voluntary health agencies, initiating early nutrition investigations, and establishing milk stations and school lunch programs in large cities to supplement the food of the poor and to combat the high rates of morbidity and mortality of infants and children. During the 20th century, demographic changes; advances in nutrition science and technology; and social, political, and economic changes influenced the growth and development of public health nutrition services. Such changes included the high rates of disease and deaths among mothers and children; food shortages during the wars; an increasing number of children in day care as more mothers went to work; the development of new programs to serve special groups such as the mentally retarded, chronically ill and handicapped, recent immigrants, and the aged; the continuing presence of poverty and hunger; the rising prevalence of behavior-related problems (eg, adolescent pregnancy and substance abuse); and a greater recognition of the benefits of health promotion and disease prevention. The number of public health nutritionists employed at national, state, and local levels increased to meet the rising demand for nutrition services. Graduate-level training programs and continuing education opportunities were developed and a broad range of nutrition standards and guidelines evolved. Throughout the 20th century, continuing threads of concern included nutrition policy and planning; development and evaluation of public health nu-

M. C. Egan is the retired associate director and chief nutritionist of the Bureau of Maternal and Child Health, Health Resources and Services Administration, Department of Health and Human Services, Rockville, MD. She is currently located in Syracuse, NY.

trition programs; organization, administration, and management of programs; quality of public health nutrition services; and the transfer and application of research into public health nutrition practice.

Through the eye of memory, we can see the trail we have made, the paths we have taken and those we have missed" (1). These words from Harry Paige capture the essence of the main objectives of this article: to describe some of the important milestones in the development of public health nutrition—with particular emphasis on nutrition services for mothers, children, and families—and to discuss some of the continuing "threads of concern" woven into the fabric of public health nutrition over the years.

From a historical perspective, two major periods will be covered: (a) the mid to late 1800s and (b) the 20th century, which consists of the early years (1900–1919), the youthful years (1920–1939), the middle years (1940–1959), the maturing years (1960–1979), and recent years (1980 to the present). Although of historical importance, only selected references will be made to the scientific advances and technological developments in foods and nutrition; to services for populations other than mothers and children, such as the aged and chronically ill adults; and to the many agencies, organizations, and institutions whose inspired leadership and professional contributions have supported the passing of the torch in public health nutrition from generation to generation.

The 1800s

Laying the foundation of public health nutrition was the primary business of the 1800s. Voluntary health agencies, particularly nursing agencies, were organized, beginning with the Visiting Nurse Association in New York City, and Boston in the 1850s. The first state department of health was established in Massachusetts in 1867. By 1877, 14 states had departments of health. In 1872, the American Public Health Association was organized.

High rates of infant mortality, epidemics of communicable disease, and many other problems associated with poor hygiene and sanitation prompted the government to act to improve conditions. Priority was given to controlling communicable disease, improving sanitation, providing health and parent education, and addressing nutrition concerns. As early as 1894, nutrition investigations were initiated in the Office of Experiment Stations of the U.S. Department of Agriculture. Milk stations were opened in New York City in 1895 and Rochester, NY, in 1897 to supplement the food of the poor and to instruct parents how to feed and care for their children. School lunch programs were also initiated in Boston in 1894 and New York City in 1889 (2).

According to Myers of Massachusetts General Hospital: "On January 1,1895, a new and interesting departure of both hospitals was made by the employment of Mrs. Ellen H. Richards and Miss S. E. Wentworth as experts to regulate the diet of the General Hospital" (3, p. 141). Richards had been the first woman to enter the Massachusetts Institute of Technology as a special student in chemistry in 1871. Considered an expert in sanitary science, she worked with the Massachusetts State Health Department on the safety of water supplies, sewage disposal, and pollution control. By 1885, she had published two books: *The Chemistry of Cooking* and *Cleaning and Food Materials and Their Adulterations* (4). Another key figure from this period was Mary Hinman Abel, who won an American Public Health Association prize in 1888 for the best essay on the subject "Practical, Sanitary and Economic Cooking Adapted to Families of Moderate and Small Means." Richards and Abel established the home economics movement through which much of the early work in public health nutrition was accomplished (4). The roots of public health nutrition can be traced back to their pioneering efforts in home economics and public health.

The Early Years (1900–1919)

The early years of the 20th century were characterized by high rates of morbidity and mortality, problems of child labor (10% of all 10- to 15-year-old children worked outside the home, eg, in textile mills, coal mines, and glass factories), and large numbers of people in poverty (2). The declaration of World War I called attention to public health concerns as many young men were rejected for selective service for health reasons.

On the positive side, many scientific advances were made during this period. Pasteurized milk was introduced in 1910, principles of growth and development were elucidated, and knowledge was expanded about the role of the nutrients in health and disease. As an outcome of the first White House Conference on Children in 1909, the U.S. Children's Bureau (CB) was created in 1912. Its mission was to investigate and report on all matters pertaining to the welfare of children and child life among all classes of people. To a large extent, the CB could be considered the mother of public health nutrition, for it took a leading role in developing and nurturing this new field (5).

During the war years, CB prepared its first nutrition publication, *Milk, the Indispensable Food for Children* (1918), to promote the feeding of young children as a priority in allocating food supplies. Because of its concern about malnourished children and the need to follow up on the 1919 Children's Year Campaign (which was launched to protect children from the effects of war), the CB arranged for Lydia Roberts, PhD, to write *What is Malnutrition?* which focused on issues of malnutrition. When Roberts revised this publication in 1927, the emphasis of the book had shifted from malnutrition to optimum development and health supervision of well children (5).

Massachusetts employed its first nutritionist in 1917 (6). Called a "health instructor in foods," she distributed educational information about nutrition by giving talks, developing pamphlets, working with various committees, and making herself available for consultation services. By 1922, a second nutritionist was hired to give nutrition courses to teachers, nurses, and other professionals.

Community nutrition work was also being done during this period by two great pioneers—Frances Stern and Lucy Gillett. They worked with pediatricians and used special nutrition clinics and classes to demonstrate that healthy growth in children can take place only when children are well fed and in good physical condition (7).

The Youthful Years (1920–1939)

Developments in public health nutrition from 1920 through 1939 were primarily a consolidation and expansion of the nutrition activities of the previous periods. The major historical event of this period—the stock market crash and the resulting economic depression—had major implications for public health nutrition. Millions of people were poor, unemployed, and suffering deprivation. High rates of immigration and an increasing diversity of cultures brought new challenges to service providers. Important social legislation was enacted and knowledge about nutrition and its role in health and disease grew by leaps and bounds (2).

In 1921, the Shepard–Towner Act created the first federal-state partnership for health services and provided states with grants-in-aid for maternal and child health. The states gave considerable attention to nutrition in their state plans for maternal and child health (8). For example, the field report of a nutritionist in Kentucky noted that "an intensive study of pellagra was made in one county, and clinics for mothers and children were held in two towns and six mining camps where the disease was prevalent. Those attending the clinics were given instructions as to the diet requirements for curing as well as preventing the disease" (5).

Many voluntary agencies, notably the American Red Cross, made major contributions to the development of public health nutrition. After the demise of the Shepard-Towner grant-in-aid funds in 1929, voluntary agencies tried to fill the gaps in nutrition services; however, the depression eventually forced them to curtail their activities.

In 1935, Congress enacted the Social Security Act to combat the serious effects of the economic depression. This historic legislation provided states with grants-in-aid for Maternal and Child Health and Crippled Children's Services (MCH) (Title V) and for Child Welfare (Title IV) (8). As a result of the MCH funds available under Title V, the field of public health nutrition grew rapidly. Before the enactment of the Social Security Act, only 3 states employed nutritionists: Connecticut, Massachusetts, and New York (5). By 1936, there were 11 positions for nutritionists in 4 states; by 1939, there were 39 positions in 24 states. To provide national leadership and direction to the development of public health nutrition services in MCH programs, the CB employed its first nutrition consultant, Marjorie M. Heseltine, MS, in 1936. Heseltine worked tirelessly with the states to include nutrition services as a part of state health programs, with professional organizations and educational institutions to develop training programs and professional standards for public health nutrition workers, and with other federal agencies to resolve nutrition problems and issues of mutual concern. Heseltine was the only nutrition consultant in the CB for several years, but she initiated a "nutrition exchange" to share information and materials among federal and state public health nutritionists.

Other important milestones of this time included the following:

- CB launched studies of the nutritional status of children in 1920;
- Iodine was added to salt in the first food fortification program in 1924;
- The federal government created the Food Distribution Program in 1935 and an experimental Food Stamp Program in 1939;
- The Milbank Memorial Fund supported the first Roundtable on Nutrition in Public Health in 1937;
- The first qualifications for nutritionists in public health were published in 1938; and
- Amendments to the Social Security Act in 1939 provided funds for special projects grants, some of which were used to support training opportunities for public health nutritionists.

The Middle Years (1940–1959)

The middle years, particularly the 1940s, seethed with rapid changes in many sectors of life. The advent of World War II meant priority had to be given to the nutritional aspects of national defense, and food supplies were rationed. Women moved into the work force to staff defense and other homefront industries. Thus, it became necessary to provide day care for children. At the same time, wondrous scientific advances were made in medicine, such as the discovery of antibiotics and the polio vaccine. In nutrition, advances were made in the enrichment of bread and flour and the fortification of milk and margarine. The population increased and shifted from rural to urban areas, thus compounding the problem of shortages and maldistribution of health personnel. Although the incomes of many families improved, there were still large numbers of poor people.

The development of public health nutrition continued at a lively pace. At their September 1940 meeting, members of the Association of State and Territorial Health Officers received suggestions for state action relative to nutrition in national defense. At the 1941 National Nutrition Conference, which focused on defense, the first Recommended Dietary Allowances were adopted (9).

In August 1944, Heseltine, the chief nutritionist of the CB, reported that "activities carried on by nutritionists are broadening. An increasing number are giving some service to institutions for care of mothers and children, including small hospitals and maternity homes . . . Service to the agencies sponsoring school lunch programs and centers for day care of preschool children seems to be on the increase. Services through industrial hygiene divisions to war industries seem to have abated as the War Food Administration has appointed regional staffs of consultants in mass feeding" (10). By 1945, all but three states included one or more nutrition consultant positions in their state health department budgets.

In 1942, the Public Health Service (PHS) began to conduct nutrition appraisals in selected states, and a few state and local health departments developed nutrition clinics. In 1944, Norman Jolliffe, MD, began a diagnostic, treatment, and training clinic for nutritional deficiency diseases at Lower East Side Health Center in New York City (11).

During this period, the nutrition of several groups in the population—premature infants, children with mental retardation, children in group care, the aged, Native Americans, and Alaskan natives—began to receive more attention. In 1946, three state health departments (Illinois, Missouri, and Maryland) established a position for consultant dietitians to institutions, and public health nutritionists had a major role in the implementation of the new National School Lunch Program. The Special Milk Program followed in 1954.

In 1943, the CB began to allocate Title V/MCH special project funds for graduate training and continuing education in public health nutrition. Additional training opportunities for public health nutritionists became available in 1956, when Title VII of the PHS Act was enacted.

The following milestones were significant in the middle years:

- CB added a second nutrition consultant, Helen Stacey, MS, to its staff in 1941;
- CB issued *Food for Young Children in Group Care* to assist day care providers;
- Title V/MCH awarded a 3-year grant to the New York City Health Department to establish a nutrition division in 1943 (11);

- The National Academy of Sciences established a Committee on Maternal Nutrition and Child Feeding in 1946;
- CB added three regional nutrition consultant positions in 1947;
- The Association of Faculties of Graduate Programs in Public Health Nutrition was formally organized in 1950;
- The Association of State and Territorial Public Health Nutrition Directors was formally organized in 1952; and
- PHS convened the National Conference on Nursing Homes and Homes for the Aged in 1958, and issued 14 recommendations to improve nutrition services (12).

The Maturing Years (1960–1979)

The period from 1960 through 1979 was characterized by considerable unrest as the nation struggled with civil rights, the war in Southeast Asia, poverty and hunger, access to health care, increasing environmental pollution, and a rising prevalence of behavior-related problems such as substance abuse, adolescent pregnancy, and sexually transmitted disease. Many cities experienced an increase in infant mortality, and rates were much higher for African Americans than for whites. The number and proportion of elderly persons grew as did the number of single-parent families.

Such events and conditions led President Johnson to declare a War on Poverty in the 1960s, which included the enactment of a massive amount of social legislation and the establishment of many new health programs targeted to low-income, high-risk populations. These programs included the special projects for Maternity and Infant Care (M&I) in 1963, the Comprehensive Health Projects for Children and Youth (C&Y) and Community Health Center and Migrant Health Programs in 1965, Family Planning Programs in 1969, the Headstart Program in 1965, the Medicare and Medicaid Programs in 1965, and the University-Affiliated Centers Program in 1963.

The number of positions for nutritionists grew rapidly as additional nutritionists were employed by these projects to provide nutrition care directly to high-risk patients and their families. For example, more than 300 nutrition positions were budgeted in the 53 M&I projects and the 58 C&Y projects (13). The concentration of nutrition services in these Title V/MCH projects greatly facilitated contributions by nutritionists to the field of public health. Public health nutritionists developed the concept of a nutrition care plan for each patient, identified the basic elements of comprehensive nutrition services, categorized nutrition problems by diagnostic code, and developed and marketed the concept of providing food assistance on the basis of health need and as an integral part of health care (14).

In 1967, Congress began a series of hearings on hunger, and a Citizen's Board of Inquiry into the extent and nature of hunger released its findings (15). To provide more information about the extent of hunger and other nutrition problems, the CB and the PHS launched several studies and surveys, including the Title V/ MCH 1968 Study of Nutritional Status of Preschool Children in the United States (16), the PHS 1970 Ten State Survey (17), and the 1971 National Health and Nutrition Examination Survey (18).

Public health nutritionists worked hard to improve food assistance to the needy, particularly high-risk pregnant women, infants, and children. The 10 years of effort that led to the development of the Special Supplemental Food Program for Women, Infants, and Children (WIC) demonstrates that long-term, continuous efforts are often required to effect change in nutrition policy and practice.

During those years, it was not uncommon to hear state public health nutrition directors say that they spent nearly 100% of their time trying to sell the WIC Program to state and local health administrators (with no support from WIC funds), or that the extra paperwork required by regulations of different agencies was driving them to despair, or that they were exhausted from helping administrators of the multiple new health programs recruit nutrition staff. The scene in public health nutrition was ever changing and fast moving, and public health nutritionists at the local, state, and federal levels went far beyond the call of duty to move these new programs from the paper stage to the arena of practice.

The following additional milestones were important during the maturing years.

- The first Conference on the Role of State Health Departments in Nutrition Research was held in 1961;
- The 1961 Survey of Home Care Programs indicated that part-time nutrition services were available in 34 of 37 programs (19);
- The Food Stamp Act passed in 1965;
- Title V/MCH awarded a grant to the National Academy of Sciences (NAS) to support the work of the Committee of Maternal Nutrition in 1968;
- The first White House Conference on Food, Nutrition, and Health was called in 1969;
- In 1970, NAS published *Maternal Nutrition and the Course of Pregnancy*, which revolutionized nutrition care practices during pregnancy (20);
- A White House Conference on Aging was convened in 1971, which led to the establishment of the Nutrition Program for the Elderly in 1973; and
- Dietary Goals for the United States were issued in 1977 (21).

Recent Years (1980 to the Present)

Important changes in the composition and mobility of the population have occurred since 1980: the number of Hispanic persons and immigrants from Southeast Asia increased, the number and proportion of older elderly persons grew, many families moved from the Northeast to the South and West, and the number of homeless persons multiplied. In addition to the health problems of the previous period, some new challenges arose, such as AIDS and Alzheimer's disease, and some reappeared, such as tuberculosis. The alarm bell about the nation's budget problems rang more frequently. Factors such as the escalating cost of health care, the continuing growth of entitlement programs, and the skyrocketing cost of interest on the public debt meant that funds for public health services were limited.

Encouraging developments during this period have included the unlocking of some of the mysteries of genetics and chronic diseases and the increasing acceptance and support for more family-centered, community-based, and comprehensive care for children with special health care needs, the chronically ill, the terminally ill, the infirm elderly, and adults with disabilities. The ethical aspects of nutrition have also received more emphasis as rapid changes in science and technology have brought more choices in the treatment and management of disease. Health promotion and disease prevention moved to the front burner, and the delineation of national health objectives made possible a more targeted approach to public health nutrition services.

The Surgeon General's 1984 Conference on Breastfeeding and Human Lactation and 1988 Conference on Nutrition and Health added impetus to the development of public health nutrition. Other national conferences and reports that had a considerable impact were *Directions for the 1980s* (22), from the National Conference on Nutrition Education; the series of reports from the Select Panel for the Promotion of Child Health (23); *Nutrition Monitoring in the United States* (24) from the Nutrition Monitoring Evaluation Committee; and *Call to Action: Better Nutrition for Mothers, Children, and Families* (25), from the MCH Interorganizational Nutrition Group.

Public health nutritionists continued to work on sharpening national and state nutrition objectives, on defining nutrition policy in both the private and public sectors, and on improving the nutrition database for program planning and evaluation. A nagging question during the period has been that of adequate financing for comprehensive nutrition services. Although a few new sources of funding for nutrition became available—Medicaid funds, Education for Handicapped funds, and Risk Reduction grants—some of the long-time sources of support, such as Title V/MCH funds, were increasingly used for other services. This meant that in some instances there was decreased support for comprehensive public health nutrition services.

Other notable milestones of this period included the following.

- Nutrition services to children with special health care needs were expanded and improved;
- The National Academy of Sciences issued guidelines for nutrition services in perinatal care (26) in 1981 and a revision in 1992;
- Legislation creating the National Nutritional Status Monitoring System was enacted;
- Human lactation and breast-feeding were successfully promoted;
- The National Academy of Sciences issued *Diet and Health: Implications for Reducing Chronic Disease Risk* (27) in 1989 and *Improving America's Diet and Health: From Recommendations to Action* (28) in 1991; and
- The Institute of Medicine reports *Nutrition During Pregnancy* (29) and *Nutrition During Lactation* were published in 1990 and 1991, respectively.

Recurring Threads of Concern

Several continuing threads of concern become evident in a review of public health services in the 20th century, including:

- nutrition policy and the planning, development, and evaluation of public health nutrition programs;
- organization, administration, and management of programs;
- quality of public health nutrition services; and
- transfer or application of research into public health nutrition practice.

Policy, Planning, Development, and Evaluation

A variety of mechanisms have been used to establish and promulgate nutrition policy: national conferences and commissions, legislation, presidential (executive) proclamations, and endorsement of recommendations from expert groups. In addition to these more visible mechanisms, budgetary decisions and technological changes have influenced policy.

Program emphasis and priorities have changed over time. In the early years, programs emphasized sanitation and hygiene, care of malnourished infants and children, parent education, and disease control. Emphasis then changed to encompass concerns related to older children and adults. Soon the nutritional aspects of treatment and rehabilitation came into focus with the growth in chronic disease control and clinical mental retardation programs and with shifts in the categories of conditions accepted for crippled children's programs. As the importance of health promotion and disease prevention was recognized, efforts were focused on the nutritional antecedents of disease: promoting changes in lifestyles, wellness programs, nutrition surveillance and assessment, and modification of food supply and dietary intake to support dietary goals. Throughout the life span of public health nutrition and regardless of the program emphasis and priority, there has been a continuing concern with policy, planning, implementation, and evaluation.

Organization, Administration, and Management

Variations in organizational philosophy, budget realities, consumer demands, program complexity, management style of administrators, and other factors have influenced the organization, administration, and management of public health nutrition services. Except for the early years when the birthing and nurturing of public health nutrition was the major goal, there has been a continuous thread of concern for organization, administration, and management. Regional and state activities also reflected this concern. For example, in Region V of the DHHS, the *Workbook on Costing Nutrition Services* (30) was prepared in 1985.

Quality of Public Health Nutrition

Approaches to quality assurance have included the development of standards and guidelines, the establishment of qualifications and support of graduate training, and the offering of continuing education opportunities. Selected illustrations of each of these approaches are provided in Figure A-1.

Development of Standards and Guidelines

Some standards and guidelines, such as the federal MCH agency guidelines for the M&I and C&Y projects, emanated from the agency administering the program. Others have been adopted from those issued by professional organizations, such as the American College of Obstetricians and Gynecologists, or expert groups, such as those convened by the Institute of Medicine. A few, such as nutrition management of the pregnant adolescent, have resulted from the work of a group of providers who worked together to reach consensus. Whatever the source, it is worthy of note that efforts have been made to update these guidelines periodically. For example, the guidelines for nutrition in pregnancy were first issued in 1950 and were revised and reissued in 1970 and in 1990.

Qualifications and Graduate Training in Public Health Nutrition

Representatives of professional organizations, employers, educational institutions, and others have met in committee over the years to delineate functions, duties, and qualifications of personnel for public health nutrition (31). In the late 1930s, the American Home Economics Association and The American Dietetic Association appointed a Joint Committee on Qualifications, Function, and Preparation of Nutritionists, whose members represented both academia and practice. Elda Robb served as chair and members were Adelia Beeuwkes, Bertlyn Bosley, Helen Hunscher, Florence McLeod, Nelle Sailor, Alice H. Smith, and Marjorie M. Heseltine.

The first graduate training program in nutrition to receive Title V/MCH funding was at the University of Tennessee under the leadership of Florence McLeod and Ruth Huenemann. In 1943, shortly thereafter, Title V/MCH funds were also awarded to the University of California at Berkeley, Case Western Reserve, University of Michigan, University of North Carolina, and Harvard. When additional funding for public health training became available under Title VII, Public Health Act, graduate training opportunities for training public health nutritionists expanded. Although the number and location of the educational programs have changed over time, a consistent base of graduate training has been maintained.

As the specialized MCH diagnostic, clinical, and comprehensive health programs were developed (eg, intensive newborn care, adolescent health, university affiliated programs, pediatric pulmonary centers, M&I, C&I), additional funds became available for special-

1920–1939	1940–1959	1960–1979	1980–Present
Development of standards/guidelines			
• Food for young children to group care (1920) • Table of average weights for height and age of children less than 6 years old (1923)	• Nutrition in national defense: suggestions for state action (1940) • Recommendations to improve nutrition services in nursing homes and homes for the aged	• Nutritional disorders of children (1966, 1977) • *Feeding the Child with a Handicap: A Guide for Professionals* (1966, 1982)	• Guide to quality assurance for ambulatory care (1983) • Nutrition screening for professionals caring for older Americans (1991)
Establishment of qualifications/support of graduate training			
• Minimum qualifications of home economists or nutritionists in health and welfare agencies *J Am Diet Assoc.* 1937; 13:340–344	• Objectives for preparation of public health nutritionists *J Home Econ.* 1950; 42:4	• Educational qualifications of nutritionists in health agencies. *Am J Public Health.* 1962; 52:1	• Personnel in public health nutrition for the 80s ASTHO Foundation (1989) • *Strategies for Success: Curriculum Guide for Graduate Programs in Public Health Nutrition NCEMCH* (1990)
Offering of continuing education programs			
• Milbank Roundtable on Nutrition in Public Health (1937)	• Workshop on dietary consultation for institutions • Workshops on nutrition and diet in relation to mental retardation	• Intensive course in pediatric nutrition initiated (1962) • Series of national seminar and regional workshops on nutrtion in pregnancy (1963–1965) • Series of regional workshops on planning and evaluation (1973–1975)	• Series of national and regional workshops on nutrition in programs for children with special health care needs • Workshop on planning and financing an integrated nutrition system • Practicum—lactation management training • Fellowships—neonatal high-risk infant nutrition

FIGURE A-1   Selected Examples of Areas of Continuing Concern Regarding Quality of Public Health Nutrition Services

ized training in MCH nutrition. To ensure that training needs were met and that training programs were responsive to the changing face and priorities in the field of practice, the federal MCH agency and the PHS have periodically convened advisory groups to review the status of training programs and to make recommendations (1964/MCH, 1984/MCH and PHS). The information in Figure A-1 illustrates the continuity of concern related to qualifications and graduate training in public health nutrition.

Continuing education

In the third approach to quality, that of continuing education, the foci depended on the events and demands of the field of practice. For example, among the factors that influenced the offerings on continuing education were the development of new programs, advances in nutrition science and technology, and political issues such as child health, chronic disease, health planning, and performance budgeting. Selected illustrations are provided in Figure A-1.

Transfer and Application of Research

More than 30 years ago, the Association of State and Territorial Public Health Nutrition Directors cited the lack of research components in nutrition programs as one of the most serious blocks to the development of vital progressive programs (32). Dr. Malcolm Merrill, State Director of Public Health in California, noted that when he entered the field of public health in 1937 it was taboo to mention research as a function of the department (33). Despite what state health departments have done or not done in research, there has always been a concern with the application of research in public health nutrition. For example, about 60 years ago, the CB cooperated with Yale University, Department of Health, and the Board of Education in New Haven, Connecticut, to evaluate various methods of assessing the physical fitness of children. The findings were widely used in child health programs across the nation to improve the assessment of growth and development (5).

Nearly 25 years ago, when the National Academy of Sciences released *Maternal Nutrition and the Course of Pregnancy* (20), public health nutritionists and other health professionals brought this landmark report to the attention of both the private and public health sectors. They worked through the health care delivery system, food assistance programs, and institutions of higher education to effect significant changes in the clinical management of pregnancy, in the priority accorded pregnant women and infants in food assistance programs, and in the standards and guidelines adopted by pacesetters in maternity care.

During the late 1950s and early 1960s, when new information about the role of nutrition in the prevention and treatment of inborn errors of metabolism became available, public health nutritionists upgraded their knowledge and skills in this area. They ensured that the information was widely disseminated and interpreted to public health practitioners, and they took steps to improve the follow-up of affected patients.

More recently, when the *Dietary Guidelines for Americans* were issued (33) and dietary recommendations began to focus on reduction of risk for chronic disease, public health nutritionists played a major role in moving this new information out of the laboratories into the realm of practice.

Application

The transfer and application of research to public health nutrition practice is essential if advances in nutrition science and technology are to benefit health care consumers in terms of the quality of care and the cost benefits to be realized. Each of the aforementioned examples underscores the important role of public health agencies in the timely transfer of research findings to health care practitioners in both the private and public sectors. Public health nutritionists can exercise leadership and open doors of opportunity in the community to positively affect nutrition practice and to improve the delivery of high-quality nutrition care.

This historical perspective should remind us that although we can learn from the past, it is essential to live in the present and look to the future. As philosopher Søren Kierkegaard said, "Life can only be understood backwards, but it has to be lived forwards (1).

The author acknowledges with appreciation the valuable assistance provided by the staff of the National Center for Education in Maternal and Child Health in the preparation of this manuscript, particularly Carol West Suitor, DSc, RD, Project Director for Nutrition, and members of the Information Publications and Administrative Services units. This information was presented at the Association for State and Territorial Public Health Nutrition Directors and the Association of Faculties of Graduate Programs in Public Health Nutrition Conference, Minneapolis, MN, June 6–9, 1993.

References

1. Paige HW. Trial by memory. *Liguorian*. 1993; January: 4–8.
2. Oglesby A, et al. History of maternal and child health. Rockville, Md: Bureau of Maternal and Child Health, Department of Health and Human Services; Unpublished manuscript.
3. Myers GW. History of the Massachusetts General Hospital, June 1872 to December, 1900. 1929. Unpublished manuscript. Mary C. Egan Reference Collection. National Center for Education in Maternal and Child Health, Arlington, Va.

4. Hunt CL. The Life of Ellen H. Richards. Washington, DC: American Home Economics Association; 1958.

5. Heseltine MM. Nutrition as a concern of the Children's Bureau. Unpublished manuscript. Mary C. Egan Reference Collection. National Center for Education in Maternal and Child Health, Arlington, Va.

6. Getting V. A modern nutrition program in a state health department. *Milbank Memorial Fund Q.* 1947; 25:3.

7. Eliot MM, Heseltine MM. Nutrition in maternal and child health programs. *Nutr Rev.* 1947; 5:33–35.

8. Lesser AJ. The origins and development of maternal and child health programs in the United States. *Public Health Rep.* 1985; 75:590–598.

9. Roberts LJ. Beginnings of the recommended dietary allowances. *J Am Diet Assoc.* 1958; 34:903–908.

10. Heseltine MM. Major activities of the nutrition unit for the year ended June 30, 1944. Mary C. Egan Reference Collection. National Center for Education in Maternal and Child Health, Arlington, Va.

11. *A Public Health Nutrition Program, Department of Health, City of New York: Retrospect, Introspect, Prospect.* New York, NY: Bureau of Nutrition, City of New York, Dept. of Health; 1968.

12. Egan MC. *Background Paper on the Recommendations of Conferences and Groups Related to National Nutrition Policy (1917–1974) for National Nutrition Policy Study Hearings.* Washington, DC: U.S. Department of Health, Education, and Welfare; 1974.

13. Egan MC. Combating malnutrition through maternal and child health programs. *Children.* 1969; 16(2):67–71.

14. Egan MC, Oglesby AC. Nutrition services in the Maternal and Children Health Program: A historical perspective. In: Sharbaugh CO, ed. *Call to Action: Better Nutrition for Mothers, Children and Families.* Washington, DC: National Center for Education in Maternal and Child Health; 1990.

15. Citizens' Board of Inquiry into Hunger and Malnutrition in the United States. *Hunger, U.S.A.* Boston: Beacon Press; 1968.

16. Owen GM, et al. A study of nutritional status of preschool children in the United States (1968–1970). *Pediatrics.* 1974; 53(Part II, Supplement): 597–646.

17. Ten State Nutrition Survey: 1968–1970. Washington, DC: U.S. Dept. of Public Health Service; 1972. DHEW Publication No. HSM 73-8130.

18. National Center for Health Statistics. *Preliminary Findings of the First Health and Nutrition Examination Survey, United States, 1971–72.* Hyattsville, Md: Public Health Service; 1975. DHEW publication no. (HRA) 75-1229,

19. Piper GM. Nutrition in coordinated home care programs. *J Am Diet Assoc.* 1961; 39:198–200.

20. Commmittee on Maternal Nutrition. *Maternal Nutrition and the Course of Pregnancy.* Washington, DC: National Academy Press; 1970.

21. *Dietary goals for the United States.* Washington, DC: U.S. Government Printing Office; 1977.

22. Dwyer J, ed. National conference on nutrition education: Directions for the 1980s. *J Nutr Educ.* 1980; 12(suppl):79–137.

23. *Select Panel for the Promotion of Child Health. Report to the United States Congress and the Secretary of Health and Human Services, Vol. I–IV.* Washington, DC: U.S. Government Printing Office; 1981. DHHS publication no. (PHS) 79-55071.

24. Joint Nutrition Monitoring Evaluation Committee. *Nutrition Monitoring in the United States: A Progress Report from the Joint Nutrition Monitoring Evaluation Committee.* Hyattsville, Md: National Center for Health Statistics; 1986. DHHS publication no. (PHS) 86–1255.

25. Sharbaugh CO, ed. *Call to Action: Better Nutrition for Mothers, Children and Families.* Washington, DC: National Center for Education in Maternal and Child Health; 1990.

26. Committee on Nutrition of the Mother and Preschool Child. *Nutrition Services in Perinatal Care.* Washington, DC: National Academy Press; 1987.

27. National Research Council. *Diet and Health: Implications for Reducing Chronic Disease Risk.* Washington, DC: National Academy Press; 1989.

28. Committee on Dietary Guidelines Implementation. *Improving American's Diet and Health: From Recommendations to Action.* Washington, DC: National Academy Press; 1991.

29. National Research Council. *Nutrition During Pregnancy: Weight Gain, Nutrient Supplements and Nutrition during Lactation.* Washington, DC: National Academy Press; 1990.

30. Splett P, Caldwell M. *Costing Nutrition Services: A Workbook.* Chicago, IL: Dept of Health and Human Services, Region V; 1985.

31. Massachusetts Department of Public Health. Conference on standardization of qualifications and salaries of nutritional workers. Unpublished report. 1920. Mary C. Egan Reference Collection. National Center for Education in Maternal and Child Health, Arlington, Va.

32. ASTPHND. Application for a research grant. 1960 Unpublished. Mary C. Egan Reference Collection. National Center for Education in Maternal and Child Health, Arlington, Va.

33. Merrill MH. *Nutrition research—what health departments can do.* Presented at the Arden House Conference on the Role of State Health Departments in Nutrition Research. 1961

34. *Nutrition and Your Health: Dietary Guidelines for Americans.* Washington, DC: U.S. Depts. of Agriculture and Health and Human Services; 1980. (Revised in 1985.)

POSITION OF THE AMERICAN DIETETIC ASSOCIATION: PROVIDING NUTRITION SERVICES FOR INFANTS, CHILDREN, AND ADULTS WITH DEVELOPMENTAL DISABILITIES AND SPECIAL HEALTH CARE NEEDS

American Dietetic Association

It is the position of the American Dietetic Association that nutrition services are essential components of comprehensive care for infants, children, and adults with developmental disabilities and special health care needs. Nutrition services should be provided throughout the life cycle in health care, educational, and vocational programs in a manner that is interdisciplinary, family centered, community based, and culturally competent. Persons with developmental disabilities and special health care needs frequently have nutrition problems including growth alterations (such as failure to thrive, obesity, and growth retardation) metabolic disorders, poor feeding skills, medication–nutrient interactions, and partial or total dependence on enteral or parenteral nutrition. Poor health habits, limited access to services, and long-term use of multiple medications are considered risk factors for additional health problems. Legislation for individuals with special needs has evolved over time, resulting in a transition from institutional facilities and programs to community living. The expansion of public access to technology and health information on the Internet challenges dietetics professionals to provide accurate scientific information for those with developmental disabilities and special health care needs. Nationally credentialed dietetics professionals are best prepared to provide appropriate nutrition information as it pertains to wellness and the maintenance of good health and quality of lifestyle.

Reprinted with permission from Elsevier Publications. Journal of the American Dietetic Association V104(1): 97–107, Cloud HH et al: "Position of The American Dietetic Association: Providing Nutrition Services for Infants, Children, and Adults with Developmental Disabilities and Special Health Care Needs." © 2004 with the permission of The American Dietetic Association.

Position Statement

It is the position of the American Dietetic Association that nutrition services are essential components of comprehensive care for infants, children, and adults with developmental disabilities and special health care needs.

Defining the Population

Individuals with developmental disabilities (1) have diagnoses and conditions that place them at nutritional risk. A developmental disability may be the result of identified etiologies (eg, chromosomal abnormalities, congenital anomalies, inherited metabolic disorders, specific syndromes, neuromuscular dysfunction) or may not be associated with any diagnosed condition. Occasionally, persons may have two or more conditions (eg, cerebral palsy and epilepsy, Down's syndrome, and congenital heart disease (2,3). Children with special health care needs are those who have or are at increased risk for a chronic physical, developmental, behavioral, or emotional condition and who also require health and related services of a type or amount beyond that required by children generally (4). A survey of children from birth to age three years with developmental delays in early intervention programs found 79% to 90% had one or more nutrition risk indicators (5,6). The Centers for Disease Control and Prevention (CDC) reported that 17% of children under 18 years of age have some type of developmental disability (7).

The majority of children with special health care needs, even those with complex medical conditions, now live to adulthood. Legislative efforts and resulting programs promoting the themes of de-institutionalization, inclusion, and individual empowerment have created the expansion of community-based residential settings and home-based services over time (8,9).

The term "developmental disabilities" includes those people whose cognitive disability or other disability is severe enough to require ongoing coordinated services and support. There are 3 to 4 million Americans with a developmental disability and another 3 million who have milder forms of cognitive disabilities or mental retardation (10,11). Mental retardation is manifest before age 18 years (12) and is defined as a substantial limitation in present functioning. It is characterized by significantly subaverage intellectual function, existing concurrently with related limitation in two or more of the following areas: communication, self-care, functional academics and home-living community use, self-direction, health and safety, leisure, work, and social skills. Mental retardation is the most common developmental disability and ranks first among chronic conditions causing major activity limitations among persons in the United States (13).

Infants born prematurely and with low birth weights have increased in numbers over the last 20 years; however, in that same period, infant and neonatal mortality rates improved dramatically. Being born too small or too soon entails high risk of serious morbidity contributing to long-term neurologic impairment. Premature infants have an increased risk for cerebral palsy, mental retardation, sensory impairment, developmental delays, and learning and school problems. Nutrition plays a key role in the prevention of prematurity and in neonatal care during hospitalization and in the follow-up period (14).

The range of health problems for individuals with developmental disabilities includes increased risk for obesity; cardiovascular disease; dental, hearing, and vision problems; and poor conditioning and fitness. The type of living arrangement is strongly linked to obesity. Fifty-five percent of individuals with mild cognitive limitations residing with their natural families were found to be obese as compared with those living in a structured setting such as a group home/community-living arrangement (15). Studies show a strong link between obesity and discrimination, along with a predisposition to heart disease.

A study investigating a population of 1,063 people 50 to 88 years of age with lifelong cognitive disability found that more than 50% of this older population had major physical problems: 17% had epilepsy, 21% musculoskeletal impairments, 14% cardiovascular disease, 32% visual problems, and 40% were overweight. Many of these problems are treatable, but there was a lack of available specialized medical care (16,17).

Legislation

Legislative support for infants, children, and adults with developmental disabilities and special health care needs has increased drastically in the last three decades (18). Recent legislative efforts and parental advocacy have driven this improvement. Along with the legislative effort, there has been an increase in the populations that meet the definition of special needs and developmental disabilities.

Historically, individuals with developmental disabilities were cared for in institutions (18). During the 1970s, landmark legislation caused the size and number of institutions to decrease, and treatment standards were imposed, including nutrition standards. Nationally, the average number of residential settings was reduced by two-thirds from 1970 to 1995. Closing and downsizing institutions are evidence of the transformation of national policy affecting individuals with developmental disabilities over the past 25 years. It has been, in part, an opportunity for dietetics professionals working in community, educational, and clinical settings (19).

Legislation that impacts services for individuals with developmental disabilities and special needs first originated in 1963 as the Developmental Disabilities Assistance and Bill of Rights Act (Figure B-1). Through this act, federal funds supported the development of state councils, protection and advocacy systems, university training programs, and projects of national significance. Nutrition training has been included in university centers and training projects (1).

The year 2000 marked the twenty-fifth anniversary of IDEA (the Individuals with Disabilities Education Act), the tenth anniversary of the Americans with Disabilities Act, and the enactment of the revised Developmental Disabilities Assistance and Bill of Rights Act (1). Current legislation emphasizes fundamental systems change, including legal services and advocacy and capacity building at the state and local levels. The focus of the legislation is on helping people with developmental disabilities and their families obtain the information, assistive technology, and support that they need to make more informed choices about where and how to live. The revised Developmental Disabilities Assistance and Bill of Rights Act continues to support university-affiliated programs to provide interdisciplinary preservice preparation of students and fellows, communications, and community services and dissemination of information and research findings (1).

---

(1) According to the Developmental Disabilities Assistance and Bill of Rights Act of 1990 (PL 101-496) 2000 (PL 106-402):

(A) IN GENERAL the term "developmental disability" means a severe chronic disability of an individual that—

  (i) is attributable to a mental or physical impairment or combination of mental and physical impairments;

  (ii) is manifested before the person attains age twenty-two;

  (iii) is likely to continue indefinitely;

  (iv) results in substantial functional limitations in three or more of the following areas of major life activity;

    (I) self-care,

    (II) receptive and expressive language,

    (III) learning,

    (IV) mobility,

    (V) self-direction,

    (VI) capacity for independent living,

    (VII) economic sufficiency; and

  (v) reflects the person's need for combination and sequence of special, interdisciplinary, or generic services, individualized supports, or other forms of services which are of lifelong or extended duration and are individually planned and coordinated,

(B) INFANTS AND YOUNG CHILDREN—Individual from birth to age 9, inclusive, who has substantial developmental delay or specific congenital or acquired condition, may be considered to have developmental disability without meeting 3 more of the criteria described in clauses (i) through (v) of subparagraph (A) if the individual, without services and supports, has a high probability of meeting those criteria later in life.

FIGURE B-1 Developmental Disabilities Assistance and Bill of Rights Act.

Infants and Children

Important legislation for infants and children with special needs first appeared in the 1920s with the passage of the Maternity and Infant Act. In 1935, Title V of the Social Security Act was passed providing for three programs: Maternal and Child Health, Crippled Children's Services, and Child Welfare. Demonstration clinical programs for children with mental retardation emerged in 1950 with workshops on nutrition and mental retardation developed to update the skills and knowledge of nutrition personnel (20). Additional legislation in the 1960s promoted programs to prevent mental retardation through improved prenatal and infancy care, children and youth projects, and training programs in the university centers. Head Start was established in 1965 with a mandate that 10% of the enrolled population must have disabilities (21). Early Head Start (ages 0 to 3 years) was created by Congress in the reauthorization of the Head Start Act in 1994. Early Head Start requires inclusion of children with disabilities, with a provision that at least 10% of the total number of enrollment opportunities be made available to them.

Children with disabilities are defined as those children who are eligible for services under Part C of IDEA (22). As a part of IDEA, children with special needs from infancy through adolescence are served by the public school system and early intervention services. Part C is the early intervention component of the legislation that provides services for the child from birth to age three years. Considerable variation exists related to which agencies within a state are involved in early intervention and how services are provided. Whether a state educational or health agency administers the program, it is recommended that a natural setting be utilized. Thus, services are provided in the home, child-care centers, or similar settings rather than bringing the child into a centrally located center (22). Nutrition services are listed as a reimbursable service in Part C of the Early Intervention component of IDEA (6).

The Child Nutrition Act of 1966 and the Special Supplemental Nutrition Program for Women, Infants, and Children (WIC) begun in 1972 provide nutrition assistance to all eligible infants, children, and adolescents, including those with special needs. Unfortunately, all WIC services are terminated at age five years. In recent years, there has been increased emphasis on the importance of ensuring that children with special needs in schools receive substitutions for the regular meal if modifications are required because of their disabilities. This is mandated by the U.S. Department of Agriculture's nondiscrimination regulations (23) as well as the regulations governing the National School Lunch Program and School Breakfast Program. The regulations require that a physician's statement be provided, listing the disability, the reason for meal modification, and the specific substitutions needed (ie, diabetic diets, phenylketonuria (PKU), lactose free, blended or pureed, and high or low calorie). The

Child and Adult Care Food Programs must provide modified meals at no extra cost for children, adolescents, and adults with special needs in residential and/or day-care settings. Additionally, the nutrition goals should be included in the child's or adolescent's Individualized Education Plan (IEP) or 504 Accommodation plans (24). For example, clients may need individualized meal plans to address specific conditions such as diabetes, dysphagia, or PKU.

Although children with special needs may be insured through their parents' coverage, commercial insurance often has coverage gaps, high premiums, and no mandate to provide benefit packages to meet their needs (25). Nutrition services are frequently not funded for individual clients through Medicaid. In 1997, the Children's Health Insurance Program (CHIP) was enacted to provide funding to states to deliver health insurance to children and families with incomes too high to qualify for Medicaid and too low to afford private health insurance. Almost all states now have CHIP programs in operation.

Adults

It is estimated that the total number of adults and children with developmental disabilities including mental retardation is from 3 to 7 million people (9,10). However, financing health care for this population has remained a problem. Medicare covers 480,000 adults with developmental disabilities, with a large percentage also enrolled in Medicaid (25). Although health care for many individuals is funded through Medicaid, many providers refuse to serve this population or limit the number of people served. For example, Medicaid does not cover dental care for adults. The medical and dental care of adults in community-based residences is no longer obtained from a centralized institution staff but from primary care providers in the community (25). Medicaid databases were not designed to identify populations with special health needs, even though most receive health care through public insurance—only 7.1% of those with developmental disabilities have insurance through their employer (25).

Characteristics of the Population, Review of Selected Conditions, and Nutritional Risk Factors

Research has demonstrated that people with developmental disabilities are at increased risk for heart disease (26), obesity, osteoporosis, seizures, mental illness and behavior disorders, hearing and vision problems, and poor conditioning and fitness. Life expectancy for these individuals has increased to the extent that younger adults with developmental disabilities are expected to demonstrate little disparity in longevity; however, for older adults, disparities continue to exist.

The severity of the nutrition problem depends on multiple factors unique to the person (ie, age, level of functioning, severity of the disability, general state of health) and to environmental, educational, training, and social conditions. The altered physical growth rate or growth stunting often seen in persons with developmental disabilities may result from prenatal, perinatal, or postnatal causes. Prenatal causes are varied and include chromosomal aberrations such as Down's syndrome and exposure to a virus such as cytomegalovirus as well as prenatal exposure to alcohol and drugs. Perinatal and postnatal conditions such as cerebral palsy, bronchopulmonary dysplasia, and congenital heart disease may result in permanent growth stunting because of associated increased energy needs, feeding difficulties, and medical conditions (27–37) (See Table B-1). Special growth charts exist for some syndromes and conditions; however, their use in nutrition assessment is limited and controversial. They were developed using very small populations, do not include all growth parameters, and some use very old and retrospective data (38,39).

Overweight/Obesity

Obesity in persons with developmental disabilities can have negative social consequences and requires greater effort from caregivers; it also contributes to the development of chronic diseases such as diabetes, hypertension, and heart disease. One study found a higher prevalence of overweight in persons with Down's syndrome than the general population (15). This prevalence of obesity among persons with Down's syndrome is a major health problem that warrants further attention from researchers as well as dietetics professionals working with this population. The common characteristic of short stature, limited mobility along with inappropriate eating practices such as pica, are seen in clients with syndromes such as Prader–Willi and Lawrence Moon–Bidel. One study recommended a reduction of energy intake for weight maintenance along with daily aerobic exercise, strict food-control procedures, and an interdisciplinary approach for behavior modification (30).

Medication–Nutrient Interaction

The long-term use of medication can result in nutrient interactions. Abnormalities in vitamin D, calcium and bone status, constipation, and gum hyperplasia have been found in persons with developmental disabilities who have limited mobility. These abnormalities are associated with the long-term use of the anticonvulsants phenytion and/or phenobarbital. A strong association between anticonvulsant use and ambulatory status was reported (40).

Many older adults with developmental disabilities take multiple medications for extended periods of time. They are at risk for com-

TABLE B-1   Selected Syndrome and Development Disabilities: Frequently Reported Nutrition Problems and Factors Contributing to Nutrional Risk

Syndrome/disability	Altered growth, underweight, obesity	Altered energy need	Constipation/ diarrhea	Feeding problems	Others
Cerebral palsy A disorder of muscle control or coordination resulting from injury to the brain during its early (fetal, perinatal, and early childhood) development. There may be associated problems with intellectual, visual, or other functions.	Growth problems	Failure to thrive	Constipation	Oral/motor Problems	Central nervous system involvement Orthopedic problems Medication/nutrient interaction related to seizure disorder
Down syndrome A genetic disorder that results from an extra #21 chromosome, causing development problems such as congenital heart disease, mental retardation, short stature, and decreased muscle tone.	Risk for obesity	Related to short stature and limited activity	Constipation	Poor suck in infancy	Gum disease Increased risk of heart disease Osteoporosis Alzheimer's
Prader-Willi syndrome A genetic disorder marked by hypotonia, short stature, hyperphagia, and cognitive impairment; when not carefully managed, characterized by obesity.	Risk for obesity	Failure to thrive in infancy	N/A	Poor suck in infancy Abnormal food-related problems	Risk of diabetes mellitus
Autism Classified as a type of pervasive developmental disorder; diagnostic criteria include communication problems, ritualistic behaviors, and inappropriate social interaction	N/A	N/A	N/A	Limited food selection Strong food dislikes	Pica Medication/nutrient interaction

Condition					
Cystic fibrosis (CF) An inherited disorder of the exocrine glands, primarily the pancreas, pulmonary system, and sweat glands, characterized by abnormally thick luminal secretions.	N/A	Increased nutrient intake Decreased food intake Decrease of nutrients related to pancreatic insufficiency and chronic pulmonary infection	N/A	N/A	Increase in secondary illnesses: Diabetes Liver disease Ostocoporosis
Spina bifida (Myeolomeningocele) Results from a midline defect of the skin, spinal column, and spinal cord. Characterized by hydrocephalus, mental retardation, and lack of muscular control.	Risk for obesity	Altered energy needs based on short stature and limited mobility	Constipation	Swallowing problems caused by the Arnold Chiari malformation of the brain	Urinary tract infections

plications caused by medication interactions. In addition, medication may have a longer half-life because of decreased lean body mass. Use of medications such as antibiotics for recurrent urinary or respiratory infections may produce gastrointestinal symptoms. Psychotropics may also increase or decrease appetite (41). Constipation is a side effect of long-term psychotropic use, which results in increased use of laxatives and stool softeners.

Attention deficit hyperactivity disorder (ADHD) is commonly treated with stimulant medications such as methylphenidate (Ritalin). Studies show that these medications depress appetite in children, resulting in a slower rate of weight gain and growth. These effects on growth may be significantly reduced by taking "vacations" from the medication during the summer or during school breaks (26).

Tricyclic antidepressants (TCAs) are used to treat depression and as a treatment for ADHD for some young adults and children over six years of age. Nutrition-related side effects of TCAs include increased appetite, nausea and vomiting, constipation, and diarrhea (26).

Energy Needs

Assessing energy requirements for this population presents a challenge because requirements differ depending on the severity of the disability, mobility status, number of medications, and feeding problems. The results of one study of adolescents with cerebral palsy found that energy requirements for both ambulatory and nonambulatory adolescents were decreased compared with a control group of normal adolescents. Fat-free mass and body weight were significantly correlated with resting energy expenditure only in the myelodysplasia group. This study suggests that the type of paralysis may affect resting energy expenditure (42,43). Another study of adults with cerebral palsy considered that the presence of athetotic movements increased the resting metabolic rate by an average of 524 kcal/day. Increased energy requirements were a result of their involuntary movements in that the subjects in this study had less fat-free mass and expended fewer calories in leisure activities than the control subjects (44).

Oral Motor/Feeding Issues

Oral motor problems, food allergies, chewing and swallowing problems, and food aversions complicate the process of implementing medical nutrition therapy (MNT). A study of 12,000 children (.5 to 3.5 years of age) with cerebral palsy examined risk factors for mortality, which included self-feeding skills and simple measures of mobility. Ninety percent of children with good to fair motor and feeding skills reached adulthood (45). Lack of self-feeding skill was associated with a six-fold increased risk in mortality, whereas severity of cerebral palsy, low birth weight, and degree of mental retardation were associated with a 1.4- to 3.0-fold increase in mortality. This suggests that feeding function may be as important an indicator of a child's health outcome as mental and/or motor capacity. A large, multicentered study of children ages two to 18 years with moderate to severe cerebral palsy assessed the relationship between feeding dysfunction, health, and nutritional status. The study showed that even those with mild feeding dysfunction had poor growth and inadequate fat stores (46). Early identification, treatment, and correction of feeding dysfunction improve the health and nutritional status in the population.

Many children and adults depend on caregivers to feed them the appropriate amount of food and fluid to achieve the client's desired weight. Weekly or, at a minimum, monthly weighings are important to evaluate whether caloric intake is adequate. The dietetics professional may need to assume the responsibility of weighing the client if the caregiver is not tracking weight. When observing a caregiver feeding a client, the dietetics professional should watch for any clinical signs of impaired swallowing function such as coughing, choking during feeding, wet sounds in throat, or changes in respiratory patterns. If any of these symptoms are noted, referral should be made to the speech therapist for further evaluation and intervention.

Tube feeding may be recommended in some patients with failure to thrive, aspiration pneumonia, dysphagia, or the inability to ingest adequate calories orally to promote growth or maintain nutritional status. A tube feeding requires ongoing monitoring and evaluation by the registered dietitian. Monitoring is critical in the group home or community setting in which the health care provider may change frequently and not be adequately trained.

Consumer and Health Care Trends

Social Changes in the United States

The goal of total inclusion for infants, children, and adults with developmental disabilities makes them a part of a rapidly changing culture and society. The racial and ethnic diversity of America's children and young adults continues to increase. In 2000, 64% of children and adolescents were white, with increasing numbers of Hispanic, black, Asian/Pacific Islanders, and American Indians. The percentage of children in two-parent homes has declined (47).

With the increasing numbers of individuals who do not speak English, providing nutrition education materials in appropriate languages and incorporating multicultural foods have become a significant need. In addition, nutrition materials related to food preparation, selection, and buying are needed for individuals with low literacy skills. Some families may have difficulty accepting the child with special needs and may require extra help to incorporate nutrition therapy and other types of intervention into their lifestyle. The proportion of children living in families with incomes below the poverty level was 16% in the year 2000; however, the poverty rate of black and Hispanic families was 30% and 27%, respectively (48). In single-parent families, the current poverty rate is 40% (48). Poverty can have a negative impact on a child's health and development through a lack of food security. Food security has been defined as access at all times to enough nourishment for an active, healthy life. At a minimum, food security includes the availability of sufficient, nutritionally adequate, and safe food and the assurance that families can obtain adequate food without relying on emergency feeding programs or resorting to scavenging, stealing, or other desperate measures to secure food (48). Adults with developmental disabilities may also suffer from poverty. Although they are capable of working in part-time or full-time jobs, opportunities are limited.

Access to health care provides reasonable assurance for obtaining medical attention needed to maintain physical well-being. Access involves both the availability of a regular source of care and the ability of the family or someone else to pay for it. Twelve percent of all children in the United States had no health insurance of any kind during 2000. Hispanic children are less likely to have health insurance than white or black children (48). National data reporting health care provision for individuals with developmental disabilities are not yet available because of difficulty in definitions and measurement.

In Healthy People 2010, the Maternal and Child Health Bureau, in partnership with the March of Dimes, American Academy of Pediatrics, and Family Voices identified six core outcomes for children with special health care needs to provide a measure of progress in making family-centered care a reality and in putting in place the systems needed. These outcomes include the following:

- the family partnering in decision making at all levels and with all services;
- all children receiving coordinated ongoing comprehensive care within a medical home;
- all families having adequate private or public insurance to pay for the services needed;
- all children receiving screening early and continuously for special health care needs;
- community-based systems organized so that families can use them easily; and
- all youths receiving the services necessary to make transitions to all aspects of adult life, including adult health care, work, and independence (49).

The concept of a medical home for infants and children with special health care needs means a source of ongoing, comprehensive, family-centered care in the child's community. The medical home should provide preventive services, immunizations, growth and developmental assessments, screening, health care supervision, and patient and family counseling about health and psychosocial issues. The need for nutrition services is apparent because previous surveys have shown that 70% to 90% of children with special health care needs have nutritional problems (5,6). The medical home concept includes a responsibility for the practitioners to be knowledgeable about all community services and organizations available to families (49).

Special Olympics provides people with mental retardation from more than 150 countries the opportunity for year-round training and competition. The nutrition section of Special Olympics is part of the Health Athletes program Health Promoter. The Special Olympics Healthy Athletes initiative provides a variety of health services designed to improve each participant's ability to train and compete.

The Special Olympics Health Athletes initiative will pilot test locally based, ongoing, health promotion programs with the goal of making good nutrition and physical fitness routine for Special Olympic Athletes. Consultations with dietitians along with other health care providers will be incorporated in the initiative (50).

Special Olympics Special Smiles is a dental screening education and referral program offered under Special Olympics, Inc. The nutrition education component offers dietetics professionals the opportunity to partner with the dental profession and demonstrate to the athlete the importance of good nutrition for overall health and fitness.

The role of technology in providing nutrition information for parents and caregivers as well as for children and adults with developmental disabilities has grown. Many parents use the Internet to search for information related to the particular syndrome or disability involving their child or young adult. Nutrition information may be questionable and possibly inaccurate but may be accepted by families seeking answers.

The need for accessible, accurate nutrition information from dietetics professionals is great. Parents purchase nutrition supplement packages of herbs, vitamins, minerals, and amino acids from information supplied on the Internet on the recommendation of family support group members, on the advice of health food store employees, and based on information in printed materials. The promise of increased growth and cognitive ability for their children or family member prompts parents to make these purchases. Unfortunately, research related to the use of these products, including safety and efficacy, is extremely limited.

Emphasis on Wellness and the Prevention of Disease

The health issues for individuals with developmental disabilities and children with special health care needs are similar to the health issues for everyone. These include physical activity, nutrition, access to health care, clinical preventive services, oral care, mental health, and family caregiving. As research in the area of human genetics increases, the incidence of genetic syndromes may eventually decrease. As genetic techniques improve to identify the tendency of an individual for chronic disease such as heart disease or diabetes, new educational strategies must be developed to work with individuals with developmental disabilities and special needs in wellness programs to prevent such disorders (51).

Effective nutritional therapy is important for children with metabolic disorders to survive infancy and avoid severe cognitive and physical problems. For example, conditions such as cystic fibrosis, phenylketonuria, and diabetes present unique nutritional challenges. The key to prevention and treatment is the early identification of the disorder as well as nutrition problems and providing services throughout the life cycle related to appropriate food intake and education on healthy eating behaviors combined with physical activity (5,6).

The importance of nutrition in the prevention of specific developmental disabilities is exemplified by the role of folic acid supplementation prior to and during pregnancy in the prevention of neurotube defects (52). The vital role of nutrition in the treatment of inborn errors of metabolism in the prevention of mental retardation and developmental disabilities is well known (53). The realization that treatment of inborn errors of metabolism is lifelong has resulted in the development of many dietary products that have enhanced treatment for these individuals and contributed to the possibility of lifelong compliance (54).

In 2001, the Centers for Disease Control and Prevention (CDC) established a new center that will focus on birth defects and disabilities. Created by the Children's Health Act of 2000, the CDC's Center on Birth Defects and Developmental Disabilities is designed to improve the health of children and adults by preventing birth defects and developmental disabilities, promoting optimal child development, and ensuring health and wellness among children and adults living with disabilities.

With the reauthorization of the Developmental Disabilities Act of 2000 (1) two new titles were authorized. One title is Family Support in which grants are provided to develop and implement statewide systems of family support services for families of children with disabilities. Nutrition services, counseling, and information should always be a part of family support services. The other new program is entitled Direct Support Workers who Assist Individuals with Developmental Disabilities. This program will develop distance learning training programs for direct support workers. Nutrition should be an appropriate part of these training modules.

Parental advocacy organizations exist for many specific syndromes such as Parent Advocates for Down Syndrome (PADS), Prader–Willi Syndrome Association, and the National PKU Organization. These organizations work for legislative changes and the provision of accurate information to the families of their members. People with developmental disabilities are becoming more connected to their regular community and each other, and are forming self-advocacy organizations to help other people with disabilities.

As the life expectancy of individuals with developmental disabilities increases, the chronic diseases associated with aging emerge and require identification and treatment. Under Medicare Part B Outpatient Services, two disorders can be treated by MNT: diabetes and renal disease (55). Traditional nutrition counseling may not be effective for the individual who is cognitively impaired, and such nutrition counseling will require collaboration among nutrition professionals, family members, care providers, and special educators to prepare effective teaching tools (56) and adequate nutritional care.

Components of Comprehensive Nutrition Services

Policy Development

Although access to health care services and equal protection of rights of all persons with developmental disabilities is guaranteed under federal law, there must be a strong working relationship between professional and advocacy groups to ensure that comprehensive nutrition services are offered. The role of nutrition in the prevention of disease and the promotion of health is included in Healthy People 2010 (49), the Surgeon General's Report on Nutrition and Health, U.S. Dept of Health and Human Services 1999 (57), and in Bright Futures (58). Healthy People 2010 lists health issues for the individual with special needs to attain as physical activity, obesity/overweight, nutrition, access to health care, clinical preventitive services, oral health, and mental health. The Third Report of the National Cholesterol Education Program (NCEP) (59), the American Diabetes Association Position Statement: Evidence-Based Nutrition Principles and Recommendations for the Treatment and Prevention of Diabetes and Related Complications (60), and the American Cancer Society and the Nutrition Screening Initiative (61) have published support for the inclusion of MNT in the prevention and treatment of disease. Individuals with special health care needs and disabilities will also benefit from the provision of these nutrition services.

Financing

Coordination among multiple agencies and disciplines is needed to foster the potential growth of the infant to a healthy adult. The Federal Interagency Coordinating Council was established in 1991 to improve collaboration between various federal agencies serving families and children and includes representatives from the National Institute of Mental Health; Bureau of Indian Affairs, Office of Special Education Programs; Division of Birth Defects and Developmental Disabilities of the Centers for Disease Control and Prevention, Maternal Child Health Bureau; Social Security Administration; and many others for early intervention programs. The Supreme Court's decision in *Olmstead v LC* charged states with developing community-based services to allow people to live as independently as is appropriate (62). Group homes in the community for both adults and children with a wide range of disabilities operate with state and local funding. The most recent trend is toward adults living independently in their own apartments, with interdisciplinary teams directing their care and services. Often the registered dietitian is not a part of this team. Dietetics professionals need to accept this challenge and seek out the agencies that provide services for these clients and advocate for the inclusion of dietetic services.

Nutrition Services

The dietetics professional's role as an effective member of the health care team is to assess the clinical, biochemical, and anthropometric measurements; dietary concerns; and feeding skills as well as understand the environmental, social, economic, and educational factors affecting the intervention plan for the client. As a team player, this includes training other disciplines, families, and caregivers on food selection and preparation. Because community-based programs have financial constraints, education of the providers/staff can influence the food selection process. The American Dietetic Association and its state affiliates often have continuing education programs to expand the knowledge of the dietetics professional in areas specific to this population.

Roles and Responsibilities of the Dietetics Professional

Services provided by the dietetics professional are essential to the health of the client with special needs. Screening may be done by another member of the health care team, who refers the client to the dietetics professional for assessment (63). Because many clients with developmental disabilities have conditions that delay physical growth, the nutrition assessment should target some of these deviations, for example, those individuals with chronic respiratory failure who require the use of a ventilator or individuals with dysphagia or feeding problems. Cognitive assessments provide understanding of the client's functional ability to develop appropriate treatment plans. Lower-level literacy programs may be appropriate for this population. A study examined the factors influencing nutrition education for persons with low literacy skills. The result of the research suggested that effective nutrition interventions must build on patients' social networks, appear in a visually based and interactive format, and be culturally appropriate (64). Evaluation of feeding skills is an important component of the assessment and treatment program. The goal of the feeding program may be to achieve independence without placing the client at nutritional risk. Occupational therapists and speech language pathologists work with the team to determine the treatment plan for the client, which may include self-help feeding devices (65–68). Often the dietetics professional is the team member who reinforces the plan and determines the food appropriate for the client.

Education

The Administration on Developmental Disabilities (ADD) is a federal program that supports a system of state-based programs designed to help people with developmental disabilities such as mental retardation live productive, independent lives in the community. ADD funds at least one University Center for Excellence (UCE) in Developmental Disabilities Research, Training, and Service in every state and most territories. The Maternal and Child Health Bureau funds Leadership Education in Neurodevelopmental Disorders (LEND) programs in many states. Previously known as University Affiliated Programs (UAPs), both the LEND and the UCE are located in universities and mandated to work in and with the communities they serve. The goal of the nationwide network is to bring validated, best-practice disability initiatives into community practice in each state. UCEs translate scientific research into practice through interdisciplinary research, training activities, and service demonstration efforts. UCEs train professionals for leadership positions and direct care workers for community services; work to ensure that systems are designed so that people with developmental disabilities have access to the services and supports they need; conduct research and validate emerging state-of-the-art practices; provide technical assistance to agencies and the community; and disseminate information to individuals with disabilities, families, public and private agencies, and policymakers. Dietetics professionals should locate the UCE in their community and investigate the services available. This is another window of opportunity for the dietetics professional seeking to provide nutritional services for this population (18).

Protocols/Standards of Care

The American Dietetic Association has not yet developed protocols for nutrition services specific to the population with developmental disabilities and special health care needs. However, many of the diseases and conditions for which protocols have been developed, such as diabetes mellitus and cardiovascular and renal disease, occur in this population. Dietetics professionals can use the MNT protocols developed by ADA for these diseases and conditions. A long-term goal to develop protocols for this population would lead the way in achieving the goal of increased reimbursement. Protocols for cystic fibrosis and high-risk prenatal care are included in the 1996 ADA publication MNT Across the Continuum of Care (69).

Recommendations

To provide comprehensive nutrition services for infants, children, and adults with developmental disabilities and special health care needs, the American Dietetic Association recommends that dietetics professionals do the following:

- develop and implement content and/or field experience that addresses the nutrition needs of persons with developmental disabilities and special health care needs in undergraduate and graduate nutrition programs;
- provide specialized interdisciplinary nutrition training for practicing dietetics professionals to address the health care needs of these persons;
- provide the opportunity for increasing the level of nutrition knowledge related to children and adults with developmental disabilities and special health care needs among all health care and human service providers;
- support programs that promote health and wellness for persons with developmental disabilities and special health care needs throughout the life cycle;
- promote and provide nutrition services, including ongoing nutrition monitoring, as an essential component of health care programs;
- support inclusion of nationally credentialed dietetics professionals experienced in the nutrition needs of persons with developmental disabilities and special health care needs in agencies developing policy in the areas of education, vocation, and health services at the federal and state levels;
- collaborate with health care providers to ensure that there are policies in place to promote family-centered, interdisciplinary, coordinated, community-based, culturally competent services;

- develop and implement evidence-based MNT protocols that address the unique needs of this population across the life cycle;
- encourage participation of nationally credentialed dietetics professionals on primary and specialty care teams and in vocation, education, and residential programs that serve this population throughout the life cycle;
- work to obtain reimbursement for MNT as part of comprehensive health care for people with developmental disabilities and special health care needs; and
- support and promote nutrition research in the areas of obesity, diabetes mellitus, hypertension, cardiac, and other diseases in an effort to continuously improve the quality of life for those with developmental disabilities and special health care needs.

References

1. Developmental Disabilities Assistance and Bill of Rights Act. PL 106–402; 2000.
2. Beange H, McElduff A, Baker W. Medical disorders of adults with mental retardation: A population study. *Am J Mental Retard.* 1995; 99:595–604.
3. Hand JE. Report of a national survey of older people with lifelong intellectual disability in New Zealand. *J Intellect Disabil Res.* 1994;38: 275–287.
4. McPherson M, Arango P, Fox H, Lauver C, McManus M, Newacheck PW, Perrin JM, Shonkogg JP, Strickland B. A new definition of children with special health care needs. *Pediatrics.* 1998;102:137–140.
5. Bayerl CT, Ries JD, Bettencourt MF, Fisher P. Nutrition issues of children in early intervention programs: primary care team approach. *Semin Pediatr Gastroenterol Nutr.* 1993;4:11–15.
6. Ekvall S, Ekvall V. Early Intervention and Nutrition. In: Stevens F, Ekvall S, eds. *Empowering Children Through Early Intervention with Good Nutrition–Focusing on Culturally Diverse Children with Special Health Care Needs.* Manual IV, MCHB. Rockville, MD: HRSA; 2001:7–20.
7. Centers for Disease Control and Prevention. Developmental Disabilities. Atlanta, GA. Available at: http://www.cdc.gov/ncbddd/dd/default.htm. Accessed August 21, 2003.
8. McFadden DL, Burke EP. Developmental disabilities and the new paradigm: Directions for the 1990s. *Ment Retard.* 1991;29:iii–vi.
9. Ireys HT, Nelson RP. New federal policy for children with special health care needs: Implications for pediatricians. *Pediatrics.* 1992;90:321–327.
10. U.S. Department of Health and Human Services. Administration on Developmental Disabilities. Fact Sheet/2002. Available at: www.acf.dhhs.gov/programs/add. Accessed September 4, 2003.

11. Kerker B. Closing the Gap: A National Blueprint for Improving the Health of Individuals with Mental Retardation. Report of the Surgeon General's Conference on Health Disparities and Mental Retardation. Washington, DC. February 2001. Available at: http://www.nichd.nih.gov/publications/pubs/closingthegap/index.htm. Accessed September 4, 2003.

12. Luckasson R, Borthwick-Duffy S, Buntinx WHE, Coulter D, Craig EM, Reeve A, Schalock RL, Snell ME, Spitalnik DM, Spreat S, Tasse MJ. *Mental retardation: Definition, classification, and systems of supports.* 10th ed. Washington, DC: American Association on Mental Retardation; 2002.

13. Pope AM, Tarlov AR. *Disability in America. Toward a National Agenda for Prevention.* Washington, DC: National Academy Press; 1991.

14. Rasmussen SA, Moore CA, Paulozzi LF, Rhodenhiser EP. Risk for birth defects among premature infants: A population-based study. *J Pediatr.* 2001;138:668–673.

15. Rubin SS, Rimmer JH, Chicoine B, Braddock D, McGuire DE. Overweight prevalence in persons with Down Syndrome. *Ment Retard.* 1998;36:175–181.

16. Rimmer JH, Braddock D, Fujiura G. Cardiovascular risk factor levels in adults with mental retardation. *Am J Ment Retard.* 1994;98: 510–518.

17. Hand JE, Reid PM. Older adults with lifelong intellectual disability in New Zealand: Prevalence disability and implications for regional health authorities. *N Z Med J.* 1996;109:118–121.

18. Cloud HH. Impact of legislation on nutrition services for individuals with developmental disabilities. *Top Clin Nutr.* 1993;8:1–4.

19. Cloud HH. Recent trends in care of children with special needs. *Top Clin Nutr.* 2001;16:28–40.

20. Egan M. Nutrition services in the Maternal and Child Health programs: A historical perspective. In: Sharbaugh CO, ed. *Call to Action: Better Nutrition for Mothers, Children and Families.* Washington, DC: National Center for Maternal and Child Health; 1991:3–22.

21. Head Start Program Performance Standards and Other Regulations. U.S. Dept. of Health and Human Services, Administration for Children and Families, Administration on Children, Youth and Families, Head Start Bureau; 1996.

22. Spiker D, Hebbeler K, Wagner M, Cameto R, McKenna P. A framework for describing variations in state early intervention systems. *Top Early Child Special Educ.* 2000;20:195–218.

23. United States Department of Agriculture. USDA and FNS Programs Nondiscrimination Statements. Washington, DC; 1999. Available at: http://www.fns.usda.gov/cr/Policy/nondiscrimination_statements.htm. Accessed on October 20, 2003.

24. Cloud HH. Clients with Special Needs. In: Owen G, Owen A, Splett P. eds. *Nutrition in the Community: The Art and Science of Delivering Services.* 4th ed. Boston, MA: WCB/McGraw Hill; 1999: 344–371.

25. U.S. Public Health Service. *Closing the Gap: A National Blueprint for Improving the Health of Individuals with Mental Retardation.* Washington, DC: The Surgeon General's Conference on Health Disparities and Mental Retardation; February 2001.

26. Rimmer JH, Braddock D, Fujiura G. Cardiovascular risk factor levels in adults with mental retardation. *Am J Ment Retard.* 1994;98: 510–518.

27. Heinrichs E, Rokusek C. *Nutrition and Feeding for Persons with Special Needs.* Pierre, SD: South Dakota University Affiliated Program University of South Dakota School of Medicine and the South Dakota Department of Education and Cultural Affairs–Child and Adult Nutrition Services; 1992.

28. Nutrition Interventions for Children with Special Health Care Needs. Washington State Department of Health; March 2001. Publication No. 961–158.

29. Wooldridge NH. Pulmonary diseases. In: Samour PQ, Helm KK, Lang CE, eds. *Handbook of Pediatric Nutrition.* 2nd ed. Gaithersburg, MD: Aspen Publishers, Inc; 1999:315–353.

30. Alexander DR. Preterm birth: Etiologies, mechanisms and prevention. *Prenatal Neonatal Med.* 1998;3:3–9.

31. Hoffman CJ, Aultman D, Pipes P. A nutrition survey of and recommendations for individuals with Prader-Willi syndrome who live in group homes. *J Am Diet Assoc.* 1992;92:823–830.

32. Ekvall S. *Pediatric Nutrition in Chronic Diseases and Developmental Disorders.* New York, NY: Oxford University Press; 1993.

33. Kao C, Chen C, Wang S, Yeh S. Bone mineral density in children with Down syndrome detected by dual photon absorptiometry. *Nucl Med Commun.* 1992;13:773–775.

34. Supulveda D, Allison D, Gomez J, Kreibich K, Brown R, Pierson R, Heymsfield S. Low spinal and pelvic bone mineral density among individuals with Down Syndrome. *Am J Ment Retard.* 1995;100:109–114.

35. Kim SH, Vlkolinsky R, Cairns N, Lubee G. Decreased levels of complex III core protein 1 and complex V β chain in brains from patients with Alzheimer's disesase and Down syndrome. *Cell Mol Life Sci.* 2000;57: 1810–1816.

36. Kim SH, Shim KS, Lubee G. Human brain nascent polypeptideassociated complex α subunit is decreased in patients with Alzheimer's disease and Down syndrome. *J Investig Med.* 2002;50: 293–301.

37. Oliver C, Crayton L, Holland A, Hall S, Bradbury J. A four-year prospective study of age-related cognitive change in adults with Down's syndrome. *Psychol Med.* 1998;28:1365–1377.

38. Center for Disease Control. 2000 CDC Growth Charts: United States. Atlanta, GA; 2000. Available at: http://www. cdc.gov/growthcharts. Accessed September 24, 2003.

39. Ekvall S. Myelomeningocele. In: Ekvall S, ed. *Pediatric Nutrition in Chronic Diseases and Developmental Disorders.* New York: Oxford University Press; 1993:107–114.

40. Baer MT, Kozlowski BW, Blyler EM, Trahm CM, Taylor ML, Hogan MP. Vitamin D, calcium and bone status in children with developmental delay in relation to anticonvulsant use and ambulatory status. *Am J Clin Nutr.* 1997;65:1042–1051.

41. Sutton E, Factor AR, Hawkins BA, Heller T, Seltzer GB, eds. *Older Adults with Developmental Disabilities. Optimizing Choice and Change.* Baltimore, MD: Paul H. Brookes Publishing Co; 1993.

42. Bandini LG, Schoeller DA, Fukagawa NK, Wykes LJ, Dietz WH. Body composition and energy expenditure in adolescents with cerebral palsy or myelodysplasia. *Pediatr Res.* 1991;29:70–77.

43. Grogan C, Ekvall S. Body composition of children with myelomeningo-cele determined by K, urinary creatinine and anthropometric measures. *J Am Coll Nutr.* 1999; 18:316–325.

44. Johnson RK, Goran MI, Ferrara MS, Poehlman ET. Athetosis increases resting metabolic rate in adults with cerebral palsy. *J Am Diet Assoc.* 1996;96:145–148.

45. Strauss DJ, Shavelle RM, Anderson TW. Life expectancy of children with cerebral palsy. *Pediatr Neurol.* 1998;18:143–149.

46. Fung EB, Samson-Fang L, Stallings VA, Conaway M, Liptak G, Henderson RC, Worley G, O'Donnell M, Calvert R, Rosenbaum P, Chumlea W, Stevenson RD. Feeding dysfunction is associated with poor growth and health status in children with cerebral palsy. *J Am Diet Assoc.* 2002;102:361–373.

47. Forum on Child and Family Statistics. America's Children: Key National Indicators of Well Being. Vienna, VA: 2001. Available at: http://child-stats.gov/ac2001/ac01.asp. Accessed August 21, 2003.

48. Forum of Child and Family Statistics. Child Poverty and Family Income, in America's Children. Vienna, VA: 2001. Available at: http://childstats.gov/ac2001/econtxt.asp#econ1a. Accessed August 21, 2003.

49. U.S. Dept. of Health and Human Services. *Healthy People 2010: Understanding and Improving Health.* 2nd ed. Washington, DC: U.S. Government Printing Office; November 2000. Stock No. 017-001-001-00-550-9.

50. Special Olympics. Special Olympics Healthy Athletes. Washington, DC. Available at: http://www.specialolympics.com/special+olympics+public+website/english/coach/coaching_guides/section+1/healthy+athletes.htm. Accessed October 16, 2003

51. Owen AL. Entering the Era of Dynamic Change. In: Owen AL, Splett PL, Owen GM, eds. *Health and Nutrition. Nutrition in the Community: The Art and Science of Delivering Services.* 4th ed. Boston, MA: McGraw Hill Companies, Inc; 1999:610–627.

52. American Academy of Pediatrics. Committee on Genetics. Folic acid for the prevention of neural tube defects. *Pediatrics.* 1999;104:325–327.

53. Winter S, Buist NR. Inborn errors of metabolism, medical and administrative orphans. *Am J Managed Care.* 1998;4:1164–1168.

54. Matalon KM. Developments in phenylketonuria. *Top Clin Nutr.* 2001; 16:41–50.

55. Medicare Coverage Policy: Decisions. Available at: http://cms. hhs.gov/mcd/viewncd.asp?ncd_ id_80-3&ncd_version_1&show_all. Accessed August 21, 2003.

56. Marcario E, Emmons KM, Sorensen G, Hunt MK, Rudd RE. Factors influencing nutrition education for patients with low literacy skill. *J Am Diet Assoc.* 1998;98:559–564.

57. U.S. Dept. of Health and Human Services. The Surgeon General's Report on Nutrition and Health; 1999. DHHS Stock No. 011-017- 024-01653-5.

58. Story M, Holt K, Sofka D. Bright *Futures in Practice: Nutrition.* 2nd ed. Arlington, VA: National Center for Education in Maternal and Child Health; 2002.

59. U.S. Dept. of Health and Human Services. Third Report of the National Cholesterol Education Program; May 2001. NH Publication No 01-3670.

60. American Diabetes Association Position Statement. Evidence-based nutrition principles and recommendations for the treatment and prevention of diabetes and related complications. *J Am Diet Assoc.* 2002;102:109–118.

61. A Physician's Guide to Nutrition in Chronic Disease Management for Older Adults. Nutrition Screening Initiative Special Chronic Disease Edition. Issue 34. Washington, DC; Winter 2002.

62. Vickery K. Community Life. *Provider.* 2001;Dec:20–34.

63. Council on Practice Quality Management Committee. Identifying patients at risk: ADA's definitions for nutrition screening and nutrition assessment. *J Am Diet Assoc.* 1994;94:838–839.

64. Macario E, Emmons KM, Sorensen G, Hunt MK, Rudd RE. Factors influencing nutrition education for patients with low literacy skills. *J Am Diet Assoc.* 1998;98:559–564.

65. Case-Smith J. Self-care strategies for children with developmental deficits. In: Christiansen C, ed. *Ways of Living: Self-Care Strategies for Special Needs.* Bethesda, MD: The American Occupational Therapy Association, Inc; 1994.

66. Pedretti L, Umphred D. Teaching and learning in occupational therapy. In: Early MB, ed. *Physical Dysfunction Practice Skills for the Occupational Therapy Assistant.* St. Louis, MO: Mosby Yearbook, Inc; 1998.

67. Mayall JK, Desharnais G. *Positioning in a Wheelchair: A Guide for Professional Caregivers of the Disabled Adult.* 2nd ed. Thorofare, NJ: Slack Inc; 1995.

68. McCuaig M. Self-care management for adults with movement disorders. In: Christiansen C, ed. *Ways of Living: Self-Care Strategies for Special Needs.* Rockville, MD: American Occupational Therapy Association, Inc; 1994.

69. The American Dietetic Association. *Medical Nutrition Therapy Across the Continuum of Care.* Chicago, IL: American Dietetic Association; 1996.

ADA position adopted by the HOD Leadership Team on May 3, 2003. This position is in effect until December 31, 2008. ADA authorizes republication of the position statement/support paper, in its entirety, provided full and proper credit is given. Requests to use portions of the position must be directed to ADA headquarters at 800/877-1600, ext 4835, or ppapers@eatright.org. Authors: Harriet Holt Cloud, MS, RD, FADA (Nutrition Matters, Birmingham, AL); Mary Ellen Posthauer, RD (M.E.P. Healthcare Dietary Services, Inc, Evansville, IN). Reviewers: Judith Amundson, MS, RD, FAMMR (University of Iowa Center for Disabilities and Development, Iowa City, IA); Cynthia Taft Bayerl, MS, RD (Massachusetts Department of Public Health, Boston, MA); Consultant Dietitians in Health Care Facilities dietetic practice group (Eileen Monahan Chopnick, MBA, RD, Jefferson Health System, Radnor, PA; Judy A. Cox, MS, RD, Renal Medicine Associates, Clovis, NM); Dietetics in Development and Psychiatric Disorders dietetic practice group (Ruth Ann Foiles, MPA, RD, dietetic consultant, Lansing, MI); Sharon Feucht, MA, RD (University of Washington, Seattle, WA); Mimi Kaufman, MPH, RD, LD (Texas Department of Health, Austin, TX); Pediatric Nutrition dietetic practice group (Molly Holland, MPH, RD, University of Vermont, Burlington, VT); Lakshman Rao, PhD, RD (South Carolina Department of Mental Health, Columbia, SC); Janet Horsley Willis, MPH, RD (Partnership for People with Disabilities, Virginia Commonwealth University, Richmond, VA); Members of the Association Positions Committee Workgroup: Barbara Emison Gaffield, MS, RD (chair); Sonja Connor, MS, RD; Betty Lucas, MPH, RD (content advisor).

POSITION OF THE AMERICAN DIETETIC ASSOCIATION: THE ROLE OF DIETETICS PROFESSIONALS IN HEALTH PROMOTION AND DISEASE PREVENTION

American Dietetic Association

Abstract

In the United States, the leading determinants of morbidity and mortality are rooted in behavioral choices related to eating habits, exercise, tobacco, alcohol consumption, and stress reduction. Scientific data consistently provide evidence that diet plays an important role in health promotion and disease prevention. Healthy eating habits—coupled with other healthful lifestyle behaviors—have the potential to reduce the risk of chronic disease.

Health care typically assumes a curative or treatment role in the United States. However, dietetics professionals are shaping an alternate view of health, which includes developing healthy public policies, creating safe and supportive environments, building communities and coalitions, and reorienting health services to include health promotion as a primary approach to delivering health care. Individual-level approaches, such as counseling and group education, have been employed most often in modifying health behaviors. However, population-level approaches that affect availability of or access to healthy foods, opportunities for physical activity, and other healthy lifestyle determinants also are important. Dietetics professionals have pivotal roles in both individual- and population-level approaches.

Reprinted with permission from Elsevier Publications. Journal of the American Dietetic Association, V102(11): 1680–1687, Hampl JS et al: "Position of The American Dietetic Association: The Role of Dietetics Professionals in Health Promotion and Disease Prevention." © 2002 with the permission of The American Dietetic Association.

Position Statement

It is the position of the American Dietetic Association that health promotion and disease prevention endeavors are the best population strategies for reducing the current burden of chronic disease. Dietetics professionals should be actively involved in promoting optimal nutrition in community settings and should advocate for the inclusion of healthy eating, in addition to other health-promoting behaviors, in programs and policy initiatives at local, state, or federal levels.

Environmental Mediators

Although unhealthy behaviors are the leading contributors to morbidity and mortality in the United States, the most outcome- and cost-effective ways to change community health remain unknown. Social and environmental issues are believed to play a role in fostering habits that lead to chronic disease. For example, environmental factors involved with the development of obesity include advertisements for low prices and the actual low prices of energy-dense foods, marketing of larger portion sizes and prizes, and U.S. society's increased use of convenience foods (1).

In general, lower-income and minority groups are more likely to be exposed to environmental factors that promote the use of unhealthy products, including foods high in saturated and trans-fats and tobacco. Moore et al (2) reported that alcohol and tobacco advertising are most highly concentrated in low-income neighborhoods that have a large percentage of African American residents. Also, physical structures in low-income neighborhoods are less conducive to healthy outcomes than are those in higher-income neighborhoods: lack of lighting, sidewalks, and playgrounds affects residents' physical activity, and reliance on convenience stores for shopping can result in exorbitant food costs and a limited selection of healthy food and beverage choices.

Individual characteristics—such as race—may highlight areas where environmental problems exist. Although these individual characteristics are associated with health behavior and health outcomes, they actually may be confounders in statistical or epidemiologic analyses. This would occur when environmental-level analyses are more appropriate than individual-level analyses in determining social and structural causes of illness (3).

Healthy People 2010

On January 25, 2000, the U.S. Department of Health and Human Services (DHHS) launched *Healthy People 2010*, the national health promotion and disease prevention initiative (4). Built on the foundation of the 1979 Surgeon General's Report *Healthy People* and the follow-up *Healthy People 2000*, *Healthy People 2010* has 2 primary goals: to increase the quality and years of healthy life, and to eliminate health disparities among different segments of the population (5).

During the 20th century, life expectancy—the average number of years people born in a given year are expected to live—increased greatly, from 47.3 years in the early 1900s to nearly 77 years today (6). Despite this progress, life expectancy in the United States could be extended, as evidenced by at least 18 other countries with populations of 1 million or more that have life expectancies greater than the United States (4). Native Americans and African Americans are most in need of intervention because of the considerable gap in life expectancy between these groups and whites (7).

Regarding health disparities in the United States, there is considerable variation by race and ethnicity in health care access. For example, poor diet, tobacco use, lack of physical activity during leisure time, obesity, hypertension, and lower rates of breast-feeding all are clustered in the lower socioeconomic groups (8,9). Differences in health based upon socioeconomic status are seen at all ages, with low-income groups having a greater incidence of premature and low birth weight infants, and adults having a greater risk of cardiovascular disease, stroke, and some cancers (10). Many chronic diseases can be prevented or controlled by healthy habits; however, decreased access to preventive and therapeutic care because of poverty or lack of health insurance has resulted in differential morbidity and mortality for some Americans. For example, health statistics differ greatly between African Americans and whites in the United States, with age- and gender-adjusted all-cause death rates 60% higher among African Americans (7,11). Native Americans also experience excess overall mortality, particularly related to diabetes, liver disease, and accidents, while Hispanics* have elevated hypertension and age-adjusted stroke rates compared to whites (7,12).

Leading Health Indicators

One new inclusion in *Healthy People 2010* is its use of Leading Health Indicators to categorize health objectives. These Leading Health Indicators, which reflect important health concerns in the United States at the beginning of the 21st century, were selected on the basis of their ability to motivate action and the availability of data to measure progress throughout the decade (13). Several of the Leading Health Indicators are relevant to dietetics: overweight and obesity, physical activity, tobacco use, substance abuse, mental health, and access to health care (14).

The term Hispanic in this paper refers to persons who trace their origin or descent to Mexico, Puerto Rico, Cuba, Central and South America, and other Spanish cultures.

Overweight and Obesity

The incidence of obesity is increasing rapidly, despite intense efforts concentrating on individual-level interventions. In the United States, the age-adjusted prevalence of body mass index (BMI) > 30 kg/m^2 (indicating obesity) increased from 13% to 23% between 1960 and 1994. Currently, the overall prevalence of BMI > 25 kg/m^2 (indicating overweight) among adults is 61% (15). About 14% of U.S. children are now overweight, as defined by sex-specific BMI-for-age over the 95th percentile (16), and data indicate that elevated BMI during adolescence is predictive of obesity in adulthood (17,18). Dietetics professionals working with disease prevention are concerned about obesity because of its association with a greater risk of other health problems, including type 2 diabetes, hypertension, hyperlipidemia, some cancers, menstrual disturbances, pregnancy complications, osteoarthritis, dyspnea, and varicose veins (10,19).

The causes of obesity are complex and include genetics; lack of physical activity; and high-fat, energy-dense foods, which are readily accessible, inexpensive, heavily advertised, and palatable (20,21,22). Furthermore, individuals who are overweight may not eat more than normal-weight individuals but instead may have a positive energy balance due to low-energy output (18,23). Although about 40% of the variation in body composition is estimated to be genetic (21,22), addressing genetic factors alone likely will not overcome the substantial environmental pressures for overconsumption and sedentary behavior that currently affect Americans (24).

Physical Activity

In addition to eating a healthful diet, participation in regular physical activity is one of the most important influences on health (25). Regular physical activity can lower the risk of cardiovascular disease, type 2 diabetes, colon and breast cancer, and osteoporosis, and it can help maintain healthy weight (26,27,28). Furthermore, an additive or synergistic relationship may occur in health promotion programs that incorporate both healthy eating and physical activity. Gillman et al (28) reported that increased amounts of physical activity were associated with more healthy food choices. Similarly, Eaton et al (29) showed that individuals with higher levels of activity consumed more dietary fiber, antioxidant vitamins, and calcium, while consuming less total and saturated fat.

The Centers for Disease Control and Prevention (CDC), the National Institutes of Health (NIH), the American Heart Association, and the American College of Sports Medicine all recommend that American adults accumulate at least 30 minutes of moderate-intensity physical activity on most—preferably all—days of the week, while children should accumulate 60 minutes of physical activity each day (30,31,32). However, 60% of American adults are not regularly active during their leisure time, and 25% of U.S. adults are not active at all, particularly women, older adults, African Americans, and Mexican Americans (33). Environmental issues such as neighborhood safety and reliance on motorized transportation have a strong impact on physical activity in the United States (34). Compared to years past, more time today is spent using computers, watching television, and playing videogames, particularly among children and adolescents (35). At the same time, the number of schools requiring daily physical education is declining (23); from 1991 to 1995, daily physical education among high school students dropped from 42% to 25% (33).

Tobacco Use

Cigarette smoking is a major contributor to morbidity and mortality and is strongly linked to the etiology of debilitating diseases seen in adulthood (9,26). Cigarette smoking is detrimental to health and longevity and has been estimated to increase the risk of coronary heart disease by 150% and of lung cancer by 2000% (36). There is evidence to show that smoking contributes to respiratory diseases, cardiovascular disease, ulcers, and osteoporosis (36,37,38,39). Although the relationships between smoking, dietary intake, and risk for disease are extremely complex, smokers are characterized by higher intakes of energy, fat, and cholesterol compared to nonsmokers (40,41). These dietary patterns, in turn, increase other risk factors for disease. For example, Dallongeville et al (42) reported that serum triglycerides, very-low-density lipoprotein (VLDL) cholesterol, and systolic blood pressure were significantly higher among current smokers than among nonsmokers, who had significantly higher levels of high-density-lipoprotein (HDL) cholesterol. These serum differences were the result of unhealthy patterns of food choices (eg, greater fat consumption, lower intake of fruits) and significantly greater energy intakes (42). As an acquired habit, tobacco use is preventable, and dietetics professionals can advance health promotion by including tobacco prevention and cessation in program planning (9).

Substance Abuse

Recent data indicate that alcohol use is declining in the United States (43). At the same time, the prevalence of social consequences (eg, violent behavior) and dependence symptoms has not shown a corresponding decline. Frequent drinking, related alcohol-dependence, and violence appear to be higher among Native American, African American, and Hispanic men, compared to men or women of other racial/ethnic groups (7,44). On any given day, over 700,000 people in the United States receive alcoholism treatment in either inpatient (13.5%) or outpatient (86.5%) settings (45). Although psychosocial therapies do help to reduce alcohol consumption and to maintain abstinence, 40% to 70% of patients resume drinking within 1 year of treatment (46).

For these reasons, health professionals often hesitate to discuss alcohol consumption with clients or patients (47,48). At the same time, data indicate that light to moderate alcohol consumption—defined as no more than 1 drink per day for women and older adults, and no more than 2 drinks per day for men—has a protective effect against ischemic and hemorrhagic stroke (49), coronary heart disease (50), and type 2 diabetes (51). Although the relationship between alcohol consumption and breast cancer remains equivocal (26,52), dietetics professionals may promote healthy lifestyles by reassuring the public that light to moderate alcohol consumption may have beneficial health outcomes for those who choose to drink, while heavy alcohol consumption is deleterious to health.

Mental Health

The relationships between nutrition and mental health often are overlooked (53). However, psychiatric illnesses, including mood disorders, can have a negative impact on appetite and nutritional status, and many nutrient imbalances can affect mental health (54). People with mental health problems have an additional risk of malnutrition associated with the side effects of medications, drug-nutrient interactions, poverty, social isolation, delusions regarding food, and poor food handling practices (53).

Anxiety and depression are two psychological factors known to be associated with a sedentary lifestyle (55). Also, central adiposity and type 1 and type 2 diabetes, which are important risk factors for cardiovascular disease, have been associated with increased depression and anxiety (56). Because binge eating—experienced by 10% to 30% of individuals seeking weight reduction therapy—is associated with depression, growing research in the prevention of eating disorders may lead to other avenues by which dietetics professionals can have a positive effect on promoting mental health (21).

Access to Health Care

Health care coverage continues to be an important health policy issue because health care costs consume a significant portion of our nation's economic resources (27). Household income, employment status, and years of schooling—all markers of socioeconomic status—are important predictors of access to health care and preventive measures. Public health efforts to reduce disparities in access to health care should be sure to address these social issues (57).

In the United States, non-Hispanic white adults (20 to 64 years) without diabetes are more likely (89% insured) to have health insurance than are African Americans (83% insured) or Mexican Americans (59% insured) (58). Native Americans represent < 1% of the total U.S. population. Although health care is free to many Native Americans, programs often are limited, poorly funded, and have little emphasis on disease prevention (7). To achieve the *Healthy People 2010* goals related to health disparities, dietetics professionals need to become increasingly politically savvy and mobilized at the local, state, and federal levels to ensure that all Americans have access to preventive and therapeutic health care.

Federal Support for Health Promotion and Disease Prevention

The U.S. Department of Agriculture (USDA), through the Special Supplemental Nutrition Program for Women, Infants, and Children (WIC), provides funding for most (78%) full-time equivalent public health nutritionists' salaries (59). The DHHS also provides funding for a smaller number of public health nutritionists' salaries (~ 3.4%) through its Maternal and Child Health Bureau's block grants. The USDA employs dietetic professionals through its other food assistance programs, Cooperative Extension, and the Center for Nutrition Policy and Promotion, which coordinates the review of federal dietary guidance materials and publishes the *Dietary Guidelines for Americans*, in conjunction with the DHHS (60). At the local level in counties and states, dietetics professionals are paid through federally supported programs in departments of education, public assistance, and public health.

Much of the increase in life expectancy during the 20th century occurred because of applications of public health measures to reduce infectious disease (ie, vaccinations and clean water supplies) (61). However, further research is needed to increase U.S. life expectancy and to reduce health disparities. Scientists interested in pursuing prevention-related issues have fewer sources of funding, especially at the federal level where the percentage of funds allocated toward prevention research historically has been sparse (62). Nutrition—one of the most cost-effective preventive treatments available to the American public—remains a minor priority in federal research funding, with approximately 4 cents of every $100 spent on health care in the United States directed toward nutrition research (63). Between 1965 and 1995, the proportion of health research and development funded by federal sources dropped by almost half to 37.4%, while industry's financial support increased more than twofold to 52% of the total $35.8 billion expended (64).

Recently, the National Research Council suggested that inadequate funding for competitive research has limited the potential of nutrition research (65). The largest investment in federal prevention research has been made by NIH (62), yet even within NIH, reorganization of the competitive grant review panels is slated to drop nutrition from the title of the 24 initial review groups (66). An analysis of NIH's research funding for biomedical research and training estimates that less than 4% (~$695 million) of total NIH funding is linked to nutrition, with only a small portion of this funding devoted to health promotion (63). This funding percentage has remained fairly constant over the past 10 years. The USDA also supports nutrition research, but the National Research Council reported that funding support for nutrition research from the USDA has lagged behind other USDA-funded research areas (65).

Public Policy

Federal funding certainly has an important influence on health policy, but not all public policy is determined at the national or international level. Individual circumstances—such as where people live and work—are important determinants of disease rates and, therefore, provide a fertile starting point for effective interventions to improve public health (3). To use policies and social interventions as a means to influence health behavior, dietetics professionals can be involved in policy making at the local level (eg, zoning boards, licensing and certification boards, school boards). Affiliate dietetics groups also provide opportunities to become involved in policy making and the legislative process at the local, regional, and national levels.

By adjusting the conditions in which people live, dietetics professionals can influence health behaviors and health outcomes of populations (20). For example, exposing consumers to healthy foods at the point of purchase in grocery stores or restaurants can influence food-purchasing behavior. Price incentives promoting the use of healthy items have shown promise in changing consumer purchase patterns. In addition, dietetics professionals can be involved with other community projects, such as attracting chain grocery stores to urban areas that have only convenience stores, advocating for low-lead environments for resource-constrained families, and partnering with schools and master gardeners to improve children's intakes of vegetables.

Dietetics professionals who become involved in setting policy at the local level can reap many benefits, including a quicker impact on the community, personal gratification, and opportunities to network with other policy-oriented professionals (67). One example of successful policy change at the local level is the Child and Adolescent Trial for Cardiovascular Health (CATCH) study, which demonstrated improvements in both diet and exercise among youth enrolled at participating schools (68). Changes were attributed mostly to modifications in the selections offered in the school cafeteria and the content of the physical education classes. Because changes in exercise and diet occurred only within the school setting and not while the children were at home, the school-level environmental changes were more effective than the educational components directed toward the children themselves.

Social Marketing and Behavioral Journalism

Social marketing first was introduced in 1971, when its proponents realized that the same marketing principles used to sell products to consumers could be used to "sell" ideas, attitudes, and behaviors. At the same time, social marketing is sometimes less effective than its commercial counterpart because it aims to influence people's ideas and behavior (eg, eat less saturated fat), rather than steering existing patterns of thought and behavior in a certain direction (eg, choosing one fast-food restaurant instead of another). Rather than using a "top-down" approach, public health professionals are learning to listen to the needs and desires of the target audience and to build programs based on those needs (69).

Reaching every individual in a population with an individual-level intervention is difficult and costly. Social marketing programs reach a specific audience, satisfy consumers' needs, and meet organizational objectives. For example, Reger et al (70) used a 6-week media campaign to promote consumption of 1%-fat milk and found that 34% of high-fat milk drinkers reported switching to low-fat milk and that low-fat milk sales increased from 29% of overall milk sales to 46%. Social marketing impacts the practice of dietetics by boosting consumers' awareness of health issues and healthy foods and is able to move consumers toward behavioral change.

In the United States, the media have an unparalleled ability to expose large numbers of people to health information (71), and although the media often are faulted as contributing to poor health and consumer misinformation (72, 73), proponents of "behavioral journalism" urge health professionals to work with the media to bring about lifestyle changes (74). According to the Social Cognitive Theory, imitating others is a primary mode of learning because peers are considered to be trustworthy models and are important sources of new behaviors (74,75). Behavioral journalism involves linking journalists with actual clients so that the public can follow them as they attempt behavior change and then learn from their successes and setbacks. For example, dietetics professionals could work with their local media to have weekly coverage of individuals who try different eating patterns or physical activity regimens over a period of 5 to 8 weeks. This approach allows the public to learn vicariously that healthy lifestyle patterns are achievable if attempted.

Rationale

Dietetics professionals are uniquely positioned to be the primary information resource regarding the relationships among diet, health, and disease prevention. They are trained in the relationship between food and health throughout the life cycle and thus are able to communicate this relationship to other members of the health care team, educators, policy makers, and the public.

For many years, the services of dietetics professionals were confined to clinical settings or maternal and child health clinics. However, there is now a great need for dietetics services in a variety of settings beyond traditional clinical care. If dietetics professionals are to help meet the Healthy People 2010 goals, they will need to be actively involved in day care settings, schools, community environments (eg, churches and work places), media relations, policy development, and the food and supplement industries. Dietetics professionals will need to promote nutrition wherever consumers make food decisions—grocery stores, restaurants, vending machines—to ensure the availability of safe, healthy food. Dietetics professionals will need to work actively with policy-makers to ensure that healthy eating and physical activity are included in local, state, and federal policies.

Programs and Audiences Impacted

Effective programs in health promotion and disease prevention require development of collaborative partnerships at the state, community, and provider levels to help ensure program financing and community participation. Programs should involve many types of health care providers and should incorporate federal or state programs when feasible.

A holistic approach will help communities invest in wellness and prevention. Community coalition building takes place between public health nutritionists, physicians, nurses, health educators, physical therapists, and other professionals involved in promoting physical activity, mental health services, and community outreach. In addition, community leaders and local businesses contribute to coalition building. Involving schools, worksites, churches, physician offices, hospitals, supermarkets and the food industry in designing and implementing prevention programs is important. Voluntary community organizations involved in disease prevention include the American Cancer Society, the American Heart Association, the American Diabetes Association, and the American Lung Association (76).

Dietetics Professionals

By facilitating behavior change as a community approach to promoting health and preventing chronic disease, the services of dietetics professionals are indispensable. When communities involve dietetics professionals in the design, delivery, and evaluation of health programs and services, behavior change strategies are more effective (77).

Dietetics professionals can take the lead in prevention programming because their training as counselors and educators provides skills that make them versatile members of coalitions. In addition to competencies in community nutrition or public health, dietetics professionals who develop skills in community assessment, policy development, surveillance, community-based nutrition interventions, and media and communications can be leaders in chronic disease prevention and health promotion. These skills help dietetic professionals support both individual and population changes (76).

Training dietitians concerned with health promotion and disease prevention will require shifting from a clinical focus to an emphasis on population-based public health practice. Formal training and educational programs are needed to teach the skills necessary for this area of practice. Dietitians working in community or public health nutrition must be trained to function in a team setting, develop or participate in coalitions, understand management of complex systems, comprehend the role of political entities in these areas, and interact with the media.

Other Health Professionals

Dietetics professionals have the opportunity to effect community change and foster health promotion and disease prevention by partnering with physicians, nurses, dentists, social workers, community activists, and many other public health professionals. Examples include:

- Partnering with hunger-relief agencies to reduce hunger and food insecurity and to nurture sustainable agriculture in local communities (78).
- Campaigning with obstetricians, nurse midwives, and lactation consultants to promote breast-feeding, thereby reducing the incidence of infant illnesses and, potentially, overweight in children (79).
- Reducing the number of children with early childhood caries by collaborating with dental hygienists and dentists in promoting local water fluoridation (80).

Cost Savings of Health Promotion

Nutrition services directed toward prevention can help reduce health care costs that are rising by more than 10% per year. With the leading causes of death costing at least $250 billion annually, prudent dietary choices could save billions of dollars in direct and indirect costs. Costs for cardiovascular disease, stroke, diabetes, and cancer—based on medical costs, productivity losses because of disability, and premature death—are now in excess of $70 billion (81).

Nutrition interventions that result in a 50% reduction in dietary fat intakes might eventually reduce total cancer incidence by approximately 33% for females and 17% for males in the 55- to 69-year-old age range (82). Modeling techniques estimate that if Americans reduced their intake of saturated fat by about 8 g per day, the health care system could save as much as $12.7 billion in medical costs and lost earnings annually (83). A review of 10 major studies of worksite health promotion programs found that the average cost/benefit ratio of programs ranged from 1:2.05 to 1:5.96 (84). Investment in health results in improved employee retention and company public image and increased employee allegiance.

Cost-effectiveness analyses ensure that scarce health care prevention dollars are used effectively. Determining the cost/benefit ratio of nutrition programming in chronic disease prevention requires that the intervention changes risk behavior, that risk reduction decreases morbidity or injury, and that medical costs diminish. This process is not short-term or static, and cost/benefit is not the only basis for making health promotion decisions. For example, some corporations are providing health promotion programming on the basis of improved quality of life for employees, enhanced employee satisfaction at work, and health care cost containment.

Federal Nutrition Programs

The primary food assistance programs administered by the USDA are the Food Stamp Program, the National School Lunch Program, and WIC (85). These 3 programs accounted for the majority of the $34.1 billion spent on USDA food assistance in 2001. In addition, some states offer coupons through the Farmers' Market Nutrition Programs so that WIC participants or seniors can use farmers' markets to improve their intake of vegetables and fruits (86,87). These programs were developed to assist resource-constrained individuals to acquire an adequate amount of food to help prevent chronic disease. Other USDA food assistance programs can be found at http://www.fns.usda.gov/fns/.

Projects to study the three largest food assistance programs will result in a report on the cost-efficiency of these programs sometime during 2002 or 2003 (88). Research in Missouri found that benefits paid by Medicaid in the 60 days after birth were nearly $600 more for infants who did not participate in WIC compared to WIC participants; in addition, the report found savings in newborn costs and newborn hospital lengths of stay (89). Research has also shown a positive effect of WIC on infant birth weight (90).

Role and Responsibilities of Dietetics Professionals

Changes in the health care system will have a profound effect on the number and types of jobs available to dietetics professionals, the settings in which they work, and their roles and responsibilities. The changes from a fee-for-service payment system to a prepaid capitated system and managed care are transforming the health care system. Although health promotion and prevention activities that include screenings and health education should be a top priority for health care providers and organizations, the value of these activities still is being debated. Many managed care organizations are offering preventive services, albeit mostly clinical interventions (eg, health education workshops, discounts at fitness centers) for their enrolled populations. Population-based prevention activities (such as changes in community environment to promote health) are not seen as the responsibility of private health care organizations (91).

Dietetics professionals need to become more involved in the new consumer environment—the Internet. Grocery shopping online is expected to increase over time. Online grocery shopping provides an opportunity to assist consumers with healthy food decisions through interventions designed to reach this new audience. Beyond food purchasing, numerous sites for nutrition and health advice exist; however, consumers need assistance in sorting through this maze to determine which sites provide sound nutrition and health advice as compared to those that provide inaccurate information or primarily product promotions. Web sites such as the American Dietetic Association's, http://www.eatright.org/healthy, and the USDA's, http://www.nal.usda.gov/fnic/consumersiteindex.html, provide sound nutrition guidance that can be trusted; and consumers can utilize the American Dietetic Association's Nationwide Nutrition Network, http://www.eatright.com/find.html, to find local dietetics professionals for nutrition guidance.

Although funding related to disease prevention is limited, dietetics professionals who are nutrition scientists actively need to pursue research dollars. Also, state departments of health and education should be aware of funding opportunities provided by USDA and CDC so that the best health promotion and disease prevention programs can be funded and evaluated. More locally, dietetics professionals can partner with statewide nutrition networks that participate in USDA's Food Stamp Nutrition Education Program to tap into funding and broaden nutrition education and social marketing efforts that target low-income populations (69). Dietetics professionals also are obligated to plan program evaluation as they plan program implementation and should consider submitting their results to the *Journal of the American Dietetic Association* so that all members of the Association can appreciate the breadth of impact dietetics professionals have on disease prevention and health promotion.

Dietetics professionals need to be positioned for these new settings and expanded professional roles but also need to continue to market their expertise to consumers by focusing on health promotion and disease prevention. Consumers often view dietetic professionals as providing information for those who are ill; instead, consumers should be aware that dietetics professionals are trained to provide nutrition and health-related advice to promote health and prevent disease as well. To do this, dietetics professionals need to focus their messages on healthy food choices in the language of the consumer (ie, food) and present recommendations in a positive, behaviorally appropriate manner to enhance adoption of these behaviors.

- Because of its leadership role in reaching Healthy People 2010 goals, CDC is focusing on Racial and Ethnic Approaches to Community Health (REACH 2010) to eliminate racial and ethnic health disparities in the United States. Launched in 1999, REACH 2010 has funded 36 projects that focus on diet-related issues such as cardiovascular disease, breast cancer, diabetes, and infant mortality. By empowering members of local communities, REACH 2010 encourages neighborhoods to evolve so that residents are more eager to pursue healthy behaviors and avoid unhealthy behaviors. For more information, see http://www.cdc.gov/reach2010/aag-reach.htm.

- The National 5 A Day Program was established in 1991 as a public/private partnership between the National Cancer Institute (NCI) and the Produce for Better Health Foundation. The National 5 A Day Program promotes increased consumption of fruits and vegetables as part of a healthy lifestyle. Between 1993 and 1994, state health officers in all 50 states designated a 5 A Day Program Coordinator in each state to work with NCI on this national endeavor. Since 1991, the 5 A Day Program has grown from a single public/private partnership model (the NCI and the Produce for Better Health Foundation, and their licensees) to a multiagency, shared-leadership model comprising 11 federal and non-federal organizations. Research indicates that the 5 A Day Program has been successful in increasing Americans' intakes of vegetables and fruits (92). Additional information about the program is available at http://www.5aday.gov.

FIGURE C-1   Two Examples of Success Stories that Support These Recommendations

---

References

1. French SA, Story M, Jeffery RW. Environmental influences on eating and physical activity. *Annu Rev Public Health*. 2001;22:309–335.
2. Moore DJ, Williams JD, Qualls WJ. Target marketing of tobacco and alcohol-related products to ethnic minority groups in the United States. *Ethn Dis*. 1996;6:83–98.

3. Marmot MG. Improvement of social environment to improve health. *Lancet.* 1998;351:57–60.

4. U.S. Department of Health and Human Services. Healthy People 2010. Available at http:/www.health.gov/healthypeople. Accessed December 27, 2001.

5. U.S. Department of Health and Human Services. What is its history? Available at http://www.health.gov/healthypeople/About/history.htm. Accessed December 27, 2001.

6. May RM. Science and society. *Science.* 2001;292:1021.

7. Whitfield KE, Weidner G, Clark R, Anderson NB. Sociodemographic diversity and behavioral medicine. *J Consult Clin Psychol.* 2002;70: 463–481.

8. Aguilar-Salinas CA, Vazquez-Chavez C, Gamboa-Marrufo R, Garcia-Soto N, Jesus Rios-Gonzalez J, Holguin R, Vela S, Ruiz-Alvarez F, Mayagoitia S. Obesity, diabetes, hypertension, and tobacco consumption in an urban adult Mexican population. *Arch Med Res.* 2001;32:446–453.

9. Hampl JS. Progress and plans regarding the nutritional status of smoking adolescents. *Nutrition.* 2000;16:526–528.

10. James WPT, Nelson M, Ralph A, Leather S. Socioeconomic determinants of health. The contribution of nutrition to inequalities in health. *BMJ.* 1997;314:1545–1549.

11. Carmichael SL, Iyasu S, Hatfield-Timajchy K. Cause-specific trends in neonatal mortality among black and white infants, United States, 1980–1995. *Matern Child Health J.* 1998;2:67–76.

12. Rivera JA, Barquera S, Campirano F, Campos I, Safdie M, Tovar V. Epidemiological and nutritional transition in Mexico: rapid increase of noncommunicable chronic diseases and obesity. *Public Health Nutr.* 2002;5:113–122. November 2002. Volume 102, Number 11.

13. U.S. Department of Health and Human Services. What Are the Leading Health Indicators? Available at http://www.health.gov/healthypeople/ LHI/lhiwhat.htm. Accessed December 27, 2001.

14. U.S. Department of Health and Human Services. *Healthy People 2010.* Washington, DC: Office of Disease Prevention and Health Promotion; 2001.

15. Centers for Disease Control and Prevention. Obesity trends. Available at http://www.cdc.gov/nccdphp/dnpa/obesity/trend/maps/index.htm. Accessed July 26, 2002.

16. Centers for Disease Control and Prevention. Prevalence of overweight among children and adolescents: United States, 1999. Available at http://www.cdc.gov/nchs/products/pubs/pubd/hestats/overwght99.htm. Accessed July 26, 2002.

17. Laitinen J, Power C, Jarvelin MR. Family social class, maternal body mass index, childhood body mass index, and age at menarche as predictors of adult obesity. *Am J Clin Nutr.* 2001;74:287–294.

18. Rocandio AM, Ansotegui L, Arroyo M. Comparison of dietary intake among overweight and non-overweight schoolchildren. *Int J Obes.* 2001;25:1651–1655.

19. Vuori IM. Health benefits of physical activity with special reference to interaction with diet. *Public Health Nutr.* 2001;4:517–528.

20. Cohen DA, Scribner RA, Farley TA. A structural model of health behavior: a pragmatic approach to explain and influence health behaviors at the population level. *Prev Med.* 2000;30:146–154.

21. Wadden TA, Brownell KD, Foster GD. Obesity: responding to the global epidemic. *J Consult Clin Psychol.* 2002;70:510–525.

22. Schrauwen P, Westerterp KR. The role of high-fat diets and physical activity in the regulation of body weight. *Br J Nutr.* 2000;84:417–427.

23. Hill JO, Peters JC. Environmental contributions to the obesity epidemic. *Science* 1998;280:1371–1374.

24. Egger G, Swinburn B. An "ecological" approach to the obesity pandemic. *BMJ.* 1997;315:477–480.

25. Koffman DM, Bazzarre T, Mosca L, Redberg R, Schmid T, Wattigney WA. An evaluation of Choose to Move 1999: an American Heart Association physical activity program for women. *Arch Intern Med.* 2001;161:2193–2199.

26. American Institute for Cancer Research. AICR/WCRF Expert Panel Report. Available at http://www.aicr.org/reportsummaicr.html. Accessed July 27, 2002.

27. Sevick MA, Dunn AL, Morrow MS, Marcus BH, Chen GJ, Blair SN. Costeffectiveness of lifestyle and structured exercise interventions in sedentary adults: results of project ACTIVE. *Am J Prev Med.* 2000;19:1–8.

28. Gillman MW, Pinto BM, Tennstedt S, Glanz K, Marcus B, Friedman RH. Relationships of physical activity with dietary behaviors among adults. *Prev Med.* 2001;32:295–301.

29. Eaton CB, McPhillips JB, Gans KM, Garber CE, Assaf AR, Lasater TM, Carleton RA. Cross-sectional relationship between diet and physical activity in two southeastern New England communities. *Am J Prev Med.* 1995;11:238–244.

30. NIH Consensus Development Panel on Physical Activity and Cardiovascular Health. *JAMA.* 1996;276:241–246.

31. Grundy SM, Balady GJ, Criqui MH, Fletcher G, Greenland P, Hiratzka LF, Houston-Miller N, Kris-Etherton P, Krumholz HM, LaRosa J, Ockene IS, Pearson TA, Reed J, Washington R, Smith SC, Jr. Guide to primary prevention of cardiovascular diseases. A statement for healthcare professionals from the Task Force on Risk Reduction. American Heart Association Science Advisory and Coordinating Committee. *Circulation.* 1997;95:2329–2331.

32. Pate RR, Pratt M, Blair SN, Haskell WL, Macera CA, Bouchard C, Buchner D, Ettinger W, Heath GW, King AC. Physical activity and public health. A recommendation from the Centers for Disease Control and Prevention and the American College of Sports Medicine. *JAMA.* 1995;273:402–407.

33. National Center for Chronic Disease Prevention and Health Promotion: Physical Activity and Health: A Report of the Surgeon General. Washington, DC: U.S. Dept of Health and Human Services, 1996.

34. Bell CC, Mock L, Slutkin G. The prevalence of victimization and perceptions of job neighborhood safety in a social service agency and the need for screening. *J Natl Med Assoc.* 2002;94:602–608.

35. Dowda M, Ainsworth BE, Addy CL, Saunders R, Riner W. Environmental influences, physical activity, and weight status in 8- to 16-year-olds. *Arch Pediatr Adolesc Med.* 2001;155:711–717.

36. Renaud S, de Lorgeril M. The French paradox: dietary factors and cigarette smoking-related health risks. *Ann NY Acad Sci.* 1993;686: 299–309.

37. You RX, Thrift AG, McNeil JJ, Davis SM, Donnan GA. Ischemic stroke risk and passive exposure to spouses' cigarette smoking. *Am J Public Health.* 1999;89:572–575.

38. Compston J. Secondary causes of osteoporosis in men. *Calcif Tissue Int.* 2001;69:193–195.

39. Slattery ML, Potter JD, Friedman GD, Ma KN, Edwards S. Tobacco use and colon cancer. *Int J Cancer.* 1997;70:259–264.

40. Hampl JS, Betts NM. Cigarette use during adolescence: effects on nutritional status. *Nutr Rev.* 1999;57:215–221.

41. Ma J, Hampl JS, Betts NM. Antioxidant intakes and smoking status: data from the continuing survey of food intakes by individuals 1994–1996. *Am J Clin Nutr.* 2000;71:774–780.

42. Dallongeville J, Marecaux N, Richard F, Bonte D, Zylberberg G, Fantino M, Fruchart JC, Amouyel P. Cigarette smoking is associated with differences in nutritional habits and related to lipoprotein alterations independently of food and alcohol intake. *Eur J Clin Nutr.* 1996;50:647–654.

43. Walitzer KS, Connors GJ. Treating problem drinking. *Alcohol Res Health.* 1999;23:138–143.

44. Caetano R, Schafer J, Cunradi CB. Alcohol-related intimate partner violence among white, black, and Hispanic couples in the United States. *Alcohol Res Health.* 2001;25:58–65.

45. Fuller RK, Hiller-Sturmhofel S. Alcoholism treatment in the United States. An overview. *Alcohol Res Health.* 1999;23:69–77.

46. Johnson BA, Ait-Daoud N. Medications to treat alcoholism. *Alcohol Res Health.* 1999;23:99–106.

47. Doll R. One for the heart. *BMJ.* 1997;315:1664–1668.

48. Goldberg DM, Soleas GJ, Levesque M. Moderate alcohol consumption: the gentle face of Janus. *Clin Biochem.* 1999;32:505–518.

49. Berger K, Ajani UA, Kase CS, Gaziano JM, Buring JE, Glynn RJ et al. Light-to-moderate alcohol consumption and risk of stroke among U.S. male physicians. *N Engl J Med.* 1999;341:1557–1564.

50. Wannamethee SG, Shaper AG. Type of alcoholic drink and risk of major coronary heart disease events and all-cause mortality. *Am J Public Health.* 1999;89:685–690.

51. Ajani UA, Hennekens CH, Spelsberg A, Manson JE. Alcohol consumption and risk of type 2 diabetes mellitus among U.S. male physicians. *Arch Intern Med.* 2000;160:1025–1030.

52. Ellison RC, Zhang Y, McLennan CE, Rothman KJ. Exploring the relation of alcohol consumption to risk of breast cancer. *Am J Epidemiol.* 2001;154:740–747.

53. Sullivan A, Tucker R. Meeting the nutritional needs of people with mental health problems. *Nurs Stand.* 1999;13:48–53.

54. Lacey JM, Houser RA. Dietetics and mental health counseling: time for partnership. [Letter]. *J Am Diet Assoc.* 2001;101:1313–1314.

55. Sörensen M, Anderssen S, Hjerman I, Holme I, Ursin H. The effect of exercise and diet on mental health and quality of life in middle-aged individuals with elevated risk factors for cardiovascular disease. *J Sports Sci.* 1999;17:369–377.

56. Lloyd CE, Dyer PH, Barnett AH. Prevalence of symptoms of depression and anxiety in a diabetes clinic population. *Diabet Med.* 2000;17: 198–202.

57. Escobedo LG, Giles WH, Anda RF. Socioeconomic status, race, and death from coronary heart disease. *Am J Prev Med.* 1997;13:123–130.

58. Harris MI. Racial and ethnic differences in health insurance coverage for adults with diabetes. *Diabet Care.* 1999;22:1679–1682.

59. Haughton B, Story M, Keir B. Profile of public health nutrition personnel: challenges for population/system-focused roles and state-level monitoring. *J Am Diet Assoc.* 1998;98:664–670.

60. Center for Nutrition Policy and Promotion. Nutrition and Your Health: Dietary Guidelines for Americans. Available at http://www.health.gov/dietaryguidelines/dga2000/document/frontcover.htm. Accessed December 27, 2001.

61. Bunker JP. Medicine matters after all. *J R Coll Phys Lond.* 1995;29: 105–112.

62. Griffith HM, Rabin DL. Commentary on the federal role in clinical prevention research. *Am J Prev Med.* 1998;14:293–299.

63. Sunde RA. Research needs for human nutrition in the post-genomesequencing era. *J Nutr.* 2001;131:3319–3323.

64. Rosenstock L, Lee LJ. Attacks on science: the risks to evidence-based policy. *Am J Public Health.* 2002;92:14–18.

65. National Research Council. *National Research Initiative.* Washington, DC: National Academy Press; 2001.

66. Center for Scientific Review. Recommendations for change at the NIH's Center for Scientific Review. Available at http://www.csr.nih.gov/events/summary012000.htm. 2001. Accessed December 27, 2001.

67. Mittelmark MB. The psychology of social influence and healthy public policy. *Prev Med.* 1999; 29(6 Pt 2):S24–S29.

68. Luepker RV, Perry CL, McKinlay SM, Nader PR, Parcel GS, Stone EJ, Webber LS, Elder JP, Feldman HA, Johnson CC. Outcomes of a field trial to improve children's dietary patterns and physical activity. The Child and Adolescent Trial for Cardiovascular Health. CATCH collaborative group. *JAMA.* 1996;275:768–776.

69. Hampl JS, Sass S. Focus groups indicate that vegetable and fruit consumption by food stamp-eligible Hispanics is affected by children and unfamiliarity with non-traditional foods. *J Am Diet Assoc.* 2001; 101:685–687.

70. Reger B, Wootan MG, Booth-Butterfield S. Using mass media to promote healthy eating: A community-based demonstration project. *Prev Med.* 1999;29414–421.

71. Finnegan JR, Jr., Viswanath K, Hertog J. Mass media, secular trends, and the future of cardiovascular disease health promotion: an interpretive analysis. *Prev Med.* 1999;29 (suppl):S50–S58.

72. Neumark-Sztainer D, Sherwood NE, Coller T, Hannan PJ. Primary prevention of disordered eating among preadolescent girls: Feasibility and short-term effect of a community-based intervention. *J Am Diet Assoc.* 2000;100:1466–1473.

73. Rubinstein S, Caballero B. Is Miss America an undernourished role model? *JAMA.* 2000;283:1569.

74. McAlister A. Behavioral journalism: beyond the marketing model for health communication. *Am J Health Promot.* 1995;9:417–420.

75. Field AE, Camargo CA, Jr., Taylor CB, Berkey CS, Colditz GA. Relation of peer and media influences to the development of purging behaviors among preadolescent and adolescent girls. *Arch Pediatr Adolesc Med.* 1999;153:1184–1189.

76. Owen AL, Splett PL, Owen GM. *Nutrition in the Community: the Art and Science of Delivering Services.* 4th ed. New York: McGraw-Hill; 1999.

77. Agency for Healthcare Research and Quality. Efficacy of interventions to modify dietary behaviors related to cancer risk. Available at http:// www.ahrq.gov/clinic/epcsums/dietsumm.htm. Accessed December 27, 2001.

78. Hampl JS, Hall R. Dietetic approaches to U.S. hunger and food insecurity. *J Am Diet Assoc.* 2002;102:919–923.

79. Gillman MW, Rifas-Shiman SL, Camargo CA, Jr., Berkey CS, Frazier AL, Rockett HR, Field AE, Colditz GA. Risk of overweight among adolescents who were breastfed as infants. *JAMA.* 2001;285:2461–2467.

80. Weintraub JA. Prevention of early childhood caries: a public health perspective. *Community Dent Oral Epidemiol.* 1998;26:62–66.

81. Frazão E. High costs of poor eating patterns in the United States. In: Frazão E, Ed., *America's Eating Habits: Changes and Consequences.* Washington, DC: U.S. Department of Agriculture. Agriculture Information Bulletin No. 750; 1999.

82. Prentice RL, Sheppard L. Dietary fat and cancer: consistency of the epidemiologic data, and disease prevention that may follow from a practical reduction in fat consumption. *Cancer Causes Control.* 1990;1:81–97

83. Oster G, Thompson D. Estimated effects of reducing dietary saturated fat intake on the incidence and costs of coronary heart disease in the United States. *J Am Diet Assoc.* 1996;96:127–131.

84. Joint Venture: Silicon Valley Network. Are worksite health promotion programs cost-effective? Available at http://www.jointventure.org/initiatives/health/hc-he.html. Accessed March 4, 2002.

85. Economic Research Service. Briefing room: food and nutrition assistance programs. Available at http://www.ers.usda.gov/briefing/food-nutrition assistance. Accessed January 24, 2002.

86. U.S. Department of Agriculture. WIC Farmers' Market Nutrition Program. Available at http://www.fns.usda.gov/wic/CONTENT/FMNP/FMNPfaqs.htm. Accessed March 8, 2002.

87. Anderson JV, Bybee DI, Brown R, McLean DF, Garcia EM, Breer ML, Schillo BA. 5-A-Day fruit and vegetable intervention improves consumption in a low-income population. *J Am Diet Assoc.* 2001;101:195–202.

88. Wittenburg D, Bell L, Kenyon A, Puma M, Hanchette C, Bell S, Miller C. Data development initiatives for research on food assistance and nutrition programs, phase I–ten potential data initiatives. Final Report. Electronic publications from the food assistance and nutrition research program; 2001.

89. Missouri Department of Health. WIC cost/benefit Analysis 1994. Monthly Vital Statistics. 31(4). 1997. Available at: http://www.health.state.mo.us/MonthlyVitalStatistics/ZG97.html. Accessed February 27, 2002.

90. Kowaleski-Jones L, Duncan G. The effects of WIC on children's health and development. *Pov Res News.* 2002;5(2):6–7.

91. Gordon RL, Baker EL, Roper WL, Omenn GS. Prevention and the reforming U.S. health care system: changing roles and responsibilities for public health. *Annu Rev Public Health.* 1996;17:489–509.

92. Johnston CS, Taylor CA, Hampl JS. More Americans are eating "5 A Day" but intakes of dark green and cruciferous vegetables remain low. *J Nutr.* 2000;130:3063–3067.

ADA Position adopted by the House of Delegates on October 26, 1997 and was reaffirmed on June 22, 2000. This position is in effect until December 31, 2005. ADA authorizes republication of the position statement/support paper, in its entirety, provided full and proper credit is given. Requests to use portions of the position must be directed to ADA headquarters at 800/877–1600, ext 4835, or ppapers@eatright.org.

Authors:

Jeffrey S Hampl, PhD, RD (AZ State University, Mesa, AZ)

Judith V Anderson, DrPH, RD (Michigan Department of Community Health, Lansing, MI)

Rebecca Mullis, PhD, RD (The University of Georgia, Atlanta, GA)

Reviewers:

Association of State and Territorial Public Health Nutrition Directors (Angie Tagtow, MS, RD, Iowa Department of Public Health, Des Moines, IA)

Sharleen Johnson Birkmer, PhD, RD (University of Louisville, Louisville, KY)

Karen Chapman-Novakofski, PhD, RD (University of Illinois, Urbana, IL)

Nancy Cotugna, DrPH, RD (University of Delaware, Newark, DE)

Nutrition Educators of Health Professionals dietetic practice group (Kathleen M. Rourke, PhD, RD, The Union Institute and University, Cincinnati, OH; Roger A. Shewmake, PhD, University of South Dakota School of Medicine, Sioux Falls, SD)

Oncology Nutrition dietetic practice group (Melanie R. Polk, MMSc, RD, FADA, American Institute for Cancer Research, Washington, DC; Erin Dummert, RD, Oncology of Wisconsin SC, Milwaukee, WI)

Christine Polisena, MS, MBA, RD, FADA (Whole Health Management, Cleveland, OH)

Public Health/Community Nutrition dietetic practice group (Sohailla Digsby, RD, Dept. of Health & Environment Chronic Disease/Risk Reduction, Waccamaw District, SC)

Sports, Cardiovascular and Wellness Nutritionists dietetic practice group (Denice Ferko-Adams, MPH, RD, Wellness Press, Nazareth, PA)

Members of the Association Positions Committee Workgroup:
Evelyn Enrione, PhD, RD (chair), Barbara Baron, MS, RD, Linda Nebeling, PhD, MPH, RD (content advisor)

APPENDIX D

GUIDELINES FOR COMMUNITY NUTRITION SUPERVISED EXPERIENCES, 2ND EDITION

Public Health/Community Nutrition Practice Group
American Dietetic Association 2003

The United States Department of Agriculture Food and Consumer Service provided support for development of the original Guidelines publication in 1995. Support for the second edition of the Guidelines was provided by the Public Health/ Community Nutrition Practice Group of the American Dietetic Association and the Association of Graduate Programs in Public Health Nutrition, Inc.

Acknowledgments

Guidelines for Community Nutrition Supervised Experiences was originally authored by a Core Working Committee and Review Panel representing key public health nutrition organizations. They and their organizations are acknowledged individually below.

A Revision Committee, also representing key public health nutrition organizations and dedicated to bringing the Guidelines into the 21st century, undertook the revision of Guidelines for Community Nutrition Supervised Experiences. These professionals contributed their considerable expertise and thoughtful consideration to the revision. They too are recognized individually below.

The Revision Committee acknowledges Dr. Jan Dodds, who chaired the development of the 2nd edition, for her leadership in accessing and uniting the breadth of expertise involved in the revision process. Her skill in public health practice permeates her professional demeanor. Sincere thanks and acknowledgement go to Heather Mixon, Project Coordinator, who organized the review, detailed changes, and ensured the integrity of the revisions.

Original Guidelines Authors

Project Director, Helene Kent, MPH, RD
Coordinator, Janice B. Carlton, MS, RD, LDN
Project Coordinator, Janice Dodds, EdD, RD
ADA Coordinator, Aurelia McCoy

Individual	**Organization Represented**
Erlinda Binghay, MPH, RD	American Public Health Association Food and Nutrition Section
Ted Fairchild, MPH, RD, CD	American Dietetic Association Public Health Nutrition Practice Group
Cathy Franklin, MS, RD, CD	National Association of WIC Directors
Betsy Haughton, EdD, RD, LDN	Association of Faculties of Graduate Programs in Public Health Nutrition
Lyn Konstant, PhD, RD	Society for Nutrition Education
Michele Lawler, MS, RD	United States Department of Agriculture Food and Consumer Services
Margaret Tate, MS, RD	Association of State and Territorial Public Health Nutrition Directors

Original Guidelines Reviewers

Individual	Organization Represented
Kristin Biskeborn, MPH, RD	Association of State and Territorial Public Health Nutrition Directors
Brenda Lisi, RD, MPA, MS	United States Department of Agriculture Food and Consumer Services
Jean Collins Norris, MS, MPH, RD	Bureau of Maternal and Child Health Services Department of Health and Human Services
Patricia L. Splett, PhD, MPH, RD	Society for Nutrition Education
Merryjo J. Ware, MPH, RD	National Association of WIC Directors
Collette Zyrkowski, MPH, RD	Centers for Disease Control

Guidelines 2nd Edition

Chair

Jan Dodds, EdD, RD
Professor of Nutrition and Maternal
and Child Health
University of North Carolina
School of Public Health
4101 McGavran Greenberg Bldg, CB 7461
Chapel Hill, NC 27599-7461
Phone: 919-966-7229 Fax: 919-966-8392
Jan_dodds@unc.edu

Coordinator

Heather Mixon, MS, RD
Public Health Nutrition Consultant
1229 Highland Drive
Chattanooga, TN 37405
Phone: 423-266-1362
hmixon@earthlink.net

Review Committee

Indivdual	Contact Information	Organization Represented
Anne Bennett Internship Director Tri-County Health Department	4857 S. Broadway Englewood, CO 80110 Phone: 303-783-7148 Fax: 303-761-1528 bennett@tchd.org	**American Dietetic Association** Public Health/Community Nutrition Practice Group
Susanne Gregory, MPH Public Health Nutrition Consultant	204 Melwood Lane Richmond, VA 23229 Phone: 804-282-1355 Fax: 804-282-7801 susannegregory@yahoo.com	**Society for Nutrition Education**

Indivdual	Contact Information	Organization Represented
Ellen Harris, DrPH Asst. Director, Nutrition Monitoring Beltsville Human Nutrition Research Ctr.	ARS, USDA, Bldg. 005, Rm. 117 Beltsville, MD 20705 Phone: 301-504-0610 Fax: 301-504-0698 eharris@rbhnrc.usda.gov	**American Public Health Association** Food and Nutrition Section
Betsy Haughton, EdD, RD, LDN Associate Professor Director, Public Health Nutrition Department of Nutrition College of Education, Health and Human Sciences The University of Tennessee	1215 Cumberland Avenue Knoxville, TN 37996-1920 Phone: 865-974-6267 Fax: 865-974-3491 Haughton@utk.edu	**Association of Graduate Programs in Public Health Nutrition, Inc.**
Michele Lawler, MS, RD Maternal and Child Health Bureau HRSA Department of Health and Human Services	Parklawn Building, Room 18-05 5600 Fishers Lane Rockville, MD 20857 Phone: 301-443-2204 Mlawler@hrsa.gov	**Department of Health and Human Services** Maternal and Child Health Bureau
Barbara Polhamus, PhD, MPH, RD National Center for Chronic Disease Prevention and Health Promotion, Division of Nutrition and Physical Activity	Mail stop K-25 4770 Buford Highway, NE Atlanta, GA 30341-3717 Phone: 770-488-5657 Fax: 770-488-5369 bfp9@cdc.gov	**Centers for Disease Control and Prevention**
Sally Swartz, MS, RD Community Education Coordinator Nutrition Division Tri-County Health Department	7000 E. Belleview, Suite 301 Greenwood Village, CO 80111 Phone: 303-846-6273 Fax: 303-220-9208 swartz@tchd.org	**American Dietetic Association** Public Health/ Community Nutrition Practice Group
Margaret Tate, MS, RD Chair, Office of Nutrition Services and Chronic Disease Prevention Programs Arizona Dept of Health	1740 West Adams, Room 203 Phoenix, AZ 85007 Phone: 602-542-2829 Fax: 602-542-1890 mtate@hs.state.az.us	**Association of State and Territorial Public Health Nutrition Directors**

Indivdual	Contact Information	Organization Represented
Peggy Trouba, RD, MPH State WIC Director Office of Family Health Nebraska Dept. of Health & Human Services	P.O. Box 95044 301 Centennial Mall South Lincoln, NE 68509-5044 Phone: 402-471-2781 Fax: 402-471-7049 peggy.trouba@hhss.state.ne.us	National WIC Association
Judy Wilson, Director Nutrition Services Staff Office of Analysis, Nutrition and Evaluation Food and Nutrition Service USDA	Office of Analysis, Nutrition and Evaluation, Food and Nutrition Service USDA Judy.Wilson@fns.usda.gov	U.S. Department of Agriculture Food and Nutrition Service

Guidelines for Community Nutrition Supervised Experiences

Purpose

In 1995 the American Dietetic Association's Public Health Nutrition Practice Group responded to demand for guidance on training experiences from those working in public health nutrition. *Guidelines for Community Nutrition Supervised Experiences* was offered as the first comprehensive curriculum for enhancing the capacity of public health nutrition personnel to respond to the broad range of responsibilities demanded from this field.

The purpose of *Guidelines for Community Nutrition Supervised Experiences 2nd Edition* is to update the guidelines in consideration of the changes in public health nutrition over the past decade. This purpose maintains the original intent, which was to provide guidelines for supervised experiences for community nutrition personnel in community nutrition programs that promote the health and well being of individuals, families, and communities. These guidelines are the essential starting point for personnel working in community nutrition programs who seek to enhance their level of practice, be they Nutritionists, Community Nutrition Educators, or Clinical Nutritionists and whether or not they are a Registered Dietitian or Dietetic Technician Registered. Enhanced education and training are considered critical to recruiting and retaining qualified community nutrition professionals.

Guidelines for Community Nutrition Supervised Experiences is intended to help community nutrition personnel not only enhance their current practice for client-focused personal nutrition services, but also transition to a practice that will be more population/systems focused. Although the rate at which this transition occurs will vary across the country, it is imperative that public health and community nutrition personnel clearly understand and assume their responsibilities consistent with public health's mission, to assure conditions in which people can be healthy.

Target Audience

These supervised experience guidelines are intended for Bachelor's- and Master's-level Registered Dietitians (RDs), Associate-level Dietetic Technician Registered (DTR) and Bachelor's-level personnel who lack training and/or supervised experiences in community nutrition, but who work in community nutrition positions providing primarily client-focused, individual nutrition services. The supervised experiences are intended to assist these personnel in acquiring needed community nutrition skills. In addition, education of future dietetic personnel in the Community Nutrition Training Areas will ensure a qualified incoming workforce.

The three audiences most likely to benefit from *Guidelines for Community Nutrition Supervised Experiences* are:

- Nutrition personnel, Registered Dietitians, and Dietetic Technicians Registered seeking additional preparation in public health;
- Public health and nutrition administrators striving to employ qualified nutrition personnel in their community programs and agencies; and
- Dietetic Program Directors, Dietetic Internship Directors, Public Health Nutritionists, and others who educate future dietetic professionals on community nutrition topics.

Personnel in Public Health Nutrition for the 1990's (1), published in 1991, does not describe a position title for Bachelor's-prepared community nutrition personnel who are not Registered Dietitians. Therefore, in recognition that many community nutrition programs employ skilled personnel with Bachelor's degrees to provide nutrition education and counseling for low risk clients, a position title of *Community Nutrition Educator* is used to identify individuals with this academic preparation (please see the Glossary of Terms in Appendix D-1).

The supervised experience guidelines are not intended for Master's-level Registered Dietitians who have specialized public health training that includes graduate course work in biostatistics, epidemiology, environmental sciences, public health policy and administration, social/behavioral sciences and education, and advanced nutrition consistent with the curriculum outlined in *Strategies for Success: Curriculum Guide for Graduate Programs in Public Health Nutrition* (2) and recently revised competencies for entry-level Public Health Nutritionists (3). The training described in this document provides knowledge and skills to work primarily with population/systems-focused nutrition programs and services. Consistent with the terminology described in *Personnel in Public Health Nutrition for the 1990's* (1), the term 'public health' in nutrition titles is reserved for positions requiring this academic public health preparation.

Introduction

Public health and community nutrition professionals are members of community health agency staffs and community health programs, who are responsible for nutrition services that emphasize community-wide health promotion and disease prevention and address the needs of individuals. The programs include a variety of nutrition personnel, each of whom has different functions that can be described along a continuum of emphasis from population/systems focus to the client or individual focus. This continuum is described in *Personnel in Public Health Nutrition for the 1990's* (1). These nutrition professionals establish linkages with related personnel involved with the broad range of human services, including child care agencies, services to the elderly, educational institutions, and community-based research. They focus on promoting health and preventing disease in the community using a population/systems focus and a client-focused, or personal nutrition service, approach.

Over the past decade myriad and dramatic changes have occurred that impact how the work of public health nutrition is accomplished. These include changes in the demographic profile in the United States; changes in food purchasing and preparation habits; food production practices; availability and use of technology; and our understanding of nutritional biochemistry and molecular biology. Demographic data show the U.S. population is aging, becoming increasingly obese and culturally diverse (4). The poorest Americans are becoming poorer, with approximately one fifth of American children living in poverty (5,6). Dramatic changes in how America eats occurred during the last 35 years. Almost half of family food purchases are for foods eaten away from home, with a full one third for fast foods (7). Biotechnology and sustainable agriculture influence food production in the United States (8). The information technology revolution has enhanced the availability of nutrition and health information to consumers, professional communications, and our ability to advocate for effective nutrition policies. Perhaps most amazingly, completion of the sequencing of the human genome by the Human Genome Project may soon enable individuals to regulate their genes at the molecular level through dietary factors such as phytochemicals (9). To assimilate and advance these emerging trends, public health nutritionists must have up to date expertise and experience in a broad range of topic areas.

According to the Institute of Medicine in *The Future of Public Health*, the mission of public health is to assure conditions in which people can be healthy (10). To accomplish this mission three core functions will need to be emphasized, and community nutrition professionals will shift from a client-focus to a population/systems focus. The population/systems approach demands competence in program planning, skills in coalition-building, assets mapping, behavior change strategies, and cultural competency, including sensitivity to both the resources and needs of population groups from different cultures, religions, and socioeconomic and educational strata. These competencies help ensure that community-based interventions are designed to meet community needs and priorities effectively by enlisting community resources. Public health practice will require technical expertise in using community-based data sets to monitor and evaluate health status and outcomes, establish practice guidelines, and monitor and promote quality systems of care. Tools such as the Geographic Information System (GIS) will allow users to map resources and assets in relation to where community groups live, work, and play. Public health nutritionists must be policy and advocacy experts, as they develop and promote policies to address nutrition concerns for the population. The shift from a client to a population/systems focus will occur at different rates. In communities where access to clinical preventions and therapeutic services is limited, the transition will be slow. Public health and community nutrition professionals will need to be proactive and creative in assuming their responsibilities.

Assumption of these responsibilities requires an understanding of the core public health functions and how they are related to community nutrition practice. These functions can be described as:

1) *assessing* the nutrition problems and needs of the population, monitoring the nutritional status of populations and related systems of care, and processing information back into the assessment functions;
2) *developing* policies, programs, and activities that address highest priority nutritional problems and needs; and
3) *assuring* the implementation of effective nutrition strategies.

The core functions are interrelated and accomplished through essential services, as reflected in Figure D-1.

Assessment activities include surveillance, needs and resource identification, collection and interpretation of data, identification of population needs, monitoring using diverse and multiple data sets, forecasting trends, estimation of threats to the food supply, and evaluation of outcomes. Geographic Information Systems will facilitate a better understanding of how resources, assets, environmental factors, and health concerns are related within neighborhoods and communities. Assessment also includes evaluation of how interrelated sys-

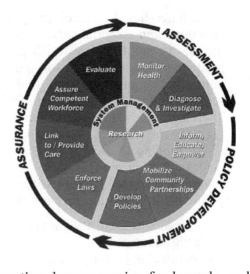

FIGURE D-1 Core Functions and Essential Services of Public Health (11)

tems, such as health, education, human service, food supply, and financial or insurance systems, impact communities' health status.

Policy development in public health nutrition includes setting priorities, developing and implementing community nutrition plans, assuming leadership in developing policies that relate to nutrition goals and objectives, and advocating, convening, negotiating, and brokering for nutrition components in new and existing programs. Administrative roles, such as fiscal management, supervision, and program administration, are important parts of policy development.

Assurance involves access and quality in the implementation of public health and community nutrition plans. It implies the development and maintenance of services and activities needed to maintain safety, access, and adequacy of the food supply for optimal nutrition and health of populations. It includes maintaining the capacity to respond to food and nutrition crises, as well as supporting crucial services such as nutrition monitoring and surveillance; population-based, culturally competent nutrition education; individual and group nutrition services to high risk, under-served, and culturally diverse populations; nutrition counseling for individuals with nutrition-related conditions and disease; mobilizing nutrition resources; emergency preparedness; marketing; provision of public information about nutrition issues; and encouragement of private and public sector action concerning nutrition issues through incentives and persuasion. Assurance includes setting standards and maintaining quality assurance for services and activities that are provided in both private and public sectors. It also includes setting standards for nutrition personnel in recognition that different levels of education and credentialing are necessary for different position responsibilities. Finally, assurance includes maintaining accountability to the community by setting objectives and reporting progress.

Science-based research provides the foundation for these core functions and essential services of public health. New insights and innovative solutions to health problems are critical to success in public health and result from rigorous investigative processes. Collaboration among academic and public health nutrition practice sectors can lead to applied research to benefit the population served. Therefore, study design, implementation, and data analysis are integral in the training of public health personnel.

In *Moving to the Future* (12) Probert lists the essential public health nutrition services, which support the Core Functions and Essential Services of Public Health outlined in Figure D-1. Essential public health nutrition services include:

- assessing the nutritional status of specific populations or geographic areas;
- identifying target populations that may be at nutritional risk;
- initiating and participating in nutrition data collection;
- providing leadership in the development of and planning for health and nutrition policies;
- recommending and providing specific training and programs to meet identified nutrition needs;
- raising awareness among key policy makers of the potential impact of nutrition and food regulations and budget decisions on the health of the community;
- acting as an advocate for target populations on food and nutrition issues;
- planning for nutrition services in conjunction with other health services, based on information obtained from an adequate and on-going data base focused on health outcomes;
- identifying or assisting in development of accurate, up-to-date nutrition education materials;
- ensuring the availability of quality nutrition services to target populations, including nutrition screening, assessment, education, counseling, and referral for food assistance and follow-up;
- participating in nutrition research, demonstration, and evaluation projects;
- providing expert nutrition consultation to the community;
- providing community health promotion and disease prevention activities that are population-based;
- providing quality assurance guidelines for personnel dealing with food and nutrition issues;
- facilitating coordination with other providers of health and nutrition services within the community; and
- evaluating the impact of the health status of populations who receive public health nutrition service.

Background

High employment levels reported by nutritionists participating in a recent American Dietetic Association membership survey demonstrate the continued demand for food and nutrition services (13). Of the 49,000 jobs held by nutritionists and dietitians in 2000, more than 1 in 10 were in state and local government—mostly health departments. According to the U.S. Bureau of Labor Statistics, the employment of dietitians is expected to grow through 2010 at the same rate as the average for all occupations. This growth will result from increasing emphasis on disease prevention through improved dietary habits. "A growing and aging population will increase the demand for meals and nutritional counseling in community health programs and home healthcare agencies. Attrition presents another occupational flux. Job openings will result from the need to replace experienced workers who leave the occupation" (14). Employment by social service agencies is expected to grow quickly, although employment growth for dietitians and nutritionists may be somewhat constrained by employers' utilizing other workers, such as health educators and dietetic technicians.

Personnel Availability and Expertise
The field of public health nutrition and community nutrition is currently suffering from both a shortfall in the number of personnel and a lack of training in public health and community-based nutrition. In 1994 there were approximately 2,393 full time public health nutritionists working in the U.S. (15). "The recommended staffing ratio is 1 public health nutritionist per 50,000 people (1). Application of this ratio to the 1990 population residing in the states and territories that participated in this census survey, suggests that 4,379 public health nutritionists with population/systems-focused responsibilities are needed for the United States, an 83% increase from the current level" (15).

While the Supplemental Nutrition Program for Women, Infants, and Children (WIC) accounts for the vast majority of the public health and community nutrition workforce, public health nutrition expertise within the WIC workforce is limited. Preliminary results of the 2000 Association of State and Territorial Public Health Nutrition Directors (ASTPHND) Work Force study show that of those working in WIC, 19% have Bachelor's degrees in a *variety of disciplines outside nutrition*, including family and consumer sciences and health education among others. Fifty-four percent have Bachelors degrees in *nutrition* or *dietetics* and 12% have Master's degrees in *nutrition* or *dietetics*. Less than 7% of the WIC nutrition workforce has a Bachelor's or Master's degree in *public health nutrition* or *community nutrition*. Of the non-WIC public health nutrition workforce, 26 % have Bachelor's degrees in fields *other than nutrition*. Seventy percent have Bachelor's degrees in *nutrition* or *dietetics* and 28% have Master's degrees in *nutrition* or *dietetics*. Two percent and 14% of the non-WIC public health nutrition workforce have a Bachelor's degree or a Master's degree in *public health nutrition* or *community nutrition*, respectively (16). There is likely some overlap between those with Master's degrees and those with Bachelor's degrees in public health or community nutrition. The shortage of professional staff at WIC agencies is expected to worsen in the coming years, because a large portion of the experienced WIC workforce will retire in the next few years (17).

Preliminary results on the sources of funding for public health and community nutrition positions from the 2000 Association of State and Territorial Public Health Nutrition Directors Workforce study (16) indicate that WIC funded 81% of public health and community nutrition positions in state and local government, up from 78% reported in 1994. Title V Maternal and Child Health Block Grants continued to decline as a funding source funding only 1.9% of the positions, down again from 3.4% reported in 1994 and 8% to 9% reported in 1987 (16,18). This continuing trend is notable because, "although WIC is an important public health nutrition program, it focuses on direct services for a select population subgroup" (15). Funding for chronic disease prevention is also declining, as evidenced by the decline in FTE positions funded by preventive health and health services block grants to .6% of all FTE positions. "If official health agencies are to shift to public heath core functions that are population-based and system-focused, then a notable proportion of the public heath nutrition workforce must not only change how they practice but they must also obtain the knowledge and skills to perform these functions" (15).

A competent workforce depends on didactic and continuing education that is sensitive to the core knowledge and ancillary skills needed for public health and community nutrition. Preliminary research findings from the ASTPHND 2000 Public Health Nutrition Workforce Study (16) indicate the top ten training needs include:

1. nutrition for children with special health care needs
2. breastfeeding
3. infant and preschool nutrition
4. prenatal nutrition
5. nutrition counseling, behavior change, and client education
6. high-risk clients, including HIV and addiction
7. childhood nutrition
8. eating disorders
9. supplemental and alternative dietary therapies
10. use of current information technology, including computers.

While these training needs are predominantly nutrition content-related, additional emerging areas requiring expertise have been defined in a recent General Accounting Office report (17). They include, for example, navigating the changing health and welfare system under managed care, and assessing clients' levels of readiness for changing health behaviors. Public health and community nutrition training needs are clear; it is the provision of training that is limited. This General Accounting Office report (17) also indicates that while WIC regulations require state agencies to provide in-service training, a more defined commitment from the U.S. Department of Agriculture (USDA) to improve training opportunities for WIC staff is forthcoming. In order to alleviate selected staff training issues, USDA has recently created the 'WIC Works' website as a resource for WIC staff and is developing online learning modules for WIC staff that address a variety of nutrition and program related issues.

Recruitment and Retention

Recruitment and retention of qualified staff is essential to maintaining the quality of community nutrition services. Well-trained nutritionists are important to the public health community because they contribute to the mission of public health and attainment of health objectives for the U.S. population, such as *Healthy People 2010: Understanding and Improving Health* (19). Staff retention and recruitment is one of the top emerging areas of concern for state and territorial agency nutrition units (16).

Barriers to recruiting and retaining community nutrition professionals include a low level of job satisfaction related to salary levels and inadequate benefit packages, which are lower and more inadequate than those of other allied health professionals and nutrition professionals in other roles. Although the estimated median annual income for dietitians working in community nutrition increased by 8.9% since 1997, at $37,990 community nutritionists continue to earn substantially less than RDs in food and nutrition management, consultation and business, and education and research (13). "Personnel skilled in population-focused responsibilities find limited opportunities in public health agencies for professional growth and development" (15). It has been hypothesized that qualified candidates do not apply for WIC positions due to the routine nature of the work and the rural locations of many agencies (17).

The *Recruitment Strategies for Public Health and Community Nutritionists Workshop* (20), held in January 1994 and sponsored by government and private organizations, provided an impetus to develop strategies to address difficulties the state and local agencies were experiencing in recruitment and retention. One of the priority recommendations of the national, interorganizational workshop, *Call to Action: Better Nutrition for Mothers, Children, and Families*, was to increase the number and improve the quality of personnel (professional and paraprofessional) providing nutrition services (21). Despite efforts to improve the situation, recruitment and retention of qualified public health and community nutrition staff continues to be a growing concern a decade after the Maternal and Child Health Interagency Nutrition Group (MCHING) and Recruitment Strategies workshops. In fact as recently as 1998 approximately half of all WIC agencies reported having difficulty recruiting and hiring professional staff (17).

The most recent comprehensive WIC workforce data were collected in 1994 and are outdated. While updated workforce survey results are pending (16), no information on the demand for nutritionists and dietitians in underserved areas will be provided. For these reasons, the General Accounting Office (GAO) capstone report, *Food Assistance: WIC Faces Challenges in Providing Nutrition Services*, includes a recommendation to "conduct an assessment of the staffing needs of state and local WIC agencies." The GAO hopes that the resulting data will assist Congress and the USDA in identifying strategies to address challenges relating to recruiting and retaining qualified staff (17).

Community Nutrition Practice

Public health and community nutrition practice ranges from a population/systems focus to a client focus. This is reflected in the public health and community nutrition team positions described by Kaufman (22). Very few community nutrition practices focus exclusively on public health services; most provide a combination of public health and personal nutrition services.

Prevention plays a prominent role in community nutrition practice. In this document, prevention is defined comprehensively to include a wide array of interventions, which can be categorized as three essential components of prevention:

- individually-based,
- community-based, and
- systems-based.

Each component has a distinct role, importance, and focus. Individually-based efforts deal with prevention issues at the personal level. Community-based prevention messages are targeted at groups. Prevention at the systems level focuses on changing policies and law so that the goals of prevention practices are achieved. Community nutrition practice involves making appropriate and coordinated use of each.

For each of the three components of prevention, there are three levels of prevention.

- Primary prevention involves health promotion to maintain a state of wellness and focuses on changing or enhancing the environment, community, family, and individual life styles and behaviors.

- Secondary prevention consists of risk appraisal and reduction and includes interventions that include screening, detection, early diagnosis, treatment, and follow-up.
- Tertiary prevention is directed at managing and rehabilitating persons with diagnosed health conditions to extend their years of productivity.

Table D-1 presents the three essential components of prevention and provides examples for the three levels of prevention in community nutrition practice.

Kaufman's 'Conceptual Framework for Public Health,' shown in Appendix D-3, adds a third dimension to the delivery of prevention in public health nutrition practice—that of 'stages in life' (22). The framework thereby demonstrates how public health and community nutrition services are delivered across the lifecycle and are focused at primary, secondary, and tertiary levels of prevention at each of these stages. In this model, the delivery mode for preventive services also follows a continuum ranging from those delivered to individuals to services focused at communities or a population/systems focus. For example, in WIC a prenatal woman might meet with the Community Nutrition Educator about how to feed her baby. This would be an example of primary prevention delivered to a prenatal woman and using an individual delivery mode. The National High

TABLE D-1   Essential Components and Levels of Prevention in Public Health and Community Nutrition Practices

	Components of Prevention		
Levels of Prevention	**Personal**	**Community**	**System**
Primary Prevention	Food Guide Pyramid education at health fair	Local "5 a Day" campaign in association with the farmers' market, schools and grocery stores Use of local produce in school lunch program	School lunches required by law to be consistent with the Dietary Guidelines for Americans Folic acid fortification of foods
Secondary prevention	Work site nutrition education for highrisk employees Nutrition education for high-risk WIC clients	Health fairs with screening and referrals to primary care providers	Food labels required to include information on particular nutrients, including calories
Tertiary Prevention	Medical nutrition therapy	Diabetes classes offered by local health departments	Legislation requiring medical nutrition therapy for identified diseases

Source: Adapted from AL Owen, PL Splett, GM Owen. *Nutrition in the Community: The Art and Sciences of Delivering Services.* Boston: WCB/McGraw-Hill; 1999.

Blood Pressure Education Program might develop national public service announcements targeting adults across the United States. This would be an example of secondary prevention with a national adult population focus. A hospital may establish a summer camp for youth learning to live with diabetes, which would be an example of tertiary prevention for the adolescent population at the city or county level.

The process in which nutrition care is provided across the three levels of prevention and at the personal and community levels is described by the American Dietetic Association's nutrition care process (Standardized Nutrition Care Process and Model, March 1, 2003, American Dietetic Association). This process includes nutrition screening/referral, nutrition assessment, nutrition diagnosis, nutrition intervention, nutrition documentation, nutrition outcomes, and outcomes and management systems. It is a standard process for nutrition care that can be applied by dietetics professionals who are Registered Dietitians and Dietetic Technicians, Registered, in a variety of public health and community practice settings including, for example, primary prevention for health promotion and individual or group nutrition education for secondary prevention.

It is necessary for community nutrition professionals to be aware of all levels and components of preventive practices and to incorporate them into their daily work activities. Coordinating the various levels and components of prevention will result in the following:

- prevention of unnecessary duplication of services;
- promotion of the broad concept of prevention as one that includes a range of services and programs that affects individuals, communities, and systems; and
- increased cost effectiveness of combined individual preventive services as they influence the general health of the population; for example, maintaining nutritional status of at risk clients may make them less likely to contract communicable diseases.

Curriculum Development

The Community Nutrition Training Areas are listed on page 16. The Guide for Curriculum Development, which begins on page 18, lists expected target behaviors, suggested work-related and learning activities, and examples of resources for each of the Community Nutrition Training Areas. It is assumed that the trainee and supervisor will use appropriate textbooks and other recognized resources related to the training area. A self-assessment, like the one in Appendix D-2, provides the practitioner and supervisor information on the practitioner's strengths and weaknesses.

Application of the Guidelines

Training and Length

Guidelines for Community Nutrition Supervised Experiences is designed to provide ideas for supervised community nutrition experiences. Training areas are to be used selectively by the individual supervising the particular trainee. For example, a Registered Dietitian working with high risk prenatal women will have different needs and responsibilities compared to a Bachelor's level non-Registered Dietitian working with food stamp nutrition education participants. The training should be individualized for the trainee, taking into account his/her nutrition/dietetic education or experience. The length of the training is determined jointly by the supervisor and trainee and will vary according to the specific needs and strengths of the trainee.

Supervision

The supervisor of the trainee should be a Public Health Nutritionist who is willing to provide leadership and direction to enable the trainee to fulfill his/her training goals. It is recommended that the supervisor have at least two years experience in public health nutrition.

Evaluation

The Self-Assessment Tool for Public Health Nutritionists (Appendix D-2) can be used at the beginning and end of the training as a useful evaluation for the trainee. The supervisor and trainee may identify other evaluative methods to complete during and at the conclusion of the training.

Suggestions for Use

To summarize, the intended audiences for *Guidelines for Community Nutrition Supervised Experiences* are:

- Nutrition personnel, Registered Dietitians, and Dietetic Technicians Registered seeking additional preparation in public health and community nutrition;
- Public health and nutrition administrators striving to employ qualified nutrition personnel in their community programs and agencies; and
- Dietetic Program Directors, Dietetic Internship Directors, Public Health Nutritionists, and others who educate future dietetic professionals on community nutrition topics.

With the roles of public health nutritionists becoming more complex and the population/systems focus expanding, practicing community nutrition professionals may come to recognize the need to increase their own skills in a broad range of public health topic areas. The training areas will assist them in developing plans for continuing education. Similarly, public health nutrition professionals who are Registered Dietitians may access the training areas to fulfill their continuing education requirements using the Commission on Dietetic Registration's new Professional Development Portfolio system. By selecting training areas that will further their professional abilities, RDs will have a pre-developed set of target behaviors, learning activities and resources to accomplish professional continuing education requirements. Because specialty certification is not required for various aspects of dietetics, Registered Dietitians will move between clinical, food service, and community nutrition practice positions. Utilizing the Community Nutrition Training Areas will serve to smooth this transition. A self-assessment tool, such as the one found in Appendix D, will aid in identifying priority areas for training.

Competencies have been successfully used in the public health sector to write Public Health Nutrition position descriptions. By connecting performance evaluations to the training areas, agencies are able to justify continuing education expenses and evaluate individual accomplishment using the training areas as objective measures (23). State or locally conducted assessment of training needs may indicate a need for continuing education in the public health-related areas of food and nutrition science, research and evaluation, communication and culture, and management and leadership. The training areas defined and detailed in this publication offer professionals and their supervisors guidance for the development and completion of successful comprehensive inservice training experiences, helping to ensure qualified nutrition personnel. The training areas may be used in their entirety or may be used to tailor experiences for agency divisions or individual staff members.

Educators responsible for preparing future nutrition professionals have used this document with both dietetic interns and students at undergraduate and graduate levels to ensure required experiences cover the basics of public health and community nutrition (23–27). Used in conjunction with the Commission on Accreditation of Dietetics Education's Community Emphasis Competencies (28), the Community Nutrition Training Areas detailed in this publication offer specific ideas for relevant experiences (25, 27).

Distribution of the Guidelines

Guidelines for Community Nutrition Supervised Experiences is available in electronic (.pdf) format on the American Dietetic Association's Public Health/ Community Nutrition Practice Group Website at www.phcnpg.org. Guidelines for Community Nutrition Supervised Experiences will be of interest to public health and community nutrition personnel, educators, and administrators. Announcements via listserve and organizational newsletters and inservice events, as well as hyperlinks on public health and nutrition agencies' and organizations' websites will serve to inform potential users of this resource.

The User Survey in Appendix D-3 will allow for future updates of Guidelines for Community Nutrition Supervised Experiences to address real-world applications and issues to better prepare public health and community nutrition personnel for their role in assuring the health of Americans through nutrition, public health, and social/behavioral sciences and education.

Bibliography

1. Dodds, JM, Kaufman, M. *Personnel in Public Health Nutrition for the 1990's.* Washington, DC: The Public Health Foundation; 1991.

2. Endres, J (Ed). *Strategies for Success: Curriculum Guide for Graduate Programs in Public Health Nutrition.* Carbondale, IL: Southern Illinois University, in association with Association of the Faculties of Graduate Programs in Public Health Nutrition; 1990.

3. *Strategies for Success. Curriculum Guide. Graduate Programs in Public Health Nutrition.* Second Edition. Association of Graduate Programs in Public Health Nutrition, Inc., 2002. http://nutrition.utk.edu/resources/StrategiesForSuccess.pdf.

4. Johnson RK, Kennedy E. The 2000 Dietary guidelines for Americans: What are the changes and why were they made? *J Am Diet Assoc.* 2000;100:769774.

5. Shapiro I, Greenstein R. *The Widening Income Gulf.* Washington DC: Center on Budget and Policy Priorities; 2000.

6. U.S. Census Bureau. *Poverty in the United States, 1999.* Available at: www.census.gov/hhes/www/povty99.html

7. Frazao E. *America's Eating Habits: Changes and Consequences.* Food and Rural Economics Division, Economic Research Service. Agriculture Information Bulletin No. 750. Washington, DC: U.S. Department of Agriculture; 1999.

8. Alternative Farming Systems Information Center. *Sustainable Agriculture Resources.* Available at: http://warp.nal.usda.gov/afsic/agnic/agnic.htm

9. Johnson DB, Eaton DL, Wahl PW, Gleason C. Public health nutrition practice in the United States. *J Am Diet Assoc.* 2001;101:529–34.

10. Institute of Medicine. *The Future of Public Health.* Washington, DC: National Academy Press; 1989.

11. U.S. Department of Health and Human Services. *Public Health in America.* Available at: www.health.gov/phfunctions/public.htm.

12. KL Probert. *Moving to the Future: Developing Community-Based Nutrition Services.* Washington, DC: Association of State and Territorial Public Health Nutrition Directors; 1996.

13. Bryk JA, Kornblum T. Report on the 1999 membership database of the American Dietetic Association. *J Am Diet Assoc.* 2001;101: 947–53.

14. U.S. Department of Labor. *Occupational Outlook Handbook,* 2002–03 Edition. Available at: http://stats.bls.gov/oco/home.htm. Accessed 7/02.

15. Haughton B, Story M, Keir B. Profile of public health nutrition personnel: Challenges for population/system-focused roles and state-level monitoring. *J Am Diet Assoc*. 1998;6:664–670.

16. Kier B. *Survey of the Public Health Nutrition Workforce 1999–2000*. ASTPHND Annual Meeting, Cleveland, OH; 2002.

17. U.S. General Accounting Office. Report to Congressional Committees. *Food Assistance: WIC Faces Challenges in Providing Nutrition Services*. (GAO-02–142) Washington; 2001. Available at: www.gao.gov/new.items/d02142.pdf. Accessed 9/02.

18. Kaufman M, Lee S. Nutrition services in state and local public health agencies: how do we measure up in 1987? *J Am Diet Assoc*. 1988;88: 1576–1580.

19. U.S. Department of Health and Human Services. *Healthy People 2010: Understanding and Improving Health*. 2nd ed. Washington, DC: U.S. Government Printing Office, November 2000. Available at: www.health.gov/healthypeople.

20. United States Department of Agriculture, Food and Nutrition Service. *Recruitment Strategies for Public Heath/Community Nutritionists. Final Report*. Alexandria, VA United States Department of Agriculture; 1995.

21. Sharbaugh, C, Ed. *Call to Action. Better Nutrition for Mothers. Children, and Families*. Washington, DC: National Center for Education in Maternal and Child Health; 1990.

22. Kaufman, M. *Nutrition in Public Health: A Handbook for Developing Programs and Services*. Rockville, MD: Aspen Publishers; 1990.

23. Binghay E. Winfield Moody Health Center Nutrition Director, Chicago, IL. Personal communication, August 2002.

24. Bennett A, Tri-County Health Department Internship Director, Englewood, CO. Personal communication, July 2002.

25. Moreau-Stodola D, Ad Hoc Professor, University of Wisconsin, Green Bay, WI. Personal communication, July 2002.

26. Schilling J, California Department of Health Services, Childhood Lead Poisoning Prevention Program, Oakland, CA. Personal communication, July 2002.

27. Silverstein S, Dietetic Internship Director, Virginia Department of Health, Richmond, VA. Personal Communication, July 2002.

28. Commission on Accreditation for Dietetics Education, American Dietetic Association, *CADE Accreditation Handbook;* 2002.

Community Nutrition Training Topic Areas

Nutrition Training Topic Areas

1. Knows issues related to establishing nutrient requirements and dietary recommendations
2. Assesses and prioritizes nutritional problems of individuals from various age and population groups using appropriate anthropometric, biochemical, clinical, dietary, and socioeconomic assessment techniques

3. Uses nutrition and physical activity research findings in developing and/or implementing nutrition programs

4. Knows and applies factors that impact the accessibility, adequacy and safety of the food supply system (production, processing, distribution and consumption) and the relationship of those factors to community health

5. Knows the principles of food science, preparation and management and translates them to meet food needs of various population groups

6. Knows how to evaluate emerging and controversial food and nutrition claims for accuracy and practical implications

Public Health Training Topic Areas

7. Knows federal, regional, state and local governmental structures and the processes involved in the development of public policy, legislation, and regulations that influence and relate to nutrition and health services

8. Participates in organized advocacy efforts for health and nutrition programs

9. Understands political and ethical considerations within and across organizations and their impact on agency planning, policy, and decision-making

10. Knows management principles for effective community assessment, program planning, implementation, and evaluation and applies them to community-based public health nutrition programs

11. Knows how nutrition services are integrated into overall mission, goals, and plan of the health agency

12. Understands resource management, including grant application, identifying funding sources, and reading fiscal reports

13. Knows the principles of personnel management, including recruiting, staffing, supervising, performance appraisal, staff development, and conflict resolution

14. Understands descriptive statistics, principles of data collection and management, monitoring and surveillance reports, and basic computer applications for data compilation and analysis

15. Knows the principles of an epidemiologic approach to assess the health and nutrition problems and trends in the community

16. Knows principles of research and evaluation

17. Knows relationships of the environment to public health, risk assessment, and biological, physical, and chemical factors that effect the nutritional status of the public

18. Knows processes of monitoring, technical assistance, guidance, consultation, and collaboration within and across agencies and organizations

19. Selects and appropriately uses group process and group facilitation techniques (brainstorming, focus groups, nominal group process) to achieve goals and objectives of food and nutrition programs and services

20. Is familiar with the role and operation of agency and/or community boards, committees, task forces, coalitions, and partnerships in public health

21. Develops skills in functioning as a multidisciplinary and interdisciplinary team member or leader within and across disciplines

Social/Behavioral Sciences and Education Training Topic Areas

22. Knows and applies skills in selecting and/or developing nutrition education materials and approaches appropriate for individuals or small groups within the target population

23. Effects behavior change through knowledge and application of behavioral, social, and education theories

24. Communicates accurate, scientifically based information—both oral and written—at levels appropriate for various audiences: clients, general public

25. Uses media strategies in various print, broadcasting, and telecommunications channels, such as video and the Internet, to reach population groups

Revised from:
Public Health Nutrition Practice Group of the American Dietetic Association. Guidelines for Community Nutrition Supervised Experiences. Chicago, IL: American Dietetic Association; 1995.

Guide for Training Program Development

Training Topic Area	Example Target Behaviors	Suggested Work-Related & Learning Activities	Example Resources
1. Knows issues related to establishing nutrient requirements and dietary recommendations	• Uses appropriate resources for dietary recommendations to determine nutrient requirements for specific populations	• Analyze menus to determine if they meet the relevant needs of specific populations • Investigate the Dietary Guidelines for Americans to determine the strengths and weaknesses of the recommendations • Study the *Dietary Guidelines for Americans* to become familiar with the interrelationships between nutrition and physical activity • Analyze individual dietary intake of a pregnant or breastfeeding woman and make dietary change recommendation • Compare the Dietary Guidelines for Americans to specific consumption patterns of a population group or community	• Dietary Reference Intakes. Food and Nutrition Board, National Academy of Sciences. www.nal.usda.gov/fnic/etext/000105.html • *Dietary Guidelines for Americans* 5th ed. USDA and U.S. Department of Health and Human Services. USDA Home and Garden Bulletin No. 232. Washington, DC: USDA, 2000. www.usda.gov/cnpp/Pubs/DG2000/Index.htm or www.health.gov/dietaryguidelines/dga2000/dietgd.pdf • Dietary assessment software: www.nal.usda.gov/fnic/etext/000053.html Interactive Healthy Eating Index: www.usda.gov/cnpp • Food Guide Pyramid: www.usda.gov/cnpp/pyramid2.htm www.pueblo.gsa.gov/cic_text/food/food-pyramid/main.htm www.nal.usda.gov/fnic/Fpyr/pyramid.html • Food Pyramid for Children 2–5: www.usda.gov/cnpp/KidsPyra/index.htm or www.usda.gov/cnpp/using.htm • *Celebrating Diversity: Approaching Families Through their Food*. DC Eliades, CW Suitor. Arlington, VA: National Center for Education in Maternal and Child Health; 1994. • *Bright Futures in Practice: Nutrition*. National Center for Education in Maternal and Child Health: www.brightfutures.org/

Training Topic Area	Example Target Behaviors	Suggested Work-Related & Learning Activities	Example Resources
2. Assesses and prioritizes nutritional problems of individuals from various age and population groups using appropriate anthropometric, biochemical, clinical, dietary, and socioeconomic assessment techniques	• Interprets and compares growth data to standard growth curves • Interprets and compares dietary assessment results to norms • Uses appropriate dietary assessment methodology • Completes feeding assessments and recommends appropriate intervention • Completes physical activity assessment and recommends appropriate action • Demonstrates appropriate anthropometric measurement techniques • Understands dependence of surveillance on accurate individual assessment • Uses the American Dietetic Association's Nutrition Care Process and Model for personal health care community nutrition activities (RDs only)	• Review health records of various age and population groups, e.g., medical and school records • Evaluate anthropometric and biochemical measures of various age and population groups • Review standardized anthropometric measurement techniques • Apply quality assessment standards, e.g., Pediatric Practice Groups Standards • Utilize surveillance data, e.g. Pediatric Nutrition Surveillance System (PedNSS) data, for internal quality assurance and improvement • Complete online training on CDC growth charts and Dietary Guidelines for Americans • Reviews the American Dietetic Association's Nutrition Care Process and Model	• Patient/client records • Vital records • Journal of the American Dietetic Association • Handbook of Lab Values: MT Daily: Medical Transcription Networking Center www.mtdaily.com/mt1/lab.html • Nutrition Throughout the Life Cycle. Worthington-Roberts B, Williams Sr. 4th Ed. Boston: McGraw Hill; 2000. • Software for nutrient analysis: www.nal.usda.gov/fnic/etext/000053.html Interactive Healthy Eating Index: www.usda.gov/cnpp • Bright Futures in Practice: Nutrition. National Center for Education in Maternal and Child Health: www.brightfutures.org/ • Maximizing Resources for Results! Extending Bright Futures Through Community-Based Nutrition Planning. S Gregory; 2001. http://nutrition.he.utk.edu/max_resources/maximize/ • Bright Futures in Practice: Physical Activity: www.brightfutures.org/physicalactivity/pdf/index.html • CDC Growth Chart training: www.cdc.gov/growthcharts. • Lacey K, Pritchett E. Nutrition care process and model: ADA adopted road map to quality care and outcomes management. J Am Diet Assoc. 103: 1061–1072; 2003.

2, *continued*

Assesses and prioritizes nutritional problems of individuals from various age and population groups using appropriate anthropometric, biochemical, clinical, dietary, and socioeconomic assessment techniques

- *Moving People and Communities - Applying Bright Futures in Practice: Physical Activity.* H Mixon; 2002. http://nutrition.he.utk.edu
- *Kids Count.* www.aecf.org/kidscount/rightstart/index.htm;
- *Kids Count 2000.* www.aecf.org/kidscount/kc2001/
- Community Health Status Indicator Project. U.S. Department of Health and Human Services, Health Resources and Services Administration. www.communityhealth.hrsa.gov/
- Child Health USA. MCH Information and Resource Center. www.mchirc.net/
- FedStats: www.fedstats.gov/
- *Cross Cultural: A Guide for Nutrition and Health Counselors.* Alexandria, VA: USDA/USDHHS, Publication No. FNS-250; 1986.
- *Diversity Rx:* Promoting language and cultural competence in healthcare: www.diversityrx.org
- CDC Surveillance Systems: www.cdc.gov/nccdphp/dnpa/surveill.htm
  - Behavioral Risk Factor Surveillance System (BRFSS) Youth Risk Behavior Surveillance System (YRBSS)
  - Pediatric Nutrition Surveillance System (PedNSS)
  - Pregnancy Nutrition Surveillance System (PNSS)
- CDC Division of Nutrition and Physical Activity: www.cdc.gov/nccdphp/dnpa/physicalactivity.htm
- *Dietitian's Desk Reference.* A Bennett. Tri-county Health Department; 1999.

Training Topic Area	Expected Outcomes	Suggested Learning Activities	Example Resources

3. Uses nutrition and physical activity research findings in developing and/or implementing nutrition programs	• Recognizes elements of sound research and evaluation
	
	• Applies sound research when developing nutrition interventions
	
	• Implements a community project, e.g., 5-A-Day for Better Health Program, as part of the agency nutrition plan
	
	• Recognizes the interrelationship between nutrition and physical activity in promoting health and preventing disease
	
	• Understands and demonstrates in practice the interrelationships between nutrition and physical activity in promoting health and preventing disease
		• Review research applicable to a specific population group
		
		• Choose ongoing community project and determine if program components are based on science-based research
		
		• Conduct a literature search for a specific target population, e.g.,
		
		  – Preliminary research demonstrates an association between antioxidant vitamins and cancer
		
		  – An epidemiological study further demonstrates that increased consumption of fruits and vegetables reduces the risk of certain types of cancer
		
		  – Demonstration projects are designed and implemented to increase fruit and vegetable consumption
		
		• Complete case study from current, published literature on a community-based intervention
			• Research articles in peer reviewed publications
			
			• Nutrition interventions based on scientific research, e.g., National 5-A-Day for Better Health Programs
			
			  – 5-A-Day Program Evaluation Report: http://cancercontrol.cancer.gov/5ad_exec.html and http://cancercontrol.cancer.gov/5aday_12–4–00.pdf
			
			  – National Institutes of Health: www.NIH.gov
			
			  – CDC 5 A Day Web page: www.cdc.gov/nccdphp/dnpa/5ADay/index.htm
			
			• USDA Center for Nutrition Policy and Promotion: www.usda.gov/cnpp
			
			• Kids Walk to School: www.cdc.gov/nccdphp/dnpa/physicalactivity.htm
			
			• Increasing Physical Activity: A Report on Recommendations of the Task Force on Community Preventive Services. MMWR—Physical Activity Comprehensive Guide: www.cdc.gov/mmwr/preview/mmwrhtml/rr5018a1.htm
			
			• Bright Futures in Practice: Physical Activity, National Center for Education in Maternal and Child Health: www.brightfutures.org/physicalactivity/pdf/index.html
			
			• Wise Woman: www.cdc.gov/wisewoman
			
			• Blueprint for Breastfeeding: www.cdc.gov/breastfeeding/report-blueprint.htm
			
			• USDA Food and Nutrition Services Website: www.fns.usda.gov/fns/

| 4. Knows and applies factors that impact the accessibility, adequacy and safety of the food supply system (production, processing, distribution and consumption) and the relationship of those factors to community health | • Describes the food supply system including grocery stores, farmers markets, etc.
• Identifies family assistance resources available to population groups, e.g., social service programs
• Knows eligibility rules and benefits for food assistance programs
• Knows rules and location of emergency food systems
• Understands the Thrifty Food Plan
• Uses information about nutrients and contaminants in the food supply and relates these factors to community health indicators
• Interprets food and nutrition surveys and relates these factors to community health indicators | • Analyze availability, cost and quality of foods in food stores in various geographic areas of the community
• Compare food costs and food access of neighborhoods with a variety of incomes, available transportation, ethnicities
• Compare cost of comparable foods available at food stores, restaurants, and fast food
• Analyze Thrifty Food Plan for adequacy
• Develop weekly menus for a culturally diverse population
• Evaluate impact of schoolbased Child Nutrition Programs, Food Stamps, WIC, day care homes or nursing centers, congregate feeding on adequacy of food supply for family | • Restaurant/ fast food menus and nutrient analysis
• Thrifty Food Plan: www.usda.gov/cnpp or www.usda.gov/cnpp/FoodPlans/TFP99/Index.htm
• Family Economics and Nutrition Review: www.usda.gov/cnpp/FENR.htm
• National Center for Health Statistics: www.cdc.gov/nchs
• National Health and Nutrition Examination Survey (NHANES): www.cdc.gov/nchs/nhanes
• Hispanic Health and Nutrition Examination Survey (HHANES): www.cdc.gov/nchs/fastats/hisfacts
• Dietary Reference Intakes. Food and Nutrition Board, National Academy of Sciences: www.nal.usda.gov/fnic/etext/000105.html
• Dietary Guidelines for Americans. 5th ed. USDA and U.S. Department of Health and Human Services. USDA Home and Garden Bulletin No. 232. Washington, DC: USDA, 2000. www.usda.gov/cnpp/Pubs/DG2000/Index.htm
• Head Start Program Performance Standards: http://headstartinfo.org/publications/publicat.htm
• FDA guidelines for processed foods and seafood: www.fda.gov |

Training Topic Area Continued	Example Target Behaviors	Suggested Work-Related & Learning Activities	Example Resources
4, continued Knows and applies factors that impact the accessibility, adequacy and safety of the food supply system (production, processing, distribution and consumption) and the relationship of those factors to community health	• Utilizes federal and state food safety resources, e.g., Extension, Food and Drug Administration, Food Safety and Inspection Service	• Use data from the Current Population Survey and its Household Food Security Questionnaire to understand the coping strategies of those who are food insecure and/or hungry.	• USDA meat and produce inspection guidelines www.usda.gov
			• State Extension Service: www.reeusda.gov/1700/statepartners/usa.htm
			• National Nutrition Monitoring Data: www.cdc.gov/nchs
		• Plan a monthly family budget, including rent, transportation, food and welfare resources, e.g., Food Stamps, WIC, Housing, School Food Service, etc.	• Food Surveys Research Group: www.barc.usda.gov/bhnrc/foodsurvey/home.htm
			• American Public Health Association: www.apha.org
		• Accompany environmental health specialist to a day care center, grocery store, and restaurant to observe inspections	• American Academy of Pediatrics: www.aap.org
			• *Caring for Our Children: National Health and Safety Performance Standards: Guidelines for Out of Home Child Care Programs.* American Academy of Pediatrics, National Resource Center for Health and Safety in Child Care, American Public Health Association, United States Maternal and Child Health Bureau. 2nd Ed. Elk Grove Village, IL; 2002. http://nrc.uchsc.edu/CFOC/
		• Visit with food and drug administration enforcement officer or USDA food safety education specialist	
			• CDC growth charts: www.cdc.gov/growthcharts
		• Analyze a food facility's HACCP plan with an environmental health specialist	• *USDA's Guide to Measuring Household Food Security:* www.fns.usda.gov/fsec/FILES/FSGuide.pdf

5. Knows the principles of food science, preparation and management and translates them to meet food needs of various population groups

- Demonstrates an understanding of the cultural and developmental priorities, needs, and assets of the various population groups and is able to apply to practice

- Evaluates shopping and food preparation skills of homemakers and makes appropriate recommendations in practice

- Applies the principles of food science, preparation, and management to meet the food needs of the population served

- Participate in training on cultural food habits/dietary habits

- Participate in training on agespecific and developmental issues related to food intake and food safety

- Develop Hazard Analysis Critical Control Points (HACCP) plan for a day care center feeding site

- Participate in community-based field experiences, e.g., food banks, homeless shelters, soup kitchens, congregate feeding program or child care feeding site

- Develop a one-week set of menus for a congregate feeding program or child care feeding site

- Modify a recipe to meet a special nutritional need of the target population and test it for acceptability

- Develop a one-week set of menusfor a pregnant teen in an alternative school for pregnant teens

- Develop a one-week set of menus for a family receiving both food stamps and WIC benefits

- State and Licensing standards for Day Care and Long Term Care Facilities

- Head Start Program Performance Standards http://headstartinfo.org/publications/publicat.htm

- *Food Service Organization: A Managerial and Systems Approach.* 4th Ed. Spears, MC. New York: Macmillan Publishing Company; 2000.

- Food and Nutrition Information Center: www.nal.usda.gov/fnic

- Community-Based programs, e.g., Expanded Food and Nutrition Education Program (EFNEP), Head Start, food banks, congregate food sites

- Agency video tapes and training materials, Hazard Analysis Critical Control Points (HACCP) manual

- National Food Service Management Institute: www.olemiss.edu/depts/nfsmi/

- The Provider's Guide to Quality and Culture. Management Sciences for Health. http://erc.msh.org/quality&culture

- Nutrition Education for New American Populations. Dept of Anthropology and Geography, Georgia State University. http://monarch.gsu.edu/nutrition

Training Topic Area	Example Target Behaviors	Suggested Work-Related & Learning Activities	Example Resources
6. Knows how to evaluate emerging and controversial food and nutrition claims for accuracy and practical implications	• Uses standard criteria to evaluate claims and literature • Defines clearly the difference between food and nutrition fact and fiction • Presents a cogent argument to refute inappropriate claims • Differentiates between what are safe and unsafe food and nutrition practices • Presents scientific rationale clearly	• Review literature on supplements and botanicals • Interview providers and promoters of nutrition supplements • Survey health food store products and claims • Investigate and respond to health and nutrition information and misinformation (TV, radio, newspapers, books, Internet) in a proactive manner • Review popular diets/nutrition practices and determine recommendations, providing rationale • Identify sources of reliable nutrition information	• American Dietetic Association's National Center for Nutrition and Dietetics: www.eatright.org/ncnd.html • State Health Department Nutrition Programs • National Council Against Health Fraud: www.ncahf.org/ • *The Health Robbers: Close Look at Quackery in America.* S Barrett. Buffalo, NY: Prometheus Books; 1995. • *The Vitamin Pushers: How the 'Health Food' Industry Is Selling America a Bill of Goods.* S Barrett, V Herbert. Amherst, NY: Prometheus Books; 1994. • Clinical Indications of Drug-Nutrient Interactions and Herbal Use. Roche Labs. Order from www.rochedietitians.com • Learning Resource for Classroom and Independent Study. Roche Labs. Order from www.rochedietitians.com • National Center for Alternative and Complementary Medicine: http://nccam.nih.gov/

7. Knows federal, regional, state and local governmental structures and the processes involved in the development of public policy, legislation, and regulations that influence and relate to nutrition and health services			
• Has strong familiarity with federal nutrition and health programs	• Visit federal government nutrition and health Websites	• USDA Food and Nutrition Services: www.fns.usda.gov/fns/
• Understands the system used to develop legislation, regulation, and public policy and to appropriate funding	• Review organizational charts at federal, state, and local levels	• USDHHS Maternal and Child Health Bureau: www.mchdata.net
	• Access educational resources on how to deal effectively with legislators	• *Guidelines for Comprehensive Programs to Promote Healthy Eating and Physical Activity:* www.astphnd.org/programs/00Nupawgfm.pdf
• Explains legislation accurately to consumers and other professionals	• Identify where authority lies for nutrition and food programs at Federal, State and local levels	• Legislative newsletters
• Is able to participate actively in support of nutrition related legislation	• Observe a committee meeting in state legislature	• American Dietetic Association's Policy Initiatives and Advocacy Web page: www.eatright.com/gov/
• Understands how policies can be designed to support nutrition and health related programs	• Read and write comments on proposed nutrition-related regulations from the Federal Register	• Federal Register www.gpo.gov
	• Attend a Board of Health meeting	• National Conference of State Legislatures: www.ncsl.org
	• Track a bill through passage to implementation	• State or local personnel manual
	• Identify specific agency activities that support Healthy People 2010 objectives	• *Nutrition and the Community.* A Owen, P Splett, and G Owen. Boston, McGraw Hill, 1999.
	• Review regulations of food and nutrition programs available in agency, e.g., WIC, Food Stamps	• *Healthy People 2010: Understanding and Improving Health.* 2nd ed. USDHHS. Washington, DC: U.S. Government Printing Office, November 2000. www.health.gov/healthypeople
	• Identify policies that support or promote improved nutrition and regular physical activity	• League of Women Voters Organization www.lwv.org/

Training Topic Area	Example Target Behaviors	Suggested Work-Related & Learning Activities	Example Resources
7. Knows federal, regional, state and local governmental structures and the processes involved in the development of public policy, legislation, and regulations that influence and relate to nutrition and health services	• Has strong familiarity with federal nutrition and health programs • Understands the system used to develop legislation, regulation, and public policy and to appropriate funding • Explains legislation accurately to consumers and other professionals • Is able to participate actively in support of nutrition related legislation • Understands how policies can be designed to support nutrition and health related programs	• Visit federal government nutrition and health Websites • Review organizational charts at federal, state, and local levels • Access educational resources on how to deal effectively with legislators • Identify where authority lies for nutrition and food programs at Federal, State and local levels • Observe a committee meeting in state legislature • Read and write comments on proposed nutrition-related regulations from the Federal Register • Attend a Board of Health meeting • Track a bill through passage to implementation • Identify specific agency activities that support Healthy People 2010 objectives • Review regulations of food and nutrition programs available in agency, e.g., WIC, Food Stamps • Identify policies that support or promote improved nutrition and regular physical activity	• USDA Food and Nutrition Services: www.fns.usda.gov/fns/ • USDHHS Maternal and Child Health Bureau: www.mchdata.net • *Guidelines for Comprehensive Programs to Promote Healthy Eating and Physical Activity*: www.astphnd.org/programs/00Nupawgfm.pdf • Legislative newsletters • American Dietetic Association's Policy Initiatives and Advocacy Web page: www.eatright.com/gov/ • Federal Register www.gpo.gov • National Conference of State Legislatures: www.ncsl.org • State or local personnel manual • *Nutrition and the Community.* A Owen, P Splett, and G Owen. Boston, McGraw Hill, 1999. • *Healthy People 2010: Understanding and Improving Health.* 2nd ed. USDHHS. Washington, DC: U.S. Government Printing Office, November 2000. www.health.gov/healthypeople • League of Women Voters Organization www.lwv.org/

8. Participates in organized advocacy efforts for health and nutrition programs

- Understands agency advocacy policy
- Is familiar with strategies to influence the awareness and thinking of public stakeholders and policy makers
- Is able to identify advocacy opportunities and initiate action
- Knows basic food and nutrition issues and their impact on nutrition programming, as well as impact of physical activity on nutritional status

- Participate in an activity (forum, telephone tree, letter writing campaign) for individuals or groups to bring issues to the public for support and influence legislative and public policy, for example, breastfeeding support through public assistance programs
- Assess agency and community for nutrition advocacy opportunities
- Develop talking points on a selected topic area

- Local social and welfare agencies and advocacy groups
- Nutrition Week, Community Nutrition Institute Newsletter, Consumer Reports
- Legislative newsletter, American Dietetic Association: www.eatright.org
- *National Conference of State Legislators:* www.ncsl.org
- *Increasing Physical Activity: A Report on Recommendations of the Task Force on Community Preventive Services:* www.cdc.gov/mmwr/preview/mmwrhtml/rr5018a1.htm
- *Bright Futures in Practice: Physical Activity,* National Center for Education in Maternal and Child Health: www.brightfutures.org/physicalactivity/pdf/index.html
- *The Community Tool Box.* University of Kansas: http://ctb.lsi.ukans.edu/
- Food Research and Action Center: www.frac.org
- Bread for the World: www.bread.org
- Center for Science in the Public Interest: www.cspinet.org

Training Topic Area	Example Target Behaviors	Suggested Work-Related & Learning Activities	Example Resources
9. Understands political and ethical considerations within and across organizations and their impact on agency planning, policy, and decision-making	• Understands the development and/or policy approval process • Understands types of skills to influence policy • Able to develop or assist in developing nutrition policy • Understands the consequences of policy actions at the individual, family, and community levels	• Identify key player(s) responsible for agency/program planning • Review agency policy manual • Assess political milieu of organizational structure • Attend political briefing in agency • Attend community coalition meeting • Interview agency staff responsible for involving community in planning, policy and needs assessment • Apply a model like the Socio-Ecological Framework to a program decision	• Organizational charts • Agency and program plans • Agency policy manuals • *Nutrition and the Community*. A Owen, P Splett, and G Owen, Boston, McGraw Hill, 1999. • *Community Tool Box*. University of Kansas: ctb.lsi.ukans.edu • *Moving to the Future: Developing Community-Based Nutrition Services* (Workbook and Training Manual). KL Probert, ed. Washington, DC. Association of State and Territorial Public Health Nutrition Directors. 1997. Order from www.astphnd.org • American Public Health Association—Code of ethics: http://apha.org • American Dietetic Association—Code of ethics: www.eatright.org

10. Knows management principles for effective community assessment, program planning, implementation, and evaluation and applies them to community-based public health nutrition programs

- Applies effective management principles in the implementation of community-based public health nutrition program
- Demonstrates the importance of obtaining and utilizing customer/community input and feedback in the assets mapping and needs assessment processes

- Identify short and long term priorities in the management process
- Participate in annual or other short-range planning as well as strategic planning that utilizes surveillance data for decision making
- Observe and interview various individuals involved in the planning process, including agency and community representatives
- Compile information on the community food, nutrition and health programs
- Identify criteria for implementing a Continuous Quality Improvement plan for the local agency and/or community
- Define customer service and identify examples in community based public health nutrition programs

- Interdisciplinary team members
- Community-based programs
- Resources on effective management strategies, e.g., Total Quality Management, Continuous Quality Improvement
- Local newspapers
- Community Needs Assessment Guides
- County profile data
- State profiles—DHHS Bureau of Maternal and Child Health: www.mchdata.net/Reports_Graphs/summenu.htm
- CDC Surveillance Systems: www.cdc.gov/nccdphp/dnpa/surveill.htm
- *Building Communities from the Inside Out.* JP Kretchmann and JL McKnight. Chicago: Northwestern University; 1993.
- *Mobilizing for Action through Planning and Partnership* (MAPP). National Org of City & County Health Officials: http://mapp.naccho.org/MAPP_Home.asp
- *Healthy People 2010 Toolkit:* www.health.gov/healthypeople/state/toolkit/default.htm

Training Topic Area Continued	Example Target Behaviors	Suggested Work-Related & Learning Activities	Example Resources
10, *continued* Knows management principles for effective community assessment, program planning, implementation, and evaluation and applies them to community-based public health nutrition programs		• Participate in a community-based planning process that includes assets mapping, needs assessment, and establishing community priorities • Conduct a simple cost analysis of a nutrition service • Develop an evaluation plan for a community program based on Framework for Program Evaluation in Public Health • Observe meeting of a local health council and interview members	• *Framework for Program Evaluation in Public Health.* Centers for Disease Control and Prevention. MMWR Sept 17, 1999/ Vol 48 No RR11;1 www.cdc.gov/eval/framework.htm or www.cdc.gov/mmwr/preview/mmwrhtml/rr4811a1.htm or http://search.cdc.gov/search97cgi/s97is.dll • *Cost-Effectiveness Analysis for the Real World.* A Ellis, M Green, B Haughton. http://nutrition.he.utk.edu/cea • *Costing Nutrition Services: A workbook.* Splett P, Caldwell M; 1985. • *Moving to the Future: Developing Community-Based Nutrition Services.* KL Probert, ed. Washington, DC: Association of State and Territorial Public Health Nutrition Directors; 1996. • *Maximizing Resources for Results! Extending Bright Futures Through Community-Based Nutrition Planning.* S Gregory; 2001. http://nutrition.he.utk.edu/max_resources/maximize/ • *A Program Evaluation Tool Kit: Excerpt—Program Logic Model.* The Community Health Research Unit, University of Ottawa. www.uottawa.ca/academic/med/epid/excerpt.htm • *Nutrition and the Community.* A Owen, P Splett, and G Owen. Boston, McGraw Hill, 1999.

11. Knows how nutrition services are integrated into overall mission, goals, and plan of the health agency

- Participate in developing mission, vision, and goal statement for nutrition unit that are consistent with the organization
- Compares nutrition plan with agency plan
- Understands nutrition's role, mission and goals in agency

- Review the mission, vision statement and goals of the health agency
- Compare the mission, vision, and goals statement of nutrition services or programs to the agency goals
- Assess integration of nutrition in various programs within the agency

- Strategic plans from state agency, health departments, and nutrition programs
- Workshops on planning, including development of mission statements, vision statements, and goals
- Written materials on planning
- *Guidelines for Comprehensive Programs to Promote Healthy Eating and Physical Activity:* www.astphnd.org/programs/00Nupawgfm.pdf

Training Topic Area	Example Target Behaviors	Suggested Work-Related & Learning Activities	Example Resources
12. Understands resource management, including grant application, identifying funding sources, and reading fiscal reports	• Demonstrates ability to apply several financial management principles • Knows potential funding sources	• Read a financial statement • Interview a program development manager to investigate resource management • List potential funding sources for nutrition programs • Assist with writing a grant application • Participate in reviewing grant applications • Complete a sample program budget	• Agency's grants, financial statements • Federal Register • Foundations Directory • University faculty and their respective research offices • *Program Planning and Proposal Writing*. Expanded Version. NJ Kiritz. Los Angeles: Grantsmanship Center; 1980. • Nutrition.gov 'Funding Agency' Web page: www.nutrition.gov/framesets/ frameset.php3?topic=resources&subtopic=funding%20agencies • Nutrition.gov 'Grant Opportunities' Web page: www.nutrition.gov/framesets/ frameset.php3?topic=research&subtopic=grant%20opportunities • Food Stamp Nutrition Education Grants: www.nal.usda.gov/foodstamp/program_facts.html#grants • Team Nutrition Training Grants: www.fns.usda.gov/tn/Grants/index.htm • Seniors Farmers' Market Nutrition Program (SFMNP) grants: www.fns.usda.gov/wic/CONTENT/SFMNP/SFMNP menu.htm • Fundraising and Grant Writing Resources www.fundsnetservices.com/grantwri.htm • The Grantsmanship Center: www.tgci.com/

13. Knows the principles of personnel management, including recruiting, staffing, supervising, performance appraisal, staff development, and conflict resolution	• Understands the relationships between positions in a unit or agency	• Draw an organizational chart	• Administrative manual
	• Knows the components of a job description	• Write a job description	• Performance expectations used by agency/organization
		• Participate in an interview of nutrition staff candidate	• *Self-Assessment Tool for Public Health Nutritionists.* Public Health Nutrition Practice Group of the American Dietetic Association; 1988.
		• Develop sample interview questions for a position	
	• Writes and conducts performance appraisals with subordinates	• Review criteria for and role-play a performance appraisal	• *Personnel in Public Health Nutrition for the 1990s.* J Dodds, M Kaufman. Washington, DC: The Public Health Foundation; 1991.
	• Is knowledgeable about training	• Develop a training plan for growth and development of subordinates	• Current performance appraisal form used by agency/organization
	• Understands Affirmative Action and organization's corrective disciplinary procedures	• Develop staff in-service program using a presentation software program, such as Microsoft PowerPoint, based on documented training needs	• Agency's Affirmative Action Plan
		• Assess own public health & community nutrition training needs and develop own plan for professional development	• *First Things First: To Live, To Love, To Learn, To Leave a Legacy.* SR Covey, AR Merrill, RR Merrill. New York: Simon and Schuster; 1994.
	• Demonstrates one or more conflict resolution techniques	• Read Affirmative Action plans of agency	• *The Seven Habits of Highly Effective People.* SR Covey. New York: Simon and Schuster; 1989.
		• Attend conflict resolution workshops	• *SSNAPS.* J Dodds. Chapel Hill, NC: University of North Carolina-School of Public Health; 1996.
		• Identify and bring a conflict to surface, and work toward insight resolution	• *Difficult Conversations. How to Discuss What Matters Most.* D Stone, B Patton, S Heen. New York: Penguin Books; 1999.
			• *Nutrition and the Community.* A Owen, P Splett, and G Owen. Boston, McGraw Hill, 1999.

Training Topic Area	Example Target Behaviors	Suggested Work-Related & Learning Activities	Example Resources

14. Understands descriptive statistics, principles of data collection and management, monitoring and surveillance reports, and basic computer applications for data compilation and analysis	• Identifies and prioritizes nutritional problems of various age and population groups
	
	• Understands how data are used in developing program plans
	
	• Evaluates quality of data
	
	• Understands basic descriptive statistics
		• Interview statistics and/or epidemiology personnel at a local and a state health agency
		
		• Review published morbidity and mortality data; identify areas that have nutrition components
		
		• Design and implement a simple survey; conduct analysis of the data
		
		• Devise a systematic data collection process in routine nutrition services
		
		• Review surveillance data, e.g., Pediatric and Pregnancy, Behavioral Risk Factors Surveillance System (BRFSS), National Health and Nutrition Examination Survey (NHANES), Cancer, etc.
		
		• Use online resources from related sites to determine national and state health issues
		
		• Complete online training modules on basic statistics
			• Short courses in biostatistics
			
			• *Morbidity and Mortality Weekly Reports*: www.cdc.gov/mmwr
			
			• County profile data
			
			• WIC participant and program data
			
			• Breastfeeding data
			
			• Epi-info 2000: www.cdc.gov/epiinfo/
			
			• Data sets of various groups
			
			  – Community Childhood Hunger Identification Project: www.frac.org/html/publications/pubs.html
			
			  – National Health and Nutrition Examination Survey: www.cdc.gov/nchs/nhanes
			
			  – Continuing Survey of Food Intakes by Individuals: www.barc.usda.gov/bhnrc/foodsurvey/Cd98.html
			
			• Online data training modules: www.sph.unc.edu/toolbox/
			
			• CDC Surveillance Systems: www.cdc.gov/nccdphp/dnpa/surveill.htm
			
			  – Behavioral Risk Factor Surveillance System
			
			  – Youth Risk Behavior Surveillance System
			
			  – Pediatric Nutrition Surveillance System
			
			  – Pregnancy Nutrition Surveillance System
			
			• Title V Information System: www.mchdata.net

15. Knows the principles of an epidemiologic approach to assess the health and nutrition problems and trends in the community	• Understands basic epidemiologic concepts and processes • Assesses nutritional risks of a specific population group	• Review existing epidemiologic data from the community • Complete a literature review of nutrition risk factors (i.e., obesity) within a selected population group • Identify major nutrition problems of selected risk groups in the population served • Interview an epidemiologist • Conduct a case study on an outbreak of food borne illness	• Centers for Disease Control and Prevention: www.cdc.gov • University of North Carolina online training modules: www.sph.unc.edu/toolbox/ • CDC WONDER: http://wonder.cdc.gov • Epi-Info 2000: www.cdc.gov/epiinfo/ • National Center for Health statistics (NCHS): www.cdc.gov/nchs • State and local health departments (use online resources) • Prevalence of Overweight among Children and Adolescents: United States, 1999. National Center for Health Statistics, Centers for Disease Control and Prevention, 2001. www.cdc.gov/nchs/products/pubs/pubd/hestats/overwght99.htm

Training Topic Area	Example Target Behaviors	Suggested Work-Related & Learning Activities	Example Resources
16. Knows principles of research and evaluation	• Critiques research (outcomes evaluation) projects in an applied setting, e.g.: – case studies – chart/record review – analysis of surveillance or other data – research designs • Has knowledge of the purposes of and differences between research and evaluation • Assesses how to incorporate a new research article into an existing body of evidence	• Compare and contrast several published research findings – Examine study methodology and strengths and weaknesses of research • Review available or potential resources of data: – surveillance – written records – local and state prevalence data – morbidity and mortality data • Select a program or project to evaluate. Develop a statement clarifying the purpose of the evaluation and the evaluation questions • Review an evidence-based prevention guideline (eg, obesity, hyperlipidemia from U.S. Preventive Services Task Force • Evaluate one new research article related to the evidencebased guideline reviewed	• Published research articles • Food and Nutrition Information Center, National Agriculture Library: www.nal.usda.gov/fnic • *Research: Successful Approaches.* E Monsen, ed. Chicago, IL: American Dietetic Association; 1003. • *Costing Nutrition Services: A Workbook.* Splett P, Caldwell M. 1985. • *Framework for Program Evaluation in Public Health.* Centers for Disease Control and Prevention. MMWR 1999; 48(No. RR-11). www.cdc.gov/mmwr/PDF/rr/rr4811.pdf • *Cost-Effectiveness Analysis for the Real World.* A Ellis, M Green, B Haughton. http://nutrition.he.utk.edu/cea • Myers EF, Pritchett E, Johnson EQ. Evidence-based practice guides vs. protocols: What's the difference? *J Am Diet Assoc* 2001;101:1085–1090.

17. Knows relationships of the environment to public health, risk assessment, and biological, physical, and chemical factors that effect the nutritional status of the public

- Knows state and local environmental issues and notes argument pros and cons
- Discusses and evaluates issues based on current scientific knowledge
- Understands the types of preventive measures and plans that can be implemented to increase preparedness in the event of emergency or natural disaster

- Meet with staff who work on environmental issues
- Read case studies of environmental topics
- Read case studies in the following areas:
  - Physical—natural disaster, sanitation, E coli outbreak
  - Biological/Biotechnical— genetically engineered foods, bovine growth hormone, food safety and bioterrorism
  - Chemical—food additives such as BHT or guar gums
- Prepare a press release on a chemical food additive, e.g., BHT or guar gums, for a community-based publication

- Epi-Info 2000: www.cdc.gov/epiinfo
- CDC WONDER: http://wonder.cdc.gov
- Food Safety Website: http://foodsafety.gov
- State and local health departments
- Public Health Emergency Preparedness and Response: www.bt.cdc.gov/
- Biological Incidents: Health and Human Services Preparedness and Response: Department of Health and Human Services www.hhs.gov/hottopics/healing/biologi cal.html

Training Topic Area	Example Target Behaviors	Suggested Work-Related & Learning Activities	Example Resources
18. Knows processes of monitoring, technical assistance, guidance, consultation, and collaboration within and across agencies and organizations	• Knows appropriate situations to use monitoring, technical assistance, guidance, consultation, and collaboration • Determines appropriate action in response to nutrition consultation	• Define and compare monitoring, technical assistance, guidance, consultation, and collaboration processes • Observe and interview nutritionist in community carrying out these tasks • Read selected materials on these processes • Read a written report and provide response to a nutrition consultation on a public health project/program • Participate in a community intervention project, collaborating with other agencies	• *The Competitive Edge.* KK Helm, JC Rose. Chicago, IL: American Dietetic Association; In Print, 2002. • *Nutrition in the Community: the Art and Science of Delivering Services* 4th edition by A Owen, P Splett and G Owen, 1999. McGraw-Hill Publishers, Boston. • *Flawless Consulting.* P Block. San Francisco, Jossey-Bass Pfeiffer, 2000. • *Coordination Strategies Handbook: A Guide for WIC and Primary Care Professionals.* Washington, DC: U.S. Department of Agriculture, Food and Nutrition Service; 2000. • *Consulting on the Inside.* B Scott. American Society for Training and Development, Alexandria, VA, 2000. www.astd.org

19. Selects and appropriately uses group process and group facilitation techniques (brainstorming, focus groups, nominal group process) to achieve goals and objectives of food and nutrition programs and services	• Successfully demonstrates knowledge of group process and group facilitation techniques	• Observe individuals using specific techniques
		• Complete a project using selected techniques
		• Complete online module on qualitative methods
			• Articles and text on Nominal Group Process, Focus Groups
			• *Focus Groups: A Practical Guide for Applied Research.* RA Krueger. Thousand Oaks, CA: Sage Publications; 1994.
			• Qualitative methods:
			  – www.worldbank.org/poverty/impact/methods /qualita.htm
			  – www.sph.unc.edu/toolbox/
			• *The Skilled Facilitator: Practical Wisdom for Developing Effective Groups.* R Schwarz. San Francisco, CA: Jossey-Bass Inc. 1994.
			• *Essential Manager's Manual.* R Heller, T Hindle, London, England: Dorling Kindersley. 1998.

Training Topic Area	Example Target Behaviors	Suggested Work-Related & Learning Activities	Example Resources

20. Is familiar with the role and operation of agency and/or community boards, committees, task forces, coalitions, and partnerships in public health	• Understands role and importance of coalitions in public health nutrition programming
	
	• Describes techniques for successful networking or coalition building
	
	• Lists allies that might be mobilized around key food and nutrition issues
		• Attend a wide variety of political, community and professional meetings, conferences, and social events,
		  – Maternal and Child Health Conference,
		  – Healthy Mothers Healthy Babies,
		  – hunger groups,
		  – breastfeeding coalition, etc.
		• Provide written or verbal analysis of various community coalitions
		• Develop and present a nutrition related program to a board, task force, or community agency committee
			• Human and Nutrition Service directories
			• Advocacy groups, e.g., Food Research and Action Center: www.frac.org; Children's Defense Fund: www.childrensdefense.org
			• *Healthy Communities. New Partnerships for the Future of Public Health.* Executive Summary. Committee on Public Health, Institute of Medicine. Washington, DC: National Academy Press; 1996.
			• *The Community Tool Box.* University of Kansas. http://ctb.lsi.ukans.edu/
			• *A Manual for Building Local Leadership for Community Nutritional Health.* M. Crave, 1996. University of Wisconsin-Extension-Family Living Program
			• *Healthy People 2010 Toolkit: A Field Guide to Health Planning.* www.health.gov/healthypeople/state/toolkit/default.htm
			• *Moving to the Future: Developing Community-Based Nutrition Services* (Workbook and Training Manual). KL Probert, ed. Washington, DC. Association of State and Territorial Public Health Nutrition Directors. 1997. Order from www.astphnd.org

21. Develops skills in functioning as a multidisciplinary and interdisciplinary team member or leader within and across disciplines	• Understands how nutrition services are integrated into comprehensive health and social services • Recognizes importance and value of areas of public health, community, and society outside of nutrition • Understands role of case manager and paraprofessionals in coordination and collaboration	• Assess and analyze agency to identify multidisciplinary program and approaches to delivery of services • Participate in team assessments/case conferences with other health care providers, the client/patient, and family members • Interview members of team, including paraprofessionals; write a description of roles and responsibilities • Provide appropriate client referrals to other team members and other health care and social service agencies • Conduct an in-service for other members of the health care team • Participate in/lead team building within and across disciplines	• Other members of health care team • Professional organizations with which other team members are affiliated • *Personnel in Public Health Nutrition for the 1990s.* JM Dodds, M Kaufman. Washington, DC: The Public Health Foundation; 1991. • Comprehensive Nutrition and Physical Activity: www.astphnd.org and www.astphnd.org/programs/00Nupawgfm.pdf • *Coordination Strategies Handbook: A Guide for WIC and Primary Care Professionals.* Washington, DC: U.S. Department of Agriculture, Food and Nutrition Service; 2000. • *WIC and Head Start, Partners in Promoting Health and Nutrition for Young Children and Families.* USDA, USDHHS, October 1999.

Training Topic Area	Example Target Behaviors	Suggested Work-Related & Learning Activities	Example Resources
22. Knows and applies skills in selecting and/or developing nutrition education materials and approaches appropriate for individuals or small groups within the target population	• Accesses research-based, field-tested nutrition education materials • Selects and develops nutrition education materials appropriate for the target population • Successfully utilizes a variety of communication techniques, e.g., interviewing, counseling, presenting an educational session • Utilizes a variety of current technologies in materials development and presentations • Understands the different roles & responsibilities of public health nutrition personnel based on educational preparation & credentials	• Evaluate appropriateness of education materials to client's culture, diagnoses and family needs • Evaluate agency's nutrition education materials using standard criteria • Develop and implement nutrition education program for clients/patients to include strategy, materials development, field testing, and evaluation • Determine the appropriate literacy level for the population and how to determine level • Participate in training on adult learning theory • Use presentation software program such as Microsoft Power Point, to develop a presentation to individuals and families • Use desktop publishing software to update or create a nutrition pamphlet or publication for a target population • Evaluate the reading level of a client education material	• Food and Nutrition Information Center: www.nal.usda.gov/fnic • Client education materials • Computer programs to evaluate literacy level • *Teaching patients with Low Literacy Skills.* CC Doak, LG Doak, JH Root. Philadelphia: JP Lippincott Company; 1996. • *Evaluating Nutrition Education Materials.* Bureau of Nutrition & WIC, Iowa Department of Public Health. www.nal.usda.gov/wicworks/Sharing_Center/RQNS/rqns_15.pdf • *Diversity Rx:* Promoting language and cultural competence in healthcare: www.diversityrx.org • *Writing and Designing Print Materials for Beneficiaries: A Guide for State Medicaid Agencies.* DHHS. Oct 1999, HCFA Pub # 10145. • *Clear & Simple,* National Institutes of Health, Publication #95–3594. • *The Provider's Guide to Quality and Culture.* Management Sciences for Health: http://erc.msh.org/quality&culture

22, *continued*
Knows and applies skills in selecting and/or developing nutrition education materials and approaches appropriate for individuals or small groups within the target population

- Accesses research-based, field-tested nutrition education materials
- Selects and develops nutrition education materials appropriate for the target population
- Successfully utilizes a variety of communication techniques, e.g., interviewing, counseling, presenting an educational session
- Utilizes a variety of current technologies in materials development and presentations
- Understands the different roles & responsibilities of public health nutrition personnel based on educational preparation & credentials

- Evaluate appropriateness of education materials to client's culture, diagnoses and family needs
- Evaluate agency's nutrition education materials using standard criteria
- Develop and implement nutrition education program for clients/patients to include strategy, materials development, field testing, and evaluation
- Determine the appropriate literacy level for the population and how to determine level
- Participate in training on adult learning theory
- Use presentation software program such as Microsoft Power Point, to develop a presentation to individuals and families
- Use desktop publishing software to update or create a nutrition pamphlet or publication for a target population
- Evaluate the reading level of a client education material

- Food and Nutrition Information Center: www.nal.usda.gov/fnic
- Client education materials
- Computer programs to evaluate literacy level
- *Teaching patients with Low Literacy Skills.* CC Doak, LG Doak, JH Root. Philadelphia: JP Lippincott Company; 1996.
- *Evaluating Nutrition Education Materials.* Bureau of Nutrition & WIC, Iowa Department of Public Health. www.nal.usda.gov/wicworks/Sharing_Center/RQNS/rqns_15.pdf
- *Diversity Rx:* Promoting language and cultural competence in healthcare: www.diversityrx.org
- *Writing and Designing Print Materials for Beneficiaries: A Guide for State Medicaid Agencies.* DHHS. Oct 1999, HCFA Pub # 10145.
- *Clear & Simple,* National Institutes of Health, Publication #95–3594.
- *The Provider's Guide to Quality and Culture.* Management Sciences for Health: http://erc.msh.org/quality&culture

Training Topic Area	Example Target Behaviors	Suggested Work-Related & Learning Activities	Example Resources
23. Effects behavior change through knowledge and application of behavioral, social, and education theories	• Applies effective counseling and group facilitation techniques • Uses appropriate instructional and learning theories in nutrition education • Demonstrates knowledge of psychosocial theories of health behavior and their application to eating behavior • Uses appropriate theories of cognitive, social, and emotional development in nutrition education • Applies appropriate theories and techniques from the behavioral sciences for modifying behavior such as: • attitude-change theories • persuasive communication concepts • social learning and other cognitive-behavioral theories • behavior modification techniques • concepts of social marketing • client-centered strategies	• Use a counseling checklist while observing a counselor • Observe and critique a nutrition education session • Videotape a nutrition education session or case study; evaluate counseling and identify positive and negative aspects • Practice/ explore alternate interviewing approaches, such as motivational interviewing • Assess the education needs of a target population using appropriate methodologies, e.g., focus groups, interviewsurveys • Review methodologies for assessing education needs of a population • Review social behavior theories: Health Belief Model, Stages of Change, Social Marketing, Precede-Proceed, Diffusion Theory	• Counseling guidelines • Workshops on marketing and education • *Nutrition Centered Counseling Skills for Medical Nutrition Therapy.* LG Snetsalaar. MD Gaithersburg. Aspen Publishers, Inc; 1997. • *A Handbook for Developing Multicultural Awareness.* P Pedersen. Alexandria, VA: American Counseling Association; 2000. • *How to make nutrition education more meaningful through facilitated group discussion.* R Abusabha, J Peacock, C Achterberg. J Am Diet Assoc. 1999;99:72–76. • *Health Behavior and Health Education: Theory, Research and Practice.* 3rd Ed. K Glanz, FM Lewis, BK Rimer (Eds). San Francisco: Jossey Bass Publishers; 2002. • *Celebrating Diversity: Approaching Families Through Their Food.* DC Bliades, CW Suitor. Arlington, VA: National Center for Education in Maternal and Child Health; 1994. • WIC Works Resource System: www.nal.usda.gov/wicworks • Motivational interviewing videotapes: www.motivationalinterview.org/training/videos. html

23, *continued*
Effects behavior change through knowledge and application of behavioral, social, and education theories

- Assesses current marketing strategies to develop education programs for targeted audiences
- Uses culturally appropriate education strategies
- Discusses social behavior theories in relation to public health nutrition interventions

Training Topic Area	Example Target Behaviors	Suggested Work-Related & Learning Activities	Example Resources
24. Communicates accurate, scientifically based information—both oral and written—at levels appropriate for various audiences: clients, general public	• Identifies accurate, scientifically based nutrition information and incorporates content into nutrition education strategies • Selects and develops effective strategies to best communicate message to the target population	• Research and write a nutrition article/communiqué on a selected nutrition issue • Assess appropriate literacy and cultural preferences • Develop a press release • Assist a public health nutritionist in planning and presenting a series of family-centered nutrition classes for parents of young children in a local community • Develop and present an education session to target audience	• Case studies • Food Guide Pyramid: www.usda.gov/cnpp/pyramid2.htm • Media tapes • *Making Health Communication Programs Work: A Planner's Guide.* U.S. Department of Health and Human Services, Public Health Service, National Institutes of Health. NIH Publication #92–1493; 1992. https://cissecure.nci.nih.gov/ncipubs/details.asp?pid=209 • *Communicating as Professionals.* R Chernoff, ed. Chicago, IL: American Dietetic Association; 2nd ed., 1994. • International Food Information Council: www.ific.org • CDCynergy: www.cdc.gov/cdcynergy/ • National Council Against Health Fraud: www.ncahf.org

25. Uses media strategies in various print, broadcasting, and telecommunications channels, such as video and the Internet, to reach population groups

- Demonstrates ability to identify media strategies appropriate to target population groups
- Utilizes effective media strategies to reach target population

- Participate in various public education campaigns that emphasize community health promotion and disease prevention, e.g., breastfeeding promotion, 5-A-Day for Better Health, food labeling, etc.
- Describe the key points or objectives for a promotional topic and three facts you want the public to remember
- Practice a media interview with the American Dietetic Association's state media representative and videotape for critique

- Public relations firms
- *Healthy People 2010: Understanding and Improving Health.* 2nd ed. USDHHS. Washington, DC: U.S. Government Printing Office, November 2000. www.health.gov/healthypeople
- *Introduction to Media Relations.* ASTPHO and Public Health Foundation www.trainingfinder.org/search.cgi?action=view_course&course_id=10920
- *Media Advocacy and Public Health: Power for Prevention.* L Wallack, L Dorfman, D Jernigan, M Themba. Newbury Park: Sage Publications; 1993.

Additional References

Documents and Web sites considered pertinent to the Guidelines are cited below. Please note that some of the documents are currently being revised and are updated continually. Therefore, the reader is encouraged to seek revised publications when available. Particularly, *Moving to the Future* is in revision by the Association of State and Territorial Public Health Nutrition Directors (ASTPHND), as is *The Competitive Edge* by the American Dietetic Association. The Institute of Medicine will soon release *Assuring the Health of the Public in the 21st Century*, which will replace *The Future of Public Health*.

Coalitions and Partnerships

Berkowitz B. "Collaboration for Health Improvement: Models for State, Community, and Academic Partnerships." *Journal of Public Health Management and Practice.* 2000;6:67–72.

Fawcett SB, Francisco VT, Paine-Andrews A, Schultz JA. "A model memorandum of collaboration: a proposal." *Public Health Reports.* 2000;115:174–9.

Green L, Daniel M, Novick L. "Partnerships and Coalitions for Community-Based Research." *Public Health Reports.* 2001;116:20S1–31S1.

Holmes M. *Promising Partnerships: How To Develop Successful Partnerships in Your Community.* Alexandria, VA. National Head Start Association; 1996.

Linial G. "Effective Coalition Building" *Healthcare Executive.* 1995;10:45.

Nelson JC, Raskind-Hood C, Galvin VG; Essein JD, Levine LM. "Positioning for Partnerships. Assessing Public Health Readiness." *American Journal of Preventive Medicine.* 1999;16:103S-17S.

Parker EA, Eng E, Laraia B, Ammerman A, Dodds J, Margolis L, Cross A. "Coalition building for prevention: lessons learned from the North Carolina Community-Based Public Health Initiative." *Journal of Public Health Management and Practice.* 1998;4:25–36.

Roussos ST, Fawcett SB. "A Review of Collaborative Partnerships as a Strategy for Improving Community Health." *Annual Review of Public Health.* 2000;21:369–402.

Wilson JL. "Leadership Development: Working Together to Enhance Collaboration." *Journal of Public Health Management and Practice.* 2002;8:21–6.

Wolff T. "The Future of Community Coalition Building." *American Journal of Community Psychology.* 2001;29:263–8.

Ethics

Callahan D, Jennings B. "Ethics and Public Health: Forging a Strong Relationship." *American Journal of Public Health.* 2002;92:169–76.

Childress JF, Faden RR, Gaare RD, Gostin LO, et al. "Public Health Ethics: Mapping the Terrain" *Journal of Law, Medicine and Ethics.* 2002;30:170–178.

Fornari A. "Approaches to Ethical Decision Making." *J Am Diet Assoc.* 2002;102:865–6.

Kass NE. "An Ethics Framework for Public Health." *American Journal of Public Health.* 2001;91:1776–82.

Roberts MJ, Reich MR. "Ethical Analysis in Public Health." *Lancet.* 2002;359:1055–9.

Thomas JC, Sage M, Dillenberg J, Guillory VJ. "A Code of Ethics for Public Health." *American Journal of Public Health.* 2002;92:1057–9.

Nutrition Education in Public Health

Armitage CJ, Conner M. "Reducing Fat Intake: Interventions Based on the Theory of Planned Behaviour." *Changing Health Behavior: Intervention and Research with Social Cognition Models.* Philadelphia; 2002:87–104.

Black DR, Blue CL, Coster DC. "Using Social Marketing to Develop and Test Tailored Health Messages." *American Journal of Health Behavior.* 2001;25:260–71.

Breastfeeding Promotion and Support: www.nal.usda.gov/wicworks/ Learning_Center/Breastfeeding.html

Donovan RJ. "Steps in planning and developing health communication campaigns: A comment on CDC's framework for health communication." *Public Health Reports.* 1995;110:215–7.

Dooley D, Soll L. "Scripting Public Service Announcements for Radio." *Journal of Nutrition Education.* 1999;31:239–240.

Fu S, Fancher M, Snyder D. "Mass Media and National Communications." *5 A Day For Better Health Program.* Bethesda, MD: National Institutes of Health, National Cancer Institute; 2001:83–98. Available at: www.5aDay.gov

Institute of Medicine, Committee on Health and Behavior: Research, Practice and Policy, Board on Neuroscience and Behavioral Health. *Health and Behavior: The Interplay of Biological, Behavioral, and Societal Influences*; National Academy Press, Washington, DC; 2001.

Kristal AR, Glanz K, Curry SJ, Patterson RE. "How Can Stages of Change Be Best Used in Dietary Interventions?" *J Am Diet Assoc.* 1999;99;679–84.

National Center for Education in Maternal and Child Health. Bright Futures in Practice: *Nutrition.* Available at: www.brightfutures.org/

National Center for Education in Maternal and Child Health. *Bright Futures in Practice: Physical Activity.* Available at: www.brightfutures.org/ physicalactivity/pdf/index.html

Schwarzer R, Renner B. "Social-Cognitive Predictors of Health Behavior: Action Self- Efficacy and Coping Self-Efficacy." *Health Psychology.* 2000;19:487–495.

Slater MD. "Integrating application of media effects, persuasion, and behavior change theories to communication campaigns: A stages-of-change framework." *Health Communication.* 1999;11:335–354.

Smedley BD, Syme SL, (Eds). Institute of Medicine, Committee on Capitalizing on Social Science and Behavioral Research to Improve the Public's Health, Division of Health Promotion and Disease Prevention. *Promoting Health: Intervention Strategies from Social and Behavioral Research.* Washington, DC: National Academy Press; 2000.

USDA Infant Nutrition: www.nal.usda.gov/wicworks/Topics/Infant_Nutrition.html

USDA Online Nutrition Education Materials
 Educator Materials
  www.fns.usda.gov/tn/Educators/index.htm
  www.nal.usda.gov/fnic/pubs/bibs/gen/ethnic.html
 Materials for All Audiences
  www.fns.usda.gov/tn/Resources/index.htm
 Native American Materials
  www.fns.usda.gov/fdd/programs/fdpir/fdpir_pubs.htm
 Parent Materials
  www.fns.usda.gov/tn/Parents/index.htm
 Spanish Materials
  www.fns.usda.gov/tn/Resources/index.htm
 Student Materials
  www.fns.usda.gov/tn/Students/index.htm

USDA Nutrition Education Research and Studies: www.fns.usda.gov/oane/MENU/Published/nutritioneducation/nutritioneducation.htm

USDA Report to Congress: "Nutrition Education in FNS: A Coordinated Approach for Promoting Healthy Behaviors." Available at: www.fns.usda.gov/oane/menu/published/nutritioneducation/Files/CongressNutEd(2-2002).pdf

USDA Team Nutrition: www.fns.usda.gov/tn/

Wallack L, Dorfman L, Jernigan D, Themba M. *Media Advocacy and Public Health: Power for Prevention.* Newbury Park: Sage Publications; 1993.

Public Health and Public Health Training and Practice

American Dietetic Association Website: www.eatright.org

Association of Graduate Programs in Public Health Nutrition, Inc: http://nutrition.he.utk.edu/AGPPHN/mission.htm

Association of Schools of Public Health: www.asph.org

Bruening KS, Mitchell BE, Pfeiffer MM. "2002 Accreditation Standards for Dietetics Education." *J Am Diet Assoc.* 2002;102:566–77.

Centers for Disease Control and Prevention, 2000 CDC Growth Charts: www.cdc.gov/growthcharts

Centers for Disease Control and Prevention. CDCynergy. Available at: www.cdc.gov/cdcynergy/

Child Care Nutrition Resource System: www.nal.usda.gov/childcare/index.html

Dodds JM, Kaufman M. *Personnel in Public Health Nutrition for the 1990s.* Washington, DC: The Public health Foundation; 1991.

Durch JS, Bailey LA, Stoto MA, Eds. Institute of Medicine, Committee on Using Performance Monitoring to Improve Community Health. *Improving Health in the Community: A Role for Performance Monitoring.* Washington, DC: National Academy Press; 1997.

Endres J (Ed) . *Strategies for Success: Curriculum Guide for Graduate Programs in Public Health Nutrition.* Carbondale, IL: Southern Illinois University in association with Association of the Faculties of Graduate Programs in Public Health Nutrition; 1990.

Federal Nutrition Programs Website: www.nutrition.gov

Harris-Davis E, Haughton B. "Model for Multicultural Nutrition Counseling Competencies." *J Am Diet Assoc*; 2000;100:1178–85.

Healthy School Meals Resource System: http://schoolmeals.nal.usda.gov/index.html

Hess AMN, Haughton B. "Continuing education needs for public health nutritionists." *J AmDiet Assoc.* 1996;96:716–718.

Institute of Medicine. *Assuring the Health of the Public in the 21st Century.* Washington, DC: National Academy Press; 2002. Available at: www.iom.edu/IOM/IOMHome.nsf/Pages/Assuring+the+Health+of+the+Public

Kim Y, Canfield A. "How to Develop a Service Learning Program in Dietetics Education." *J Am Diet Assoc.* 2002;102:174–6.

Olmstead-Schafer M, Story M, Haughton B. "Future training needs in public health nutrition: Results of a national Delphi survey." *J Am Diet Assoc.* 1996;96:282–3.

Probert KL, (Ed). *Moving to the Future: Developing Community-Based Nutrition Services* (Workbook and Training Manual). Washington, DC: Association of State and Territorial Public Health Nutrition Directors; 1997. Order from www.astphnd.org

Public Health/ Community Nutrition Practice Group of the American Dietetic Association. *Self-Assessment Tool for Public Health Nutritionists.* Chicago, IL: American Dietetic Association; 1988.

Public Health/Community Nutrition Practice Group of the American Dietetic Association Website: www.phcnpg.org

Ralston PA. "The MEMS Program: Increasing Minority Professionals in the Food and Nutritional Sciences." *J Am Diet Assoc.* 2000;100:1449–50.

Spangler AA, Spear B, Plavcan PA. "Dietetics Education by Distance: Current Endeavors in CAADE-Accredited/Approved Programs. *J Am Diet Assoc.* 1995;95:925–9.

Stevens RH. "Public Health Practice in Schools of Public Health: Is There a Fit?" *Journal of Public Health Management and Practice.* 2000;6:32–7.

Tufts University. Tufts Nutrition Navigator—A Guide to Rating Nutrition Web Sites. Available at: www.navigator.tufts.edu/

U.S. Department of Agriculture (USDA) and U.S. Department of Health and Human Services. *Dietary Guidelines for Americans.* 5th ed. USDA Home and Garden Bulletin No. 232. Washington, DC: USDA; 2000. Available at: www.usda.gov/cnpp/Pubs/DG2000/Index.htm or www.health.gov/dietaryguidelines/dga2000/dietgd.pdf

USDA Food and Nutrition Service. *WIC Nutrition Services Standards.* Available at: www.nal.usda.gov/wicworks/Learning_Center/WICnutStand.pdf

USDA Report to Congress: "A Decline in Food Stamp Participation." Available at: www.fns.usda.gov/oane/MENU/Published/FSP/FILES/Participation/PartDecline.htm

U.S. Department of Health and Human Services. *Healthy People 2010: Understanding and Improving Health.* 2nd ed. Washington, DC: U.S. Government Printing Office; November 2000. Available at: www.health.gov/healthypeople

WIC Works Resource System: www.nal.usda.gov/wicworks/index.html

Staffing, Recruitment, and Retention

Bryk JA, Kornblum T. "Report on the 1999 membership database of the American Dietetic Association." *J Am Diet Assoc.* 2001;101:947–53.

Chance KG, Green CG. "The Effect of Employee Job Satisfaction on Program Participation Rates in the Virginia WIC Program (Special Supplemental Nutrition Program for Women, Infants, and Children)." *Journal of Public Health Management and Practice.* 2001;7:10–20.

Dodds, JM, Kaufman, M. *Personnel in Public Health Nutrition for the 1990's.* Washington, DC: The Public Health Foundation; 1991.

Green CG, Harrison M, Henderson K, Lenihan A. "Total Quality Management in the Delivery of Public Health Services: a Focus on North Carolina WIC Programs." *Journal of Public Health Management and Practice.* 1998;4:72–81.

Greenwald HP, Davis RA. "Minority Recruitment and Retention in Dietetics: Issues and Interventions." *J Am Diet Assoc.* 2000;100:961–6.

Hatner-Eaton C. Public Health Departments and the Quality Movement: a Natural Partnership?" *Clinical Performance and Quality Health Care.* 1995;3:35–40.

Haughton B, Story M, Keir B. "Profile of public health nutrition personnel: Challenges for population/system-focused roles and state-level monitoring." *J Am Diet Assoc.* 1998;98:664–70.

Kornblum TH. "Professional demand for dietitians and nutritionists in the year 2005." *J Am Diet Assoc.* 1994;94:2l–22.

Oleckno WA, Blacconiere MJ. "Job Satisfaction in Public Health: a Comparative Analysis of Five Occupational Groups." *Journal of the Royal Society of Health.* 1995;115:386–90.

U.S. Department of Agriculture. *Revitalizing Quality Nutrition Services in WIC.* Available at: www.fns.usda.gov/wic/CONTENT/RQNS/RQNS.htm

Appendix D-1

Glossary of Terms

The following are definitions of terms used in this document.

Community Nutrition

Community Nutrition is the branch of nutrition that addresses the entire range of food and nutrition issues related to individuals, families, and special needs groups living in a defined geographical area. Community nutrition programs include those programs that provide increased access to food resources, food and nutrition education, and healthrelated care in a culturally competent manner.

Community Nutrition Educator

A Community Nutrition Educator is defined as an individual with a baccalaureate degree with a minimum of 15 hours course work in nutrition from a regionally accredited college or university.

Community Nutritionist/Dietitian

A Community Nutritionist/Dietitian is defined as an individual with a baccalaureate degree and is a Registered Dietitian or registration eligible.

Registered Dietitian

A Registered Dietitian has completed a baccalaureate degree in dietetics or a related area at an accredited U.S. college or university, completed a supervised clinical experience, and passed a national examination administered by the Commission on Dietetic Registration, which is recognized by the National Commission for Certifying Agencies. To retain RD status, continuing education activities are required. Registered Dietitians are qualified to perform nutrition screening, assessment, and treatment.

Public Health Nutritionist

The title Public Health Nutritionist is reserved for positions that require dietetic registration status, and graduate-level public health preparation in biostatistics, epidemiology, social-behavioral sciences, environmental sciences, health program planning, management, and evaluation. The term is usually used for an individual with a Master's degree in Public Health Nutrition.

Appendix D-2

Self-Assessment Tool for Public Health Nutritionists

> The public health nutritionist is that member of the public health agency staff who is responsible for assessing community nutrition needs and planning, organizing, managing, directing, coordinating and evaluating the nutrition component of the health agency's services. The public health nutritionist establishes linkages with community nutrition programs, nutrition education, food assistance, social or welfare services, child care, services to the elderly, other human services, and community based research.*

This tool is designed to help me implement the ADA Standards of Practice (#4) and objectively assess my expertise in the five general areas of public health nutrition and then use the assessment to develop a career development plan. It is important to complete each item even though the particular skill or knowledge may not be required in my present job.

For the purpose of this self-assessment, the following definitions are used for guidance:

Prepared by the Department of Nutrition and the Learning Resources Center, School of Public Health, University of North Carolina at Chapel Hill. Public Health Nutrition Practice Group of the American Dietetic Association, (c) 1988

*From Kaufman, M. Ed. et al *Personnel in Public Health Nutrition for the 1980s*, Washington, DC, ASTHO Foundation, 1982

1. Expert—possess this knowledge/skill as a result of training and/or experience and feel able to speak and act with authority in this area.
2. Competent—feel knowledge/skill exceeds the average but is less than the level of "expert".
3. Adequate—consider knowledge/skill is satisfactory or average.
4. Beginner—feel knowledge/skill is characterized by uncertainty and lack of confidence.
5. Unqualified—assess knowledge/skill as inadequate and performance in area would be difficult without technical assistance; assistance would be needed if required to apply this knowledge/skill.

I. Nutrition and Dietetics Practice

	Expert ←——→ Unqualified				
• Knowledge of the principles and practice of nutrition throughout the life cycle					
— normal nutrition	1	2	3	4	5
— therapeutic nutrition	1	2	3	4	5
— meal planning, food selection, preparation, processing andservice for individuals and groups	1	2	3	4	5
• Knowledge of human behavior, particularly health and diet-related behaviors	1	2	3	4	5
• Knowledge of techniques for effecting behavior change	1	2	3	4	5
• Skill in process of interviewing and counseling	1	2	3	4	5
• Knowledge of the cultures and lifestyles of ethnic and socioeconomic groups represented in the community	1	2	3	4	5
• Knowledge and skill in nutrition assessment techniques:					
— anthropometric	1	2	3	4	5
— biochemical	1	2	3	4	5
— clinical	1	2	3	4	5
— dietary	1	2	3	4	5
— socio-economic	1	2	3	4	5
• Skill in the interpretation and use of data from nutrition assessment for:					
— individuals	1	2	3	4	5
— populations	1	2	3	4	5

II. Communications

	Expert ⟷ Unqualified				
	1	2	3	4	5

- Skill in communicating scientific information at levels appropriate for different audiences, both orally and in writing:

  – consumers/public
  – health professionals
  – the media

- Skill in using various communication channels and working with the media:

	1	2	3	4	5
– printed media (newspapers, magazines, newsletters)	1	2	3	4	5
– radio	1	2	3	4	5
– films/videos	1	2	3	4	5
– television	1	2	3	4	5

- Knowledge of methods to outreach to prospective clients to enhance their participation in health and nutrition programs   1   2   3   4   5

- Knowledge of the principles of social marketing for use in health and nutrition programs   1   2   3   4   5

- Skill in negotiation and use of group process techniques (brainstorming, focus groups, nominal group process) to achieve goals and objectives   1   2   3   4   5

- Skill in participating effectively as a member of agency and/or community boards, committees, and task forces   1   2   3   4   5

- Skill in using the consultation process   1   2   3   4   5

III. Public Health Science and Practice

	Expert ⟷ Unqualified				

- Skill in communicating scientific information at levels appropriate for different audiences, both orally and in writing:

  — consumers/public
  — health professionals
  — the media

	Expert				Unqualified
	1	2	3	4	5

- Skill in using various communication channels and working with the media:

  — printed media (newspapers, magazines, newsletters)   1 2 3 4 5
  — radio   1 2 3 4 5
  — films/videos   1 2 3 4 5
  — television   1 2 3 4 5

- Knowledge of methods to outreach to prospective clients to enhance their participation in health and nutrition programs   1 2 3 4 5

- Knowledge of the principles of social marketing for use in health and nutrition programs   1 2 3 4 5

- Skill in negotiation and use of group process techniques (brainstorming, focus groups, nominal group process) to achieve goals and objectives   1 2 3 4 5

- Skill in participating effectively as a member of agency and/or community boards, committees, and task forces   1 2 3 4 5

- Skill in using the consultation process   1 2 3 4 5

IV. Management

	Expert ←———→ Unqualified

	Expert				Unqualified
• Skill in community organization.	1	2	3	4	5
• Skill in translating community assessment data into agency program plan for nutrition services, including:					
– prioritizing goals	1	2	3	4	5
– development of measurable objectives	1	2	3	4	5
– development of achievable action plans	1	2	3	4	5
– use of quality control measures	1	2	3	4	5
– development of evaluation systems	1	2	3	4	5
• Skill in integrating plan for nutrition services into overall mission and plan of the health agency	1	2	3	4	5
• Skill in organizing and prioritizing work	1	2	3	4	5
• Knowledge of quality assurance methodology, including the writing of measurable health outcomes and nutrition care standards	1	2	3	4	5
• Skill in applying the principles of personnel management, including:					
– recruiting	1	2	3	4	5
– staffing	1	2	3	4	5
– supervising	1	2	3	4	5
– performance appraisal	1	2	3	4	5
– staff development	1	2	3	4	5
• Skill in applying principles of financial management of health services, including:					
– forecasting of fiscal needs	1	2	3	4	5
– budget preparation and justification	1	2	3	4	5
– reimbursement systems	1	2	3	4	5
– control of revenues and expenditures	1	2	3	4	5
• Knowledge of available funding sources for public health and public health nutrition programs	1	2	3	4	5
• Skill in grant and contract management, including:					
– preparation	1	2	3	4	5
– negotiation	1	2	3	4	5
– monitoring	1	2	3	4	5
• Skill in applying principles of cost/benefit and cost effectiveness analysis	1	2	3	4	5

V. Legislation and Advocacy

	Expert ← → Unqualified				
• Knowledge of current and emerging public health and nutrition problems	1	2	3	4	5
• Skill in identifying economic and societal trends which have implications for the health and nutritional status of the population	1	2	3	4	5
• Knowledge of the political considerations involved in agency planning and decision making	1	2	3	4	5
• Knowledge of the legislative base for public health and public health nutrition programs	1	2	3	4	5
• Knowledge of federal, state, and local governmental structures and the processes involved in the development of public policy, legislation, and regulations that influence nutrition and health services	1	2	3	4	5
• Knowledge of the purposes, function, and politics of organizations in the community, which influence nutrition and health	1	2	3	4	5
• Skill in participating in organized advocacy efforts for health and nutrition programs	1	2	3	4	5

My Career Development Plan

To help me implement The American Dietetic Association Standards of Practice this outline for a career development plan will aid me in planning to strengthen the areas I identified as needing improvement. The relative priority to work on any item will be determined by my individual needs and career goals. Setting a target time frame for each area will be based on my priorities. Establishing a time frame will enhance the usefulness of this tool for my professional growth and development as a public health nutritionist.

1. My personal career goal is: _____

2. As I review my responses on the self-assessment tool, I
   identify three items that are most critical to my career goals.

My first priority is: _____

My plan will include the following courses, activities, consultations.	My time frame(s)
1.	
2.	
3.	
Notes:	

My second priority is: _____

My plan will include the following courses, activities, consultations.	My time frame(s)
1.	
2.	
3.	
Notes:	

My third priority is: _____

My plan will include the following courses, activities, consultations.	My time frame(s)
1.	
2.	
3.	
Notes:	

References

Association of State and Territorial Public Health Nutrition Directors, Model State Nutrition Objectives, 1988, unpublished.

Baird, S.C. and Sylvester, J. Role Delineation and Verification for Entry-level positions. In *Community Dietetics*, Chicago: The American Dietetic Association, 1983.

Committee on Professional Education, The American Public Health Association, The educational qualifications of nutritionists in health agencies, *J Amer Diet Assoc* 22:1,41–44,1946.

Curriculum and Membership Committee, Association of Faculties of Graduate Programs In Public Health Nutrition. A Description of Graduate Programs in Public Health Nutrition, 1980, unpublished.

Egan, MC. Public health nutrition services: Issues today and tomorrow, *J Amer Diet Assoc* 77:4,423–27,1980.

Kaufman, M. Ed. et al, Personnel in Public Health Nutrition for the 1980's, Washington, DC: ASTHO Foundation (Association of State and Territorial Health Officials Foundation), 1982.

Kaufman, M., Preparing public health nutritionists to meet the future, *J Amer Diet Assoc* 8&4, 511–514, 1986.

Nutrition services in state and local health agencies, *Public Health Rep.* 98:7, 1983.

Peck, E.B. The public health nutritionist-dietitian An historical perspective, *J Amer Diet Assoc* 64:6,642–47,1974.

The American Dietetic Association, Standards of Professional Practice. The American Dietetic Association. Adopted October 1997. http://www.eatright.org/Member/83_9468.cfm. (Accessed October 20, 2003).

Appendix D-3

Guidelines for Community Nutrition Supervised Experiences

User Survey

Please complete and return to the ADA Public Health/Community Nutrition Dietetic Practice Group, C/O ADA Practice Team, 120 South Riverside Plaza, Suite 2000, Chicago, IL 60606-6995.

1. Individual completing survey _____
   (Name; Credentials; Title):_____
   _____

2. Agency/ organization name: _____
   address: _____
   _____
   telephone: _____
   FAX: _____

3. The Guidelines lend themselves to a wide variety of applications. How were they used in your situation? Please select all that apply.
   ___ (1) Training curriculum development to ensure qualified nutrition personnel
   ___ (2) Student or new employee orientation
   ___ (3) One time or periodic reference document
   ___ (4) Other: _____

4. Which of the following best describes the individual who supervised the community nutrition supervised experience?
   ___ Public health nutrition practitioner seeking specialty training
   ___ Public health employers seeking to ensure qualified nutrition personnel
   ___ Practitioners and educators providing community nutrition training
   ___ Other: _____

5. Which of the following best describes the individual who used the guidelines to enhance his/her competence?
   ___ Public health nutrition practitioner seeking specialty training
   ___ Registered Dietitian seeking continuing education
   ___ Dietetic student seeking ADA registration eligibility
   ___ Other: _____

HELPFUL NUTRITION WEBSITES

Aim for a Healthy Weight
Patient and public education materials from the National Heart, Lung, and Blood Institute.
www.nhlbi.nih.gov/health/public/heart/obesity/lose_weight/recommend.htm

CDC Health Topics: Nutrition
Fact sheets on various nutrition topics, from the Centers for Disease Control and Prevention.
www.cdc.gov/health/nutrition.htm

CDC's Nutrition and Physical Activity Program
Addresses the role of nutrition and physical activity in health promotion and the prevention and control of chronic diseases.
www.cspinet.org

Center for Science in the Public Interest
Health and nutrition information.
www.cspinet.org

Consumer Nutrition and Health Information
Nutrition and health information from the Food and Drug Administration.
www.cfsan.fda.gov/~dms/lab-cons.html

Dietary Guidelines for Americans
Recommended Dietary Guidelines from the U.S. Department of Health and Human Services and the U.S. Department of Agriculture.
http://www.health.gov/dietaryguidelines

Food and Nutrition Information Center
FNIC, located at the National Agricultural Library, collects and disseminates information about food and human nutrition.
http://www.nal.usda.gov/fnic

Health Information: Weight Loss and Control
The National Institute of Diabetes and Digestive and Kidney Diseases of the National Institutes of Health provides information on obesity, weight control, physical activity, and nutrition.
www.niddk.nih.gov/health/nutrit/nutrit.htm

Healthfinder: Obesity
Links to a variety of sites on obesity.
www.healthfinder.gov/scripts/SearchContext.asp?topic=592

MEDLINEplus: Nutrition
http://www.nlm.nih.gov/medlineplus/nutrition.html

MEDLINEplus: Obesity
http://www.nlm.nih.gov/medlineplus/obesity.html

MEDLINEplus: Weight Loss and Dieting
http://www.nlm.nih.gov/medlineplus/obesity.html

Nutrition.gov
A guide to nutrition and health information on federal government websites.
www.nutrition.gov

Obesity Education Initiative Website
Information for health professionals and the public, from the National Heart, Lung, and Blood Institute.
www.nhlbi.nih.gov/health/public/heart/obesity/lose_wt

Overweight and Obesity
Information on trends and health consequences of obesity, from the Centers for Disease Control and Prevention.
www.cdc.gov/nccdphp/dnpa/obesity/index.htm

The American Dietetic Association
An organization of food and nutrition professionals, ADA's mission is to promote optimal nutrition and well-being for all people.
http://www.eatright.org

Weight Loss and Nutrition Myths
Corrections to common myths about dieting and nutrition.
www.niddk.nih.gov/health/nutrit/pubs/myths/index.htm

Public Health Nutrition List
Preventive and primary nutrition services and public health nutrition core functions. Message: subscribe PHNUTR-L your-name.
subscribe to: listproc@u.washington.edu

APPENDIX F

STATE HEALTH DEPARTMENT WEBSITES

- Alabama—www.adph.org/
- Alaska—www.hss.state.ak.us/dph/
- Arizona—www.hs.state.az.us/
- Arkansas—www.healthyarkansas.com/
- California—www.dhs.cahwnet.gov/
- Colorado—www.cdphe.state.co.us/cdphehom.asp
- Connecticut—www.state.ct.us/dph/
- Delaware—www.state.de.us/dhss/dph/index.htm
- District of Columbia—dchealth.dc.gov/index.asp
- Florida—www.doh.state.fl.us/
- Georgia—www.ph.dhr.state.ga.us/
- Hawaii—www.state.hi.us/health/
- Idaho—www2.state.id.us/dhw/
- Illinois—www.idph.state.il.us
- Indiana—www.state.in.us/isdh/
- Iowa—www.idph.state.ia.us/default.asp
- Kansas—www.ink.org/public/kdhe/
- Kentucky—chs.ky.gov/publichealth/
- Louisiana—www.dhh.state.la.us/
- Maine—www.state.me.us/dhs/boh/index.htm
- Maryland—www.dhmh.state.md.us/
- Massachusetts—www.state.ma.us/dph/dphhome.htm
- Michigan—www.michigan.gov/mdch
- Minnesota—www.health.state.mn.us/
- Mississippi—www.msdh.state.ms.us/
- Missouri—www.health.state.mo.us/
- Montana—www.dphhs.state.mt.us/
- Nebraska—www.hhs.state.ne.us/
- Nevada—www.hr.state.nv.us/
- New Hampshire—www.dhhs.state.nh.us/
- New Jersey—www.state.nj.us/health/
- New Mexico—www.health.state.nm.us
- New York—www.health.state.ny.us/
- North Carolina—www.state.nc.us/DHR/
- North Dakota—www.health.state.nd.us/

- Ohio—www.odh.state.oh.us/
- Oklahoma—www.health.state.ok.us/
- Oregon—www.ohd.hr.state.or.us/
- Pennsylvania—www.health.state.pa.us/
- Rhode Island—www.health.state.ri.us/
- South Carolina—www.scdhec.net/
- South Dakota—www.state.sd.us/doh/index.htm
- Tennessee—www.state.tn.us/health/
- Texas—www.tdh.state.tx.us/
- Utah—hlunix.hl.state.ut.us/
- Vermont—www.healthyvermonters.info/
- Virginia—www.vdh.state.va.us/
- Washington—www.doh.wa.gov/
- West Virginia—www.wvdhhr.org/
- Wisconsin—www.dhfs.state.wi.us/
- Wyoming—wdhfs.state.wy.us/wdh/

2004 TEAM NUTRITION TRAINING GRANT APPLICATION

Cover Sheet

2004 Team Nutrition Training Grant
CFDA # 10.574

State(s): _____

State Director(s): _____
    E-mail address: _____

Grant Contact Person/Project Director: _____
    E-mail address: _____
    Phone: _____
    Fax: _____

Return your application *on or before 5:00 p.m. Eastern Daylight Time, April 16, 2004.*

No. 0584-0512
Attachment G—Sample Team Nutrition Training Grant Proposal Format

A successful grant proposal is one that is thoroughly planned, well prepared, and concisely packaged. There are, generally, eight basic components in a solid proposal package:

1. Proposal summary
2. Introduction to the organization
3. Problem statement (or needs assessment)
4. Proposal objectives
5. Proposal methods or design
6. Project assessment
7. Proposal budget narrative
8. Appendices

Proposal Summary or Synopsis

- Appears at the beginning of the proposal and outlines the project. It should be brief, no longer than two or three paragraphs.
- It is often helpful to prepare the summary after the proposal has been developed. This makes it easier to include all the key points necessary to communicate the objectives of the project.
- The summary or synopsis becomes the foundation of the proposal. The first impression it gives will be critical to the success of the venture. This synopsis will be used on the TN website to describe a grant project.

Introduction to the Organization

- The information should be relevant to the goals of the grant and should establish the applicant's credibility.
- Required—Identify project director and other key staff of the project. Key staff should include anyone that will have direct responsibility for the implementation of project activities.
- Required—Include resumes of project director and other key staff. Resumes must be no more than 2 pages per person. Simplify project director and key staff's resume to include experiences and qualification that pertain to implementation of this grant project.
- Background in nutrition, food service, and planning for the project director is highly recommended. If a project director has not yet been identified, a position description should be provided that describes duties, responsibilities, and knowledge required for the position.

- Required—Include letters of commitment from the project director, project director's supervisor, and key staff. A letter of commitment for at least 33% of time from the proposed project director and a letter of commitment from his/her current supervisor are required. If the project director is a contracted employee, a letter of commitment from the State representative overseeing the contractor is required. Letters of commitment should include the percent-of-time commitment as well as an understanding of the duties for which the staff will be responsible.
- If coordination exists among partners, collaborators, and/or other State agencies, letters of agreement/support must be supplied with the application that provide evidence of coordination and clear understanding of relationships.

Problem Statement (Needs Assessment)

- It should be a clear, concise, well-supported statement of the problem to be overcome or the needs to be addressed by the grant.
- Zero-in on a specific problem you want to solve or the training you want to provide.
- An applicant should include data collected during a needs assessment that would illustrate the problems to be addressed and/or target audience and number to be trained.
- Use statistics to support existence of your problem or issue.
- Set up the delivery of your goals and objectives.

Project Goals and Objectives

- Project goals and objectives should be clearly stated.
- Goals are general and offer the reviewer an understanding of the thrust of your program.
- Objectives are specific, measurable outcomes. They should be realistic and attainable. Be realistic.
- Applicants should explain the expected results and benefits of each objective.

Project Methods or Design

- The project method outlines the rationale of tasks or activities that will be accomplished with the available resources to meet the proposal objectives.
- Describe in detail the activities that will take place in order to achieve desired objectives.
- Make sure your methods are realistic and cost effective.
- If sub-grants or mini-grants are to be awarded to schools and/or childcare centers, the specific criteria for the funding should be stated as well as how the State agency plans to provide oversight.
- It is helpful to structure the project method or design as a timeline, with tasks or activities laid out in a schedule over the grant period, and persons responsible for each task. This will allow reviewers to consider what personnel, materials, and other resources will be needed to complete the tasks or activities.

Project Assessment

- Applicants should develop criteria to assess progress toward objectives and goals. It is important to define carefully and exactly how success will be determined.
- If you have a problem developing your evaluation process, take another look at your objectives.
- Be ready to begin evaluation as soon as you begin your project.

Project Budget Narrative

- A detailed, itemized budget is required along with supporting narrative and justification for each budget category.
- The budget justification must provide detailed summaries, which clearly itemize the costs associated with the respective line items. For example, for "travel," list total costs of all travel paid for with TN Training Grant funds and itemize costs by number of individuals traveling, number of trips involved, lodging, per diem, mileage, etc. Another example would be when providing a breakdown of personnel charges, identify personnel by title and name (if known), percentage of time allocated to the project, and the individual annual salaries or a pro-rated amount. Please indicate if fringe benefits are to be treated as part of an approved indirect cost rate.

- The budget should demonstrate consistency with project activities. Divide the budget into categories, such as personnel salaries and benefits, travel, equipment, supplies, contract costs, etc.
- Identify when salaries of key staff will be provided as in-kind contribution.
- When providing other sources of funding for the proposal, please note that SAE funding is not State funding.

Appendices

- Resumes of project director and other key staff, letters of commitment from the project director, project director's supervisor and key staff, and letter of agreement/support from partners, collaborators, and/or other State agencies, if applicable, must be included in the Appendices section.
- Please do not include information not specifically relevant or requested by this Request for Application.

LEARNING ACTIVITIES

Carol E. O'Neil, PhD, MPH, LDN, RD

Theresa A. Nicklas, DrPH

Learning Activities

1. Learn more about the science behind the U.S. Dietary Guidelines for Americans and how to teach the guidelines to the public through the on-line course: http://www.dga2000training.usda.gov/welcome.htm. Then work with your instructor to develop a lesson plan to deliver (and evaluate) to a community group, such as a school. This is called service-learning. To find out more about service-learning, go to The National Service-Learning Clearinghouse: http://www.servicelearning.org or to your university's service-learning office. If you do work with children, check out this website for ideas for nutrition and kids: http://www.nal.usda.gov/fnic/etext/000100.html or food safety and kids: http://www.cdc.gov/nchs/data/misc/nutri98.pdf.

2. It's easy for nutrition students and health professionals to understand the food label and to monitor changes. It's not so easy for most consumers to understand the nuances, and it's not so easy for students or entry-level practitioners to explain it. To be sure you understand the label and everything it has to offer, go to http://www.cfsan.fda.gov/~dms/foodlab.html; then design, execute, and evaluate a lesson to another community group. You could also work with a local high school to teach the food label. At http://ific.org/publications/other/tnfl.cfm, a food label education program for high school students is available from the International Food Information Council. You could also help the high school group learn how to teach a younger group.

3. What else could you do? Work with your instructor to write up this experience for publication! For example, *The American Biology Teacher* is a nationally recognized journal that provides specific how-to suggestions for the classroom and

laboratory, field activities, interdisciplinary programs, and articles on recent advances in biology and life science. You, your group, and your teacher could write about this project for publication. Your paper might just be part of the science base that is used to set nutrition policy.

4. A lot of time in this chapter was devoted to discussing nutrition policy—how it is developed and how it is changed. In a class presentation, choose a policy to explain to a group— your classmates or community stakeholders—and discuss how this policy has changed or can be changed to reflect current science and consumer issues.

5. Discuss the importance of the food label as a health education tool. Explain how scientific evidence is used to support each health claim that can be used on a food label and why it is so difficult to have health claims added to labels for given foods. Could (should) this process be shortened? For validated claims, think about how you would integrate specific foods into a client's diet or into consumer health messages.

6. Read and evaluate the article by Dr. Marlene Most (*J Amer Diet Assoc* 2003;103:729-735) on controlled feeding studies. She provides information on the knowledge and skills that dietetics professionals must have to do these studies, including suggestions for working with study participants. Discuss how you would work with clients that you would be counseling.

7. DASH and DASH sodium were landmark studies on how behavioral change can improve hypertension and, subsequently, health. Explain the science behind the DASH diet, what other potential beneficial effects this blood pressure–lowering diet can have, and how you can bring the DASH diet home to your clients.

8. Many agencies promulgate similar recommendations. Prepare a table or chart looking at the similarities and differences in the recommendations of the American Heart Association, the National Cancer Institute, The National Cholesterol Education Program, Healthy People 2010, and the 2005 U.S. Dietary Guidelines. Explain how some of the differences are tailored to each agency's specific target audience.

INDEX

Numerics

"1% or less" campaign, 198–199
5 A Day program, 61, 70–72, 175–176, 182
5 As (mnemonic), 400
5 to 9 a Day program, 71
10-step planning model, 562–563

A

AAP (American Academy of Pediatrics), 203
academic courses and programs, 773
academic preparation. *See* education of
    practitioners
acceptable macronutrient distribution range
    (AMDR), 51
access to food, 121, 133, 149–152
    collaboration with networks, 721
    ensuring sufficient. *See* food insecurity
    FNS (Food and Nutrition Service), 268–271
        Action for Health Kids initiative, 705
        WIC. *See* WIC program
    food variety, 96–97, 319
        school meals, 321–322
    fruits and vegetables, 207
    modifying with policy, 240, 246–247
    safeguarding. *See* safeguarding food
        supply; security of food supply
access to healthcare, 129–130, 134
accountability, 90
accreditation, group care, 425
acids as food additives, 465
acting out behavior, 324–325
Action for Health Kids initiative, 565–569,
    571, 705
action plans, 570, 760
actual cost fee-for-service, 618
ADA (American Dietetic Association),
    642–646, 702–703
    membership in, 773
    professional networking, 725
additives to food, 461–467
    chronic health effects, 469
    safety regulations, 446–447
    sweeteners, 464
adequate intake (AI), 49–51
    adolescents, 325
    children, 313
adjourning stage (group development), 712
Administration on Aging (AoA), 380–385
administrative staff
    earning support from, 757–765

government programs, 647
group care, 432–433
adolescents, 322–328. *See also* children
    micronutrient intake, 313–315
    pregnancy of, 302–303
adult outplacement homes, 427
Adult Treatment Panel (ATP), 356
advertising, 156, 159, 213–214, 745–747
    to children, 214, 217, 322
    DAP (Division of Advertising Practices),
        441, 443
advocacy, 770. *See also* politics and political
    support
    grant writing, 160–162, 595, 614, 616,
        625–627, 764–765
        Internet resources, 764
    importance of, 253–254
    infrastructure of support, building,
        261–264
    media, working with, 162–164
    physical education, 155
    policy. *See* public policy
    political parties and groups, 258–260
    programs. *See* social programs
aerosol weaponization, 548
AFHK (Action for Healthy Kids), 565–569,
    571, 705
aflatoxins, 458–459
after-school programs, 173
age. *See* baby boomers; children; seniors
age, segmenting market by, 740
agencies, role of, 247–248
agency administration, 757–765
Agency for Healthcare Research and Quality
    (AHRQ), 23
agenda setting, 242, 255–256
agents of bioterrorism, 525–526, 528–533, 546
aggregation of data. *See* analysis of
    quantitative data
aging population, 375–377
agricultural chemicals, 467
agricultural policy, 240. *See also* policy
Agricultural Research magazine, 280
Agricultural Research Service (ARS),
    274–281, 440
agroterrorism. *See* bioterrorism
AHEI (Alternate Health Eating Index), 348
AHRQ (Agency for Healthcare Research and
    Quality), 23, 395–397
AI (adequate intake) levels, 49–51
    adolescents, 325
    children, 313